The Ureter

Your bonus with the purchase of this book

With the purchase of this book, you can use our "SN Flashcards" app to access questions free of charge in order to test your learning and check your understanding of the contents of the book. To use the app, please follow the instructions below:

1. Go to **https://flashcards.springernature.com/login**
2. Create an user account by entering your e-mail adress and assiging a password.
3. Use the link provided in one of the first chapters to access your SN Flashcards set.

MOREMEDIA

Your personal SN Flashcards link is provided in one of the first chapters.

If the link is missing or does not work, please send an e-mail with the subject "**SN Flashcards**" and the book title to **customerservice@springernature.com**.

Mahmoud Abdel-Gawad • Bedeir Ali-El-Dein
John Barry • Arnulf Stenzl
Editors

The Ureter

A Comprehensive Review

Springer

Editors
Mahmoud Abdel-Gawad
Belqas
Elnagar Urology Center
Mansoura City, Egypt

John Barry
Department of Urology and Department of Surgery
Oregon Health & Science University
Portland, OR, USA

Bedeir Ali-El-Dein
Urology Department
Urology and Nephrology Center
Faculty of Medicine
Mansoura University
Mansoura, Egypt

Arnulf Stenzl
Department of Urology
Universitatsklinikum Tubingen
Tübingen, Baden-Württemberg, Germany

ISBN 978-3-031-36214-9 ISBN 978-3-031-36212-5 (eBook)
https://doi.org/10.1007/978-3-031-36212-5

This Springer imprint is published by the registered company Springer Nature Switzerland AG
The registered company address is: Gewerbestrasse 11, 6330 Cham, Switzerland

Paper in this product is recyclable.

Contents

List of Contributors

Mahmoud Abdel-Gawad Toshka Urology and Endoscopy Center, Mansoura, Egypt

Ahmed Abdelhalim Urology Department, Urology and Nephrology Center, Faculty of Medicine, Mansoura University, Mansoura, Egypt

Bedeir Ali-El-Dein Urology Department, Urology and Nephrology Center, Faculty of Medicine, Mansoura University, Mansoura, Egypt

Fahad Alyami King Saud University, College of Medicine, King Faisal Specialist Hospital and Research Centre, Riyadh, Saudi Arabia

Stefan Aufderklamm Department of Urology, Eberhard Karls University, Tübingen, Germany

Mohamed A. Baky Fahmy Pediatric Surgery, Al-Azhar University, Cairo, Egypt

John M. Barry Division of Abdominal Organ Transplantation, Oregon Health and Science University, Portland, OR, USA

Mario Basulto-Martínez Endourology, Laparoscopy, and Robotic Surgery Fellow, Schulich School of Medicine and Dentistry, Division of Urology, Western University, London, ON, Canada

Rohan Batra Consultant Urologist, Muljibhai Patel Urological Hospital, Nadiad, Gujarat, India

Swati Bhardwaj, MD Anatomic and Clinical Pathology, Department of Pathology, Icahn School of Medicine, The Mount Sinai Hospital, New York, NY, USA

Adel Bondok Anatomy and Neuroscience, Faculty of Medicine, Mansoura University, Mansoura, Egypt

Leslie Charondo Department of Urology, University of California San Francisco, San Francisco, CA, USA

Ben H. Chew The Stone Centre at Vancouver General Hospital, Department of Urologic Science, University of British Columbia, Vancouver, BC, Canada

John Denstedt Professor of Urology Schulich School of Medicine and Dentistry, Western University, London, ON, Canada

Zachary Dovey, MBBS General Urology, Robotics, and Uro-oncology, Milton and Carroll Petrie Department of Urology, Icahn School of Medicine, The Mount Sinai Hospital, New York, NY, USA

Mohamed Elawdy Consultant Urologist, Ministry of Health, Muscat, Oman

Tarek A. El-Diasty Consultant of diagnostic radiology, medical imaging and interventional radiology, Radiology Department, Urology and Nephrology Center, Mansoura University, Mansoura, Egypt

Mostafa El-Ksas Specialist of diagnostic radiology, medical imaging and interventional radiology, Radiology Department, Urology and Nephrology Center, Mansoura University, Mansoura, Egypt

Ahmad M. Eliwa Urology Department, Zagazig University, Zagazig, Egypt

Ahmed M. Eliwa Urology and Andrology, Urology Department, Zagazig University, Zagazig, Egypt

Francisco Escobedo Department of Urology, University of California Los Angeles, Los Angeles, CA, USA

Hashim Farg Fellow of diagnostic radiology, medical imaging and interventional radiology, Radiology Department, Urology and Nephrology Center, Mansoura University, Mansoura, Egypt

Eduardo González-Cuenca Endourology, Laparoscopy, and Robotic Surgery Fellow, Schulich School of Medicine and Dentistry, Division of Urology, Western University, London, ON, Canada

Raghav Gupta, MD Milton and Carroll Petrie Department of Urology, Icahn School of Medicine, The Mount Sinai Hospital, New York, NY, USA

Ashraf T. Hafez Mansoura Urology and Nephrology Center, Mansoura University, Mansoura, Egypt

Fadl Hamouche Department of Urology, University of California San Francisco, San Francisco, CA, USA

Ahmed M. Harraz Mansoura Urology and Nephrology Center, Mansoura University, Mansoura, Egypt

Roman Herout The Stone Centre at Vancouver General Hospital, Department of Urologic Science, University of British Columbia, Vancouver, BC, Canada

Pavan Surwase Jain Fellow in Endourology, Muljibhai Patel Urological Hospital, Nadiad, Gujarat, India

Dirk Lange The Stone Centre at Vancouver General Hospital, Department of Urologic Science, University of British Columbia, Vancouver, BC, Canada

Moritz Maas Department of Urology, Eberhard Karls University, Tübingen, Germany

Ziad M. Nakshabandi National Center for Health Workforce Planning, SCFHS, Riyadh, Saudi Arabia

Leslie Ojeaburu Department of Urology, University of California Los Angeles, Los Angeles, CA, USA

Helmy Omar Urology Department, King Fahad Specialist Hospital Dammam, Dammam, Saudi Arabia

Yasser Osman Mansoura Urology and Nephrology Center, Mansoura University, Mansoura, Egypt

Dhruti Patel, MD General Urology, Robotics, and Uro-oncology, Milton and Carroll Petrie Department of Urology, Icahn School of Medicine, The Mount Sinai Hospital, New York, NY, USA

Parth Patel Department of Urology, University of California Los Angeles, Los Angeles, CA, USA

Niramya Pathak Fellow in Endourology, Muljibhai Patel Urological Hospital, Nadiad, Gujarat, India

Abhijit Patil Department of Urology, Muljibhai Urological Hospital, Nadiad, India

Adriana M. Pedraza, MD Clinical Urologic Oncology, Milton and Carroll Petrie Department of Urology, Icahn School of Medicine, The Mount Sinai Hospital, New York, NY, USA

Alina Reicherz The Stone Centre at Vancouver General Hospital, Department of Urologic Science, University of British Columbia, Vancouver, BC, Canada

Ravindra Sabnis Consultant Urologist, Muljibhai Patel Urological Hospital, Nadiad, Gujarat, India

Osama Sarhan Urology and Nephrology Center, Faculty of Medicine, Mansoura University, Mansoura, Egypt

Kemal Sarica Department of Urology, Biruni University, Medical School, Istanbul, Turkey

Kymora B. Scotland Department of Urology, University of California Los Angeles, Los Angeles, CA, USA

Bilge Turedi Sezer Konya City Hospital, Konya, Turkey

Akash Shah, MBBS, MCh Department of Uro-oncologic Surgery, Kokilaben Dhirubhai Ambani Hospital, Achutrao Patwardhan Marg, Four Bungalows, Mumbai, India

Doaa Sharaf, Ass. Prof. Dr. MD. EDiUR Radiology Department, Urology & Nephrology Center, Mansoura University, Mansoura, Egypt

Haytham Shebel, Prof. Dr., MD. EDiUR Radiology Department, Urology & Nephrology Center, Mansoura University, Mansoura, Egypt

Arnulf Stenzl Division of Abdominal Organ Transplantation, Oregon Health and Science University, Portland, OR, USA

Department of Urology, Eberhard Karls University, Tübingen, Germany

Marshall Stoller Department of Urology, University of California San Francisco, San Francisco, CA, USA

Ashutosh Tewari, MBBS, MCh Milton and Carroll Petrie Department of Urology, Icahn School of Medicine, The Mount Sinai Hospital, New York, NY, USA

Sapna Thaker Department of Urology, University of California Los Angeles, Los Angeles, CA, USA

Vinayak Wagaskar, MBBS Milton and Carroll Petrie Department of Urology, Icahn School of Medicine, The Mount Sinai Hospital, New York, NY, USA

Yasin Yitgin Department of Urology, Istinye University, Istanbul, Turkey

Chapter 1
Introduction

Mahmoud Abdel-Gawad, Bedeir Ali-El-Dein, Arnulf Stenzl, and John M. Barry

Flashcard access code: BF062-DBFBE-14D2E-0D887-A135E Flashcard short URL: ▶ https://sn.pub/vbTnwP
Test your learning and check your understanding of this book's contents: use the "Springer Nature Flashcards" app to access questions. To use the app, please follow the instructions below:
1. Go to https://flashcards.springernature.com/login
2. Create a user account by entering your e-mail address and assigning a password.
3. Use the following link to access your SN Flashcards set: ▶ https://sn.pub/vbTnwP
If the link is missing or does not work, please send an e-mail with the subject "SN Flashcards" and the book title to customerservice@springernature.com

M. Abdel-Gawad
Departments of Urology and Surgery, Division of Abdominal Organ Transplantation, Oregon Health and Science University, Portland, OR, USA

Elnagar Urology, Toshka Urology and Endoscopy Centers, Mansoura, Egypt

B. Ali-El-Dein
Departments of Urology and Surgery, Division of Abdominal Organ Transplantation, Oregon Health and Science University, Portland, OR, USA

Urology Department, Urology and Nephrology Center, Faculty of Medicine, Mansoura University, Mansoura, Egypt

A. Stenzl
Departments of Urology and Surgery, Division of Abdominal Organ Transplantation, Oregon Health and Science University, Portland, OR, USA

Department of Urology, Eberhard-Karls-University Tuebingen, Tuebingen, Germany
e-mail: Arnulf@stenzl.net

J. M. Barry (✉)
Departments of Urology and Surgery, Division of Abdominal Organ Transplantation, Oregon Health and Science University, Portland, OR, USA
e-mail: barryj@ohsu.edu

M. Abdel-Gawad et al. (eds.), *The Ureter*,
https://doi.org/10.1007/978-3-031-36212-5_1

The Ureter: A Comprehensive Review is an entire book devoted to a tube that transports urine from its production site in the kidney to its storage site in the bladder. Come, join us for a fascinating journey from embryology to anatomy to physiology and pharmacology to the diagnosis and treatment of disease states with clever imaging, instrumentation and surgical techniques. There's something for students, residents, fellows, urologists and curious patients within its pages. Open this book to a random page and read a paragraph; you'll be hooked.

Chapter 2
Embryology and Congenital Anomalies

Osama Sarhan and Helmy Omar

Abstract In this chapter we discuss the embryology and the possible congenital anomalies of the ureter. The ureter originates from the ureteric bud that grows from the caudal end of the mesonephric duct. During embryological development, alterations in the number or position of the ureteric buds can cause anomalies such as duplication, triplication or even ectopic insertion of the ureter. Congenital ureteric obstruction may occur in the ureteropelvic or ureterovesical junction and lead to ureteropelvic junction obstruction or megaureter. Other rare anomalies of the ureter, such as ureteral atresia, ureteral diverticulum and the retrocaval ureter, are described. Brief notes on vesicoureteric reflux and ureterocele are also included.

Keywords Ureter · Embryology · Ureteric bud · Anomalies · Duplication · Ectopic ureter · Retrocaval ureter · Ureterocele · Ureteric obstruction

2.1 Embryology of the Ureter

The embryology of the ureter is a part of the embryology of the urinary and genital systems which develop mainly from the intermediate mesoderm [1]. Ureters originate from the mesonephric duct and protrude laterally from the Wolffian duct at the end of the 4th week of gestation to finally insert into the metanephric blastema (primitive kidney) and branches recurrently to form the renal pelvis, calyceal system, and collecting tubules. Understanding the embryology of the ureter and its

Test your learning and check your understanding of this book's contents: use the "Springer Nature Flashcards" app to access questions. To use the app, please follow the instructions in Chapter 1.

O. Sarhan (✉)
Urology and Nephrology Center, Faculty of Medicine, Mansoura University, Mansoura, Egypt

H. Omar
Urology Department, King Fahad Specialist Hospital Dammam, Dammam, Saudi Arabia

M. Abdel-Gawad et al. (eds.), *The Ureter*,
https://doi.org/10.1007/978-3-031-36212-5_2

disorders explains many of the encountered anomalies in pediatric urologic practice and offers clues to the appropriate approach and management of these conditions.

2.1.1 Phases of Kidney and Ureter Development (Pronephros, Mesonephros, and Metanephros)

During the 4th week of the embryo's development, there are three nephric structures that develop in succession from the intermediate mesoderm. The first pronephros, which appears in the cervical portion and rapidly regresses, does not form any nephron-like structures. Consequently, the development of the mesonephros by the appearance of tubular structures in the midportion (thoracic and lumbar sections) of the intermediate mesoderm.

The mesonephric or Wolffian ducts form lateral to this region and grow downward to enter the lateral wall of the cloaca. These primitive renal units have capillary tufts at the proximal ends of simple nephrons and possibly begin functioning at between 6 and 10 weeks, producing small quantities of urine. At nearly 10 weeks of human gestation, these lower parts of the mesonephros degenerate, leaving the upper nephrons, which will contribute to the development of the genital duct system.

At the beginning of the 5th week of gestation, a diverticulum appears on the posteromedial aspect of the lower portion of the mesonephric ducts. This structure, the ureteric bud, grows in a cranial direction and penetrates the metanephric blastema which is a portion of the intermediate mesoderm where an important process of induction occurs at this point. Induction indicates that adjacent tissues influence each other with the development of a "biochemical crosstalk." The ureteral bud induces the metanephric blastema to transform it from an indifferent mesenchyme to form the specialized nephrons and that continues throughout gestation and is complete at 36 weeks (Fig. 2.1).

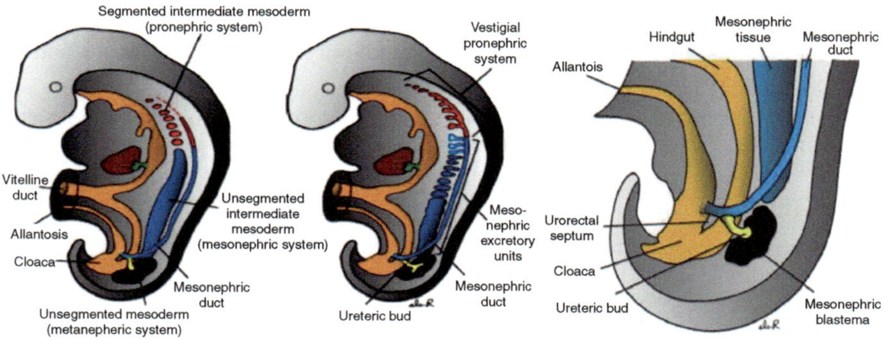

Fig. 2.1 5 week embryo with the origin of the ureteric bud from the mesonephric duct

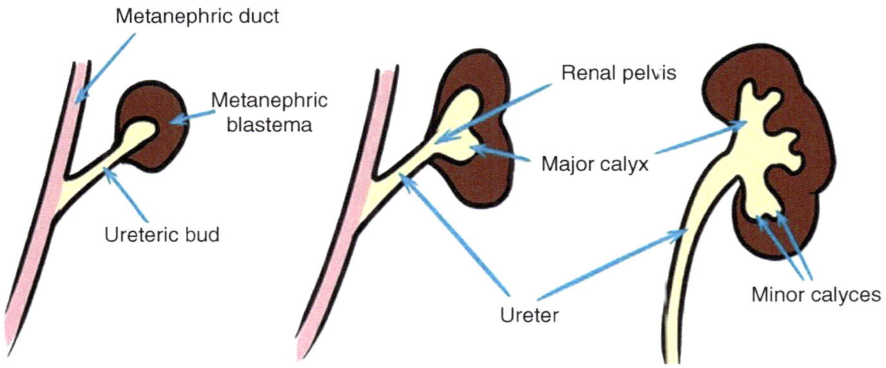

Fig. 2.2 The origin of the ureteric bud from the mesonephric duct with the formation of the renal pelvis and calyces

The tip of the ureteric bud dilates to form the renal pelvis, and then it begins to branch dichotomously: The first four generations coalesce to form the major calyces, and the sixth to eighth generations similarly fuse to form the minor calyces (Fig. 2.2). The next eight generations form the definitive collecting tubules. Blastema cells collect around the tip of each collecting duct and form nephrons, comprising a Bowman capsule, proximal convoluted tubule, the loop of Henle, and distal convoluted tubule. The branching of the ureteric bud is complete by about 14 weeks, but new generations of nephrons continue to be produced within the parenchyma throughout the remainder of gestation [2].

At about 6 weeks, the mid ureter is a solid cord that recanalizes in both directions and canalization starts from the midportion and extends cranially and caudally [3]. A theory has suggested that the ureteropelvic and ureterovesical areas are the last to recanalize so, most ureteral hypoplastic adynamic segments occur at these two sites. Other authors indicate this solid cord recanalization process does not involve ureteropelvic areas. A more plausible explanation is that in human fetuses histologic differentiation of ureteral mural smooth muscle begins at the bladder and proceeds toward the kidney where such muscle is evident by 16 weeks of gestation. It is logical to us that premature arrest of ureteral wall musculature development leads to an aperistaltic hypoplastic ureteral adynamic segment at the UPJ region.

By the time the ureteric buds appear (28 days), the partitioning of the cloaca starts. An ingrowth of mesoderm from the allantois progresses toward the cloacal membrane forming an advancing septum in the hindgut that divides the cloaca into an anterior primitive urogenital sinus, which receives the mesonephric ducts, and a posterior rectum. This division is complete when the advancing edge of the urorectal septum reaches the cloacal membrane during the 6th week, dividing it into an anterior urogenital and a posterior anal membrane [4]. The urogenital membrane breaks down during the 7th week, beginning continuity between the developing urinary tract and the amniotic cavity. The upper part of the primitive urogenital sinus between the allantois and the mesonephric ducts is called the vesicourethral canal; it will form the definitive bladder. The allantois remains attached to the apex of the fetal bladder and extends into the umbilical root; it loses its patency and persists as the median umbilical ligament which is otherwise known as the urachal remnant. By the 13th week, the intermingling circular and longitudinal strands of the smooth muscle of the trigone are apparent. By 16 weeks, these are refined into discrete inner and outer longitudinal layers and a middle circular layer; at this time, continence may be possible. The definitive urothelium is observable by 21 weeks of gestation. During the process of cloacal septation, the mesonephric ducts distal to the ureteric bud origins widen and become incorporated into the posterior aspect of the primitive urogenital sinus. The ureteric orifices arrive on the surface of this posterior wall early and become separated from the mesonephric duct orifices. As further incorporation of the lower mesonephric ducts occurs, the ureteric orifices move in a superolateral direction to the mesonephric duct orifices. The epithelia of both ducts fuse in the midline, and the triangular area between them and the ureteric orifices outlines the trigone of the bladder [5, 6].

2.1.2 Ureteral Duplication

When two ureteric buds occur on one side a duplex kidney is induced with upper and lower renal moieties. If a single bud divides close to its origin, the result is an incomplete duplex kidney with a common distal ureter. If two separate buds form, the kidney is drained by two separate ureters. As it reaches the urogenital sinus, the lower ureter migrates laterally and crosses the upper ureter. The Weigert-Meyer law states that when complete ureteral duplication exists, the medial and caudal ureteral orifice is that of the ureter to the upper pole of the kidney (Fig. 2.3). The lower moiety of the kidney is, therefore, more prone to reflux while the upper pole ureter is the one that is more prone to end ectopically [7, 8].

2.1.2.1 Incidence

In an autopsy population, ureteral duplication occurs in 1 in 125 patients (0.8%) and constitutes the most frequent ureteral anomaly [9, 10]. The right and left kidneys are affected equally. Bilateral duplication occurs in about 20–40% of cases. There are twice as many girls as boys with duplications [11, 12].

2.1.2.2 Origin

Duplication may be transmitted as an autosomal dominant trait with incomplete penetrance. When an index child with a duplication is found in a family, the frequency of a sibling with a duplication increases. An increased incidence of other urinary tract anomalies has been associated with ureteral duplication that includes

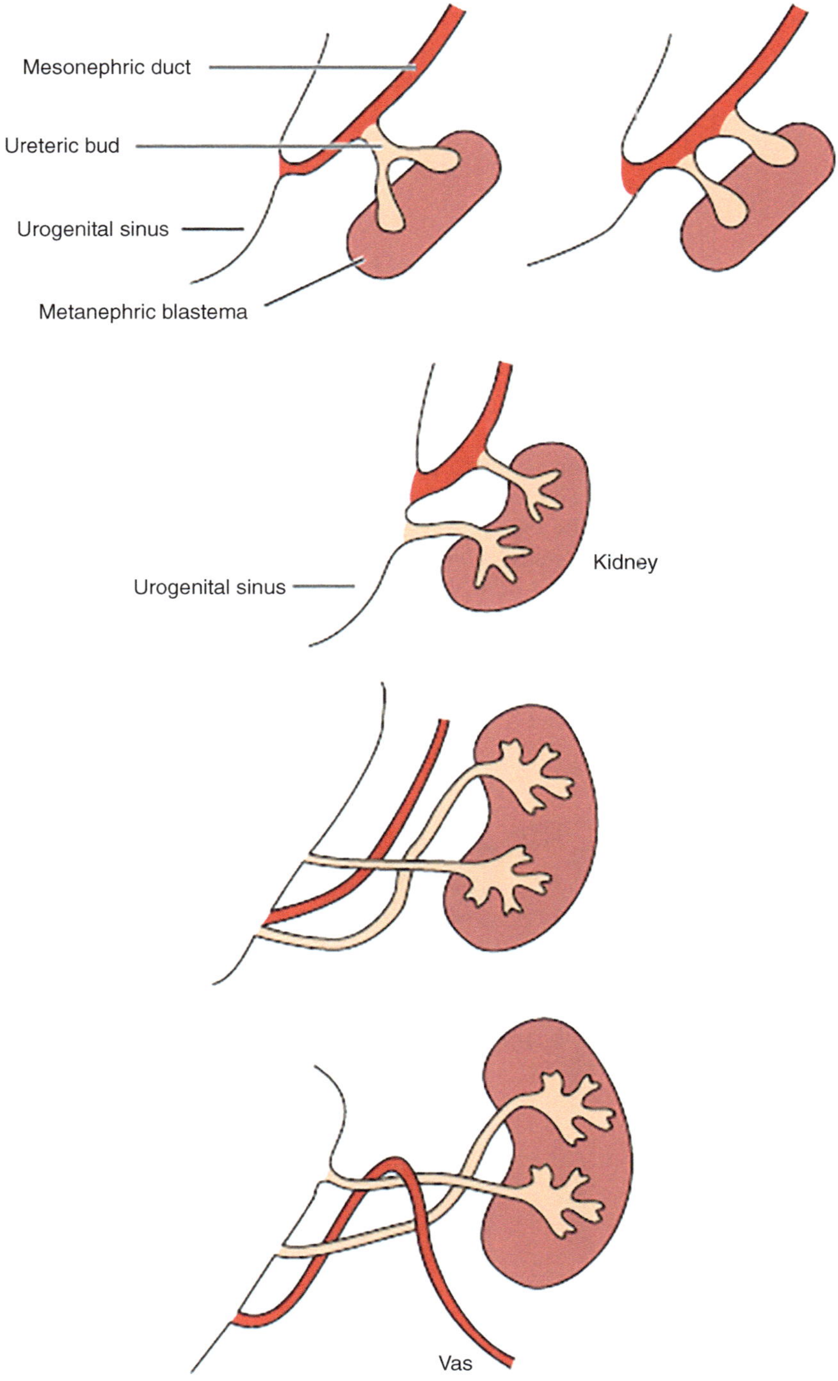

Fig. 2.3 Embryogenesis of ureteric duplication with evidence of Weigert-Mayer law

obstruction, reflux, or renal scarring. In children who present with UTIs and are found to have ureteral duplication, associated ectopic ureteroceles are present in 6% to 20% of children. On histological level, renal hypoplasia or dysplasia and pyelonephritic scarring have an increased incidence [11, 12].

2.1.2.3 Types

The type of duplication depends on whether the ureteric bud duplicates from its origin from the mesonephric duct or bifurcates after its formation [7, 13].

1. **Complete Duplication**

   Two ureteric buds originate from the mesonephric duct simultaneously. The formation of two ureteric buds from the start gives origin to a completely duplicated ureter (Fig. 2.4).

   Clinical Presentation: Urinary tract infection (UTI) is the most common mode of presentation, and the incidence of childhood UTIs is increased with duplications, as might be expected with the associated increased incidence of reflux or obstruction. A study of more than 700 children presenting with UTIs found that 8% had ureteral duplication. In one clinical series of patients with urinary symptoms, there was a much higher incidence of duplication: 2–4%.

   Diagnosis is established by intravenous pyelogram (IVP) or fluoroscopy showing the ureteral reflux. A CT urogram or MRU can help in diagnosis. A voiding cystourethrogram (VCUG) is essential to eliminate ureteral dilation due to VUR.

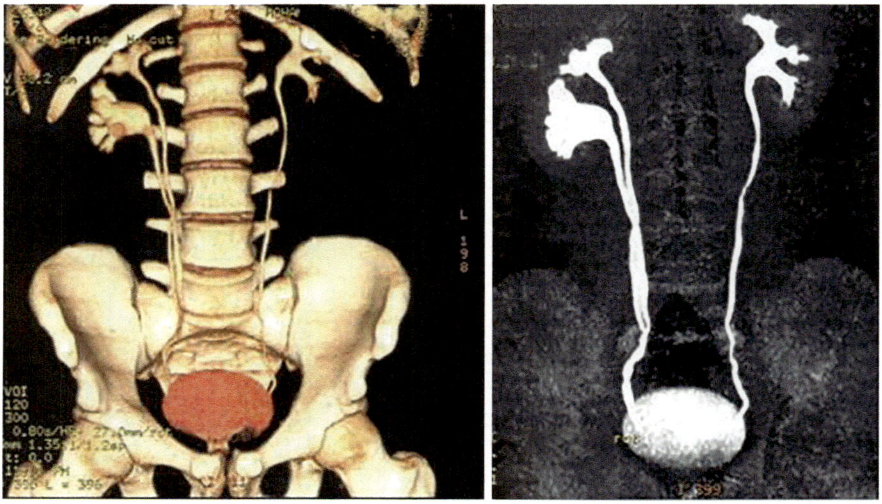

Fig. 2.4 CT urography with complete duplex right kidney. From the courtesy of Dr Bedeir Ali-El-Dein

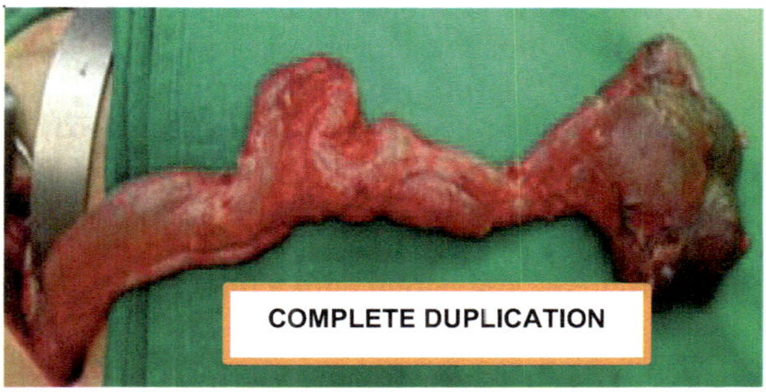

Fig. 2.5 Intraoperative picture of complete duplication. From the courtesy of Dr Bedeir Ali-El-Dein

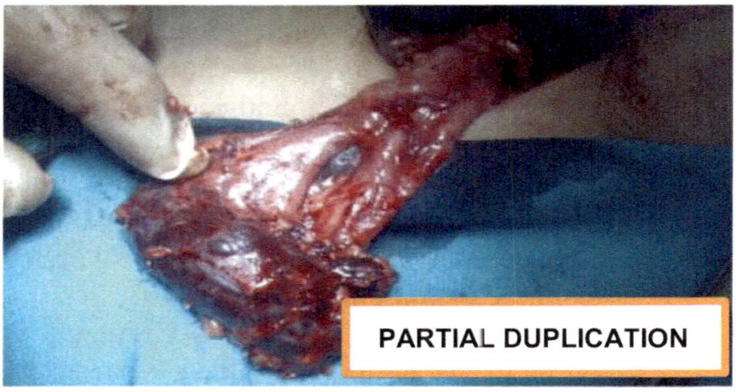

Fig. 2.6 Intraoperative picture of partial duplication. From the courtesy of Dr Bedeir Ali-El-Dein

Management: The presence of a ureteral duplication by itself is not an indication for intervention because many duplications may be incidentally noted (Fig. 2.5). Consideration of a surgical procedure is indicated based on the presence of associated abnormalities such as VUR, ureterocele, ectopic ureter, obstruction, or nonfunctional moiety [14].

2. **Incomplete Duplication (Y Ureter)**

A ureteral bud that bifurcates early results in an incomplete duplication. A bifid renal pelvis is the result of the most proximal anatomic level of bifurcation and occurs in about 10% of the population. Of the other incomplete duplications, approximately 25% each are found to divide in the proximal or distal third of the ureter, and the remaining 50% divide in the middle section (Fig. 2.6). Most partial duplications are discovered incidentally; however, with a Y junction in the ureter, it is possible for urine to be passed down to the junction and then, in a retrograde fashion, up the other side of the Y. This "yo-yo" ureteral reflux is most common when the bifurcation is at a low position but is rare if the duplication ends in the intramural portion of the ureter.

Clinical Presentation: In incomplete duplication, there may be associated urinary stasis, infection, ureteral dilation, or flank discomfort, but these findings are not common.

Management: When surgery is necessary in case of incomplete duplication, and the duplication is very low, a conversion to complete duplication with reimplantation of the ureters into the bladder with separate ureteral orifices may be possible. In cases with a higher duplication and single ureteral obstruction, a ureteropyelostomy or ureteroureterostomy at the kidney level with excision of most of the distal obstructed ureter is curative [15, 16]. Occasionally, ureteropelvic junction obstruction of the lower moiety may be associated with incomplete duplex systems and poses interesting reconstructive problems. Usually, the lower pole ureter is short, and a side-to-side anastomosis of the obstructed lower pole pelvis to the upper pole ureter is required.

3. **Incomplete Duplication with a blind-ending ureter**

   If a ureteral bud bifurcates, but only one limb induces the associated metanephric blastema, a rare form of incomplete duplication with one blind-ending ureteral branch is generated. Most of these duplications are in the middle or distal right ureter and affect females three times more often than males. Occasionally, a long blind-ending ureter may end in the bladder and be confused with a periureteral diverticulum because of the frequent association of VUR.

   Clinical Presentation: The blind-ending ureter rarely causes symptoms, but it may induce flank pain when associated with infection or calculi.

   Diagnosis: A retrograde ureterogram may be required for diagnosis because in the blind-ending duplication the blind duplication may not fill on IVP.

   Management: Treatment comprises surgical excision of the blind-ending ureter or entire duplication if clinically indicated.

4. **Incomplete Duplication (inverted Y Ureter)**

   When two separate ureteral buds arise from the mesonephric duct but fuse before penetrating the metanephric ridge, an inverted Y ureter is generated. This is a very rare anomaly and has been seen almost exclusively in girls. If one limb is distally ectopic, urinary incontinence may result. **Management:** Treatment is directed at problems caused by the ectopic limb and resection is usually required.

2.1.3 Ureteral Triplication

Ureter triplication is an extremely rare congenital anomaly of the urinary system with approximately 100 cases reported in the literature since it was first described in 1870 [17]. Ureteral triplication is more common in females and is commonly located on the left side. It is classified into 4 types and is frequently associated with ipsilateral or contralateral urological anomalies [18]. Associated congenital anomalies with ureteral triplication include ureteral duplication, ureteral ectopia, renal dysplasia, occasionally ureterocoele or vesicoureteric reflux, fusion anomalies, and rarely syndactyly, angiomas, or sex organs malformation [19–21].

2.1.3.1 Origin

Normally the ureter arises as a metanephric diverticulum (ureteric bud) in the 4-week embryo from the Wolffian duct. The ureteric bud grows dorsally and cranially and the dilated distal end differentiates into the renal pelvis and the major and minor calyces during the 6th to 8th weeks. Ureteric duplication and triplication have been explained by multiple ureteric buds arising independently from the Wolffian duct, and/or early fusion of one or more ureteral buds. Most cases of ureteral duplication conform to the Weigert-Meyer law, which states that the ureter from the upper pole of the kidney is incorporated into the bladder or the distal derivatives of the Wolffian duct more caudally and medially than the lower pole ureter [22]. However, the Weigert-Meyer principle does not apply to all patients with ureteral triplication. This lack of conformity has been postulated by Ireland and Chute as being due to the early splitting of a single ureteric bud [23].

2.1.3.2 Classification

Smith classification is used to classify ureter triplication into the following four subtypes (Fig. 2.7): (1) Complete triplication: where three ureters from the kidney drain separately into the bladder or ectopically. This is the most common type, accounting for 35% of all triplications. (2) Double ureter with one bifid: where there are three ureters from the kidney and two join draining into two ureteric orifices in the bladder. This accounts for 21% of triplications. (3) Trifid ureters: where the three ureters join into a single ureteral orifice seen in 31% of triplications. (4) Double ureters from the kidney, with one bifurcating as an inverted Y draining into three orifices in the bladder [18].

2.1.3.3 Clinical Presentation

Paucity of symptoms often leads to a delayed or missed diagnosis. Triple ureters may be responsible for recurrent UTIs, incontinence, enuresis, or flank pain caused by ureterocele but most of the time this anomaly is asymptomatic and detected incidentally during the investigation of other conditions, and this can explain its late presentation [21, 24].

2.1.3.4 Diagnosis

Urinary tract ultrasound and computed tomography are useful in the diagnosis of triplicate ureters, but intravenous urography or CT urography may be more useful in completely defining the anatomy (Fig. 2.8). Other investigations include VCUG, nuclear scans, and MRI. Cystoscopy and retrograde studies can prove the presence of one to three ureteric orifices according to the type of triplication [19, 25].

2.1.3.5 Management and Prognosis

The basic problem of triplication is its own correct diagnosis because it occurs in different forms, and it may be misdiagnosed as duplication. Sometimes it is even diagnosed incidentally during intraoperative dissection. Management depends on the presenting symptoms and the co-existing urinary anomalies. Once ureteral

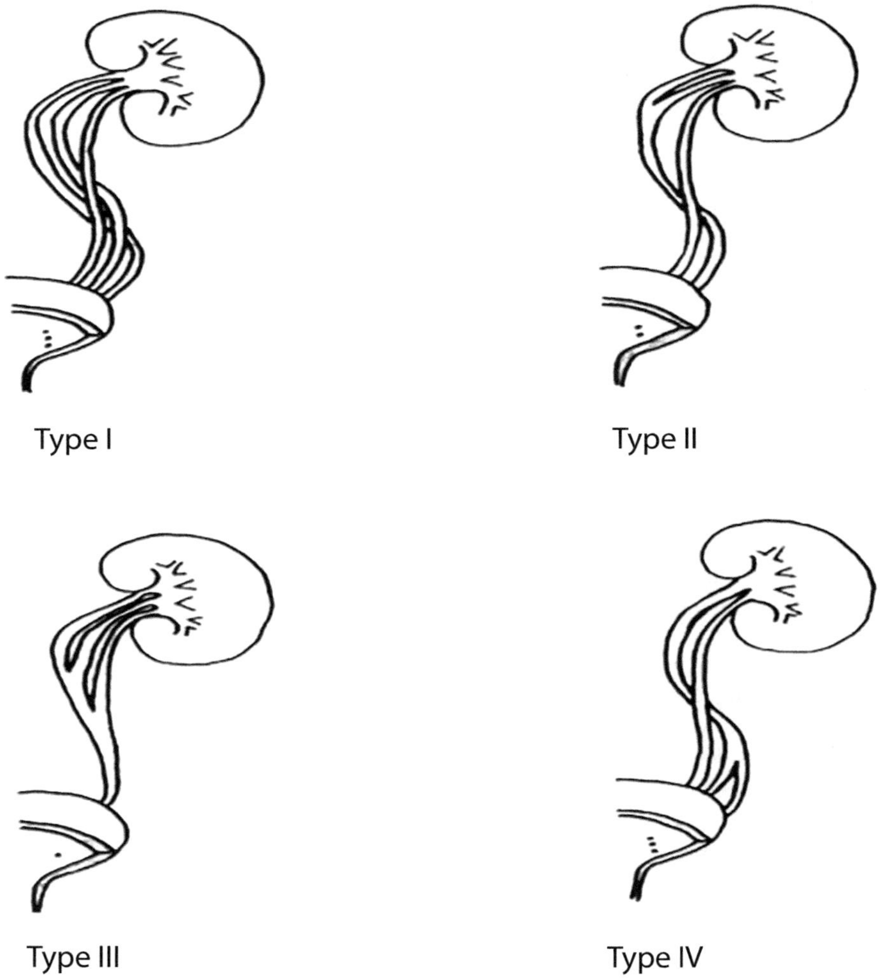

Fig. 2.7 Classification of the ureteric triplication (4 types)

triplication has been diagnosed, every patient requires an individual strategy for management and treatment [26, 27].

2.1.4 Ectopic Ureter

2.1.4.1 Definition

a ureter that does not open in its normal position in the superolateral aspect of the trigone.

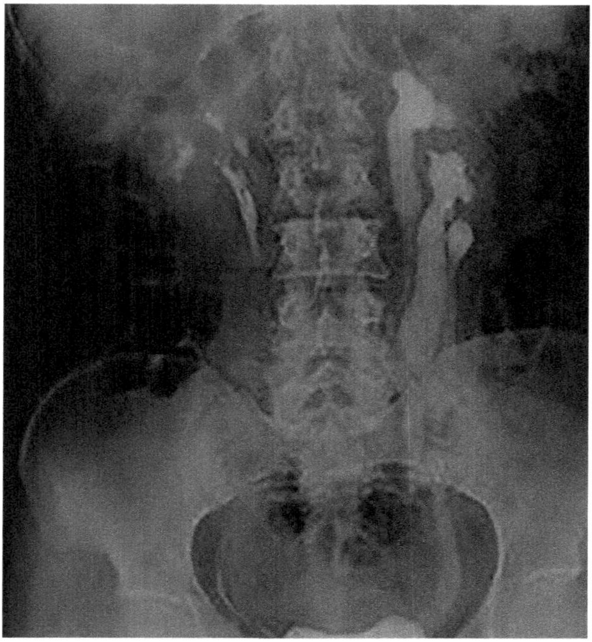

Fig. 2.8 IVP image of the left ureteric triplication

2.1.4.2 Embryology

When a ureteral bud originates slightly higher than normal on the mesonephric duct, it is incorporated into the urogenital sinus lateral than normal. This results in a shorter cranial and lateral migration, producing a minor displacement of the ureteral orifice caudally and medially toward the bladder neck. When the ureteral bud originates significantly higher than normal on the mesonephric duct, it might fail to incorporate into the bladder altogether and ends in the urethra or mesonephric remnants [28–30].

2.1.4.3 Sites

In males, an ectopic ureter can open into the epididymis, vas deferens, ejaculatory duct or seminal vesicle. An ectopic ureter always terminates above the level of the external urethral sphincter, so urinary incontinence is uncommon.

In females, by contrast, an ectopic ureter commonly exits below the sphincteric control, creating constant wetting from the ectopic ureter and normal voiding of urine from other ureters terminating in the bladder. In females, the ectopic ureter may open anywhere from the bladder neck to the perineum and into the vagina, uterus and even rectum. It may be associated with a cyst of the Gartner duct which is the distal remnant of the mesonephric duct that runs from the broad ligament of the uterus along the lateral wall of the vagina to end at the hymen. A very high origin of the ureteral bud in the female could end anywhere along this duct and, with secondary rupture of the duct into the vagina, resulting in a vaginally ectopic ureter [28–32].

2.1.4.4 Incidence

The incidence of ectopic ureters in the autopsy series is 1 in 1900 (0.05%). Ectopic ureters are much more common in girls, with only about 15% of ectopic ureters occurring in boys. In 80% of all ectopic ureters, the ureter is connected to the upper pole of a duplicated renal system. The percentage of ectopic ureters associated with duplication in girls is even higher than 80%; however, in boys, an ectopic ureter drains a single system more commonly. About 10% of ectopic ureters are bilateral. When an ectopic ureter is part of a duplex system, the contralateral system is duplicated in about 80% of cases, and 21% of these have contralateral ectopy as well [28–32].

Renal hypoplasia or dysplasia constitutes the most frequently encountered anomaly associated with an ectopic ureter. Generally, the degree of ureteral ectopy away from the bladder correlates with the degree of renal abnormality, although this correlation is more apparent for duplex systems than for single systems. Severe ectopy with an orifice in the genital system is almost always associated with nonfunctioning renal parenchyma. Some series have shown a higher incidence of other associated anomalies, especially imperforate anus, in single-system than in duplex ectopy [32, 33].

Ectopic Ureter in Girls

The essential gender difference in ureteral ectopy is that in girls the ectopic ureter can terminate at a level distal to the external sphincter and cause urinary incontinence. About one-third of ectopic ureters open at the level of the bladder neck or slightly more distally in the proximal urethra. With a higher orifice, there is a lesser chance of associated urinary incontinence; however, obstruction is more common because a higher ectopic ureter traverses the bladder neck and drains only during voiding when the continence mechanism is open. VUR occurs in 75% or more of these higher ectopic ureteral orifices, producing the paradox of reflux and obstruction. By having the bladder neck repeatedly open, the cyclic VCUG provides an opportunity for the obstructed ectopic ureter to drain before contrast material is voided, and increases the likelihood that the contrast material will reflux into the ectopic system. When the ectopic ureter enters at the level of the external sphincter or lower, reflux is less commonly present. One-third of ectopic ureters in girls terminate in the area of the vaginal vestibule closely around the urethral orifice. This area marks the terminal end of the Gartner duct, the mesonephric duct remnant in the female. Infrequently, an ectopic ureter enters what appears to be in a urethral diverticulum, but which is actually a Gartner duct cyst. In about 25% of ectopic ureters in girls, the orifice opens into the proximal vagina. More rarely, an ectopic ureter can end at a higher site along the course of the Gartner duct with an opening at the level of the cervix or uterus (5%). These uterine, cervical, or vaginal ectopic ureters probably result from rupture of the Gartner duct into the uro-vaginal canal along their common wall. Ureteral ectopy into the rectum is very uncommon but has been reported [33, 34].

Clinical Presentation: About one-half of girls with ectopic ureters present with a classic history of continuous dribbling of urine despite what seems to be a normal voiding pattern. Sometimes, parents may not note the abnormal character of continuous incontinence in a preschool-aged girl, and commonly the problem in the female goes not documented until adulthood. If the associated ureter is very dilated, the child may be continent when supine, and the pattern may be daytime wetting wrongly indicative of stress incontinence or bladder overactivity. Occasionally, girls may present with a persistent foul-smelling vaginal discharge. If the ureter ends in a Gartner duct cyst, the child may present with a mass on the anterior vaginal wall. When the ectopic orifice is quite high, and there is significant obstruction or reflux or both, urinary infection is frequent and is the most common presentation for an ectopic ureter in a small child. The evaluation of prenatal hydronephrosis is another form of presentation. An infant may present with an abdominal mass resulting from a severely obstructed ectopic ureter. There are well-documented cases of girls with ectopic ureters entering the vestibule or distal urethra without incontinence, presumably owing to obstruction of the ureter as it traverses the continence mechanism with emptying only during voiding.

Diagnosis: The diagnosis of an ectopic ureter in a girl may be somehow difficult. Ultrasound may be especially useful, detecting the dilated ectopic ureter behind the bladder (Fig. 2.9). If there is little dilatation of the ectopic upper pole system, diagnosis may depend on recognizing the absence of an upper pole calyx or an apparent excessive thickness of the renal tissue on the medial aspect of the upper pole. Computed tomography (CT) or renal scintigraphy may aid in making this diagnosis. Magnetic resonance imaging (MRI) has been used to delineate the fluid-filled ureter and its anatomy (Fig. 2.10). Bilateral ectopic ureters occur in about 10% of cases, and diagnosis frequently requires a high index of suspicion. If the ectopic ureter is single and beyond the continence mechanism, the associated renal tissue frequently is poorly functioning, and the diagnosis may be rendered even more difficult by the fact that the associated kidney itself may be ectopic or even crossed and fused. Renal function may be inadequate to permit visualization by either IVP or renal scan (Fig. 2.11).

During cystoscopy, the finding of a hemitrigone may lead to the erroneous diagnosis of renal agenesis. Physical examination with close observation of the area around the urethral meatus and distal vagina may reveal a recurring drop of liquid over a very small opening that can be probed and retrogradely injected to confirm the location of an ectopic ureter. Vaginograms carried out by occluding the introitus with a Foley balloon may show reflux into a vaginal ectopic ureter. The ectopic ureter alternatively may be visualized at vaginoscopy. The presence of an ectopic ureter may be suggested if the bladder is filled with methylene

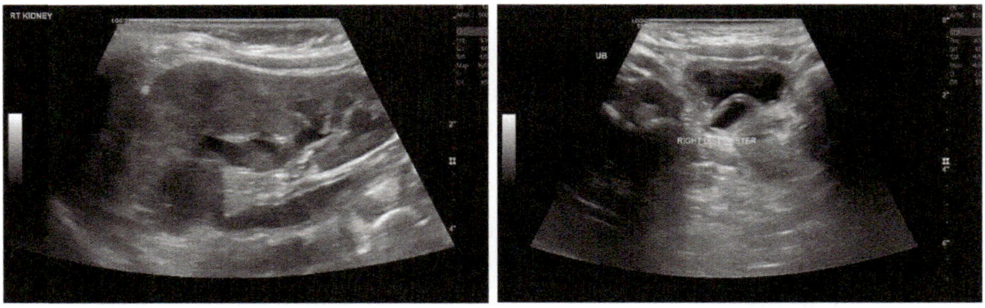

Fig. 2.9 Ultrasound photos of duplex right kidney with atrophic upper moiety and ectopic ureter of the upper moiety (dilated lower end of the ectopic ureter of upper moiety elevate the bladder base; pseudoureterocele)

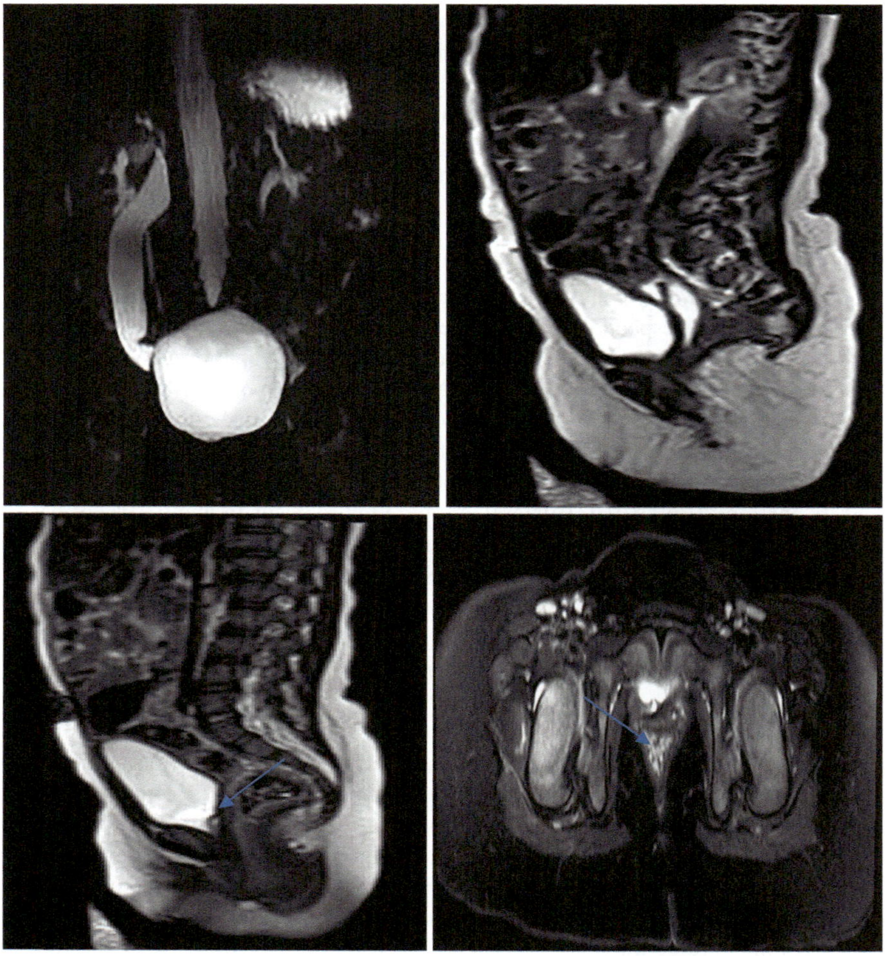

Fig. 2.10 MRU finding of the ectopic ureter of duplex right kidney with ectopic ureter ending in the bladder neck (arrow)

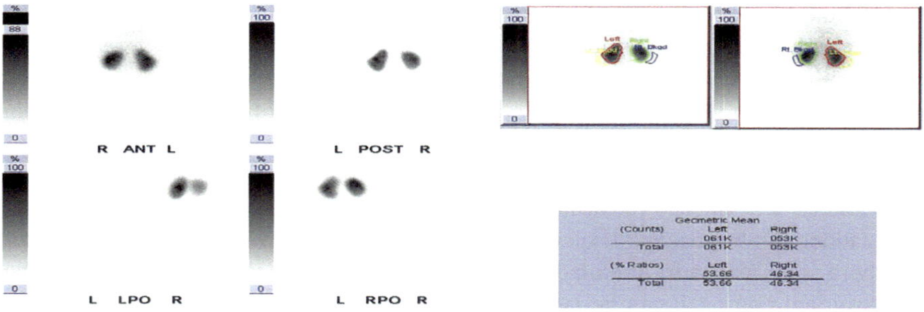

Fig. 2.11 DMSA scan of a patient with duplex right kidney with ectopic right upper moiety ureter showing nonfunctioning upper moiety

blue-stained saline solution via a Foley catheter and observation of the perineum reveals a continued slow drip of clear urine. Phenazopyridine hydrochloride (Pyridium) seems to be a better color marker excreted by poorly functioning renal tissue than methylene blue or indigo carmine, and if a cotton swab is left high in the vagina overnight and stains orange, it suggests the diagnosis of a vaginally ectopic ureter. Vaginoscopy with attention to the superior lateral aspect of the vagina may reveal the vaginal ectopic ureter. Exerting pressure on the anterior vaginal wall may produce a jet of cloudy fluid or pus from the ectopic orifice, revealing its presence. There are cases, however, in which exploratory surgery is required to look just above the bladder for the ureter. When found, the ureter can be traced upward to its associated renal unit.

Management: The surgical treatment of an ectopic ureter in a girl depends on the associated ipsilateral renal function. If the function of the ectopic ureter is worth saving, another option is ureterovesical reimplantation with tailoring as the ureter is usually dilated.

A single-system ectopic ureter to the genital system usually has a poor function, and a nephroureterectomy is appropriate, either by an open or a laparoscopic approach [35]. With a single-system ectopic ureter to the bladder neck or urethra, the function may justify ureterovesical reimplantation. Endoscopic injection with a bulking agent for VUR of an ectopic ureter with its orifice at the bladder neck has been attempted with a dismal 14% success rate. When the ectopic ureter is associated with the upper pole of a duplex renal unit, the function of the upper pole is usually poor, and an upper pole partial nephroureterectomy is generally performed. Rarely, the upper pole functions enough, and a ureteropyelostomy or ureteroureterostomy to drain the ectopic system into the lower pole system is appropriate. In the case of the lower pole pelvis being intrarenal and the lower pole ureter non-dilated, this approach is technically challenging [36, 37].

Management of the terminal ureteral stump in the case of an ectopic ureter is still controversial. If an ectopic ureter enters into the introitus or vagina, the entire distal ureter usually needs not to be removed because the distal ureteral segment is a rare source of later problems. If the distal segment becomes a source of stasis and infection, marsupialization of the ureter, usually a Gartner duct cyst, into the vagina corrects the problem. If nephroureterectomy without distal ureterectomy is performed in an ectopic ureter ending in the bladder neck or urethra, reflux of voided urine into the residual ureteral stump is likely to occur. The ureteral stump may lead to a small amount of dribbling incontinence after micturition or, more commonly, recurrent urinary infection. Plaire and colleagues reported the need for additional surgery to remove the ureteral stump in 12% of patients with ectopic ureter previously treated with an upper tract approach [38]. Removal of the ureteral stump is more likely to be needed for urinary ectopic ureters. Although the dissection behind the bladder can be tedious, if dissection is kept immediately on the wall of the ureter, there is no reason for the bladder neck or external sphincter to be damaged. The transtrigonal approach can be very useful. In a postpubertal girl, excision may be accomplished transvaginally. If the ectopic ureteral stump is not too large, its lining can be destroyed endoscopically using a Bugbee electrode to obliterate the ureteral lumen. Laparoscopic removal of distal ureteral stumps also has been described.

Ectopic Ureter in Boys

Ectopic ureters in boys may end in the bladder neck, posterior urethra to the level of the verumontanum, or mesonephric duct derivatives: epididymis, seminal vesicle, or vas deferens. The most common site of termination is the posterior urethra in one-half of male ectopic ureters; one-third join the seminal vesicle [29, 30, 38, 39, 40].

Clinical Presentation: In males, the presentation does not include incontinence, but rather infection and pain of the affected organs. Symptoms of flank pain and UTIs are more common. An ectopic ureter to the male genital tract may manifest as epididymitis. Any prepubertal boy with epididymitis requires evaluation for an ectopic ureter. In some boys, symptoms caused by a genitally ectopic ureter do not manifest until the onset of sexual activity. At that time, a man may present with epididymitis, prostatitis, seminal vesiculitis, or occasionally an infected seminal vesicle cyst that may lead to pain with a bowel movement or tenderness on rectal examination. A dilated single-system ectopic ureter into the prostatic urethra may elevate the bladder neck, causing outlet obstruction.

Diagnosis: A high index of suspicion is required to diagnose an ectopic ureter in a boy. An ectopic ureter entering the genital tract is often single and drains a nonfunctioning renal unit. Ultrasonography may show a dilated ureter and its associated renal element. In the case of an ectopic ureter associated with a duplex renal unit, the indirect signs of hydroureteronephrosis of the upper pole unit. The greatest diagnostic difficulties arise in duplex renal units when there is a tiny upper pole unit draining into a minimally obstructed ectopic ureter with little dilation. Most ureters ectopic to the urethra or bladder neck reflux, and careful examination of the oblique views from a VCUG and use of the cyclic voiding technique may enable the diagnosis to be made. In boys, as in girls, ectopic ureters at the level of the sphincters may show the paradoxical finding of obstruction and reflux. Occasionally, when the ectopic ureter is outside the urethra, the ejaculatory duct is so dilated as to permit reflux. MRI may be useful for showing the ectopic ureteral anatomy. The advent of fast-scan MRI technology should improve the utility of this diagnostic study in pediatric patients. The function of the affected renal unit should be assessed before the initial management using nuclear scans usually done by DMSA imaging. Cystoscopy and examination under anesthesia are useful in establishing the diagnosis of ectopic ureter. A mass may be palpated in the area of the seminal vesicle, or elevation of the bladder floor over a cyst ("pseudoureterocele") may be noted at cystoscopy. The ectopic ureteral orifice may be seen at the bladder neck or urethra, or there may be an enlarged ejaculatory duct that permits a retrograde study to establish the diagnosis. When there is single ureteral ectopy, a hemitrigone is present. Occasionally, a vasogram is useful in defining the anatomy.

Management: Treatment of an ectopic ureter associated with duplex units in boys usually involves removal of the associated poorly functioning renal unit. Rarely, the function is adequate to justify a diverting ureteropyelostomy or uretero-ureterostomy. Because the ectopic ureter is usually dilated, reimplantation of the duplex ectopic ureter into the bladder is a less attractive alternative. These issues arise only rarely in boys because most duplex ectopic ureters occur in girls. With a single-system ectopic ureter, a functioning renal unit worthy of salvage occurs more frequently with ectopy to the urinary tract. In contrast, when the single ectopic ureter enters a mesonephric remnant, the kidney usually functions poorly, and a nephroureterectomy is appropriate. When an ectopic ureter enters the male genital duct, it may be unfit for the passage of sperm, and ligation of the vas may be required to avoid recurrent epididymitis.

Bilateral Single Ectopic Ureters

Bilateral single ectopic ureters are rare, and when present at the level of the urethra or more distally are usually associated with a poorly developed bladder with an absent trigone with a poorly developed bladder neck. Very rarely, there is bladder agenesis. Associated genital and anal anomalies are very common with bilateral single ectopic ureters, as are associated renal dysplasia or hydronephrosis [41, 42]. Girls most commonly are found to have bilateral single ectopic ureters located in the distal urethra. Infant girls usually present with UTIs and continuous incontinence. Older girls most commonly present with incontinence. Girls generally have worse bladders and more severe renal anomalies than those seen in boys with bilateral single ectopic ureters. Because some urine enters the bladder in boys, it is often of slightly larger capacity than the bladder seen in girls. Although enough urine may enter the bladder in boys to permit some voiding to occur, boys may also present with incontinence. When bilateral single ectopic ureters are present at the bladder neck level, children may present with infection and upper urinary tract dilation from obstruction or reflux or both, but the bladder neck is generally better formed, and continence is more likely. When one ureter is ectopic to the urethra and one is ectopic at the bladder neck, there is an intermediate condition, but incontinence is usually present.

Diagnosis of bilateral single ectopic ureters is usually established by a carefully executed IVP and VCUG. The associated renal units may show very poor function.

The VCUG shows a small bladder with an open bladder neck. If the ectopic ureters are in the urethra, reflux is commonly present, and the VCUG usually makes the diagnosis. If the ureters are further down the ectopic pathway than the urethra, they usually are not shown by the VCUG. Ultrasound or MRI may be useful. A retrograde flush vaginogram with a Foley balloon occluding the introitus may similarly detect refluxing vaginally ectopic ureters. At cystoscopy, a child with bilateral single ectopic ureters usually is noted to have a poorly defined, funnel-shaped bladder neck and a small bladder capacity. In boys, the ureteral orifices are usually located in the distal bladder neck or urethra, but in girls, they may be more ectopic and more difficult to locate. A child who is incontinent with bilateral single ectopic ureters presents a major challenge to reconstructive surgery. In the case in which bladder capacity seems to be adequate, reimplantation of the ureters into the bladder and a Young-Dees-Leadbetter type of reconstruction of the bladder outlet may be appropriate. If bladder capacity is inadequate, it may be feasible to turn the entire bladder into a long detrusor tube to provide continence and to create an adequate reservoir by augmentation cystoplasty with antirefluxing anastomoses of the ureters to the bowel segment. The difficulty of creating a continent bladder outlet in this patient population frequently leads to eventual bladder neck closure and appendicovesicostomy to achieve continence [41, 42].

2.1.5 Ureteral Atresia

Ureteral atresia represents an extremely rare congenital malformation of the ureter, which is often associated with a dysplastic non-functioning kidney [43, 44]. Its combination with another urinary abnormality is even rare [45, 46]. The atresia may be unilateral or bilateral, short or long, and may involve any part of the ureter with the distal one more frequently affected than the proximal [44, 47]. There is no incidence data about ureteral atresia in each of its possible forms up to date.

2.1.5.1 Origin

The development of ureteral atresia is thought to be a result of relative or total ischemia that might occur during the migration of the developing kidney with changes in the distribution of regional blood supply to the ureter. This theory is based on experimental studies on intestinal atresia and might be extrapolated to explain ureteral stenosis and postnatal involution of the multicystic dysplastic kidney (MCDK) (Fig. 2.12). It is also hypothesized that the atresia could be caused by a failure of canalization of a segment of the ureter during the development and elongation of the ureteric bud [44, 48, 49].

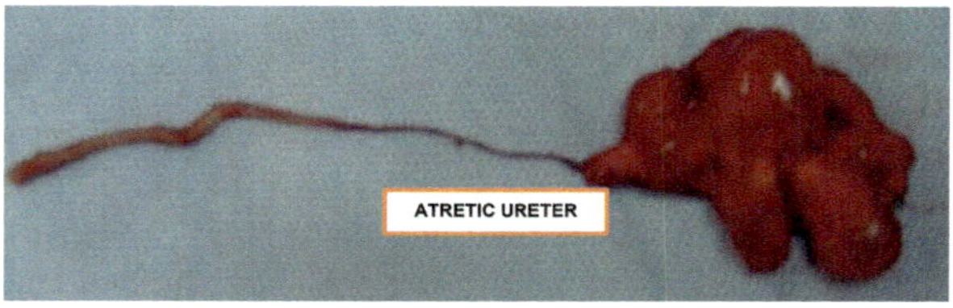

Fig. 2.12 Picture of the multicystic dysplastic kidney (MCDK) with the atretic upper ureter. from the courtesy of Dr Bedeir Ali-El-Dein

2.1.5.2 Types

Ureteral atresia may be unilateral or bilateral, distal or proximal, complete or partial, short or long. The ureter may be absent entirely, or it may end blindly after extending only part of the way to the flank.

2.1.5.3 Clinical Presentation

Ureteral atresia may be associated with an absent kidney or MCDK. The MCDK is usually unilateral, asymptomatic, and of no clinical significance. Rarely, it could be associated with hypertension, infection, or tumor. The distal atresia is more frequent and is associated with kidney dysplasia, even if cases of renal function recovery, after removal of the obstruction, are described [46, 50, 51].

2.1.5.4 Diagnosis

Ureteral atresia is often a cause of prenatal hydronephrosis, due to the obstruction of urine from the kidney. Prenatal diagnosis is possible and cases are detected by routine ultrasounds screening during pregnancy. Postnatally, renal ultrasound, CT, or even MRI, and nuclear scans are valuable radiological imaging for diagnosis. The MCDK has special radiological characteristics while other cases might be associated with either absent kidneys or hydronephrosis. Contralateral VUR is common, and many clinicians recommend a voiding cystourethrogram (VCUG) as a part of the initial workup [51].

2.1.5.5 Management

It depends on the associated anomalies. In cases of MCDK or absent kidneys, management is conservative in the majority of cases. In cases of distal ureteral atresia, only 11 cases were reported and among those, 4 of them had successful preservation of the renal function.

2.1.6 *Ureteral Diverticulum*

A ureteral diverticulum is a rare urological condition with only 45 cases described in the literature [52]. These previously reported cases vary in their presentation, diagnosis, and management and there is no consensus in the literature on the best diagnostic tool available. It may present as an incidental finding or by a secondary complication [53–55]. Diagnosis is usually made using a retrograde study. Conservative management is the mainstay of management and surgical management is only advocated in complicated cases.

Origin: It may arise from an abortive bifid ureter that ends blindly or is acquired from secondary obstruction (stone or iatrogenic).

2.1.6.1 Classification

Ureteral diverticulum is classified into 3 categories [56]

1. Abortive ureteral duplications as disordered ureteral budding
2. True congenital ureteral diverticulum comprised of the layers of a normal ureter
3. Acquired diverticulum secondary to ureteral obstruction representing a mucosal herniation.

2.1.6.2 Clinical Presentation

Ureteral diverticula might be entirely asymptomatic and only appear on imaging as an incidental finding or can present with hematuria, flank pain, urinary tract infection, and fever.

2.1.6.3 Diagnosis

Radiological imaging is the mainstay of diagnosis using ultrasound and CT [57]. The antenatal diagnosis was made by ultrasound in a congenital diverticulum. When associated with ureteral obstruction, a stone may be discovered with a proximal hydroureteronephrosis. A retrograde uretero-pyelogram is the most affirmative tool for diagnosis (Fig. 2.13).

2.1.6.4 Management

The majority of reported cases were managed conservatively. Only symptomatic cases associated with ureteral obstruction necessitated surgical intervention. Reconstructive surgery including segmental resection with the restoration of ureteral continuity was reported either by open, laparoscopic, or even robotic approach [58, 59].

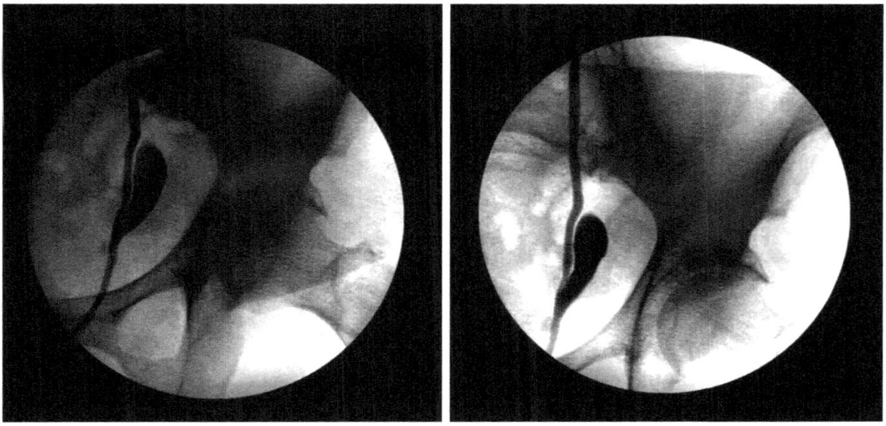

Fig. 2.13 A retrograde study showing distal ureteral diverticulum

2.1.6.5 Prognosis

In asymptomatic uncomplicated cases, the prognosis is usually excellent. The outcome after surgical management was also favorable. Very rarely, perforation of the diverticulum or malignancy has been reported [55, 60].

2.1.7 Retrocaval Ureter

Retrocaval ureter (RCU), also known as circumcaval ureter or pre-ureter vena cava, involves the right ureter and was first described in 1893 [61]. It is a rare congenital anomaly that occurs due to anomalous development of inferior vena cava (IVC) and not ureter with a reported incidence of one in 1500 at autopsy. The incidence of RCU in males is approximately four times higher than that in females [62]. Associated anomalies have been reported in up to 20% of patients with RCU. These congenital anomalies include cardiovascular anomalies, genitourinary anomalies such as horseshoe kidney, absent or ectopic opposite kidney, agenesis of vas or uterus, Turner syndrome, and imperforated anus [63]. Therefore, all patients with RCU should be screened for these disorders.

2.1.7.1 Origin

Embryologically, the condition occurs due to the anomalous development of vena cava wherein the right subcardinal vein persists and forms the inferior vena cava (IVC), which remains ventral to the ureter; consequently, the ureter passes behind the IVC and then turns around the IVC to attain the final lateral position. This results in an anomalous relationship between the IVC and the ureter.

2.1.7.2 Types

Huntington and McClure (1920) described 15 different types of pre-ureteral vena cava; 12 of these types have been documented in animals. In 1959, Nelson described five different variants in human beings [61]. The first type is unilateral right-sided single preureteral vena cava is caused due to the persistence of the right subcardinal vein and or the disappearance or failure of development of the right supracardinal vein. The second group is unilateral right-sided double IVC and the ureter lies between the two veins is caused because of the persistence of the right supracardinal vein and right posterior cardinal vein. The third group consists of bilateral, single IVC of which the right is preureteric and the left is postureteric is due to the persistence of the right posterior cardinal vein and left supracardinal vein. The fourth type is bilateral single preureteric IVC arises because of the persistence of the right and left posterior cardinal veins. The fifth group is double right vena cava, ureter between the two veins, and single postureteric left vena cava occurs because of the persistence of the right supracardinal and posterior cardinal veins and left supracardinal vein [64].

Radiologically Bateson and Atkinson (1969) classified RCU into Type I and Type II; 90% of the retrocaval ureter is Type 1 [65]. Type I is characterized by a typical S-shaped, "fish hook" or "shepherd crook" deformity and is associated with moderate-to-severe hydronephrosis (Fig. 2.14). In these cases, the ureter passes behind the IVC at the level of the third lumbar vertebral segment. The majority of the patients with Type 1 RCU are obstructed and symptomatic. Type II RCU is a rare subtype associated with a gentler curve and appears as sickle-shaped on IVU/CT urogram. Most patients with Type II are asymptomatic.

2.1.7.3 Clinical Presentation

The condition is usually associated with the obstructed ipsilateral pelvicalyceal system. RCU is either atretic or kinked, leading to obstruction [66]. Although the pathology is congenital, a majority of cases present in the third to fourth decade of life. Clinical presentation of the patients may vary from incidental detection to flank pain, pyelonephritis, renal stone disease, and rarely gross hematuria. The patients typically present with flank pain secondary to obstruction, pyelonephritis, or with urolithiasis requiring surgical intervention.

2.1.7.4 Diagnosis

The initial investigation of choice is ultrasound; subsequently all patients underwent CT urogram with 3D reconstruction. CT urogram facilitates precise anatomical delineation of the pelviureteral junction, the relation of the lower ureter with the IVC, and the presence of any other aberrant vessels [67]. This facilitates the planning of definitive surgery. Authors of previous case series recommend RGP in all

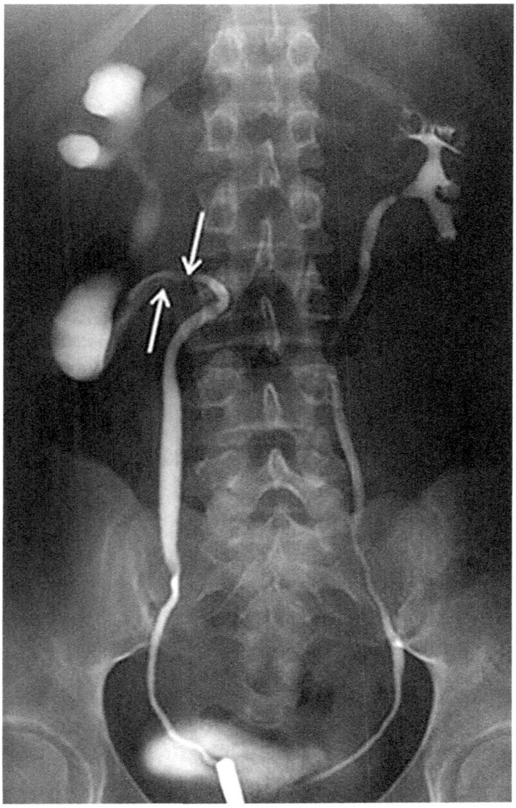

Fig. 2.14 Fish-hook sign of retrocaval ureter

patients before definitive repair. MRI can demonstrate the course of RCU and could give more detailed anatomy which is less invasive when compared with CT and RGP.

2.1.7.5 Management

Symptomatic patients or patients with obstruction require surgical intervention. The obstruction has traditionally been treated with pyelopyelostomy, pyeloureterostomy, and ureteroureterostomy after ureteral division (Fig. 2.15). Anderson and Hynes originally described the necessity of dismembering the ureter in a patient with RCU in 1949 [68]. However, open surgery has now been largely replaced by laparoscopy [69, 70]. Nonetheless, the laparoscopic techniques for retrocaval ureter are technically challenging due to the complex relationship of the ureter with the IVC. Currently, laparoscopic repair is the procedure of choice; however, the approach, that is, retroperitoneal or transperitoneal, would depend on the surgeon's preference [71–73]. The first case of transperitoneal laparoscopic repair

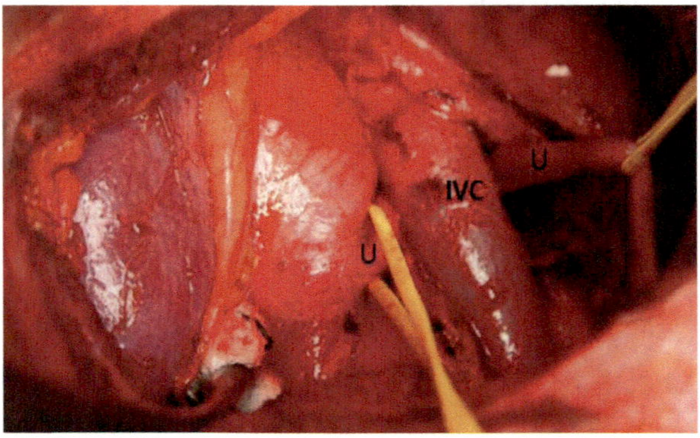

Fig. 2.15 Intraoperative photo of retrocaval ureter. From the courtesy of Dr Bedeir Ali-El-Dein

for RCU was reported in 1994 by Baba et al.; the procedure lasted around 9 h [69]. Extracorporeal anastomosis has been suggested as a means to reduce the operative time. Robotic repair of the RCU was reported with a good success rate [74, 75].

2.1.8 Vesicoureteric Reflux (VUR)

2.1.8.1 Definition

VUR is a permanent or intermittent retrograde flow of bladder urine into the upper urinary tract. In normally developed ureters, the ureteric insertion point is tunneled obliquely within the bladder muscular layer in a length-to-diameter ratio of 5:1. If the insertion was ectopic or the insertion ratio was not matched; VUR is due to happen.

2.1.8.2 Types

It occurs either as a primary abnormality in an anatomically normal bladder or secondary to another cause of urine flow impairment or bladder pathology.

2.1.8.3 Incidence

The incidence in the general pediatric population is 1% to 2%, and it is usually diagnosed in infants being investigated for urinary tract infection. The associated predisposition to infection can lead to significant morbidity due to scarring and chronic renal dysfunction [76]. VUR accounts for approximately 10% of all instances of prenatally diagnosed hydronephrosis, although bilaterally dilated ureters and bladder may be seen in severe cases. It is not possible to make a definitive diagnosis in utero. More than 80% of children with prenatally diagnosed reflux are boys. In contrast, the postnatal incidence of reflux has a female-to-male ratio of 5:1. The increased voiding pressure required in boys, which in utero may distort the ureterovesical junction, is a possible explanation for this. VUR may be associated with other renal abnormalities, in particular, ureteroceles in duplex kidneys, PUJ anomalies, multicystic dysplastic kidneys, and unilateral renal agenesis.

2.1.8.4 Diagnosis

Prenatal sonography may not be able to assess VUR cases definitively, so all infants should be carefully assessed in the postnatal period. For prenatally diagnosed VUR, the dilatation may be confirmed postnatally with ultrasound, but this is not reliable. A micturating cystourethrogram (MCUG) should be carried out to confirm the presence of VUR and to grade it (Fig. 2.16). If reflux is suspected, it is important to proceed postnatally to a DMSA isotope scan, so that individual renal function and the presence of renal scarring can be assessed [77]. Approximately 60% of kidneys with significant degrees of reflux show an abnormal renogram within the first 4 weeks of life before a urinary tract infection had occurred in the majority of cases. These data suggest that abnormalities in renal development with reflux occur during intrauterine life. A top-down approach with A DMSA first then MCUG, if there is an abnormal finding, is also available [78].

2.1.8.5 Management

Management options of VUR include conservative medical treatment, endoscopic correction, and anti-reflux surgery [79–81]. There is no consensus on the optimal management of VUR, VUR treatment options, or the most effective timing of treatment, and because of the complexity of VUR cases and their variable presentations, the clinical management should be individualized [82]. Conservative treatment refers to active surveillance and antibiotic prophylaxis. Patient compliance plays a crucial role in this therapeutic option and, the patient's parent or guardian needs to understand that compliance is the cornerstone throughout the therapeutic journey of their child [83].

Surgical treatment can be classified into two main groups. The first group includes endoscopic surgeries, which refers to the endoscopic sub ureteric injection of bulking agent to create support to the intravesical ureters without obstructing the urine's antegrade flow, at the same time allowing maturation and elongation of the ureter's intramural tunnel [81, 84]. The second group includes ureterovesical reimplantation via open, laparoscopic, and robotic approaches.

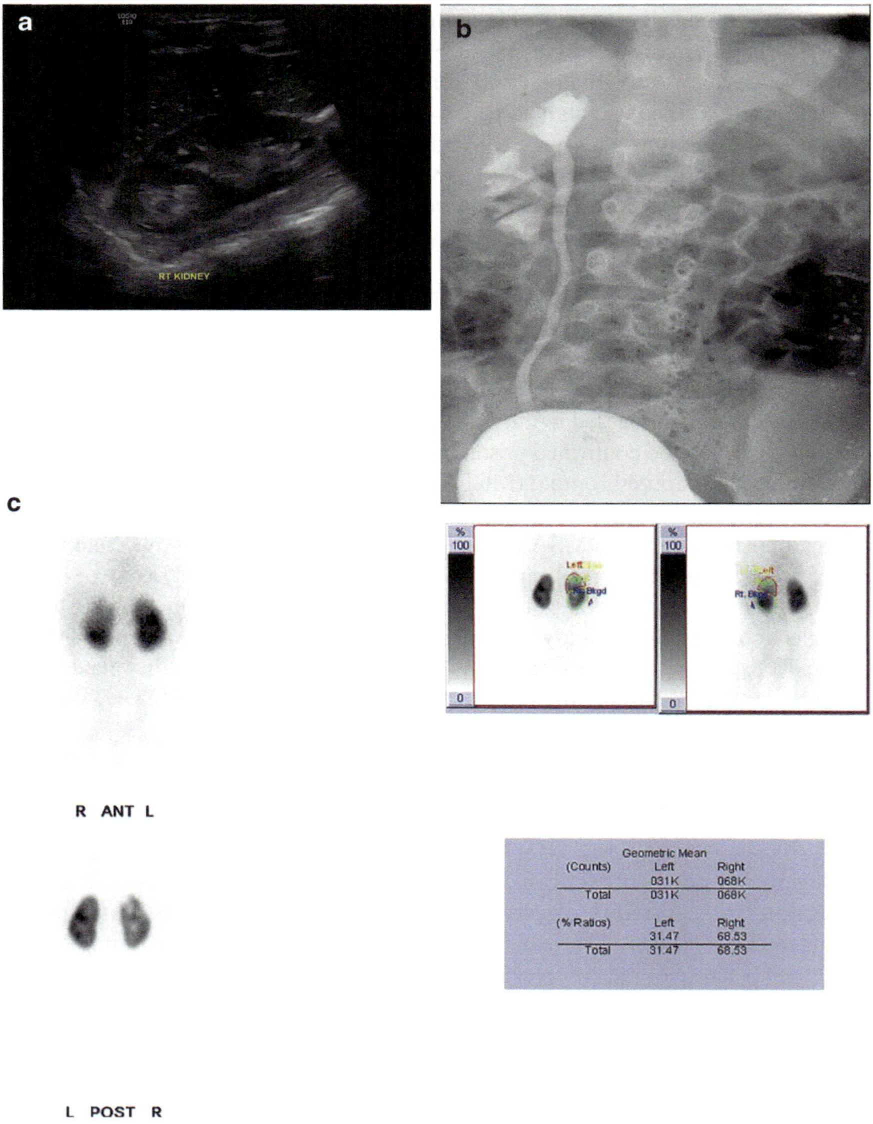

Fig. 2.16 Images of a case of VUR with duplex right kidney. Ultrasound image showed duplex right kidney with no Hydronephrosis (**a**). VCUG showed G3 VUR in both upper and lower moieties (**b**). DMSA scan showed evidence of scarring in both moieties (**c**)

2.1.9 *Ureteropelvic Junction Obstruction (UPJO)*

2.1.9.1 Definition

UPJO is a dilatation of the renal pelvis and calyces without ureteral dilatation.

2.1.9.2 Incidence

It is the most common cause of congenital hydronephrosis, accounting for 35% of prenatally detected uropathies, with an incidence of 1 in 2000 live births. Males are more commonly affected with a 2:1 male: female ratio. The majority of cases occur unilaterally and are more common on the left side. The incidence of bilateral UPJO is between 10 and 40% [85, 86].

2.1.9.3 Etiology

It is of unknown etiology, however, there are three theoretical causes of PUJ obstruction: extraluminal, luminal, and intraluminal. Luminal anomalies are the most common type and are caused by an abnormal distribution of the muscular and collagen fibers at the level of the PUJ. Extraluminal anomalies are less common and can be caused by aberrant vessels, kinks, bands, adhesions, and arteriovenous malformations, spanning the PUJ and reducing the urine flow intermittently. In these cases, the dilatation of the pelvis and symptoms are often intermittent. Intraluminal anomalies are rare and are mainly due to ureteral valves or benign fibroepithelial ureteral polyps [85–87].

2.1.9.4 Associated Anomalies

It is essential to define whether the PUJ anomaly is an isolated condition or is associated with other anomalies. Twenty-five percent of cases are associated with other renal abnormalities, including renal agenesis, multicystic dysplastic kidney (MCDK), VUR, ureteric hypoplasia, partial or complete ureteric duplication, and horseshoe kidney. Some cases have extra-renal abnormalities, such as anorectal anomalies, congenital heart disease, or VATER syndrome.

2.1.9.5 Diagnosis and Management

A definitive diagnosis of PUJ anomaly cannot be made until after birth. However, the diagnosis may be suspected prenatally if renal pelvis dilatation is seen without ureteric dilatation, and with a normal bladder appearance. Amniotic fluid volume is usually normal. Differential diagnoses include MCDK, megaureter, renal cysts, and perinephric urinomas. As obstruction progresses, the renal cortex becomes thinner, and associated dysplasia may manifest with increased cortical echogenicity or cortical cysts, or both. Serial ultrasound scans are recommended during pregnancy to assess the degree and progression of dilatation, because this may correlate with postnatal renal function [88].

The outcome is generally good for both unilateral and bilateral affection. Serial sonography during pregnancy may help to inform both parents and pediatricians as to the likelihood of requirement for surgical intervention, but ultimately this decision will be undertaken after postnatal investigation (Figs. 2.17 and 2.18). After delivery, the infant should be placed on prophylactic antibiotics while these tests are carried out, to minimize the risk of urinary tract infection. Almost one-third of cases required surgical intervention and is usually by pyeloplasty through an open, laparoscopic or robotic approach [68]. Indications for intervention include worsening hydronephrosis on serial ultrasound, deteriorating differential renal function on diuretic renogram, and symptomatic cases.

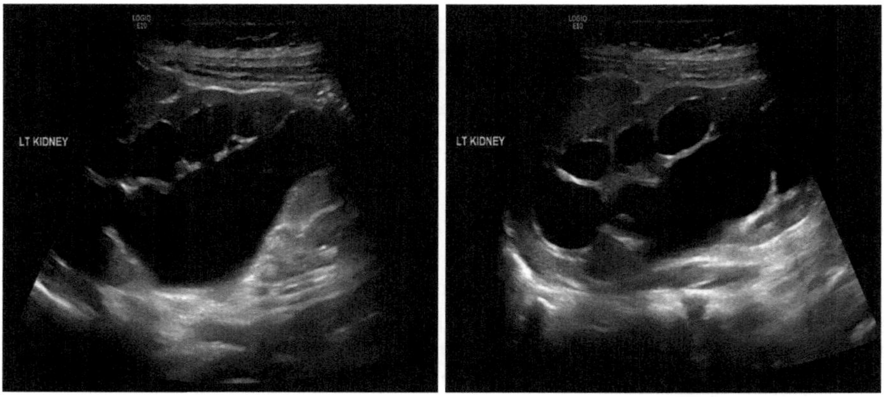

Fig. 2.17 Ultrasound image of a girl with antenatal hydronephrosis showing postnatal left G4 hydronephrosis with non-dilated upper ureter; a picture of left UPJO

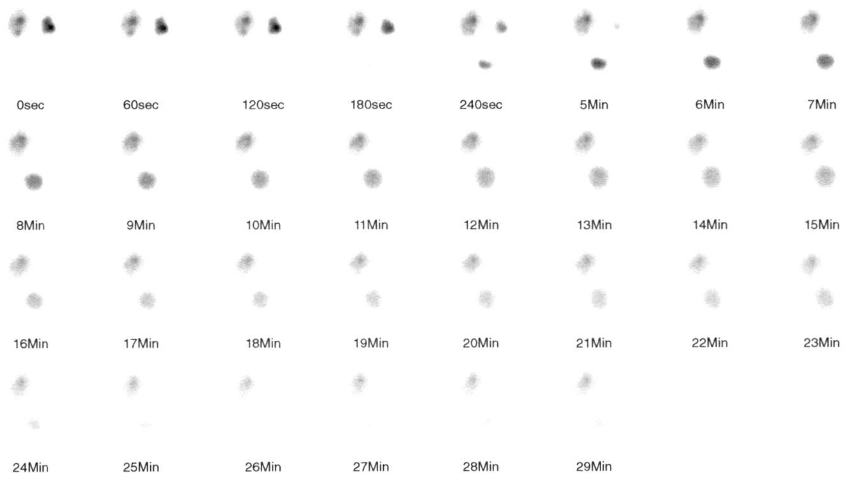

Fig. 2.18 MAG3 image showing obstructed left kidney with delayed excretion of radiocontrast

2.1.10 Ureterocele

2.1.10.1 Definition

A ureterocele is a cystic dilatation of the distal part of the ureter.

2.1.10.2 Incidence

Ureteroceles are known to happen roughly in 1 in 4000 children, being most common in Caucasians. They are more frequently seen in females and the left side is more to be affected. Bilateral ureteroceles can occur in up to 10% of patients. A ureterocele may occur isolated in single ureter systems or is usually associated with the ureter of the upper pole of a duplex kidney in 80% of cases. Incidence of an ectopic ureterocele has been seen almost four times as compared to the intravesical ureterocele [39, 89, 90].

2.1.10.3 Etiology

It is a cystic dilatation of the submucosal segment of the intravesical ureter with consequent narrowing of the ureteral orifice. Etiology is related to uretero-trigonal development error. Proposed etiologies include ureteral meatal obstruction, incomplete muscularization of the distal ureter, and excessive dilatation of the ureter as it incorporates into the bladder.

The embryology of all ureteroceles cannot be explained by one model. In the embryo, Chwalla described a two-cell layer ureteral membrane that is present at the time the ureteral bud arises from the mesonephric duct and later recedes. If this membrane does not completely break down, an obstructed ureteral-meatal orifice could result, leading to the formation of a ureterocele. The ureteroceles seen with stenotic orifices or associated with muscular hypertrophy of the ureteral wall support Chwalla's model. Stephens and others have described cases, however, in which ureteroceles are found to have large patulous ureteral orifices that are difficult to explain with Chwalla's model. Alternatively, it has been suggested that the distal ureteral segment may be acted on by the same forces that cause the expansion of the urogenital sinus to form the bladder. Tanagho's model suggests that delay in establishment of the lumen of the ureteral bud with that of the mesonephric duct could result in ureteral expansion secondary to the same process that results in expansion of the urogenital sinus into the bladder. If this model were a complete explanation for ureterocele formation, all caudal ectopic ureters should be associated with a ureterocele, which is not the case. Renal tissue associated with ectopic ureters and ureters joining ureteroceles is frequently dysplastic or hypoplastic.

2.1.10.4 Classification

The simplest system is either intravesical or extravesical (ectopic) ureterocele. In each category, additional features can be described as follows:

1. Stenotic: The orifice is very tiny and difficult to identify.
2. Sphincteric: The orifice is situated within the urethral sphincter zone.
3. Caecoureterocoele: The orifice is in the bladder and there is a caudal extension in the submucosal plane of the urethra.
4. Blind ureterocoele: There is atrophy of the ureter distal to the ureterocoele.

2.1.10.5 Clinical Presentation

Presentations are related to obstruction, infection, and urinary incontinence.

- Acute obstruction occurs at the bladder outflow tract and is caused by ectopic ureterocoeles extending into the urethra. This represents the most common cause of bladder outlet obstruction in girls and is the second most common cause in boys after posterior urethral valves. The clinical presentation is that of a distended, palpable bladder with failure to pass urine.

- A prolapsing ureterocoele presents as a purplish mass protruding from the urethral orifice, showing congestion and edema. The urethral opening can usually be identified and catheterized.
- Obstruction can also lead to hydronephrosis, which in severe cases presents with an abdominal mass.
- Urinary tract infection (UTI) occurs in 50% of cases. Patients present with flank pain and fever, indicating pyelonephritis. This may also be associated with failure to thrive and nonspecific abdominal pain [39, 91].

2.1.10.6 Diagnosis

Ureteroceles may be identified prenatally by the detection of an echolucent circular rim within the fetal bladder. Occasional non-visualization of a ureterocele in a bladder, particularly during fetal life may be due to its compression. They may exist and be imaged outside the bladder simulating a fetus with such cystic masses as an ovarian cyst or anterior meningocele [39, 91, 92].

On postnatal ultrasound, the ureterocele is usually imaged as a thin-walled cystic structure seen within the bladder (Fig. 2.19). One report suggested they could simulate a pseudo-septated bladder. Also, a dilated upper pole of a duplex system or a dilated single system may be identified.

A micturating cystourethrogram (MCUG) is carried out in all cases where the US has demonstrated a dilated upper tract or the presence of a ureterocoele. The MCUG may show reflux into the lower moiety of a duplex system and thus delineate the dilated ureter (Fig. 2.20). The dimercaptosuccinic acid (DMSA) scan is useful to identify the functioning renal tissue and to assess the presence of renal scarring which helps in the management decision. Endoscopic evaluation is the final element of diagnosis to check the urethra, bladder neck, trigone, and the location of ureteric orifices and the ureterocele [91, 92].

2.1.10.7 Management

Management strategy may vary from patient to patient and is prejudiced by various factors such as age, presenting complaints, presence of any reflux, the function of each renal segment in case it is associated with a duplex system, and complications like urinary tract infection. Basic measures are taken to preserve renal function. Over the last few decades there have been many different surgical approaches, and yet there still is no consensus among pediatric urologists regarding the optimal surgical strategy [92, 93]. In 2010, Merguerian et al. surveyed pediatric urologists to determine practice patterns in the management of intravesical ureteroceles arising from the upper pole of a duplicated system. They found a significant variation in practice and also noted that most participants saw fewer than 10 cases per year [94].

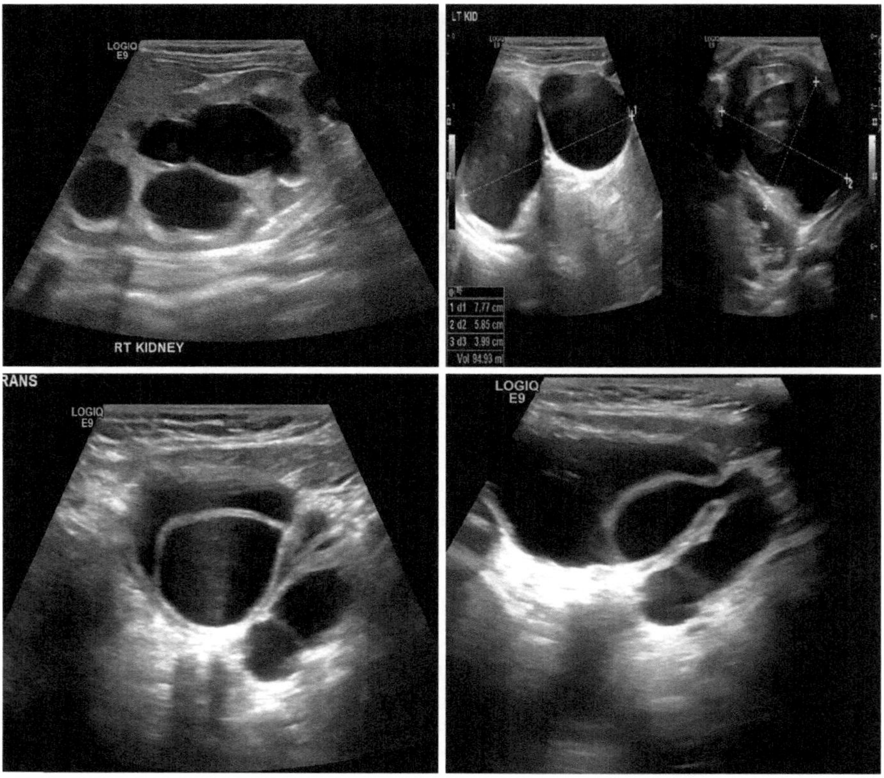

Fig. 2.19 Ultrasound of a boy with antenatal bilateral hydronephrosis showing evidence of left ureterocele in a duplex left kidney with bilateral hydroureteronephrosis

Primarily, these cases were managed by a transurethral incision of the ureterocele which is an easy, minimally invasive, and practicable option for dealing with patients who have ureteroceles. Endoscopic puncture of the ureterocele was initially proposed to be a definitive procedure, but subsequent studies have shown this was often not the case; however, it was very effective when used as a temporizing measure in cases of bilateral obstruction or infection, followed by lower tract reconstruction. The risk of VUR development after incision varies from 0–50% depending on the method, and type of the ureterocele. Secondary surgery is more common with extravesical ureteroceles and with lower pole VUR [39, 93, 95].

In case of a non-functioning upper pole: a total reconstruction of both upper and lower tracts in the form of upper pole nephrectomy, ureterocele excision, and reimplantation of the lower pole ureter was performed via two incisions (flank and suprapubic) then by laparoscopic upper pole partial nephrectomy and Pfannenstiel incisions. The reported success rates were good but it is uncertain if it is appropriate for most children. In case of a functioning upper pole with a ureterocele, the management is by lower

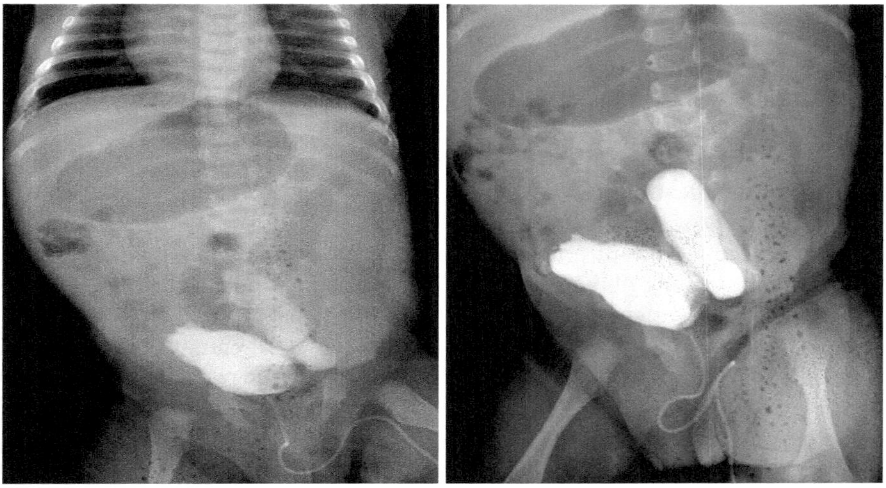

Fig. 2.20 VCUG of a boy with left ureterocele in duplex left kidney showing the filling defect of ureterocele and left G5 VUR in the lower moiety of duplex left kidney

urinary tract reconstruction (ureterocele excision and common sheath ureteric reimplantation) or via pyeloureterostomy or uretero-ureterostomy [39, 96, 97].

Observational management was also adopted in carefully selected patients with ureterocele but is controversial [98]. If there is no obstruction on the diuretic renogram, a non-functioning upper moiety with a limited degree of VUR in the lower pole ureter, there is a good chance of resolution of the upper pole dilatation and the lower pole VUR. The challenge is in counseling families regarding this approach.

2.1.11 Megaureter

The term megaureter is a descriptive term that was first described by Caulk in 1923 as megaloureter. It is an uncommon cause of severe hydronephrosis [99, 100].

2.1.11.1 Definition

A megaureter is a ureteral dilatation of 7 mm or more irrespective of the cause [101, 102].

2.1.11.2 Incidence

VUJO anomalies account for about 10% of prenatally detected instances of upper tract dilatation, with an approximate incidence of 1 in 6500 live births. The male-to-female ratio is approximately 2:1, and up to 25% of cases are bilateral [99–102].

2.1.11.3 Etiology

Primary due to intrinsic stenosis or secondary due to bladder pathology e.g. neurogenic bladder or bladder outlet obstruction.

2.1.11.4 Classification

Belman defined 3 types of primary megaureter: obstructed, refluxing, and nonrefluxing nonobstructing [99]. The exact etiology of these is unknown.

The obstructed variety is really caused by a functional obstruction theoretically of similar etiology to the UPJ obstruction but at the distal end of the ureter (i.e., deficiency of ureteral smooth muscle fibers leading to limited peristalsis). A catheter can be placed through the UVJ proving it to be a functional rather than true anatomic obstruction. It usually involves the distal 2 cm (0.5–4 cm) of the ureter. The abnormal ureter is of normal caliber. More proximal ureter, usually the distal third, but at times the entire ureter and even the pelvis are dilated. The ureteral orifice and the submucosal tunnel are normal.

Refluxing megaureter may be caused by a short or absent intravesical ureter or a paraureteric diverticulum.

The nonobstructing nonrefluxing megaureter is caused neither by reflux or stenosis and is the most common type of megaureter in neonates.

A more practical classification was given by King in 1980 as refluxing, obstructed, not refluxing, not obstructed, and both refluxing and obstructed [100].

2.1.11.5 Clinical Presentation

The majority of cases are diagnosed by an antenatal screening (around 80%) are asymptomatic. Presenting symptoms include UTIs, abdominal pain, and hematuria.

2.1.11.6 Diagnosis

Prenatal sonography shows a dilated ureter, which may be seen communicating with the dilated renal pelvis. The bladder appearance and Amniotic fluid volume are normal. The main differential diagnoses are VUR and ureteric obstruction due to ureterocele associated with a duplex kidney. Coexisting urologic abnormalities occur in about 15% of cases and include PUJO, MCDK, ectopic pelvic kidney, renal agenesis, and VUR.

Postnatal sonography usually shows a markedly dilated ureter behind the bladder with varying degrees (Fig. 2.21). Further imaging information is necessary to exclude secondary causes of megaureter such as posterior urethral valves, urethral stricture, ureterocele, or neurogenic bladder [101]. Voiding cystourethrography

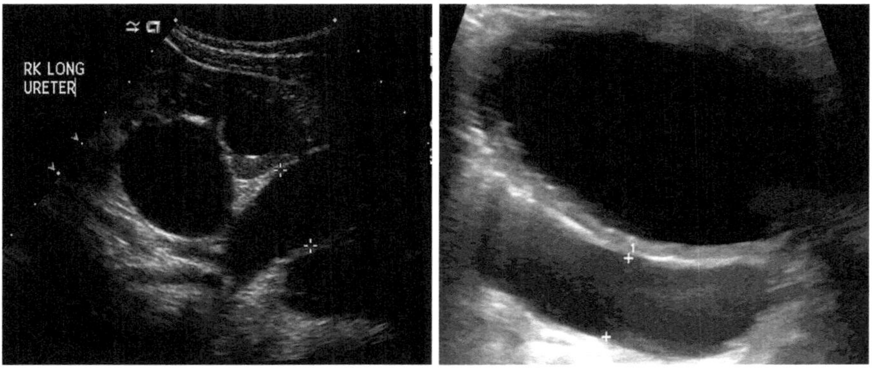

Fig. 2.21 Ultrasound image of obstructed right megaureter

Fig. 2.22 VCUG image of refluxing left megaureter

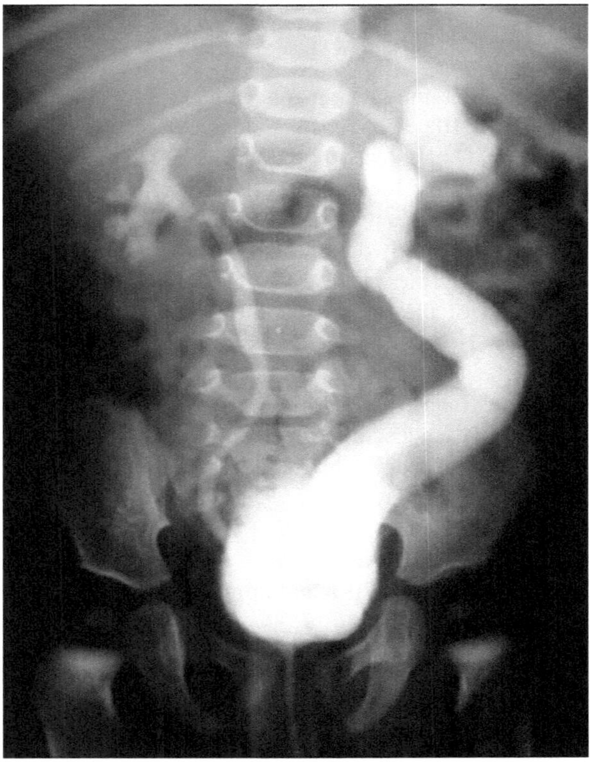

(VCUG) will exclude reflux (Fig. 2.22). Perfusion nuclear medicine studies with diuretic renography help denote the position of and degree, if any, of obstruction or relative obstruction. At least 50% of cases are treated conservatively.

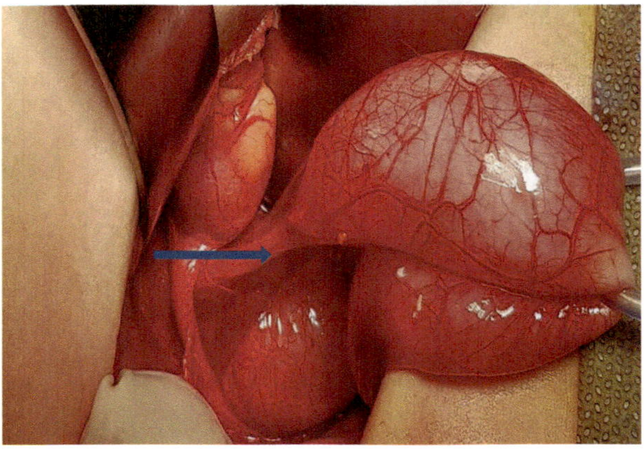

Fig. 2.23 The intraoperative image of obstructed megaureter showing an atretic distal segment of the distal ureter. From the courtesy of Dr Bedeir Ali-El-Dein

2.1.11.7 Management

Most cases of non-refluxing megaureter have a benign course and resolve spontaneously [102, 103]. The time and degree of resolution depend on the degree of ureteral dilatation. Ureters with more than 10 mm dilatation are more prone to develop complications with a low probability of resolution. Indications for intervention include symptomatic cases with recurrent febrile UTIs or progressive unremitting dilatation or most importantly deteriorating differential renal function on a diuretic renogram. Definitive treatment is by excision of the abnormal segment with tailoring and reimplantation of the ureter into the bladder in a non-refluxing fashion (Fig. 2.23). Tailoring is achieved by either plication, folding or excisional tapering. The approach can be either open, laparoscopic or even robotic and it can be either intravesical, extravesical or combined [51, 104–106].

Recently, endoscopic management has emerged as a minimally invasive alternative for primary obstructive megaureters. The most common endoscopic approaches were cystoscopy + high-pressure balloon dilation + double-J ureteral stent placement, cystoscopy + incisional ureterotomy + double-J ureteral stent placement, and cystoscopy with only double-J ureteral stent placement. The success rate is around 70% and approximately one-third of patients require surgical re-intervention [107].

Questions

1. At what gestational time point does the ureteric bud development begin?
    (a) 20th day
    (b) 24th day
    (c) 28th day
    (d) 32nd day

Answer: (c)

2. Which of the following statements is NOT TRUE about The Weigert-Meyer law?

   (a) It occurs when complete ureteral duplication exists.
   (b) The ureter of the upper moiety opens medial and caudal.
   (c) The ureter of the lower moiety opens lateral and proximal.
   (d) The upper moiety ureter is more prone to reflux.

Answer: (d)

3. In males, an ectopic ureter can most commonly open into

   (a) The epididymis.
   (b) The vas.
   (c) The seminal vesicle.
   (d) The proximal urethra.

Answer: (d)

4. Ureteral atresia represents an extremely rare congenital malformation of the ureter, which is often associated with

   (a) Multicystic dysplastic kidney.
   (b) Unilateral Renal Agenesis.
   (c) Ureteropelvic junction obstruction.
   (d) Vesicoureteral Reflux.

Answer: (a)

5. Which of the following statements is TRUE about a ureteral diverticulum?

   (a) It is usually symptomatic.
   (b) Surgical intervention is necessitated in most cases.
   (c) The ureter of the lower moiety is commonly involved.
   (d) A retrograde study is the most affirmative tool for diagnosis.

Answer: (d)

6. Retrocaval ureter results from:

   (a) persistence of posterior cardinal veins.
   (b) persistence of anterior cardinal veins.
   (c) duplication of inferior vena cava.
   (d) aberrance of lumbar veins.
   (e) retro aortic renal veins.

Answer: (a)

7. All of the following contribute to a refluxing ureter EXCEPT:

   (a) lateral ureteral insertion.
   (b) lax bladder neck.
   (c) poorly developed trigone.
   (d) gaping ureteral orifice.
   (e) short intramural tunnel.

Answer: (b)

8. Surgical reconstruction of ureteropelvic junction obstruction requires:

   (a) a funnel-shaped anastomosis between the renal pelvis and the ureter.
   (b) dependent drainage.
   (c) water-tight anastomosis.
   (d) tension-free anastomosis.
   (e) all of the above.

Answer: (e)

9. What is the preferred method for endoscopic ureterocele management?

   (a) Resection of the roof of the ureterocele
   (b) Puncture of the ureterocele's urethral extension
   (c) Puncture of the roof of the ureterocele
   (d) Transverse incision at the base of the ureterocele
   (e) Resection of the base of the ureterocele only

Answer: (d)

10. Which of the following is the most serious complication to ureteral tailoring in Megaureter reconstruction?

   (a) Gradual tapering can cause a sudden change of the ureteral caliber with subsequent kinking.
   (b) A too-short tunnel can cause vesicoureteral reflux
   (c) Compromise of the vasculature of the ureter with subsequent fibrosis
   (d) Stenotic ureteral orifice
   (e) Bladder dysfunction

Answer: (c)

References

1. Rosenblum ND. Developmental biology of the human kidney. Semin Fetal Neonatal Med. 2008;13(3):125–32.
2. Cebrián C, Borodo K, Charles N, Herzlinger DA. Morphometric index of the developing murine kidney. Dev Dyn. 2004;231(3):601–8.
3. Alcaraz A, Vinaixa F, Tejedo-Mateu A, Forés MM, Gotzens V, Mestres CA, Oliveira J, Carretero P. Obstruction and recanalization of the ureter during embryonic development. J Urol. 1991;145(2):410–6.
4. Kluth D, Hillen M, Lambrecht W. The principles of normal and abnormal hindgut development. J Pediatr Surg. 1995;30(8):1143–7.
5. Marshall FF. Embryology of the lower genitourinary tract. Urol Clin North Am. 1978;5(1):3–15.
6. Batourina E, Gandhi D, Mendelsohn CL, Molotkov A. Organotypic culture of the urogenital tract. Methods Mol Biol. 2012;886:45–53.
7. Smith P, Dunn M. Duplication of the upper urinary tract. Ann R Coll Surg Engl. 1979;61(4):281–6.

8. Cooper CS, Snyder HM. The ureter. In: Gillenwater JY, Grayhack JT, Howards SS, Mitchell ME, editors. Adult and pediatric urology. 4th ed. Philadelphia: Lippincott Williams and Wilkins; 2002. p. 2155.
9. Timothy RP, Decter A, Perlmutter AD. Ureteral duplication: clinical findings and therapy in 46 children. J Urol. 1971;105(3):445–51.
10. Privett JT, Jeans WD, Roylance J. The incidence and importance of renal duplication. Clin Radiol. 1976;27(4):521–30.
11. Toka HR, Toka O, Hariri A, Nguyen HT. Congenital anomalies of kidney and urinary tract. Semin Nephrol. 2010;30(4):374–86.
12. Didier RA, Chow JS, Kwatra NS, Retik AB, Lebowitz RL. The duplicated collecting system of the urinary tract: embryology, imaging appearances and clinical considerations. Pediatr Radiol. 2017;47(11):1526–38.
13. Gearhart JG, Rink RC, Garrett R, Mouriquand PD. Pediatric urology e-book. 2nd ed. Elsevier: Saunders; 2014.
14. Sen S, Ahmed S, Borghol M. Surgical management of complete ureteric duplication abnormalities. Pediatr Surg Int. 1998;13(1):61–4.
15. Abdelhalim A, Chamberlin JD, Truong H, McAleer IM, Chuang KW, Wehbi E, Stephany HA, Khoury AE. Ipsilateral ureteroureterostomy for ureteral duplication anomalies: predictors of adverse outcomes. J Pediatr Urol. 2019;15(5):468.e1–6.
16. Chertin L, Neeman BB, Stav K, Noh PH, Koucherov S, Gaber J, Zismar A, Chertin B, Dubrov V, Bondarenko S, Neheman A. Robotic versus laparoscopic ipsilateral uretero-ureterostomy for upper urinary tract duplications in the pediatric population: a multi-institutional review of outcomes and complications. J Pediatr Surg. 2021;56(12):2377–80.
17. Li J, Hu T, Wang M, Chen S, Huang L. Ureteral triplication: the first report in China. J Pediatr Surg. 2004;39(1):E38–9.
18. Smith I. Triplicate ureter. Br J Surg. 1946;34(134):182–5.
19. Ali SN, Ali AN, Ahmad N, Ali MN. Ureteral triplication and contralateral duplication with vesicoureteral reflux. J Ayub Med Coll Abbottabad. 2014;26(2):258–60.
20. Xu Z, Li Z, Wang D, Deng G, Su C, Pan J, Li S. Ureteral triplication combined with right renal ectopia and ureteral cyst. Urol Int. 2009;83(4):476–8.
21. Al-Zubi M, Al Faqieh A, Altamimi O, Albeitawi S. Unilateral triplicate ureter with ipsilateral ureterocele a case report. Int J Surg Case Rep. 2020;70:178–81.
22. Zaontz MR, Maizels M. Type I ureteral triplication: an extension of the Weigert-Meyer law. J Urol. 1985;134(5):949–50.
23. Ireland EF Jr, Chute R. A case of triplicate-duplicate ureters. J Urol. 1955;74(3):343–7.
24. Gosalbez R Jr, Gosalbez R, Piro C, Martin JA, Jimenez A. Ureteral triplication and ureterocele: report of 3 cases and review of the literature. J Urol. 1991;145(1):105–8.
25. Singh G, Murray K. Ureteral triplication, occasionally an isolated anomaly. Urol Int. 1996;56(2):117–8.
26. Sivrikaya A, Cay A, Imamoglu M, Sarihan H. A case of ureteral triplication associated with ureteropelvic junction obstruction. Int Urol Nephrol. 2007;39(3):755–7.
27. P AS, Dumra A, Ramdev P, Kochhar G. Persistent incontinence following surgery for ureteric triplication with contralateral duplication-a management dilemma. Urology. 2019;134:221–4.
28. Gill B. Ureteric ectopy in children. Br J Urol. 1980;52(4):257–63.
29. Mandell J, Bauer SB, Colodny AH, Lebowitz RL, Retik AB. Ureteral ectopia in infants and children. J Urol. 1981;126(2):219–22.
30. Albers P, Foster RS, Bihrle R, Adams MC, Keating MA. Ectopic ureters and ureteroceles in adults. Urology. 1995;45(5):870–4.
31. Li J, Hu T, Wang M, Jiang X, Chen S, Huang L. Single ureteral ectopia with congenital renal dysplasia. J Urol. 2003;170(2 Pt 1):558–9.
32. Mikuz G. Ectopias of the kidney, urinary tract organs, and male genitalia. Pathologe. 2019;40(Suppl 1):1–8. English
33. Roy Choudhury S, Chadha R, Bagga D, Puri A, Debnath PR. Spectrum of ectopic ureters in children. Pediatr Surg Int. 2008;24(7):819–23.

34. Jain P, Sarkar D, Maiti K, Gupta S, Pal DK. Rare cases of ectopic ureter: analysis from a single centre with review of the literature. Turk J Urol. 2019;45(Supp. 1):S92–7.
35. Borer JG, Bauer SB, Peters CA, Diamond DA, Decter RM, Shapiro E. A single-system ectopic ureter draining an ectopic dysplastic kidney: delayed diagnosis in the young female with continuous urinary incontinence. Br J Urol. 1998;81(3):474–8.
36. Lee YS, Im YJ, Kim SW, Kim MJ, Lee MJ, Lim NL, Han SW. The vagaries of proper imaging in diagnosing single-system ectopic ureter in children with continuous incontinence and outcomes of simple nephrectomy. J Pediatr Surg. 2016;51(3):469–74.
37. Michaud JE, Akhavan A. Upper pole heminephrectomy versus lower pole ureteroureterostomy for ectopic upper pole ureters. Curr Urol Rep. 2017;18(3):21.
38. Plaire JC, Pope JC 4th, Kropp BP, Adams MC, Keating MA, Rink RC, Casale AJ. Management of ectopic ureters: experience with the upper tract approach. J Urol. 1997;158(3 Pt 2):1245–7.
39. Peters CA, Mendelsohn C. EU, ureterocele, and ureteral anomalies. In: Wein AJ, Kavoussi LR, Partin AW, Peters CA, editors. Campbell-Walsh urology. Philadelphia: Elsevier Saunders; 2016. p. 3087–96.
40. Glassberg KI, Braren V, Duckett JW, Jacobs EC, King LR, Lebowitz RL, Perlmutter AD, Stephens FD. Suggested terminology for duplex systems, ectopic ureters and ureteroceles. J Urol. 1984;132(6):1153–4.
41. Johnin K, Narita M, Kim CJ, Wakabayashi Y, Yoshiki T, Okada Y. Bilateral single ectopic ureters with hypoplastic bladder: how should we treat these challenging entities? J Pediatr Urol. 2007;3(3):243–6.
42. Nazer II, Alhashmi G, Sharief SN, Hefni NA, Ibrahim A, El-Desoky SM, Alsayyad AJ, Safdar OY, Kari JA. A case of urinary bladder agenesis and bilateral ectopic ureters: a case report. BMC Urol. 2018;18(1):83.
43. Floyd MS Jr, Scally J, Irwin PP. Incidental detection of a unilateral dilated blind-ending ureter, renal agenesis, and a dilated seminal vesicle. Urol J. 2012;9(4):639.
44. Bleve C, Conighi ML, Fasoli L, Bucci V, Battaglino F, Chiarenza SF. Proximal ureteral atresia, a rare congenital anomaly-incidental finding: a case report. Transl Pediatr. 2017;6(1):67–71.
45. Wu S, Xu R, Zhu X, Zhao X. Distal ureteral atresia with ureteropelvic junction obstruction in a female child: a rare case. Int J Clin Exp Med. 2015;8(1):1472–4.
46. Morozumi M, Ogawa Y, Fujime M, Kitagawa R. Distal ureteral atresia associated with crossed renal ectopia with fusion: recovery of renal function after release of a 10-year ureteral obstruction. Int J Urol. 1997;4(5):512–5.
47. Karanastasis D, Antoniou N, Tsagatakis E, Sakalis K, Stenos I. Distal ureteral atresia associated with ipsilateral renal dysplasia. Scand J Urol Nephrol. 1992;26(1):77–9.
48. Bagnara V, Castorina S, Nappo SG, Privitera G, Luca T, Caione P. Hypothesis on etiopathogenesis, congenital or acquired, of an imperforate distal ureter: a case report. J Med Case Rep. 2015;9:227.
49. Louw JH, Barnard CN. Congenital intestinal atresia; observations on its origin. Lancet. 1955;269(6899):1065–7.
50. Ashimine S, Miyazato M, Hayashi E, Morozumi M, Sugaya K, Ogawa Y. Distal ureteral atresia: recovery of renal function after relief of obstruction at ten months old. Int J Urol. 2005;12(6):578–80.
51. Riccabona M. Obstructive diseases of the urinary tract in children: lessons from the last 15 years. Pediatr Radiol. 2010;40(6):947–55.
52. McLoughlin LC, Davis NF, Dowling C, Eng MP, Power RE. Ureteral diverticulum: a review of the current literature. Can J Urol. 2013;20(5):6893–6.
53. Mejri R, Chaker K, Mokhtar B, Ben Rhouma S, Nouira Y. Ureteral diverticulum complicated by urinary lithiasis: About a case report. Urol Case Rep. 2021;39:101810.
54. Emekli E, Gündoğdu E, Özen A, Küçükay F. A rare case of ureteral diverticulum incidentally detected during angiography. Curr Med Imaging. 2021;17(4):549–51.
55. Cappellani A, Di Vita M, Zanghì A, Lo Menzo E, Conti P. Perforation of a ureteral diverticulum: a case report and review of the literature. Ann Ital Chir. 2003;74(3):349–52. discussion 352-3

56. Herndon CD, McKenna PH. Antenatally detected proximal ureteral diverticulum. Urology. 2000;55(5):774.
57. Wan YL, Hsieh ML, Hsueh C, Shum HC, Kea CL. Sonographic diagnosis of a ureteral diverticulum. J Ultrasound Med. 1996;15(6):483–5.
58. Negoro H, Inoue T, Imai K, Goto T, Sawada A, Akamatsu S, Saito R, Kobayashi T, Yamasaki T, Ogawa O. Laparoscopic excision of an acquired ureteral diverticulum: a case report. Asian J Endosc Surg. 2019;12(4):478–81.
59. Mehra K, Sreerag KS, Manikandan R, Dorairajan LN, Kalra S, Avinash J. Rare entity of proximal ureteral diverticulum managed by robotic resection and ureteroureteral anastomosis. J Endourol Case Rep. 2020;6(1):39–41.
60. Harrison GS. Transitional cell carcinoma in a congenital ureteral diverticulum. J Urol. 1983;129(6):1231–2.
61. Yarmohammadi A, Mohamadzadeh Rezaei M, Feizzadeh B, Ahmadnia H. Retrocaval ureter: a study of 13 cases. Urol J. 2006;3(3):175–8. discussion 179
62. Kenawi MM, Williams DI. Circumcaval ureter: a report of four cases in children with a review of the literature and a new classification. Br J Urol. 1976;48(3):183–92.
63. Perimenis P, Gyftopoulos K, Athanasopoulos A, Pastromas V, Barbalias G. Retrocaval ureter and associated abnormalities. Int Urol Nephrol. 2002;33(1):19–22.
64. Bartle EJ, Pearce WH, Sun JH, Rutherford RB. Infrarenal venous anomalies and aortic surgery: avoiding vascular injury. J Vasc Surg. 1987;6(6):590–3.
65. Bateson EM, Atkinson D. Circumcaval ureter: a new classification. Clin Radiol. 1969;20(2):173–7.
66. Acharya SK, Jindal B, Yadav DK, Singha S, Bagga D. Retrocaval ureter: a rare cause of hydronephrosis in children. J Pediatr Surg. 2009;44(4):846–8.
67. Murphy BJ, Casillas J, Becerra JL. Retrocaval ureter: computed tomography and ultrasound appearance. J Comput Tomogr. 1987;11(1):89–93.
68. Anderson J, Hynes W. Retrocaval ureter; a case diagnosed pre-operatively and treated successfully by a plastic operation. Br J Urol. 1949;21(3):209–14.
69. Baba S, Oya M, Miyahara M, Deguchi N, Tazaki H. Laparoscopic surgical correction of circumcaval ureter. Urology. 1994;44(1):122–6.
70. Abdessater M, El Khoury R, Elias S, Bart S, Coloby P, Sleiman W. Diagnosis and laparoscopic management of retrocaval ureter: a review of the literature and our case series. Int J Surg Case Rep. 2019;59:165–75.
71. Escolino M, Masieri L, Valla JS, Lopez PJ, Tokar B, Mushtaq I, Esposito C. Laparoscopic and robotic-assisted repair of retrocaval ureter in children: a multi-institutional comparative study with open repair. World J Urol. 2019;37(9):1941–7.
72. Gupta R, Kesar A, Mahajan A, Mehta A, Masood S. Transperitoneal laparoscopic uretero-pyeloplasty of retrocaval ureter: single surgeon experience and review of literature. Asian J Endosc Surg. 2022;15(1):90–6.
73. Li HZ, Ma X, Qi L, Shi TP, Wang BJ, Zhang X. Retroperitoneal laparoscopic ureteroureterostomy for retrocaval ureter: report of 10 cases and literature review. Urology. 2010;76(4):873–6.
74. Inoue Y, Naitoh Y, Ajiki J, Fukui A, Yamada T, Fujihara A, Yamada K, Hongo F, Ukimura O. Robot-assisted laparoscopic pyeloplasty for ureteropelvic junction obstruction due to aberrant blood vessel with ipsilateral retrocaval ureter. IJU Case Rep. 2021;4(5):273–6.
75. Hemal AK, Rao R, Sharma S, Clement RG. Pure robotic retrocaval ureter repair. Int Braz J Urol. 2008;34(6):734–8.
76. Swerkersson S, Jodal U, Sixt R, Stokland E, Hansson S. Relationship among vesicoureteral reflux, urinary tract infection and renal damage in children. J Urol. 2007;178(2):647–51. discussion 650-1
77. Routh JC, Bogaert GA, Kaefer M, Manzoni G, Park JM, Retik AB, Rushton HG, Snodgrass WT, Wilcox DT. Vesicoureteral reflux: current trends in diagnosis, screening, and treatment. Eur Urol. 2012;61(4):773–82.
78. Abdelhalim A, Khoury AE. Critical appraisal of the top-down approach for vesicoureteral reflux. Investig Clin Urol. 2017;58(Suppl 1):S14–22.

79. Tekgül S, Riedmiller H, Hoebeke P, Kočvara R, Nijman RJ, Radmayr C, Stein R, Dogan HS, European Association of Urology. EAU guidelines on vesicoureteral reflux in children. Eur Urol. 2012;62(3):534–42.
80. Peters CA, Skoog SJ, Arant BS Jr, Copp HL, Elder JS, Hudson RG, Khoury AE, Lorenzo AJ, Pohl HG, Shapiro E, Snodgrass WT, Diaz M. Summary of the AUA guideline on management of primary vesicoureteral reflux in children. J Urol. 2010;184(3):1134–44.
81. Hajiyev P, Burgu B. Contemporary management of vesicoureteral reflux. Eur Urol Focus. 2017;3(2–3):181–8.
82. Hidas G, Nam A, Soltani T, Pribish M, Watts B, Khoury AE. Primary vesico-ureteric reflux: the need for individualised risk stratification. Arab J Urol. 2013;11(1):8–12.
83. Trial Investigators RIVUR, Hoberman A, Greenfield SP, Mattoo TK, Keren R, Mathews R, Pohl HG, Kropp BP, Skoog SJ, Nelson CP, Moxey-Mims M, Chesney RW, Carpenter MA. Antimicrobial prophylaxis for children with vesicoureteral reflux. N Engl J Med. 2014;370(25):2367–76.
84. Routh JC, Inman BA, Reinberg Y. Dextranomer/hyaluronic acid for pediatric vesicoureteral reflux: systematic review. Pediatrics. 2010;125(5):1010–9.
85. Cohen HL, Kravets F, Zucconi W, Ratani R, Shah S, Dougherty D. Congenital abnormalities of the genitourinary system. Semin Roentgenol. 2004;39(2):282–303.
86. Filly R, Feldstein V. Fetal genitourinary tract. In: Callen P, editor. Ultrasonography in obstetrics and gynecology. 4th ed. Philadelphia, PA: Saunders; 2000. p. 517–50.
87. Rigas A, Karamanolakis D, Bogdanos I, Stefanidis A, Androulakakis PA. Pelvi-ureteric junction obstruction by crossing renal vessels: clinical and imaging features. BJU Int. 2003;92(1):101–3.
88. Grignon A, Filiatrault D, Homsy Y, Robitaille P, Filion R, Boutin H, Leblond R. Ureteropelvic junction stenosis: antenatal ultrasonographic diagnosis, postnatal investigation, and follow-up. Radiology. 1986;160(3):649–51.
89. Uson AC, Lattimer JK, Melicow MM. Ureteroceles in infants and children: a report based on 44 cases. Pediatrics. 1961;27:971–83.
90. Malek RS, Kelalis PP, Burke EC, Stickler GB. Simple and ectopic ureterocele in infancy and childhood. Surg Gynecol Obstet. 1972;134(4):611–6.
91. Shokeir AA, Nijman RJ. Ureterocele: an ongoing challenge in infancy and childhood. BJU Int. 2002;90(8):777–83.
92. Godinho AB, Nunes C, Janeiro M, Carvalho R, Melo MA, da Graça LM. Ureterocele: antenatal diagnosis and management. Fetal Diagn Ther. 2013;34(3):188–91.
93. Jain V, Agarwala S, Dhua A, Mitra A, Mittal D, Murali D, Kandasamy D, Kumar R, Bhatnagar V. Management and outcomes of ureteroceles in children: an experience of 25 years. Indian J Urol. 2021;37(2):163–8.
94. Merguerian PA, Taenzer A, Knoerlein K, McQuiston L, Herz D. Variation in management of duplex system intravesical ureteroceles: a survey of pediatric urologists. J Urol. 2010;184(4 Suppl):1625–30. Epub 2010 Aug 21
95. Pani E, Negri E, Cini C, Landi L, Mantovani A, Bortot G, Masieri L. Endoscopic treatment of ureterocele in children: Results of a single referral tertiary center over a 10 year-period. J Pediatr Urol. 2021:S1477-5131(21)00591-X.
96. Cohen SA, Juwono T, Palazzi KL, Kaplan GW, Chiang G. Examining trends in the treatment of ureterocele yields no definitive solution. J Pediatr Urol. 2015;11(1):29.e1–6.
97. Castagnetti M, El-Ghoneimi A. Management of duplex system ureteroceles in neonates and infants. Nat Rev Urol. 2009;6(6):307–15.
98. Coplen DE, Austin PF. Outcome analysis of prenatally detected ureteroceles associated with multicystic dysplasia. J Urol. 2004;172(4 Pt 2):1637–9. discussion 163
99. Belman AB. Megaureter. Classification, etiology, and management. Urol Clin North Am. 1974;1(3):497–513.
100. King LR. Megaloureter: definition, diagnosis and management. J Urol. 1980;123(2):222–3.
101. Shokeir AA, Nijman RJ. Primary megaureter: current trends in diagnosis and treatment. BJU Int. 2000;86(7):861–8.

102. Manzoni C. Megaureter. Rays. 2002;27(2):83–5.
103. Shukla AR, Cooper J, Patel RP, Carr MC, Canning DA, Zderic SA, Snyder HM 3rd. Prenatally detected primary megaureter: a role for extended followup. J Urol. 2005;173(4):1353–6.
104. Wilcox D, Mouriquand P. Management of megaureter in children. Eur Urol. 1998;34(1):73–8.
105. Rudin YE, Marukhnenko DV, Galitskaya DA, Aliev JK, Lagutin GV, Vardak AB. Pneumovesicoscopic ureteral reimplantation with intravesical tailoring of obstructive megaureter in pediatric patient. J Pediatr Urol. 2021;11:S1477–5131(21). 00587-8
106. DeFoor W, Minevich E, Reddy P, Polsky E, McGregor A, Wacksman J, Sheldon C. Results of tapered ureteral reimplantation for primary megaureter: extravesical versus intravesical approach. J Urol. 2004;172(4 Pt 2):1640–3.
107. Doudt AD, Pusateri CR, Christman MS. Endoscopic Management of Primary Obstructive Megaureter: A Systematic Review. J Endourol. 2018;32(6):482–7.

Further Reading

Partin AW, Peters CA, Kavoussi LR, Dmochowski RR, Wein AJ, editors. Campbell-Walsh urology 12th edition review. Amsterdam: Elsevier; 2020.
Baskin LS, Cunha G. Embryology of the genitourinary tract. In: 12th, editor. Campbell-Walsh-Wein urology. Philadelphia: Elsevier Inc; 2021. p. 305–40.
Olsen LH, Rawashdeh YF. Surgery of the ureter in children: ureteropelvic junction, megaureter, and vesicoureteral reflux. In: Campbell-Walsh-Wein urology. 12th edition. Philadelphia, PA: Elsevier; 2021.
The Developing Human: Clinically Oriented Embryology (8th Edition) by Keith L. Moore and T.V.N Persaud - Moore & Persaud Chapter 13 pp. 303–46.
Larsen's Human Embryology by GC. Schoenwolf, SB. Bleyl, PR. Brauer and PH. Francis-West. Chapter 10; pp. 261–306.

Chapter 3
Anatomy

Adel Bondok, Ahmad M. Eliwa, and Mahmoud Abdel-Gawad

Abstract The ureter is a muscular tube extending retroperitoneally from the renal pelvis superiorly to the urinary bladder inferiorly. In adults, it is about 10 in. long, 5 in. in the abdomen, and 5 in. in the pelvis. The bifurcation of the common iliac artery separates the abdominal part from the pelvic part. The ureter is crossed anteriorly by many structures on the two sides. The most crucial anterior relation is in the female pelvis, where the ureter passes behind the broad ligament of the uterus, the ovary, the ovarian vessels, and the uterine artery. The close relation of the ureter to the ovary and the uterine artery makes the ureter vulnerable to injury during oophorectomy or hysterectomy. The ureter has three sites of constrictions: (1) at the ureteropelvic (pelviureteric) junction; (2) at the bifurcation of the common iliac artery; and (3) in the wall of the urinary bladder (the intramural part). These are the common sites where ureteric stones may be arrested. On the other hand, knowledge of ureteral endoscopic anatomy is a keystone in understanding the basics of endourologic procedures of the ureter, starting from ureteroscopic stone management and endoscopic manipulation of ureteral strictures to preventing complications during

Test your learning and check your understanding of this book's contents: use the "Springer Nature Flashcards" app to access questions. To use the app, please follow the instructions in Chapter 1.

Supplementary Information The online version contains supplementary material available at https://doi.org/10.1007/978-3-031-36212-5_3.

A. Bondok
Anatomy and Neuroscience department, Faculty of Medicine, Mansoura University, Mansoura, Egypt

A. M. Eliwa
Urology Department, Zagazig University, Zagazig, Egypt

M. Abdel-Gawad (✉)
Toshka Urology and Endoscopy Center, Mansoura, Egypt

M. Abdel-Gawad et al. (eds.), *The Ureter*,
https://doi.org/10.1007/978-3-031-36212-5_3

ureteroscopy. On the other hand, applied laparoscopic surface anatomy of the ureter is very important to laparoscopic abdominal surgeons, including urologists, gynecologists, and pelvic oncologic surgeons.

Keywords Ureter anatomy · Endoscopic anatomy · Endoluminal anatomy Laparoscopic anatomy

Abbreviations

ALUT	Actual length of ureter tract
CT	Computerized tomography
IVP	Intravenous pyelography
KUB	Kidney, ureter, bladder
LD	Linear distance
UL	Ureteral length
UPJO	Ureteropelvic junction obstruction
URS	Ureteroscopy
UVJ	Ureterovesical junction

Learning Objectives

- By the end of this chapter, the reader should be able to recall basic and advanced ureteral anatomical facts and apply these data during endoscopic and surgical ureteral procedures.

3.1 Section I: Anatomy of the Ureter

Adel A. Bondok and Mahmoud Abdel-Gawad

3.1.1 Intended Learning Outcomes (ILOs)

By the end of this chapter, you should be able to know the following points and correlate the anatomical knowledge with clinical problems of the ureter:

- Length and extent of the ureter.
- Course of the ureter.
- Relations.
- Sites of constrictions.
- Arterial supply, venous drainage, and lymph drainage.
- Nerve supply and referred pain from the ureter.
- X-ray appearance of the ureter.

- Microscopic anatomy.
- Congenital anomalies of the ureter.
- References
- **Video file:** Anatomy of the Ureter
- Legend of figures
- Self-assessment (review questions).

3.1.2 Length

The ureter is a muscular tube that measures about 25 cm in length in adults (5 in. in the abdomen & 5 in. in the pelvis) (Fig. 3.1). The diameter is about 3–4 mm. In neonates, it is about 6.5–7 cm long [1].

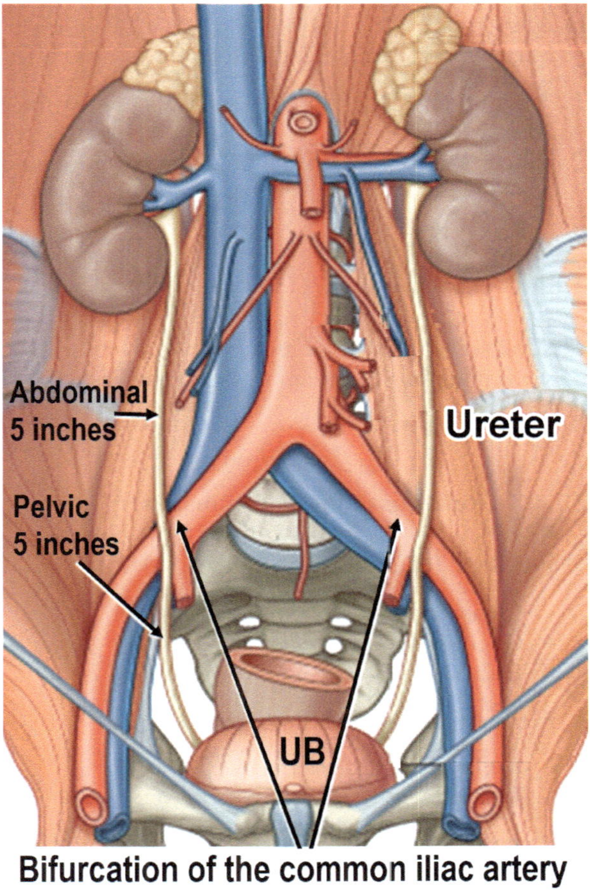

Fig. 3.1 Anatomical course and extent of the ureters

3.1.3 Extent

The ureter extends from the renal pelvis at the lower end of the kidney superiorly to the posterosuperior angle of the urinary bladder inferiorly. The renal pelvis is formed by the union of two or three major calyces, which are formed by the union of several minor calyces.

3.1.4 Course

The ureter descends behind the peritoneum (retroperitoneally) on the psoas major muscle, then crosses the bifurcation of the common iliac artery or the beginning of the external iliac artery, then crosses the sidewall of the pelvic cavity till the ischial spine, then passes forward to enter the posterosuperior angle of the urinary bladder.

The course is, therefore, **divided into two parts** (Fig. 3.1):

1. **Abdominal Part:** from the renal pelvis to the bifurcation of the common iliac artery.
2. **Pelvic Part:** from the bifurcation of the common iliac artery to the urinary bladder

3.1.4.1 Abdominal Part (5 in.)

The abdominal part of the ureter passes anterior to the psoas major muscle till the pelvic brim **opposite** the tips of the lumbar transverse processes behind the peritoneum [2].

3.1.4.2 Relations of the Abdominal Part

- **Posterior Relation:** same for the 2 sides:
  - Psoas major muscle.
  - Genitofemoral nerve.
  - Bifurcation of the common iliac artery.
- **Medial Relation:** veins
  - **Right ureter:** inferior vena cava.
  - **Left ureter:** inferior mesenteric vein.
- **Anterior Relation: the ureter is crossed anteriorly by** (Fig. 3.2 and Table 3.1):

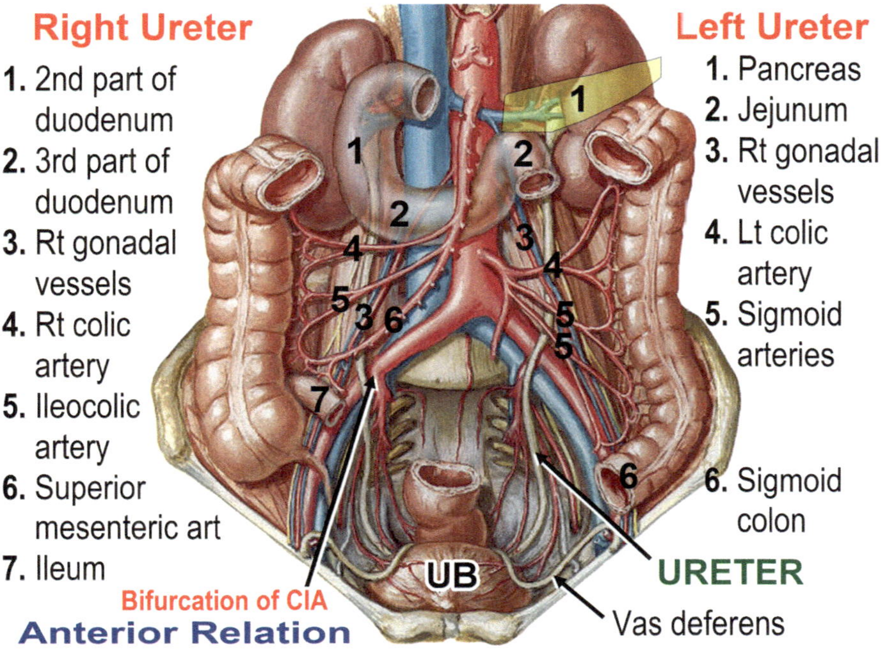

Fig. 3.2 Anterior relation of the abdominal part of the right and left ureters

Table 3.1 Anterior relation of the abdominal part of the ureter

Right ureter	Left ureter
Renal vessels in front of the renal pelvis	Renal vessels in front of the renal pelvis
Second part of the duodenum	Body of the pancreas
Third part of the duodenum	Jejunum
4 Arteries (vessels): 1. Right testicular or ovarian vessels 2. Right colic vessels 3. Ileocolic vessels 4. Superior mesenteric vessels	**4 Arteries (vessels):** 1. Left testicular or ovarian vessels 2. Left colic vessels 3. 2 sigmoid vessels
Root of the mesentery	Sigmoid mesocolon
Terminal part of the ileum	Sigmoid colon

Right Ureter

The right ureter is crossed anteriorly by the following structures, from above downward:

1. Renal vessels in front of the renal pelvis.
2. Second part of the duodenum is in front of the hilum of the right kidney and the renal pelvis.

3. Third part of the duodenum in front of the right pelvic ureteric junction.
4. It is crossed anteriorly by 4 arteries:

   (a) Right testicular or ovarian artery: from the abdominal aorta.
   (b) Right colic artery: from the superior mesenteric artery.
   (c) Ileocolic artery: from the superior mesenteric artery.
   (d) Superior mesenteric artery in the root of the mesentery.

5. Root of the mesentery.
6. Terminal part of the ileum.

Left Ureter

The left ureter is crossed anteriorly by the following structures, from above downward:

1. Renal vessels in front of the renal pelvis.
2. Body of the pancreas in front of the hilum of the left kidney and the renal pelvis.
3. Jejunum in front of the left pelviureteric junction.
4. It is crossed anteriorly by 4 arteries:

   (a) Left testicular or ovarian artery: from the abdominal aorta.
   (b) Left colic artery: from the inferior mesenteric artery.
   (c) Two sigmoid arteries: from the inferior mesenteric artery.

5. Sigmoid mesocolon.
6. Sigmoid colon.

3.1.4.3 Pelvic Part of the Ureter (5 in.)

The ureter passes on the side wall of the pelvis till the ischial spine then leaves the lateral pelvic wall and passes forward. Toward the urinary bladder to enter the posterosuperior angle of the bladder and opens in the trigone of the bladder.

In the male, the ureter is crossed anteriorly by the vas deferens.

In the female, the ureter passes behind the broad ligament of the uterus, the ovary and ovarian vessels, and the uterine artery. Before entering the urinary bladder, the ureter passes 1 cm above the lateral fornix of the vagina and about 1–4 cm lateral to the cervix [3, 4].

Clinical Consideration

The close relation of the ureter to the ovarian vessels and the uterine artery makes the ureter vulnerable to injury during oophorectomy or hysterectomy. In laparoscopic gynecologic surgery, the ureter can be identified as it crosses over the pelvic brim at the bifurcation of the common iliac artery. The most common site of operative injuries to the ureter is at the pelvic brim, where the ureter passes beneath the infundibulopelvic ligament.

3.1.5 Constrictions of the Ureter (Fig. 3.3)

There are three sites of constrictions of the ureter:

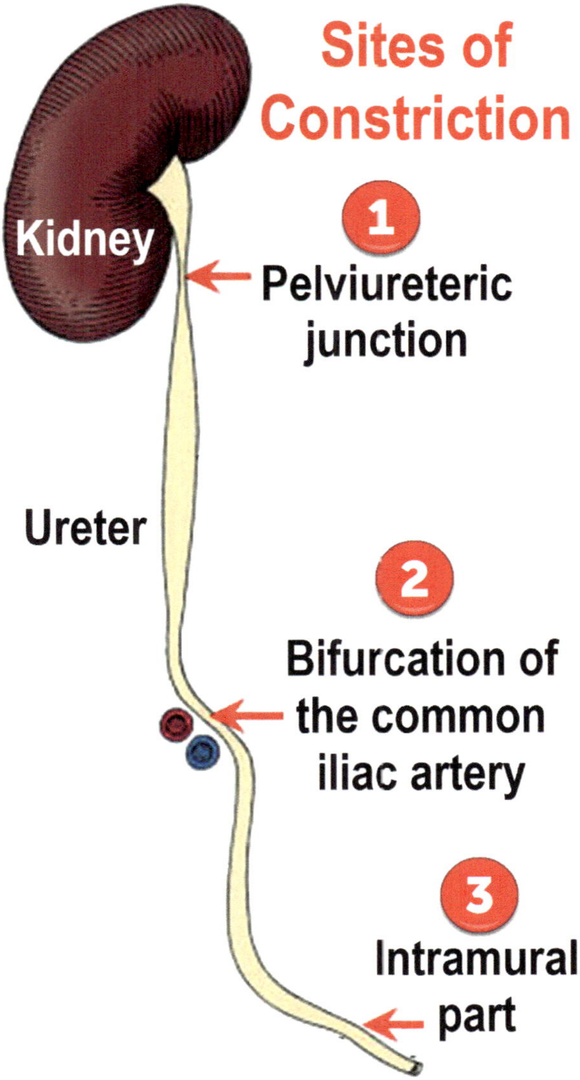

Fig. 3.3 Sites of constrictions of the ureter

1. At the ureteropelvic (pelviureteric) junction where the renal pelvis joins the ureter.
2. At the bifurcation of the common iliac artery.
3. Intramural part in the wall of the urinary bladder. According to **Anson and McVay (1984)** [5], the intravesical part of the ureter measures about 0.5–1 cm. It is the narrowest part of the ureter.

Clinical Importance of the Constrictions: they are common sites where ureteric stones may be arrested.

3.1.6 Arterial Supply of the Ureter (Fig. 3.4)

The ureter has an excellent arterial supply and a rich anastomotic network in its adventitia. It receives arterial supply from several sources along its course.

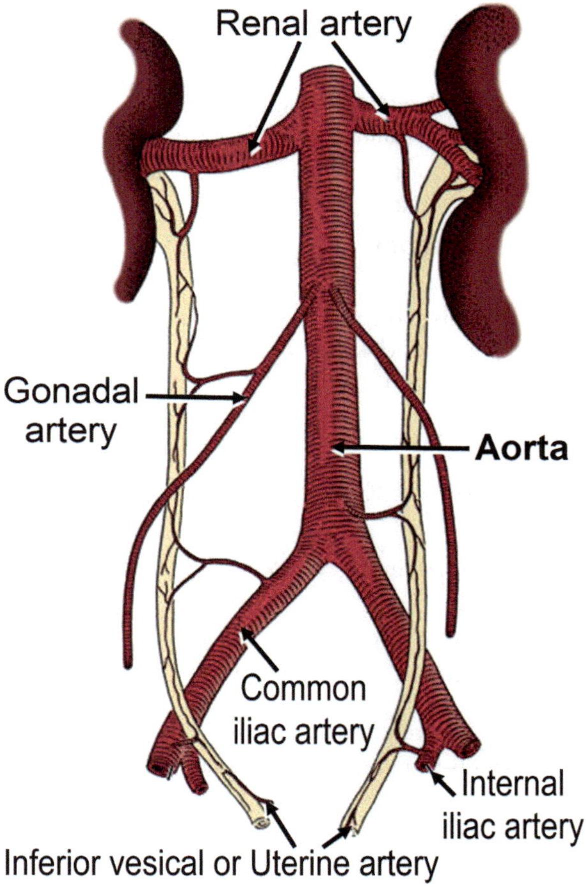

Fig. 3.4 Arterial supply of the ureter

Upon reaching the ureter, the branches divide into ascending and descending branches, which form longitudinal anastomosis around the ureter. The anastomoses of these vessels are so rich that ischemia occurs rarely [6].

1. **Upper part:** by the renal artery.
2. **Middle part:** by branches from the abdominal aorta, gonadal arteries (testicular or ovarian artery), and the common iliac artery.
3. **Lower part in the pelvis:** by branches from the internal iliac artery, superior and inferior vesical arteries in the male, and the uterine artery in the female.

According to **Redman (1996)** [7], the pelvic ureter has the richest arterial supply unlike the abdominal portion, which has the poorest arterial supply.

3.1.6.1 Clinical Consideration

It is important to maintain the integrity of the adventitia of the ureter during dissection of the ureter to prevent disruption of the longitudinal anastomosis around the ureter and prevent ischemic injury to the ureter.

3.1.7 Venous Drainage of the Ureter

The venous drainage of the ureter mirrors that of the arterial supply. The veins of the ureter begin in the submucosa and extend to the adventitia.

Veins from the upper part of the ureter drain into the renal vein or the gonadal vein.

Veins from the lower part of the ureter drain into the internal iliac vein venous network.

3.1.8 Nerve Supply of the Ureter

1. **Sympathetic:** splanchnic nerves from T12 and L1 spinal cord segments through the lowest (least) thoracic splanchnic (T12) and first lumbar splanchnic (L1) nerves. Pain fibers travel retrogradely with the sympathetic nerves and enter the spinal cord in the last thoracic and first lumbar segments.
2. **Parasympathetic:** pelvic splanchnic nerves (S2, 3, 4).

3.1.8.1 Referred Pain from the Ureter

Ureteric pain is referred to the T12 and L1 dermatomes. These skin areas include the back of the abdominal wall above the iliac crest, the suprapubic region, the scrotum in males, the labia majora in females, and the upper part of the front of the thigh (groin).

3.1.9 Lymph Drainage of the Ureter

Lymphatics follow the arterial networks to 3 groups of lymph nodes [8, 9]:

1. **Upper part:** left para-aortic lymph nodes (left ureter) and right paracaval lymph nodes (right ureter).
2. **Middle part:** common iliac lymph nodes.
3. **Lower part:** internal iliac lymph nodes.

3.1.10 X-Ray Appearance of the Ureter

In plain X-ray (Fig. 3.5), the ureter crosses the:

1. Tips of the lumbar transverse processes.
2. Sacroiliac joint.
3. Ischial spine.

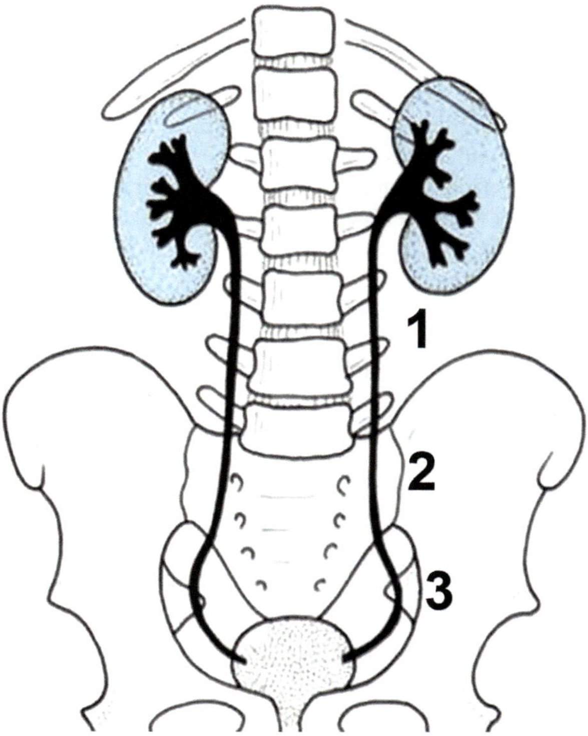

Fig. 3.5 X-ray appearance of the ureter. The ureter crosses the tips of the lumbar transverse processes (1), the sacroiliac joint (2), and the ischial spine (3)

3.1.11 *Microscopic Anatomy*

The wall of the ureter is formed of three layers [10]:

1. **Mucosa:** the inner layer. It is formed of epithelium and lamina propria:
   (a) **Epithelium:** the ureter is lined with transitional epithelium like the urinary bladder. It consists of a basal layer, middle layers of columnar cells, and apical umbrella cells. The umbrella cells are specialized to survive bathing in hypertonic urine and to stretch caused by distention of the lumen. The transitional epithelium of the ureter is derived from the mesoderm because it develops from the ureteric bud, unlike the epithelium of the urinary bladder which develops from the endoderm.
   (b) **Lamina propria:** deep to the epithelium. It is formed of elastic connective tissue.
2. **Muscle layer:** is the thickest layer of the ureter. The smooth muscles are arranged in an inner longitudinal layer and an outer circular layer (opposite to the intestine).
3. **Adventitia:** the outer fibrous layer. It contains the vascular and nerve supply.

3.1.12 *Congenital Anomalies of the Ureter*

Congenital malformations of the ureter (Fig. 3.6) are due to a disorder in the development of the ureteric bud, which arises from the mesonephric duct [11–14]. **They include:**

3.1.12.1 Ureteral atresia

The ureter may be absent or may end blindly. The atresia may occur at the entrance to the bladder. It is usually associated with renal agenesis or with a polycystic kidney.

3.1.12.2 Ureteropelvic Junction Obstruction

In ureteropelvic junction obstruction, there is a narrow connection between the ureter and the renal pelvis. A kink is almost always present causing ureteric obstruction. It can lead to significant kidney damage and gradual renal failure.

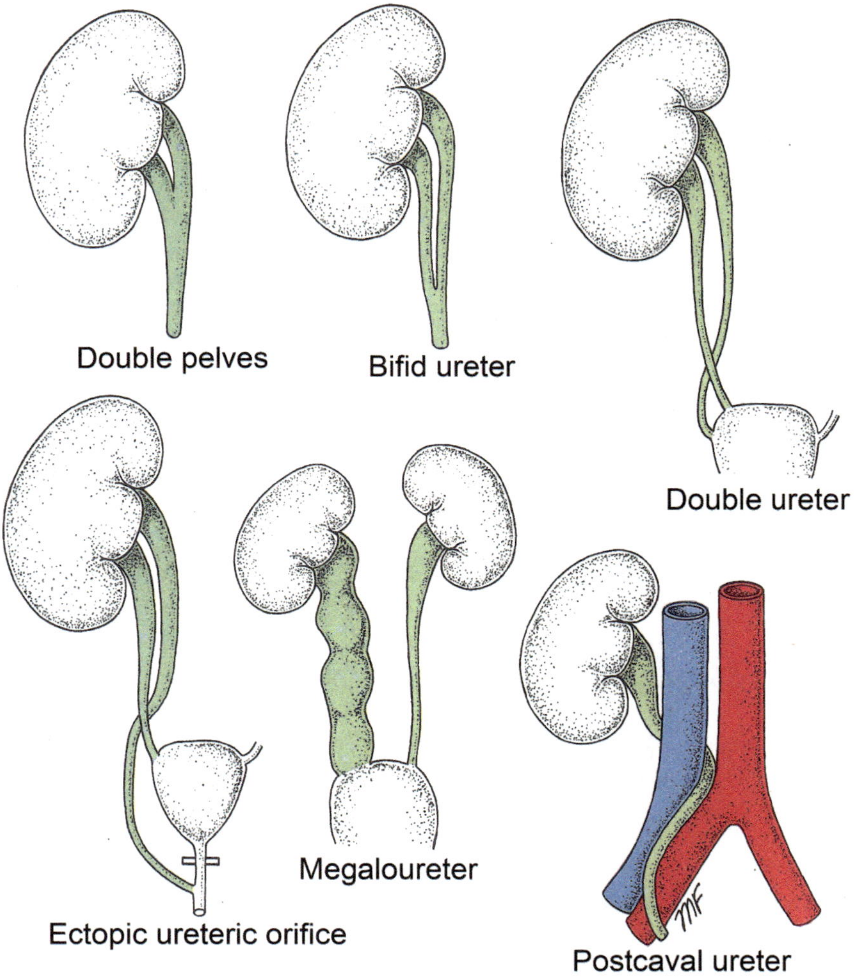

Fig. 3.6 Congenital anomalies of the ureter (Quoted from Snell, 1983) [11]

3.1.12.3 Double Ureter and Bifid Ureter

Complete duplication of the ureter is usually unilateral, and each ureter may open independently into the bladder or through a common orifice into the bladder. It is due to premature division of the ureteric bud resulting in either a double kidney or a duplicated ureter of one kidney.

Bifid Ureter and double pelves are duplications of the upper part of the ureter near the renal pelvis. The cause of the bifid ureter is a premature division of the ureteric bud near its termination.

3.1.12.4 Megaloureter

Megaloureter is a grossly dilated ureter. It may be unilateral or bilateral. The dilated segment shows a complete absence of motility. The cause is unknown; however, I suggest that it may be due to a defect in the formation of the muscle layer. Because of urinary stasis, infection is very common.

3.1.12.5 Postcaval Ureter

In the postcaval ureter, the right ureter ascends behind the inferior vena cava and may cause ureteral obstruction. It is rare (1 per 1500) and is more common in males [2, 15].

3.1.12.6 Ureterocele

Ureterocele is a cystic dilatation of the terminal part of the ureter. It is due to incomplete canalization of the ureteric bud.

3.1.12.7 Ectopic Opening of the Ureter

The ureter opens distal to its normal position; it opens in the lower part of the trigone. An ectopic ureteral orifice is caused by the failed separation of the ureteric bud from the mesonephric duct. This condition is a rare anomaly.

In males, the ectopic orifice is commonly located in the prostatic urethra, seminal vesicle, ductus deferens, or rectum. Since the opening is located above the external urethral sphincter, the patient is continent.

In females, the ectopic opening is commonly located in the urethra or the vagina. Because the ectopic opening is located below the external urethral sphincter, it is usually associated with incontinence.

3.2 Section II: Applied Endoscopic and Laparoscopic Anatomy of the Ureter

Ahmed M. Eliwa and Mahmoud Abdel-Gawad

Learning Objectives

- To understand the endoluminal course of the ureter during negotiation of the ureteroscope for endoscopic procedures.
- To elaborate on the possible difficulties during ureteroscopic procedures.
- To explain critical points and landmarks of ureteral course during laparoscopic surgery.
- To minimize ureteral injury and reduce the complications during laparoscopy and robotic surgery.

3.2.1 Introduction

The gross and microscopic anatomy has been discussed in part I of this chapter. In part II, we will discuss the detailed endoluminal and laparoscopic anatomy of the ureter pertaining to urological, laparoscopic, and robotic procedures.

3.2.2 Ureteral Length

The ureters are a pair of long muscular tubal structures localized in the retroperitoneal space. It is interpositioned between the kidney and the bladder [16]. The length ureter is approximately 22–30 cm. However, there is individual and pathophysiologic variation. The right ureter is 1 cm shorter than the left. In neonates, it is 6.5–7.0 cm long [16, 17]. The endourologist should assess the ureteric length accurately to choose the correct length of the double-J catheter. A very long catheter can cause irritative symptoms, whereas a short one may migrate toward the kidney, also knowing the ureteric length allows for proper planning of reconstructive ureteral surgery [18]. Table 3.2 illustrates different methods used to calculate both ureteral and ureteral stent length. The ureteral length is 25.36 ± 3.67 cm with no significant differences between either female and male ureters or right and left ureters.

Table 3.2 Methods used to measure the length of the ureter and the ureteral stent

	Method of measurement	Results	Equation
Forzini et al. 2019 [19]	Children ≤ 16 years 3D CT and ureter length [UL] between the ureteropelvic and ureterovesical junctions	The mean ULs on the right and left were, 9.7 and 9.91 cm at ≤1 year, 20.10 and 21.08 cm at 1-7y and 26.55 and 27.46 cm at 16y respectively	Double- J length catheter = child's age+12 cm
Paick et al. [20]	IVU 15 min view. Actual length of the ureteric tract (ALUT): ureter measured from the ureterorenal to ureterovesical junctions with a flexible ruler. Linear distance (LD) is the straight length between the same points. Ten percent was deducted to account for X-ray magnification.	The mean ALUTs right and left 23.4 ± 1.9 cm and 24.4 ± 2.0 cm, respectively, Mean LDs of the right and left were 22.1 ± 1.9 cm and 22.9 ± 2.0 cm.	Right ALUT = 0.94 × right LD+ 2.6. Left ALUT = 0.96 × left LD +2.4.
Kawahara et al. [21]	IVU and CT scan. Actual ureteral length measurement using a 5-Fr ureteral catheter.	Actual ureteral length 24.0 [23.3 (±2.0)]	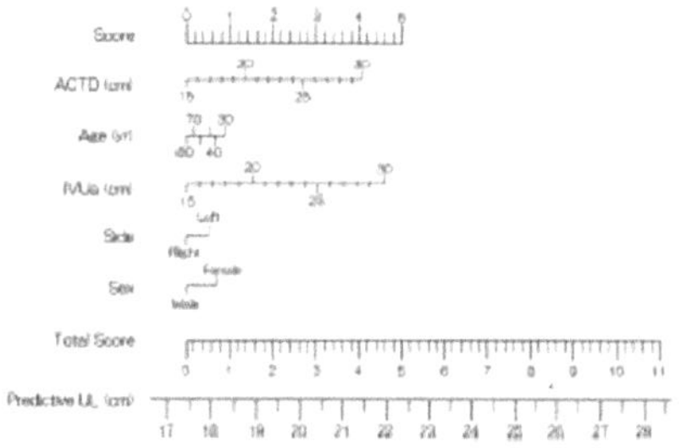

(continued)

Table 3.2 (continued)

	Method of measurement	Results	Equation
Hsu et al. [22]	Ureteral length in CT urography (ULCTU) with multiplanar reformation. Index of ureteral length measured in KUB (C-P and C-PS) and CT	ULCTU (cm) was 25.4 ± (2.3) and 24.8 ± (2.3) on the left and right ureter respectively	ULCT + C-P (measured with CT plus KUB) ULCTUL = 0.405 × ULCTL +0.626 × C-PL – 0.508 ULCTUR = 0.558 × ULCTR +0.218 × C-PR + 6.533 ULCT (measured with CT only) ULCTUL = 0.876 × ULCTL +6.337 ULCTUR = 0.710 × ULCTR +9.625 C-P (measured with KUB only) ULCTUL = 0.678 × C-PL + 4.836 ULCTUR = 0.495 × C-PR + 10.353
Shrewsberry et al. [23]	Total thickness of axial CT slices between the ureteropelvic and ureterovesical junctions adjusted up by 20%, compared with direct intraoperative measurement	Median ureteral length 25.8 cm (19.2–29.4) on the CT scan 25.5 cm (19.0–29.0) on the intraoperative measurement	Stent length = The CT straight-line ureteral length + factor of 20%.
Jeon et al. [24]	Intravenous urography (straight ureteral length; SUL) Intraoperative length with a guidewire (practical ureteral length; PUL).	Rt PUL 24.1 ± 2.0 Rt SUL 26.4 ± 2.3 Lt PUL 25.8 ± 2.1 Lt SUL 26.8 ± 2.2	PUL = 7.710 + 0.62 SUL on the right PUL = 7.792 + 0.667 SUL on the left
Pilcher et al. [25]	Stent lengths were chosen according to patient height	Stent lengths were chosen according to patient height: If the patient height is ≤5 ft. 10 in, then use 22 cm, if 5 ft. 10 in - 6 ft. 4 in, then use 24 cm, if ≥6 ft. 4 in, use 26 cm.	
Hruby et al. [26]	Ruled 5 F ureteric catheter	Mean ureteric length: 2.76 + 0.14 (height) + 0.02 (weight) – 2.44 (gender) where gender is male = 1 and female = 0.	
Bozzini et al. [27]	Graduated ureteral catheter	Between 24 and 27 cm.	A mathematical model is generated to predict female ureteral length [patient height between 161 and 181 cm]: Female expected ureteral length = 0.15 × (patient's height expressed in cm) ± 0.12 Correlation coefficient: r = 0.973
Kawahara et al. [28]	Ruled 5-Fr ureteral catheter	Actual ureteral length 23.0 cm	Choose a loop-type ureteral stent that is the same or 1 cm less than the length of the ureter when the proximal end of the stent will be in the renal pelvis

3.2.2.1 Shape and Direction

The ureter has two curves in the craniocaudal direction and the lateral direction. The ureter follows an S-shaped course from the kidney to the pelvis with a downward inferior and medial trajectory, both in the transverse and in the sagittal plane (Figs. 3.7 and 3.8). There are three ureteral inflexions: at the level of the kidney,

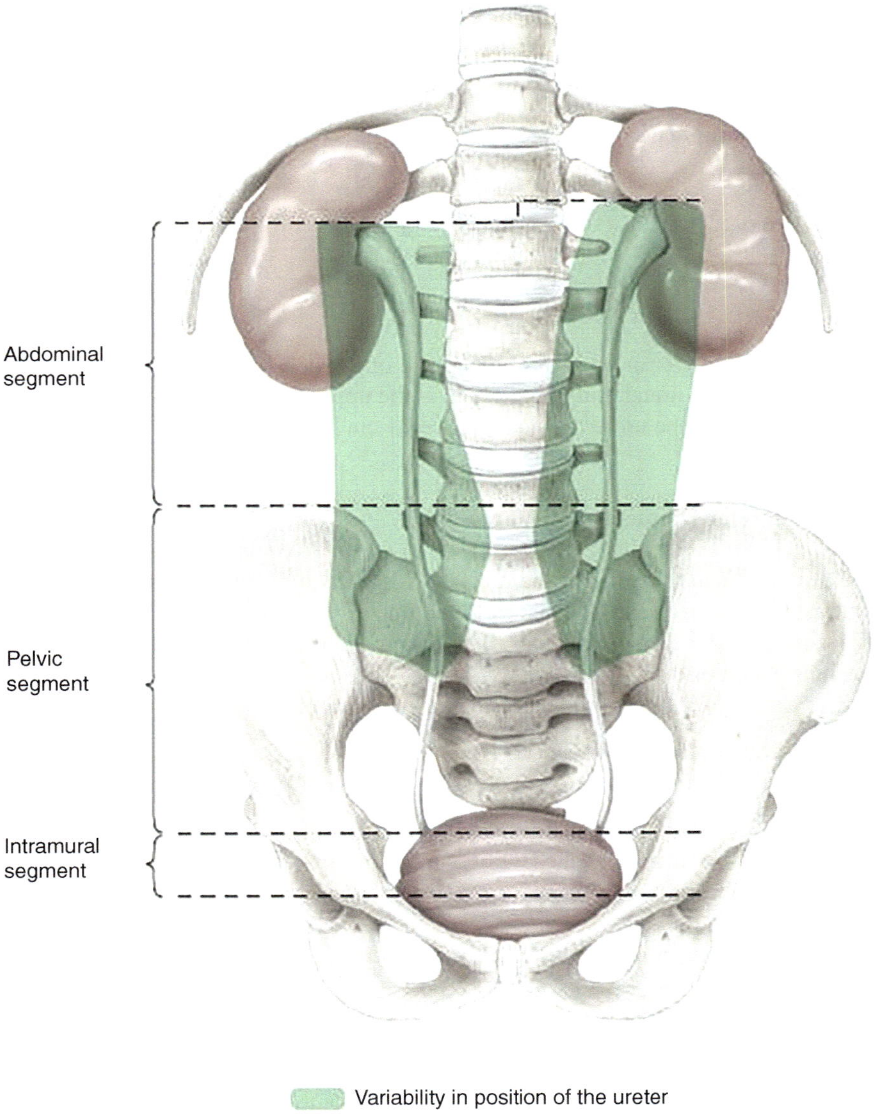

Fig. 3.7 Shaded green area represents the possibility and Variability in the Ureteral position [16]

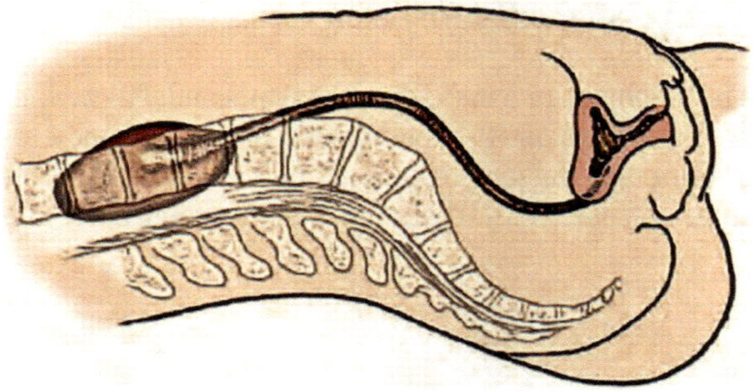

Fig. 3.8 S-shaped ureteral course [30]

Table 3.3 Diameter of the normal ureter [32]

Location	Diameter in mm	Diameter in French scale
UPJ	2–4	6–12
Upper ureter	5–6	15–18
Lower ureter	4	12
Intramural	1.5–3	5–9

crossing of the ureter at linea terminalis, and of the pelvis. There is a variable distance between the ureter and the midline: at the upper part is 4.5 cm, at linea terminalis 3 cm, and at the ureterovesical junction 1 cm [29].

3.2.2.2 Ureter Diameter and Narrowing

The normal mean diameter of the ureter is 1.8 ± 0.9 mm (range, 1–6 mm) in non-contrast CT. Zelenko and colleagues found that 96% of the diameter of the normal ureter measured 3 mm or less [31]. The normal ureteral diameter is very variable, reaching 8 mm or even more (Table 3.3).

The classic areas of natural ureteric narrowings are:

- at the ureteropelvic junction (UPJ).
- at the pelvic brim at the point of crossing over the bifurcation of the iliac vessels.
- at the ureterovesical junction (UVJ).

The areas between them are called the abdominal and pelvic spindles respectively [33].

3.2.2.3 Endoscopic and Endoluminal Landmarks of the Ureter

Trigone

The trigone is located inside the bladder neck. It is a raised, smooth triangular area with its apex at the bladder neck and its base formed by the inter-ureteric ridge that extends between the two ureteral orifices. The trigone is the most vascular and more deeply colored than the rest of the bladder. The inter-ureteric ridge is also known as "**Mercier's bar**". It is more prominent in males than females; the **ureteral orifices** are usually symmetrically located along this ridge, 1–2 cm from the midline. A characteristic mucosal vascular pattern that surrounds the ureteral orifice might be helpful in these cases. Prominent mucosal vessels are often seen coursing in an arc medial, inferior, and lateral to the orifice unless they are obscured by inflammation [34].

Ureteric Orifice Shape

Based on ureteric orifice shape and location, Lyon et al. classified the ureteral orifices into three grades (Table 3.4). As the bladder fills, the ureteral orifices are pushed out laterally and the intravesical ureter is compressed, making ureteral access more difficult [35].

Table 3.4 Various shapes of the ureteric orifice [35]

Grade 0	Grade 1	Grade 2	Grade 3
Normal cone or "Volcano" shaped	Stadium-shaped orifice	Horseshoe orifice	Golf-hole orifice
The increasing tendency to reflux			

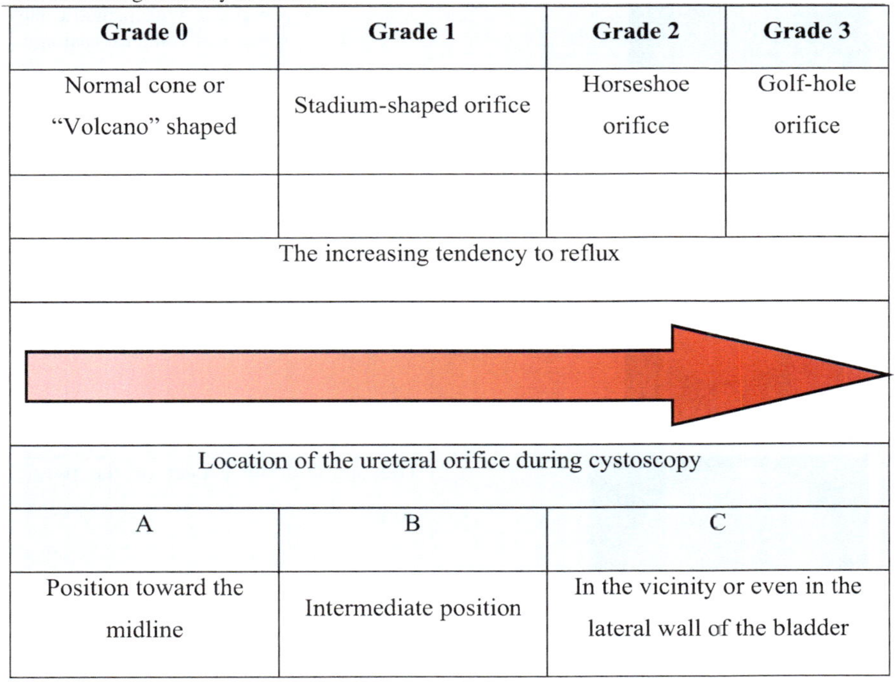

Grade 0	Grade 1	Grade 2	Grade 3
Normal cone or "Volcano" shaped	Stadium-shaped orifice	Horseshoe orifice	Golf-hole orifice
The increasing tendency to reflux			
Location of the ureteral orifice during cystoscopy			
A	B	C	
Position toward the midline	Intermediate position	In the vicinity or even in the lateral wall of the bladder	

Location of the ureteral orifice during cystoscopy		
A	B	C
Position toward the midline	Intermediate position	In the vicinity or even in the lateral wall of the bladder

Endoscopic Segments

From an endoscopic point of view (Fig. 3.9), the ureter is divided into three approximately equal segments:

- **Distal** or **pelvic segment:** consists of extravesical and intramural parts.
- **Middle segment**: between the two ends of the sacroiliac joint.
- **Proximal segment**: from the renal pelvis to the proximal end of the sacroiliac joint, at the L5 transverse process.

Endoluminal Ureteral Course

Starting from the ureteral orifice, the intravesical segment of the ureter extends for about 1.5 cm. First, the submucosal part courses posterolaterally in the bladder for about 0.5 cm, then the intramural part runs obliquely through the bladder

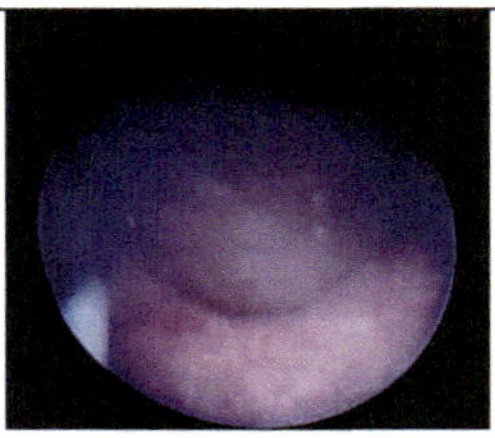	Endoscopic aspect of the interureteric bar.
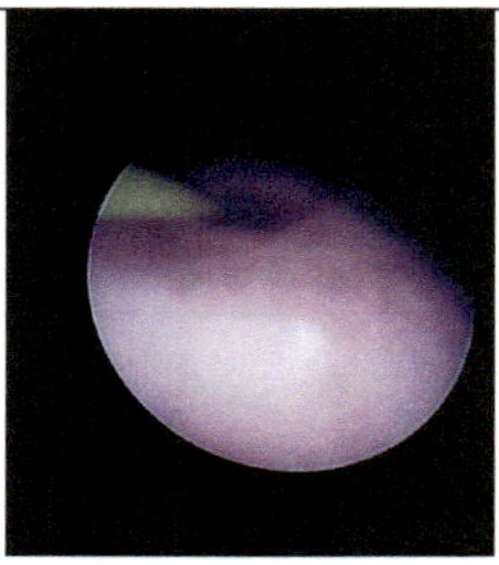	Identification and insertion of a guidewire into the ureteric orifice. Particular shapes of ureteral orifices are (a) Cone, (b) Horseshoe, (c) Golf hole, and (d) Stadium.
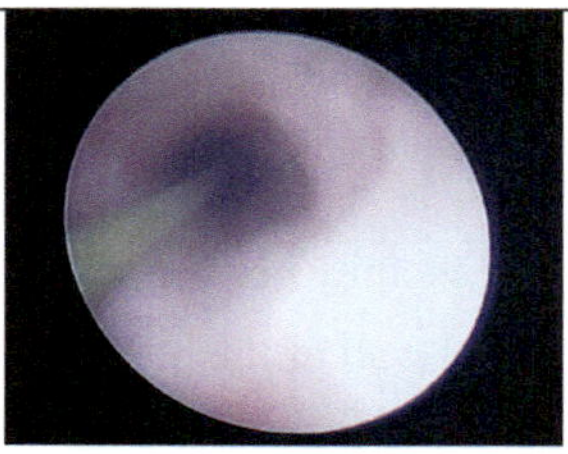	The endoluminal aspect of the pelvic ureter.

Fig. 3.9 The endoluminal landmarks and views during rigid ureteroscopy

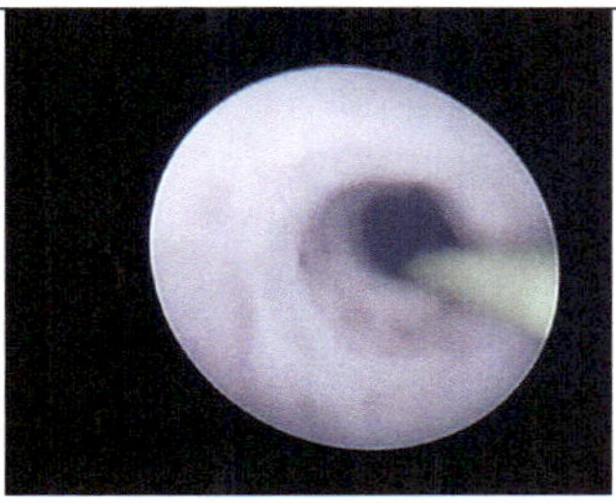	The endoluminal aspect of the iliac ureter
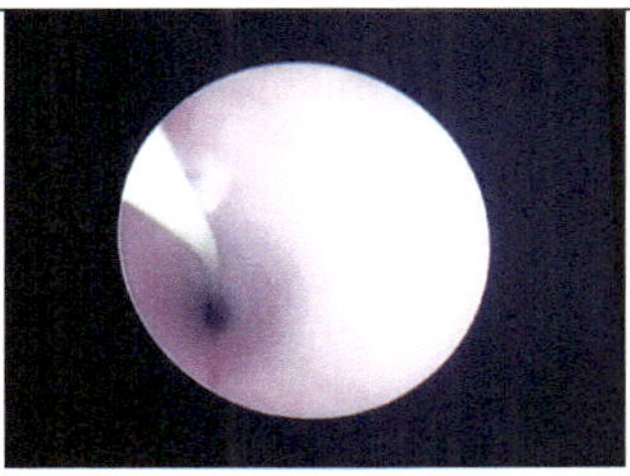	The endoluminal aspect of the lumbar ureter
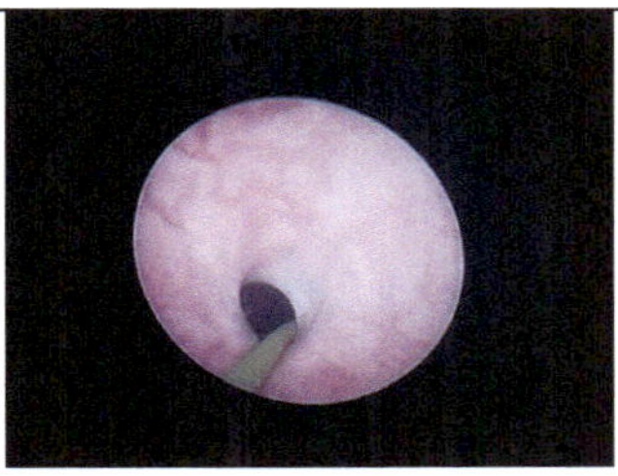	The endoluminal aspect ureteropelvic junction
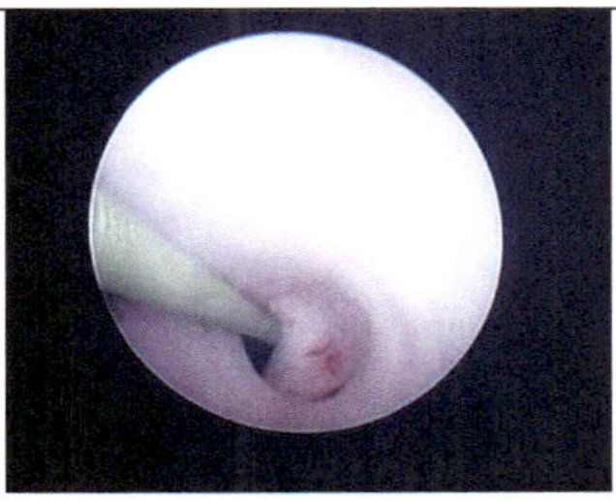	The endoluminal aspect of ureteral kink

Fig. 3.9 (continued)

musculature at the detrusor hiatus for about 1 cm [36]. At the pelvic brim is the area of the iliac vessels, which can be seen pulsating behind the ureter as this level is approached. Following this is a relatively straight section where the middle of the ureter lies on the psoas muscle. It is here that the typical stellate appearance of the non-distended ureteral lumen can be discerned. This leads to the third constriction at the ureteropelvic junction, which is identified endoscopically as a narrowing in the ureter followed by the wide renal pelvis. The uretero-infundibular angle represents the angle of deflection necessary for a flexible ureteroscope to move from the axis of the upper section of the ureter to the axis of the lower infundibulum. This was found to be 140 degrees on average, although it may range from 104 to 175 degrees [37]. The more acute this angle the more difficult for the flexible ureteroscopy to approach the lower calyx [38]. **Ureteral spasm** is also involved in the possible segmental narrowing of the lumen, observed during ureteroscopy. The short, fibrous segmental narrowing of the ureter can be dilated with balloon dilators and Teflon ureteral probes. Various pharmacological agents such as glucagon, aminophylline, and lidocaine gel can reduce the ureteral spasm.

3.2.2.4 Ureteral Narrowing and Kinking: Recent Notions [39]

The classic concept: "The ureter is naturally narrowed at the ureteropelvic junction, at the iliac vessel crossover, and the ureterovesical junction" [40]. These are considered classic teaching concepts of ureteric anatomy and surgery. The origin of this concept was attributed to the textbook, "Urology," published in 1954, without stating a clear reference to this concept (Fig. 3.10) [39, 41].

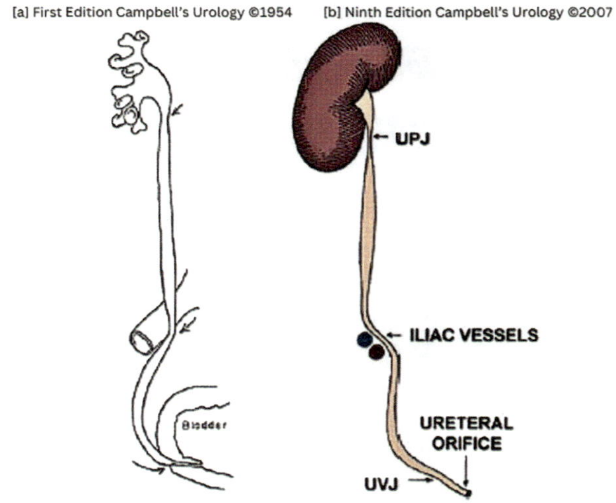

Fig. 3.10 Classic points of ureteral narrowing [39, 41, 42]

Notion of the "Crossing Point"

The widespread use of cross-sectional, 3-D reformatting and digital imaging improved the clarity and precision of urogenital imaging processing. More detailed and accurate anatomical description of the ureter could be made based on these techniques with the correlation of the anatomical narrowing areas where a stone might lodge during its passage in the ureter. Using non-contrast CT, there are two peak sites of stone locations in the ureter of patients coming to the ER with renal colic: **the upper ureter** and the **ureterovesical junction (UVJ)** [43]. Many studies reported similar results confirming the same sites [42–46]. The cause of stone impaction at these two sites could be explained as follows:

1. **The UVJ**: has a valve-like function to prevent urinary reflux and the intravesical portion of the ureter is the narrowest section of the upper urinary tract [46].
2. **At the level of the upper ureter:** the ureter inside the perirenal fat is freely mobile and when exits the perirenal fat it is fixed to the anteromedial aspect of the psoas muscle. At this point, the ureter is crossed ventrally by the gonadal vessels. This point was termed the **"crossing point"** (Fig. 3.11). This is the peak site of urinary stone impaction in the upper ureter which is due to the change in ureteral fixation at that level [47, 48].

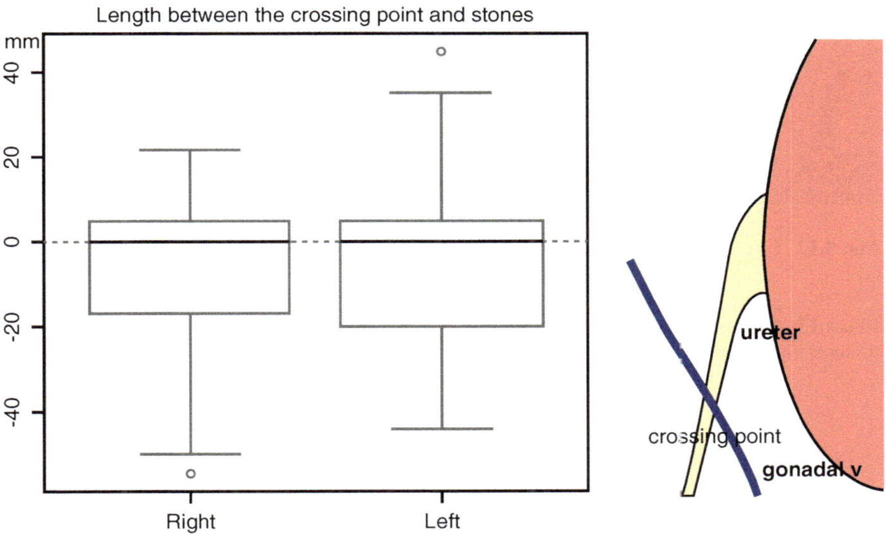

Fig. 3.11 The new concept of upper ureter narrowing, the length between the crossing point of the ureter and the gonadal vein, and the impaction site of the ureteral stone [47, 48]

Notion of Upper Ureteral Kinking

The upper ureter normally may have a kink, and this is a common clinical finding during radiologic or endourologic procedures. This finding could be explained by the previously mentioned concept of changing ureteral mobility at the crossing point from mobile upper ureter contained within the perirenal space to fixed ureter below this point. This kinking is obvious during renal descent with inspiration or other movements (Fig. 3.12) [47].

Radiologically, the upper ureter kinks are classified into three grades (Fig. 3.13):

- (Grade 1): no or mild kinking of the upper ureter.
- (Grade 2) moderate kinking containing a horizontal portion.
- (Grade 3) severe kinking containing a retrograde portion.

Grade 2 or 3 is regarded as radiologically "significant" kinking. The radiologically "significant" ureteral kinking rate is 18.4% on the right and 21.8% on the left [47].

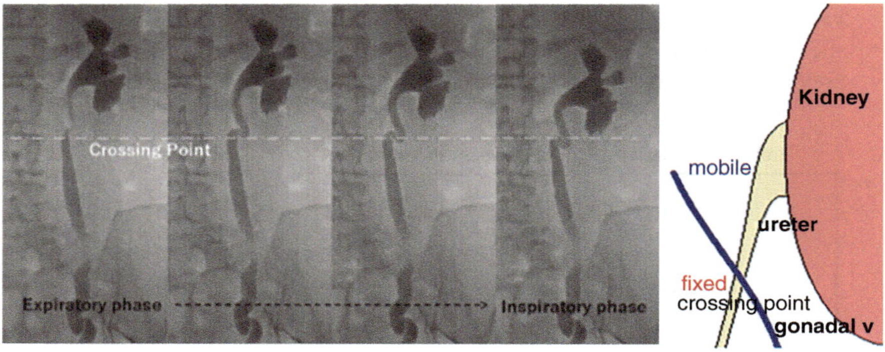

Fig. 3.12 Upper ureteral Kinking [47]

Fig. 3.13 Grades of upper ureteral kinking [47]

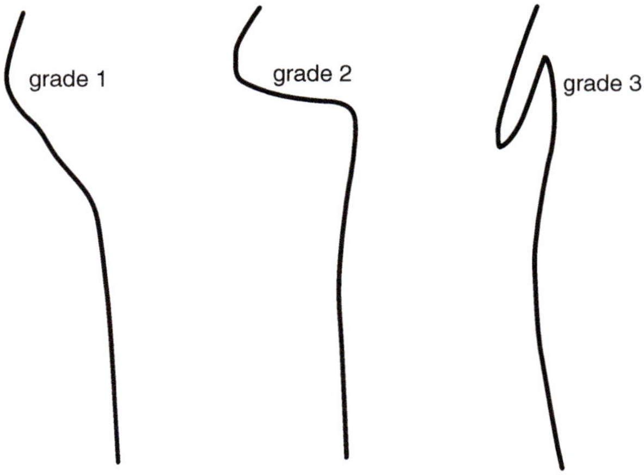

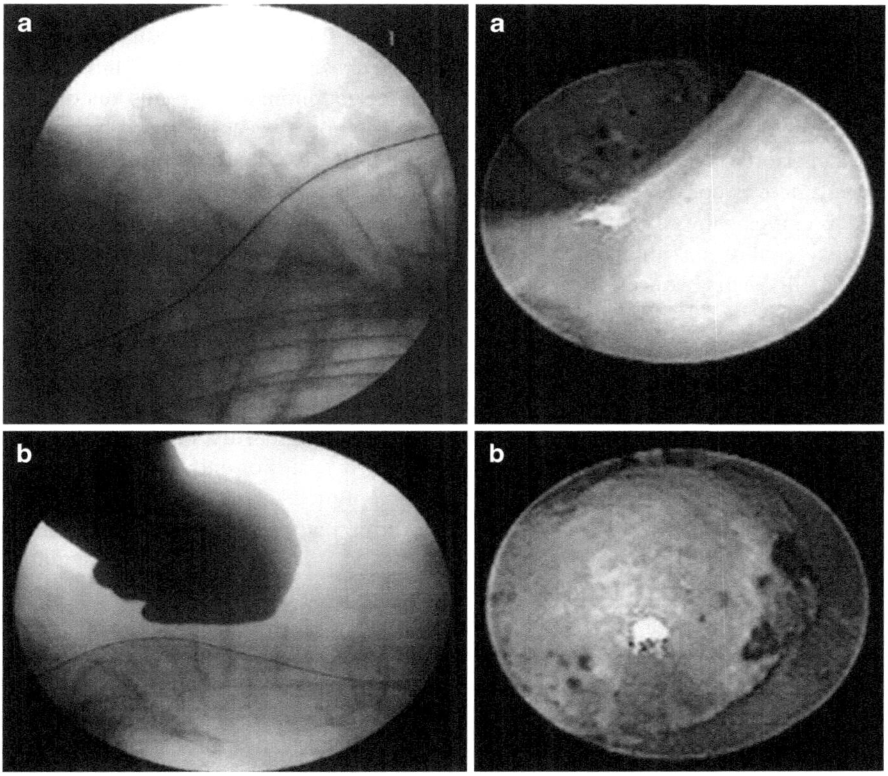

Fig. 3.14 Real time Fluroscopic image and ureteroscopy showing ureteral kink (**a**) and applying lower abdominal pressure by the surgeon's fist (**b**) facilitates passage of the semirigid ureteroscope [50]

Straightening of the severely kinked upper ureter during ureteroscopy could be made by applying cephalad and medially directed manual pressure with a closed fist on the flank this is called the **Mertz maneuver** [49]. Another maneuver described to facilitate upper ureteric access with semirigid ureteroscopy is applying lower abdominal pressure by the surgeon's fist (Fig. 3.14), which helps pass the endoscope over the iliac vessels or place the laser fiber on stones [50].

3.2.2.5 Anatomical Influence of Patient Position on the Course of the Ureter During the Endourologic Procedure

Patients are usually placed in the standard dorsal lithotomy position during ureteroscopy with the perineum flush with the edge of the operating table [51]. Difficulties in ureteroscopic access may be due to either the enlarged prostate or the narrowing at the level of the iliac bifurcation [52–54]. Surgical positions adopted for ureteroscopy include standard lithotomy, extended lithotomy, or elevation of the contralateral leg [54–56]. Fluoroscopic imaging of the ureter in an anteroposterior view has shown that the ureteral position has no relation to the degree of hip flexion. While lateral view fluoroscopy has shown that the abdominal ureter runs in a straight course while the lower ureter has two curves. The upper or sacroiliac curve is convex anteriorly with the maximal curvature anterior to the iliac bifurcation. The lower curve is convex posteriorly, following the sacrum curve behind the bladder. These curves showed maxim convexity with minimally flexed hips (as the lumbar lordosis is at its maximum and increasing degrees of hip flexion allowed for anterior pelvic tilt). This reduces lordosis of the lumber spine and straightens the ureter straightens [54, 57, 58].

3.2.2.6 Vascularization, Innervation of the Ureter and its Relation to the Endopyelotomy and Endoureterotomy Procedures

The ureter has a complex, segmental blood supply [59], and its various parts are vascularized by nearby vessels (Table 3.5). All these arterial sources form multiple anastomoses, creating a periureteral arterial plexus.

In the upper part of the ureter, the arterial sources are arranged medially, while the lower part receives the arterial sources from the lateral aspect. This arrangement and the relations of the various ureteral segments should be considered when performing endoscopic incisions. The arterial supply passes longitudinally along the ureter forming a plexus of anastomosing vessels (Fig. 3.15).

This arrangement of the ureteral vasculature is of clinical significance as it allows for the safe mobilization of the ureter during surgery when proper dissection from surrounding structures is crucial. The venous blood is drained into vessels corresponding to the arteries, which flow into the inferior cava, the iliac veins, and the vesico-genital plexus. In contrast to the native ureters, which derive their blood supply from both the renal arteries and pelvic collaterals, the transplanted ureter depends solely on the blood supplied by the branches of the renal artery that traverse periureteral tissues. This area, also known as the "**Golden Triangle**" (Fig. 3.16), contains important branches, such as the lower polar artery, which supplies the distal ureter [60].

Excessive dissection of the 'golden triangle' area should therefore be avoided during graft recovery. Damage to this triangle can lead to necrosis of the distal ureter in 70% of the cases [60–64]. The pain impulse can lead to sympathetic reflex at the kidney level, with arteriolar vasoconstriction, thus decreasing urine formation from the kidney. This mechanism is called the "**uretero-renal reflex**" [65]. The venous return, which tends to follow the arterial branches, is usually insignificant for ureteroscopy, except in rare cases of congenital venous malformations (Klippel-Trenaunay Syndrome, KTS) or retrocaval ureters [66].

Table 3.5 Segmental arterial supply of the ureter [59]

Lower suprarenal	18%
Renal	98%
Capsular	12%
Gonadal	44%
Aortic	52%
Common iliac	34%
Internal iliac	60%
Uterine	98%
Vaginal	86%
Superior vesical	92%
Inferior vesical	36%
Artery to vas	16%
Middle rectal	14%

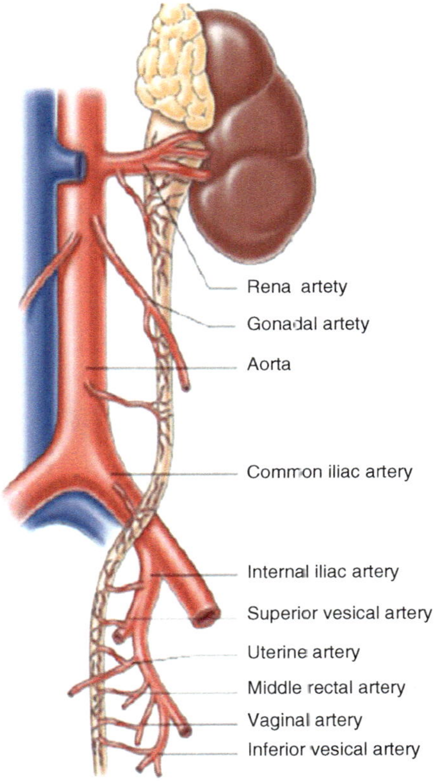

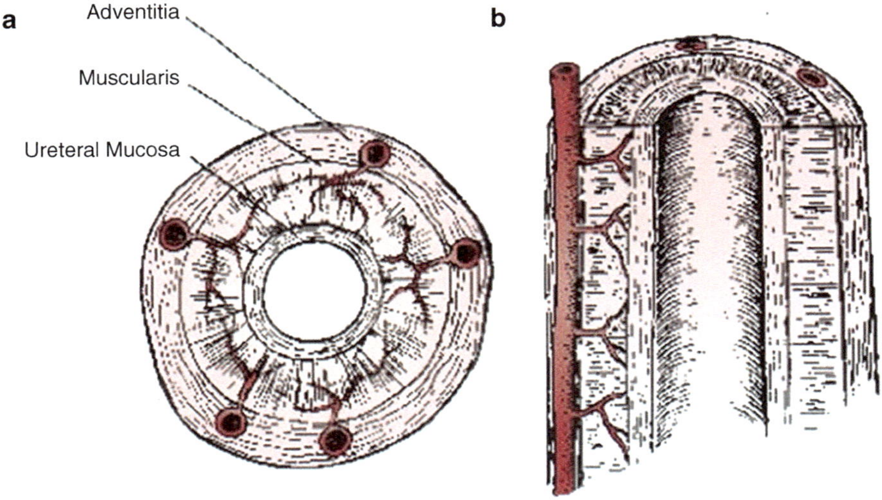

Fig. 3.15 Arrangement of arterial supply in the ureteral wall shown in transverse (**a**) and longitudinal (**b**) sections

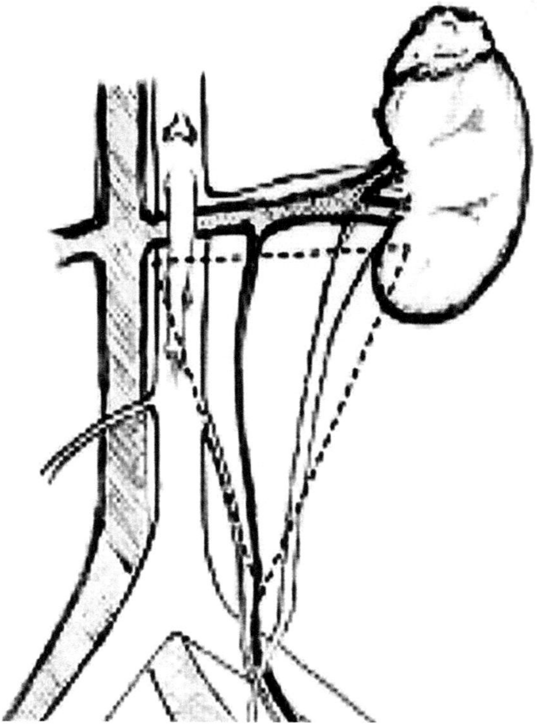

Fig. 3.16 Anatomical boundaries of the golden triangle [60]

3.2.2.7 Sites of the Endoscopic Incisions During the Endoureterotomy Procedure

The site of the endoscopic ureteral incision depends on the location of the stricture (Fig. 3.17). Proximal and middle ureteral strictures are incised on the lateral ureteral wall, while distal strictures below the iliac vessels are incised on the medial ureteral wall. Strictures at iliac vessels are incised on the anterior ureteral wall [67, 68]. If the ureteric orifice is involved, the incision is made 12 o'clock position of the ureteral orifice extending through the ureteral orifice to the stricture area [69–71]. Bleeding after endoureterotomy or endopyelotomy procedures may occur due to injury of crossing vessel [can be avoided by performing CT angiography] or incisions at wrong sites [can be avoided by air injection to define the anterior part of the ureter (12 o'clock) [72, 73].

Stricture location	Right side	Left side
At the ureteropelvic junction	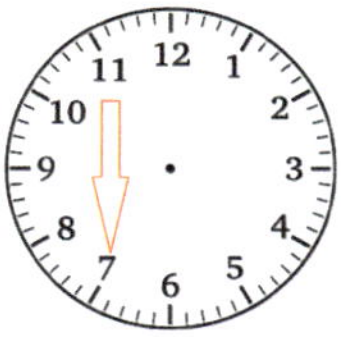	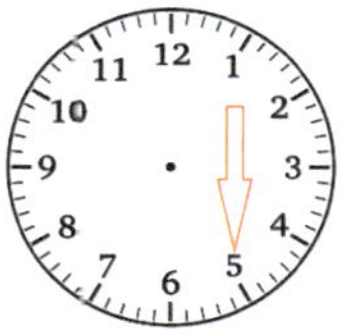
At the upper ureter	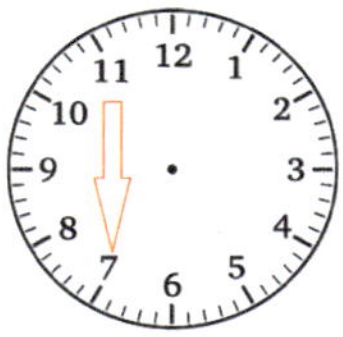	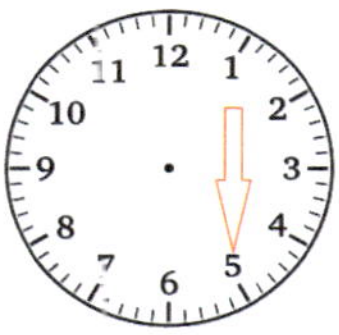
At the crossing of the iliac vessels	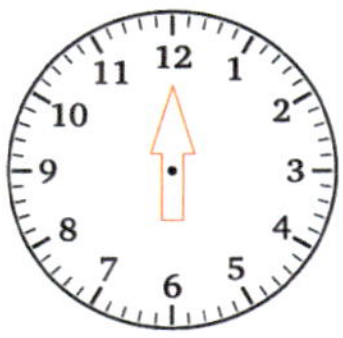	
At the pelvic ureter	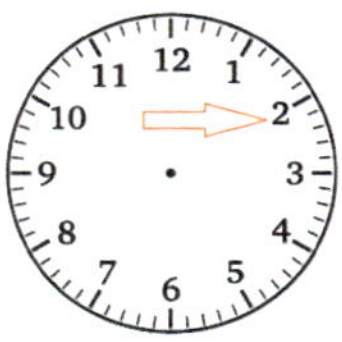	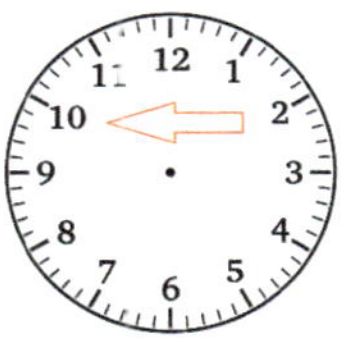

Fig. 3.17 Sites of endoureterotomy incisions according to the ureteral level if there are no anomalies [74]

3.2.2.8 Properties of Ureteral Structure

The ureter wall consists of three layers: mucosa (transitional epithelium), musculosa, and adventitia. Submucosal tunneling and false passage usually occur in the distal ureter, because the transitional layer is more redundant and bulkier, with a thick muscular backing. In contrast, ureteral perforation and avulsion usually occur in the proximal ureter, where there is less muscle wall support. The undilated ureteral mucosa appears as smooth longitudinal folds with fine vascularity. The ureteral muscle is well vascularized and will bleed with deeper perforations [29, 30]. Regarding the structural properties of the ureter, the cut section of the normal human ureter has a stellate shape. The thickness of the ureteral wall, including epithelium, lamina propria, and muscle, is approximately 1 mm. However, it significantly thickens and stiffens with age [75–77]. The intraluminal pressure of the ureter is similar to that of the renal pelvis in healthy ureters, averaging 13.5 cm H_2O in the mid-ureter, and 13 cm H_2O in the lower third of the ureter [78]. Ureteral obstruction (either internal or external) or ureteral stents increase these values substantially [79, 80]. The compliance or distensibility of the ureter wall is defined as the change in diameter in response to intraluminal pressure and it has been reported as 2 cm H_2O/mm [81]. Ureteral peristalsis is a traveling wave of contraction that directs the flow of urine from the kidneys to the bladder [82]. These waves are mostly monophasic, traveling at speeds of approximately 2–3 cm/s, with a length of 6–10 cm [81, 83]. The peristaltic wave frequency in normal humans is 1–8 times per minute and averages about three times per minute [84, 85]. Ureteral stents insertion causes ureteral a peristalsis [86, 87]. [see Chap. 10, The ureteral response to ureteral stents].

3.2.2.9 Endoscopic Anatomy of the Ureterovesical Junction and its Implication in Endoscopic Management of Vesicoureteral Reflux

The VUJ can be recognized as a small convex, bulging structure on the mucosal surface of the urinary bladder. The function of the VUJ is to allow unobstructed antegrade passage of urine bolus from the ureter into the bladder while preventing the reflux of urine from the bladder into the ureter, during both normal bladder filling and voiding. The structure and components of the VUJ include three anatomical components: the ureteral wall, the urinary bladder wall, and the ureteral sheath. Three layers cover the ureter and urinary bladder including the outer adventitia, middle muscular layer, and inner mucosal layer. At the VUJ, the middle muscle layer of the ureter is formed of longitudinally predominately orientated muscle bundles then the middle muscle layer fans out around the orifice and joins with fibers from the opposite ureter to form part of the superficial trigone. Bell's muscle represents some of the ureteric muscle fibers joining the urethra and creating a connection between the urethra and the ureter [88, 89].

Hydrodistention (HD) classification of ureteric orifice and vesicoureteric reflux [90]: Ureteral orifice (UO) hydrodistention is graded according to the extent of ureteral dilation orifice during cystoscopy (Table 3.6).

According to the grades of hydrodistention, the injection of the bulking agent is recommended as a stepwise algorithm including hydrodistention implantation technique [HIT], double HIT method, classic subureteric injection [STING], or a supra-ureteric injection (Fig. 3.18) [91].

Table 3.6 Hydrodistention classification [90]

H0	Absence of ureteral dilation: normal
H1	Dilation of the UO only: normal
H2	Visualization of the intramural ureter
H3	Visualization of the extramural ureter.

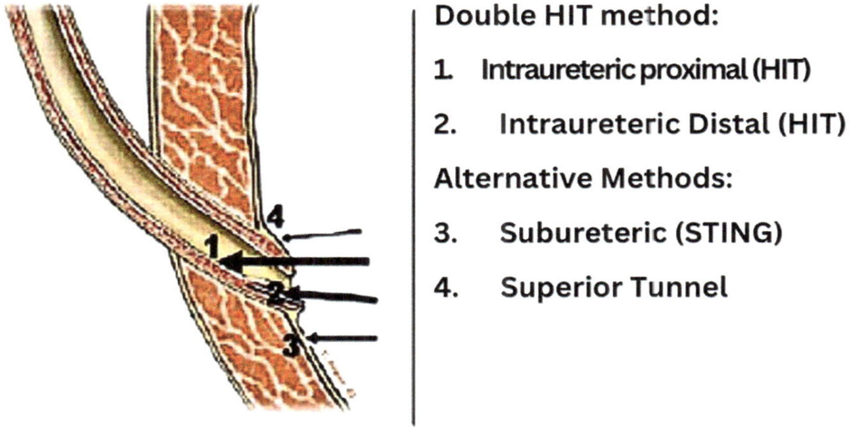

Fig. 3.18 Sites of needle insertion during endoscopic injection of bulking agents for the treatment of vesicoureteral reflux [91]

3.2.3 Applied Laparoscopic Anatomy of the ureter

From a laparoscopic point of view the ureter can be subdivided into:

3.2.3.1 Abdominal Part of the Ureter

The abdominal portion of the ureter is located at the medial border of the psoas muscle fascia overlying the genitofemoral nerve. **The right ureter** begins at the level posterior aspect of the second duodenum, descending within the retroperitoneum of the ascending colon near the right colic and ileocolic vessels, lateral to the root of the mesentery and the inferior vena cava under the ovarian vessels. Thereafter, it passes posterior to the terminal ileum and cecum. **The left ureter** descends at the lateral part of the abdominal aorta over the psoas muscle fascia and is crossed anteriorly by the left colic artery and ovarian vessels lying parallel to the inferior mesenteric vein and then passing along the posterior aspect of the sigmoid colon [92].

3.2.3.2 Pelvic Part of the Ureter

The ureters cross the bifurcation of the common iliac artery over the pelvic brim. When the ureter enters the true pelvis, it runs inferior to the ovarian vessels and goes through that path to the bladder on the posterior leaf of the broad ligament. It passes anteromedially while crossing the uterine artery (water under the bridge) afterward; it enters the ureteric tunnel (web tunnel) within the cardinal ligament. The ureter then travels laterally to the anterolateral vaginal fornix within the bladder pillar and

Table 3.7 Anatomical relations of the ureter

	Posteriorly	Anteriorly	Medially	Inferior
Abdominal ureter	Psoas muscle genitofemoral nerve common iliac vessels tips of L2-L5 transverse processes	Right ureter: 2nd duodenum gonadal vessels right colic vessels ileocolic vessels Left ureter: gonadal artery left colic artery loops of jejunum sigmoid mesentery and colon	Right ureter: IVC Left ureter: abdominal aorta inferior mesenteric vein	
Pelvic ureter	Sacroiliac joint internal iliac artery	In males: ductus deferens In females: uterine artery (in the broad ligament)	In females: Uterine cervix	In males: seminal vesicle In females: lateral fornix of the vagina

enters the trigone of the bladder. The orifices of the ureters can be seen on the postero-lateral part of the trigone. The ureters run a 1.5–2 cm course in the bladder wall [92].

3.2.3.3 Anatomical Relations (Table 3.7)

The relationships of the ureter are somewhat complex due to the differences between the left and right sides of the abdominal cavity and the differences between male and female pelvic viscera. It should be noted that the only structures that pass anteriorly across the pelvic ureter are the ductus deferens in males and the uterine artery in females [93, 94].

3.2.3.4 Surface Markings

The surface markings of the abdominal ureter can be drawn as a slightly laterally convex line, between the point of the renal pelvis [medial to the middle of the costal margin] and the point of ureteral entrance into the pelvic cavity [3 cm lateral to the mid-line on the intertubercular plane close to the point of the bifurcation of the common iliac artery] (The point of division of the common iliac artery into external and internal iliac arteries may also be marked by a point on the intertubercular plane 3 cm from the middle line). Uretero-vesical junction is represented by a point 3 cm above and lateral to the upper end of the symphysis pubis. The course of the lower part of the ureter can be drawn as a laterally convex line joining the ureterovesical junction and common iliac bifurcation points [95].

3.2.3.5 Applied Laparoscopic anatomy of the Female Pelvic Ureter: Insights into Ureteral Injuries in Gynecologic Surgeries

Avascular **spaces in the female pelvis:** Pelvic connective tissue divides the subperitoneal pelvic area into different spaces. These spaces are filled with fatty or loose areolar connective tissue, which is generally avascular. These potential spaces play a role in the functioning of the urinary, reproductive, and gastrointestinal systems. They have a crucial role in the performing of pelvic operations because knowing them exactly allows the restoration of normal anatomy and avoids injury of pelvic viscera and structures. These pelvic spaces are as follows [96]:

- Retropubic (Retzius) space.
- Paravesical space.
- Presacral (Retrorectal) space.
- Pararectal space.
- Vesicovaginal (Vesicouterine) space.
- Rectovaginal space.

The **paravesical and pararectal spaces** (Fig. 3.19) are most often encountered during pelvic oncologic procedures. These spaces are located lateral to the pelvic

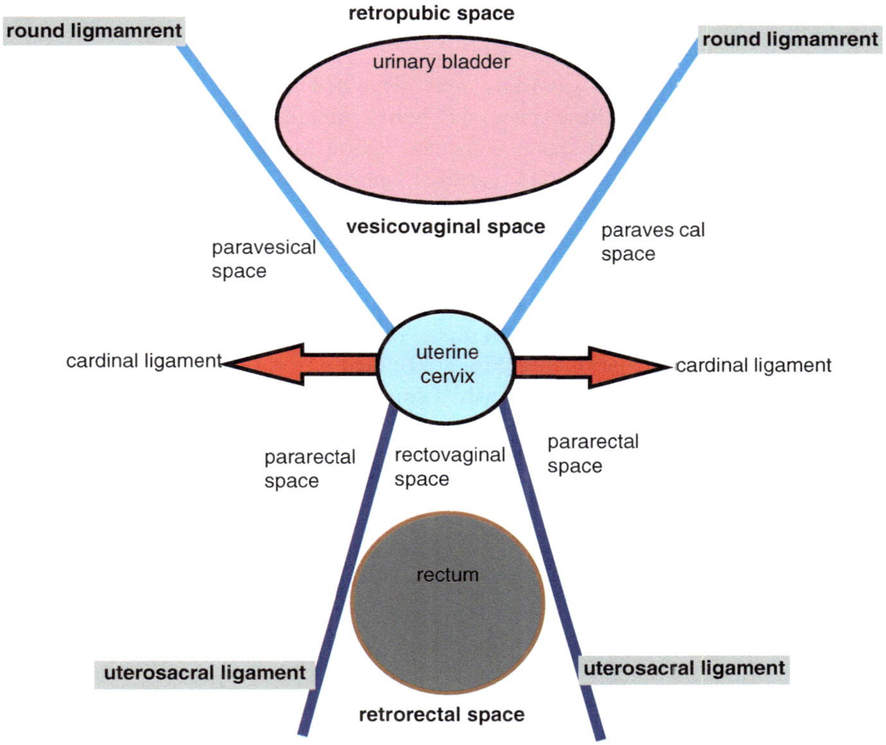

Fig. 3.19 The female retroperitoneal pelvic spaces in. B, Bladder; R, Rectum; CL, Cardinal ligament [97]

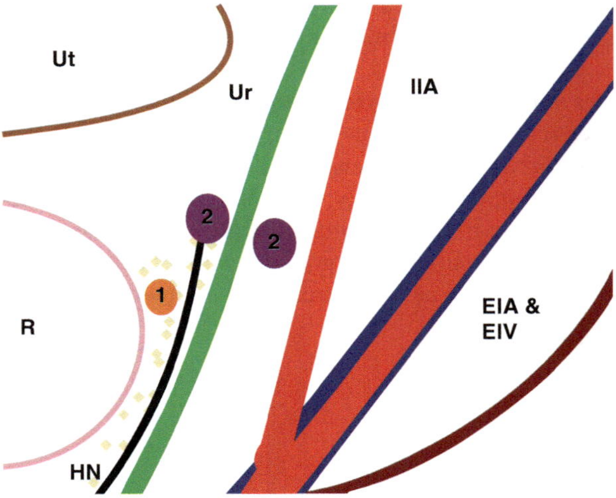

Fig. 3.20 The diagram shows the relationship between Okabayashi's pararectal space [1 orange dot] and Latzko's pararectal space [2 purple dots]. On the rectal sidewall of Latzko's pararectal space, the right ureter, and the hypogastric nerve [HN]. Okabayashi's pararectal space is medially developed between the rectum and the connective tissue plane of the ureter [Ur] and hypogastric nerve that was the rectal sidewall [R] of Latzko's pararectal space (*IIA*: Internal iliac artery, *EIA, EIV*: External iliac artery and vein, *UT*: uterus) [98]

viscera along the pelvic sidewalls and separated by the cardinal ligament. Transperitoneal access to these spaces will help in identifying the pelvic vasculature and ureters. The pararectal space is located lateral to the rectum and retrorectal space and at the posterior part of the cardinal ligament. Its boundaries are anteriorly: cardinal ligament, medially: rectal pillars, uterosacral ligament, ureter, laterally: internal iliac artery, posteriorly: sacrum, and caudally: puborectalis muscle. Both ureters pass along the medial portion of the pararectal space. The pararectal space is separated from the paravesical space by the cardinal ligament and uterine artery, and from the presacral space by the rectal septa. The pararectal space can be divided by the ureter, into two compartments (Fig. 3.20); medially is Okabayashi's space, and laterally is Latzko's space. **Okabayashi's space is t**he medial compartment of the pararectal space between the ureter and the rectouterine ligament. It can be created by opening the posterior leaf of the broad ligament. **Latzko's space is t**he lateral compartment of the pararectal space between the ureter and pelvic side wall, which is developed after the dissection of the internal iliac artery [96–98].

Exposure of the pararectal space begins by opening the broad ligament lateral and parallel to the infundibulopelvic ligament. Blunt dissection of loose areolar tissue between the external iliac artery (overlying the psoas muscle) and the ureter (found deeply on the medial leaf of the broad ligament) exposes the space [97].

An important anatomical structure during laparoscopic hysterectomy is the vesicouterine ligament (VUL) which consists of an anterior leaflet and posterior leaflet. In the anterior leaf of the VUL, the cervicovesical blood vessels are the main vascular

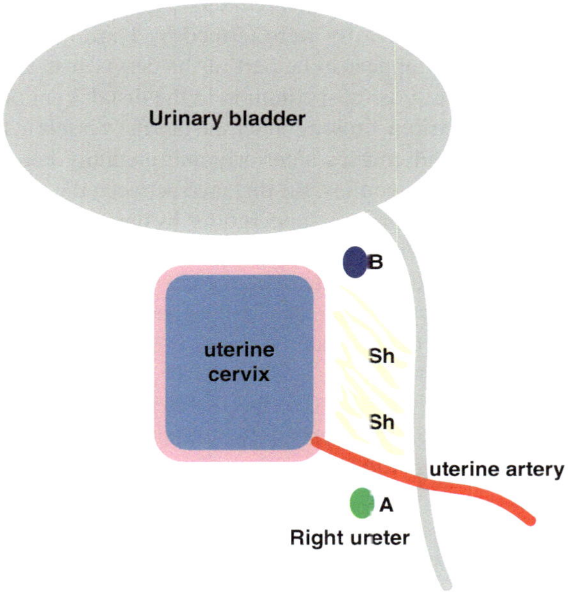

Fig. 3.21 This diagram shows the anatomical spaces around the anterior leaf of the vesicouterine ligament. The anterior leaf of the vesicouterine ligament extends from the axillary space [A green dot] to the fourth space of Yabuki [B blue dot]. Multiple "shafts" [SH] are potential avascular spaces created on the anterior leaf of the vesicouterine ligament [104]

bundles. In the posterior leaf, the middle vesical vein and inferior vesical vein draining into the deep uterine vein run from the urinary bladder to the lower cervix or vagina. There are vascular communicating branches of the middle and inferior vesical veins. Four anatomical spaces associated with the VUL were described: ureteral space, paravesical space, paravaginal space, the fourth is space of Yabuki, and the "axillary space" (Fig. 3.21). The axillary space represents the gate of the ureteral space, which is inferiorly located in relation to the uterine artery. The fourth space of Yabuki is loose avascular tissue anterolateral to the ureterovesical junction. The paravaginal space is located medial to the posterior leaf of the VUL and lateral to the vagina, while the paravesical space is the lateral margin of the posterior leaf of the VUL. These anatomical spaces allow for dissection of the ureter during laparoscopic hysterectomy, using the axillary space and other potential spaces as landmarks. Between the axillary space and the fourth space of Yabuki, several small blood vessels in the anterior aspect of the VUL cross over the ureteral space similar to vertical shafts, called **Karez**, into the ureteral space. The main goal of creating these spaces during surgery is to reduce blood loss and prevent ureteral injury [99–104].

3.2.3.6 The Proximity of the Ureter to the Uterine Cervix

Ureteral injury is one of the more serious complications of hysterectomy. This complication, which occurs in 0.1–2.5% of such operations, is mainly related to the anatomical proximity of the ureter and cervix [105–107]. Seventy percent of ureteral injuries and complications are discovered after surgical procedures, particularly laparoscopic hysterectomy. Ureters within 5 mm from the lateral cervical wall, unilaterally or bilaterally were termed by Hurd and coworkers as "**cervical ureters**" because they appear to be part of the cervix instead of the cardinal ligament [108]. Surgical injury is most common in the distal 3 cm of the ureter, as it passes through the parametrium, crosses under the uterine vessels at the ureteric canal in the cardinal ligament, and courses anteriorly and medially before its entry into the bladder. In anatomical dissections, the distance between the ureters and the cervix is 1.5–2.5 cm [109–115]. In patients undergoing hysterectomy for cervical pathology, measurement of the cervical-ureteric distance in the preoperative CT is important. The surgeon can anticipate ureteral injury and take protective measures to prevent inadvertent ureteral injury. Gemer and colleagues found that the right ureter is significantly closer to the cervix than the left (2.0 ± 0.8 cm vs. 2.2 ± 1.0 cm, $p < 0.05$). In cases with isolated cervical pathology, the right ureter was more distant than the left (2.0 ± 0.6 cm vs. 1.7 ± 0.6 cm, $p < 0.05$). At least one ureter was within 0.5 cm of the cervix in 3.6% of patients with normal CT scans and 10.3% of patients with cervical pathology. Age did not correlate with the distance of the ureters from the cervix [116].

3.2.3.7 Tips and Tricks to Avoid Ureteral Injury During Laparoscopic Hysterectomy

1. The assistant should push the uterus cephalad.
2. It is better to dissect the urinary bladder away from the vaginal fornices.
3. Early dissection of the posterior leaf of the broad ligament, therefore the ureter will fall laterally.
4. Avoid excessive coagulation of the ureter by diathermy.
5. Insertion of a ureteral stent is preferable, especially in complicated cases or expected difficulties.

Section I: Questions

1. Which of the following is correct regarding the ureter?

   (a) The abdominal part is double the length of the pelvic part.
   (b) Lies posterior to genitofemoral nerve.
   (c) Lies posterior to the iliac vessels.
   (d) Receives parasympathetic innervation from the vagus nerve.
   (e) The narrowest part is the intramural part.

Answer: (e)
Each of the abdominal and pelvic parts is 5 in. long. It passes anterior to the genitofemoral nerve and the beginning of the iliac arteries. It receives parasympathetic innervation from the pelvic splanchnic nerves (S2, 3, 4)

2. Upon investigation of a tumor of the kidney, it was noticed that the patient's left kidney has two ureters and two renal pelves. This abnormality is due to:

   (a) an abnormal division of the pronephros
   (b) an abnormal division of the mesonephros
   (c) an abnormal division of the metanephros.
   (d) an abnormal division of the mesonephric duct.
   (e) a premature division of the ureteric bud.

Answer: (e)
The ureteric bud divides normally when meets the metanephric blastema. Premature division causes duplication of the ureter and renal pelvis. In some cases, two separate kidneys may form.

3. Regarding the ureter, which of the following statements is not correct?

   (a) The right and left ureters have three constrictions.
   (b) The right and left ureters lie anterior to the corresponding sacroiliac joint.
   (c) The left ureter is crossed anteriorly by the sigmoid colon and mesocolon.
   (d) The two ureters pass anterior to the gonadal vessels (testicular or ovarian).
   (e) Both ureters receive their arterial supply from the renal arteries.

Answer: (d)
The ureters are crossed anteriorly by the testicular and ovarian vessels.

4. The lining epithelium of the ureter is derived from the:

   (a) ectoderm
   (b) mesoderm
   (c) endoderm
   (d) endoderm and mesoderm
   (e) ectoderm and endoderm

Answer: (b)
The transitional epithelium lining the ureter is derived from the intermediate mesoderm which forms the ureteric bud. The ureteric bud is a diverticulum from the mesonephric duct. This contrasts with the transitional epithelium lining the urinary bladder which develops from the endoderm.

5. Which part of the ureter has the richest arterial supply?

   (a) The renal pelvis.
   (b) The abdominal part.
   (c) The middle part.
   (d) The pelvic part.
   (e) The intravesical or intramural part.

Answer: (d)
The pelvic part is the richest part of arterial supply.

6. Ureteric pain is referred to the following dermatome:

   (a) T 10.
   (b) L 1.
   (c) L 3.
   (d) L 5.
   (e) S 2.

Answer: (b)
Pain is transmitted with the sympathetic fibers to T12 – L1 dermatomes.

7. Which of the following structures lies anterior to the left ureter?

   (a) Sigmoid arteries
   (b) Ileocolic artery
   (c) Root of the mesentery
   (d) Portal vein
   (e) Third part of the duodenum

Answer: (a)

8. Lymphatics from the upper part of the right ureter drain into the:

   (a) Celiac lymph nodes
   (b) Common iliac lymph nodes
   (c) Para-aortic lymph nodes
   (d) Paracaval lymph nodes
   (e) External iliac lymph nodes

Answer: (d)

Section II: Questions

1. You are scheduling a ureteroscopy for the right ureteral stone in a-7-year-old child and you are checking for different double J stent inventory in your endourology unit. The average ureteral length in this child and double J stent length would be:

   (a) 20 and 19 cm
   (b) 10 and 18 cm
   (c) 16 and 18 cm
   (d) 12 and 18 cm

Answer: (a)
According to Forzini et al. 2019 [4], the mean ureteral length (ULs) on the right and left are:

9.7 and 9.91 cm at ≤1 year,
20.10 and 21.08 cm at 7 year and
26.55 and 27.46 cm at 16 year respectively
Double-J length catheter = child's age+12 cm

2. You are performing urethrocystoscopy during the evaluation of hydroureteronephrosis. Which of the following ureteral orifice shape and location is highly not associated with vesicoureteral reflux?
   (a) Laterally placed golf-hole orifice
   (b) Laterally placed volcano-shaped orifice
   (c) Medially placed volcano-shaped orifice
   (d) Medially placed golf-hole orifice

Answer: (c)
Based on ureteric orifice shape and location, Lyon et al. classified the ureteral orifices into three grades. As the bladder fills, the ureteral orifices are pushed out laterally and the intravesical ureter is compressed, making ureteral access more difficult [20]. With volcano-shaped ureteral orifice approaching near midline there is decreasing tendency to reflux.

3. "Crossing point" is recently described as the point of ureteral narrowing in the upper ureter that is commonly associated with the impaction of ureteral stone. The best anatomical description of this point is:
   (a) The point of ureteral crossing iliac vessels
   (b) Ureterovesical junction
   (c) Pelvi-ureteral junction
   (d) The point between the ureter inside the perirenal and the ureter when exits the perirenal fat where it's crossed ventrally by the gonadal vessels

Answer: (d)
On non-contrast CT examination, there are two peak sites of stone locations in the ureter of patients coming to the ER with renal colic, one of them is at the level of the upper ureter where the ureter inside the perirenal fat is freely mobile, and when exits the perirenal fat it is fixed to the anteromedial aspect of the psoas muscle. At this point, the ureter is crossed ventrally by the gonadal vessels. This point was termed the "crossing point"

4. Patient with secondary right ureteropelvic junction obstruction is scheduled for endourologic management. During ureteroscopy, there is a short stricture at the ureteropelvic junction [6 mm in length] and you decided to do Ho-YAG LASER endopyelotomy, from the endourologic perspective the best site for this incision will be at:
   (a) 5 o'clock
   (b) 7 o'clock
   (c) 10 o'clock
   (d) 12 o'clock

Answer: (b)
Bleeding after endoureterotomy or endopyelotomy procedures may occur due to injury of the crossing vessel (can be avoided by performing CT angiography) or incisions performed at the wrong locations. The best location for right endopyelotomy will be at 7 o'clock according to De Coninck et al. [59].

5. Regarding ureteral proximity to uterine cervix one of the following statements is false:
   (a) Most ureteral injuries occur at the area of ureteral proximity to the cervix
   (b) In anatomical dissections, the distance between the ureters and the cervix has been measured at 1.5–2.5 cm
   (c) the right ureter is significantly further away from the cervix than the left ureter
   (d) Early dissection of the posterior leaf of the broad ligament, therefore the ureter will fall laterally is a good trick to avoid ureteral injury during laparoscopic hysterectomy

Answer: (c)
Ureteric injury is one of the more serious complications of hysterectomy. This complication, which occurs in 0.1–2.5% of such operations, is mostly related to the anatomical proximity of the ureters and cervix [90–92]. 70% of ureteral injuries and complications are discovered after surgical procedures, especially laparoscopic hysterectomy. Ureters within 5 mm from the lateral cervical wall, unilaterally or bilaterally were termed by Hurd and coworkers as "**cervical ureters**" because they appear to be part of the cervix instead of the cardinal ligament [93]. Surgical injury is most common in the distal 3 cm of the ureter, as it courses through the parametrium, crosses under the uterine vessels at the ureteric canal in the cardinal ligament, and courses anteriorly and medially before its entry into the bladder. In anatomical dissections, the distance between the ureters and the cervix has been measured at 1.5–2.5 cm [94–100]. For patients undergoing a hysterectomy for cervical pathology, measuring the cervical-ureteric distance in the preoperative CT is important. The surgeon may anticipate ureteral injury and make a protective measure that prevents inadvertent ureteral injury. It was found by Gemer and colleagues that the right ureter was significantly closer to the cervix than the left (2.0 ± 0.8 cm vs. 2.2 ± 1.0 cm, $p < 0.05$).

References

1. Fröber R. Surgical anatomy of the ureter. BJU Int. 2007;100:949–65.
2. Anderson JK, et al. Surgical anatomy of retroperitoneum, adrenals, kidneys, and ureters. In: Wein AJ, editor. Campbell-Walsh Urology, vol. 1. 9th ed. Philadelphia, PA: Saunders Elsevier; 2007. p. 3–37.
3. Barksdale PA, et al. Surgical landmarks of the ureter in the cadaveric female pelvis. Clin Anat. 1997;10:324–7.
4. Brooks JD. Anatomy of the lower urinary tract and male genitalia. In: Wein AJ, editor. Campbell-Walsh Urology, vol. 1. 9th ed. Philadelphia, PA: Saunders Elsevier; 2007. p. 38–77.
5. Anson BJ, McVay CB. Anson & McVay surgical anatomy. 6th ed. Philadelphia: WB Saunders; 1984.
6. Hinman F Jr. Atlas of urosurgical anatomy. Philadelphia: WB Saunders; 1993.
7. Redman JF. Anatomy of the genitourinary system. In: Gillenwater JY, Grayhack JT, Howards SS, Duckett JW, editors. Adult and pediatric urology. 3rd ed. St. Louis: Mosby Year Book; 1996.

8. Drake RL, et al. Gray's anatomy for students. Philadelphia: Elsevier; 2005. p. 335.
9. Kohlmann HW, Respondek M. Lympho-venous shunts and thrombosis in urinary obstruction. Pathologe. 2012;33(2):152–6.
10. Mescher AL. Ch. 19: The urinary system. In: Mescher AL, editor. Junqueira's basic histology: text and atlas. 12th ed. New York: McGraw-Hill Medical; 2010.
11. Snell RS. Clinical embryology for medical students. 3rd ed. Boston, MA: Little Brown and Company; 1983.
12. Schlussel RN, Retik AB. Ectopic ureter, ureterocele, and other anomalies of the ureter. In: Wein AJ, editor. Campbell-Walsh Urology, vol. 4. 9th ed. Philadelphia, PA: Saunders Elsevier; 2007. p. 3383–422.
13. Kogan BA. Ch. 36: Disorders of the ureter and ureteropelvic junction. Tanagho EA, McAninch JW, eds. Smith's GENERAL Urology. 17 New York, NY: McGraw-Hill; 2008.
14. Sadler TW. Langman's medical embryology. Philadelphia: Wolters Kluwer; 2018.
15. Xiaodong Z, et al. Diagnosis and treatment of retrocaval ureter. Eur Urol. 1990;18:207–10.
16. Fröber R. Surgical anatomy of the ureter. BJU Int. 2007 Oct;100(4):949–65. https://doi.org/10.1111/j.1464-410X.2007.07207.x.
17. Hickling DR, Sun TT, Wu XR. Anatomy and physiology of the urinary tract: relation to host defense and microbial infection. Microbiol Spectr. 2015;3(4) https://doi.org/10.1128/microbiolspec. UTI-0016-2012. doi:10.1128/microbiolspec. UTI-0016-2012
18. Novaes, Hugo FF, et al. Analysis of ureteral length in adult cadavers. International Braz J Urol [online]. 2013;39(2):248–56. Available from: https://doi.org/10.1590/S1677-5538. IBJU.2013.02.14. ISSN 1677–6119 https://doi.org/10.1590/S1677-5538.IBJU.2013.02.14. (Accessed 5 April 2022).
19. Forzini T, Demouron M, Uhl M, Mesureur S, Renard C, Klein C, Haraux E. Computed tomography evaluation of ureteral length in children. J Pediatr Urol. 2019;15(5):555e1–5. https://doi.org/10.1016/j.jpurol.2019.06.011. Epub 2019 Jun 21
20. Paick SH, Park HK, Byun SS, Oh SJ, Kim HH. Direct ureteric length measurement from intravenous pyelography: does height represent ureteric length? Urol Res. 2005;33(3):199–202. https://doi.org/10.1007/s00240-004-0461-3. Epub 2005 Feb 25
21. Kawahara T, Sakamaki K, Ito H, Kuroda S, Terao H, Makiyama K, Uemura H, Yao M, Miyamoto H, Matsuzaki J. Developing a preoperative predictive model for ureteral length for ureteral stent insertion. BMC Urol. 2016;16(1):70. https://doi.org/10.1186/s12894-016-0189-8.
22. Hsu JT, Tseng JS, Chen M, Sun FJ, Chen CW, Lin WR, Chiang PK, Chiu AW. Preoperative estimate of natural ureteral length based on computed tomography and/or plain radiography. Sci Rep. 2021;11(1):12202. https://doi.org/10.1038/s41598-021-91658-6.
23. Shrewsberry AB, Al-Qassab U, Goodman M, Petros JA, Sullivan JW, Ritenour CW, Issa MM. A +20% adjustment in the computed tomography measured ureteral length is an accurate predictor of true ureteral length before ureteral stent placement. J Endourol. 2013;27(8):1041–5. https://doi.org/10.1089/end.2013.0041. Epub 2013 Jul 5
24. Jeon SS, Choi YS, Hong JH. Determination of ideal stent length for endourologic surgery. J Endourol. 2007;21(8):906–10. https://doi.org/10.1089/end.2006.0476.
25. Pilcher JM, Patel U. Choosing the correct length of ureteric stent: a formula based on the patient's height compared with direct ureteric measurement. Clin Radiol. 2002;57(1):59–62. https://doi.org/10.1053/crad.2001.0737.
26. Hruby GW, Ames CD, Yan Y, Monga M, Landman J. Correlation of ureteric length with anthropometric variables of surface body habitus. BJU Int. 2007;99(5):1119–22. https://doi.org/10.1111/j.1464-410X.2007.06757.x. Epub 2007 Feb 19
27. Bozzini G, Casellato S, Viganò A, Maruccia S, Picozzi S, Carmignani L. Predicting female ureteral length: a mathematical model. J Clin Urol. 2014;7(4):265–71. https://doi.org/10.1177/2051415814520868. © British Association of Urological Surgeons 2014 Reprints and permissions: sagepub.co.uk/journalsPermissions.nav
28. Kawahara T, Ito H, Terao H, Yoshida M, Ogawa T, Uemura H, Kubota Y, Matsuzaki J. Choosing an appropriate length of loop type ureteral stent using direct ureteral length measurement. Urol Int. 2012;88(1):48–53. https://doi.org/10.1159/000332431. Epub 2011 Nov 19

29. Shnorhavorian M, Anderson KR. Anatomic and physiologic considerations in ureteroscopy. Urol Clin North Am. 2004;31(1):15–20. https://doi.org/10.1016/S0094-0143(03)00090-9.
30. Zattoni F. Chapter 36: Ureteroscopy: complications. In: Smith AD, Badlani GH, Bagley DH, Clayman RV, Docimo SG, Jordan GH, Kavoussi LR, Lee BR, Lingeman JE, Preminger GM, Joseph WS, editors. Smith's textbook of endourology. 2nd ed. London: BC Decker Inc Hamilton; 2006. p. 295.
31. Zelenko N, Coll D, Rosenfeld AT, Smith RC. Normal ureter size on unenhanced helical CT. AJR Am J Roentgenol. 2004;182(4):1039–41. https://doi.org/10.2214/ajr.182.4.1821039.
32. Omar M, Razzak A. Chapter 25: Ureteral Anatomy. In: Smith AD, Badlani GH, Bagley DH, Clayman RV, Docimo SG, Jordan GH, Kavoussi LR, Lee BR, Lingeman JE, Preminger GM, Joseph WS, editors. Smith's textbook of endourology. 2nd ed. London: BC Decker Inc Hamilton; 2006. p. 215.
33. Friedenberg RM. Excretory urography in the adult. In: Pollack HM, editor. Clinical urography. Philadelphia, PA: WB Saunders; 1990. p. 101–207.
34. Bagley DH, Huffman JL, Lyon ES. Normal anatomy of the urethra, prostate, and bladder. In: Bagley DH, Huffman JL, Lyon ES, editors. Urologic endoscopy. Boston, MA: Little Brown; 1985. p. 3–12.
35. Lyon RP, Marshall S, Tanagho EA. The ureteral orifice: its configuration and competency. J Urol. 1969;102(4):504–9.
36. Politano VA. Ureterovesical junction. J Urol. 1972;107:239–42.
37. Bagley DH, Rittenberg MH. Intrarenal dimensions. Guidelines for flexible ureteropyeloscopes. Surg Endosc. 1987;1:119–21.
38. Geavlete P, Multescu R, Geavlete B. Influence of pyelocaliceal anatomy on the success of the flexible ureteroscopic approach. J Endourol. 2007;21(Suppl. 1):A79.
39. Kamo M, Nozaki T, Horiuchi S, Muraishi N, Yamamura J, Akita K. There are no three physiological narrowings in the upper urinary tract: a new concept of the retroperitoneal anatomy around the ureter. Jpn J Radiol. 2021;39(5):407–13. https://doi.org/10.1007/s11604-020-01080-7. Epub 2021 Jan 9
40. Baggish MS. Identifying and avoiding ureteral injury. In: Baggish MS, Karram MM, editors. Atlas of pelvic anatomy and gynecologic surgery. 4th ed. Philadelphia, PA: Elsevier; 2016. p. 435–48.
41. Dodson AI. Anatomy and surgical approach to the urogenital tract in the male. In: Campbell M, editor. Urology. Philadelphia, PA: WB Saunders Company; 1954. p. 11–7.
42. Ordon M, Schuler TD, Ghiculete D, Pace KT, Honey RJ. Stones lodge at three sites of anatomic narrowing in the ureter: clinical fact or fiction? J Endourol. 2013;27(3):270–6. https://doi.org/10.1089/end.2012.0201. Epub 2012 Dec 26
43. Eisner BH, Reese A, Sheth S, Stoller ML. Ureteral stone location at emergency room presentation with colic. J Urol. 2009;182(1):165–8.
44. Song HG, Cho ST, Kim KK. Investigation of the location of the ureteral stone and diameter of the ureter in patients with renal colic. Korean J Urol. 2010;51:198–201.
45. Moon YJ, Kim HW, Kim JB, Kim HG, Chang YS. Distribution of ureteral stones and factors affecting their location and expulsion in patients with renal colic. Korean J Urol. 2015;56:717–21.
46. Arson BI, McVay CB. Ureter, great vessels, and nerves. In: Arson BI, McVay CB, editors. Surgical anatomy. 6th ed. Philadelphia, PA: W.B. Saunders Company; 1984. p. 760–77.
47. Kamo M, Nozaki T, Yoshida K, Tateishi U, Akita K. Kinking of the upper ureter in CT urography: anatomic and clinical significance. Surg Radiol Anat. 2016;38(10):1115–21. https://doi.org/10.1007/s00276-016-1689-7. Epub 2016 May 9
48. Kamo M, Nozaki T, Starkey J, Horiuchi S, Muraishi N, Hattori K, et al. The peak site of stone distribution in the upper ureter is unlikely the ureteropelvic junction: computed tomography analysis of stone lodging site concerning a newly identified area of constriction. Urology. 2017;107:31–6.
49. Schwalb DM, Eshghi M. Techniques to negotiate the tortuous ureter. J Urol. 1994;151(4):939–42. https://doi.org/10.1016/s0022-5347(17)35128-5.

50. Dagnone AJ, Blew BD, Pace KT, Honey RJ. Semirigid ureteroscopy of the proximal ureter can be aided by external lower-abdominal pressure. J Endourol. 2005;19(3):342–7. https://doi.org/10.1089/end.2005.19.342.
51. Korkes F, Lopes-Neto AC, Mattos MH, Pompeo AC, Wroclawski ER. Patient position and semi-rigid ureteroscopy outcomes. Int Braz J Urol. 2009;35(5):542–7.; discussion 548-50. https://doi.org/10.1590/s1677-55382009000500005.
52. Segura JW. Endourology. J Urol. 1984;132:1079–84.
53. Tolley DA, Beynon LL. Ureteroscopy: an alternative view. Br J Urol. 1985;57:281–3.
54. Angus DG, Webb DR. Influence of hip flexion on the course of the ureter. Ureteroscopic implications. Eur Urol. 1988;14(4):287–90. https://doi.org/10.1159/000472961.
55. Goodman T. Ureteroscopy with rigid instruments in the management of distal ureteral disease. J Urol. 1984;132:250–3.
56. Webb DR, Fitzpatrick JM. A simple aid to ureteroscopy. Eur Urol. 1985;11:57–8.
57. Davies D. Gray's anatomy. 34th ed. Harlow: Longman; 1967. p. 1538–9.
58. Woodbume RT. Anatomy of the ureterovesical junction. J Urol. 1964;92:431–5.
59. Sukumar CD, Janamala RP, Mahalakshmamma V. An anatomical study on blood supply of ureter. Int J Anat Res. 2015;3(1):970–5. https://doi.org/10.16965/ijar.2015.136.
60. Buttigieg J, Agius-Anastasi A, Sharma A, Halawa A. Early urological complications after kidney transplantation: an overview. World J Transplant. 2018;8(5):142–9. https://doi.org/10.5500/wjt.v8.i5.142.
61. Slagt IK, Ijzermans JN, Visser LJ, Weimar W, Roodnat JI, Terkivatan T. Independent risk factors for urological complications after deceased donor kidney transplantation. PLoS One. 2014;9(3):e91211. https://doi.org/10.1371/journal.pone.0091211.
62. Dinckan A, Tekin A, Turkyilmaz S, Kocak H, Gurkan A, et al. Early and late urological complications corrected surgically following renal transplantation. Transpl Int. 2007;20:702–7.
63. Krol R, Ziaja J, Chudek J, Heitzman M, Pawlicki J, et al. Surgical treatment of urological complications after kidney transplantation. Transplant Proc. 2006;38:127–30.
64. Neri F, Tsivian M, Coccolini F, Bertelli R, Cavallari G, et al. Urological complications after kidney transplantation: experience of more than 1,000 transplantations. Transplant Proc. 2009;41:1224–6.
65. Elliott Lee Hix. Uretero-renal reflex facilitating renal vasoconstrictor responses to emotional stress. Am J Physiol. 1957;192(1):191–7.
66. Hockley NM, Bihrle R, Bennett RM, Curry JM. Congenital genitourinary hemangiomas in a patient with Klippel-Trenaunay syndrome: management with the neodymium YAG laser. J Urol. 1989;141:940–1.
67. Dierks SM, Clayman RV, Kavoussi LR, et al. Intraureteral surgery: appropriate cutting modality. J Endourol. 1990;4:S114.
68. Hafez EKS, Stuart Wolf Jr J. In: Nakada SY, Pearle MS, eds. From advanced endourology: the complete clinical guide. Totowa, NJ: Humana Press Inc..
69. Yamada S, Ono Y, Ohshima S, et al. Transurethral ureteroscopic ureterotomy assisted by a prior balloon dilation for relieving ureteral strictures. J Urol. 1995;153:1418–21.
70. Hafez KS, Wolf JS Jr. Update on minimally invasive management of ureteral strictures. J Endourol. 2003;17:453–64.
71. Chandhoke PS, Clayman RV, Stone AM, et al. Endopyelolomy and endoureterotomy with the acucise ureteral cutting balloon device: preliminary experience. J Endourol. 1993;7:45–51.
72. Kim FJ, Herrell SD, Jahoda AE, Albala DM. Complications of acucise endopyelotomy. J Endourol. 1998;12:433–6.
73. Lopes RI, Torricelli FC, Gomes CM, Carnevale F, Bruschini H, Srougi M. Endovascular repair of a nearly fatal iliac artery injury after endoureterotomy. Scand J Urol. 2013;47:437–9.
74. De Coninck V, Keller EX, Traxer O. Complications of ureteroscopy. In: F Schwartz, Bradley, D Denstedt, John (eds.) Ureteroscopy. Cham: Springer, 2020. https://doi.org/10.1007/978-3-030-26649-3_12.
75. Wolf JS, Humphrey PA, Rayala HJ, Gardner SM, Mackey RB, Clayman RV. Comparative ureteral microanatomy. J Endourol. 1996;10(6):527–31. https://doi.org/10.1089/end.1996.10.52.

76. Sokolis DP. Alterations with age in the biomechanical behavior of human ureteral wall: Microstructure-based modeling. J Biomech. 2020;109:109940. https://doi.org/10.1016/j.jbiomech.2020.
77. Sokolis DP, Petsepe DC, Papadodima SA, Kourkoulis SK. Age- and region-related changes in the biomechanical properties and composition of the human ureter. J Biomech. 2017;51:57–64. https://doi.org/10.1016/j.jbiomech.2016.
78. Rattner William H, Fink S, Murphy John J. Pressure studies in the human ureter and renal pelvis. J Urol. 1957;78(4):359–62. https://doi.org/10.1016/S0022-5347(17)66448-6.
79. Cormio L, Koivusalo A, Makisalo H, Wolff H, Ruutu M. The effects of various indwelling JJ stents on renal pelvic pressure and renal parenchymal thickness in the pig. Br J Urol. 1994;74(4):440–3. https://doi.org/10.1111/j.1464-410X.1994.tb00419.x.
80. Shao Y, Shen Z-J, Zhuo J, Liu H-T, Yu S-Q, Xia S-J. The influence of ureteral stent on renal pelvic pressure in vivo. Urol Res. 2009;37(4):221–5. https://doi.org/10.1007/s00240-009-0199-z.
81. Griffiths DJ. Dynamics of the upper urinary tract: I. Peristaltic flow through a distensible tube of limited length. Phys Med Biol. 1987;32(7):813–22. https://doi.org/10.1088/0031-9155/32/7/002.
82. Rasouly HM, Lu W. Lower urinary tract development and disease. WIREs Syst Biol Med. 2013;5(3):307–42. https://doi.org/10.1002/wsbm.1212.
83. Griffiths DJ. Flow of urine through the ureter: a collapsible, muscular tube undergoing peristalsis. J Biomech Eng. 1989;111(3):206–11. https://doi.org/10.1115/1.3168367.
84. Edmond P, Ross James A, Kirkland Ian S. Human ureteral peristalsis. J Urol. 1970;104(5):670–4. https://doi.org/10.1016/S0022-5347(17)61808-1.
85. Weinberg SR, Maletta TJ. Measurement of peristalsis of the ureter and its relation to drugs. JAMA. 1961;175(1):15–8. https://doi.org/10.1001/jama.1961.0304.
86. Kinn AC, Lykkeskov-Andersen H. Impact on ureteral peristalsis in a stented ureter. an experimental study in the pig. Urol Res. 2002;30(4):213–8. https://doi.org/10.1007/s00240-002-0258-1.
87. Venkatesh R, Landman J, Minor SD, Lee DI, Rehman J, Vanlangendonck R, Ragab M, Morrissey K, Sundaram CP, Clayman RV. Impact of a double-pigtail stent on ureteral peristalsis in the porcine model: Initial studies using a novel implantable magnetic sensor. J Endourol. 2005;19(2):170–6. https://doi.org/10.1089/end.2005.19.170.
88. Gearhart JP, Canning DA, Gilpin SA, Lam EE, Goslilng JA. Histological and histochemical study of the vesicoureteric junction in infancy and childhood. Br J Urol. 1993;72:648–54.
89. Hutch JA. Theory of maturation of the intravesical ureter. J Urol. 1961;86:534–8.
90. Molitierno JA Jr., Watson JM, Kirsch AJ. Hydrodistention grading system for vesicoureteral reflux: Reproducibility and concordance. Presented at the annual AUA meeting in Anaheim, California; 2007.
91. Cerwinka WH, Scherz HC, Kirsch AJ. Dynamic hydrodistention classification of the ureter and the double hit method to correct vesicoureteral reflux. Arch Esp Urol. 2008;61(8):882–7. https://doi.org/10.4321/s0004-06142008000800005.
92. Selçuk İ, Ersak B, Tatar İ, Güngör T, Huri E. Basic clinical retroperitoneal anatomy for pelvic surgeons. Turk J Obstet Gynecol. 2018;15(4):259–69. https://doi.org/10.4274/tjod.88614. Epub 2019 Jan 9
93. Butler P, Mitchell A, Healy JC. Applied radiological anatomy. Cambridge: Cambridge University Press; 2012. Read it at Google Books - Find it on Amazon
94. Ryan S, McNicholas M, Eustace S. Anatomy for diagnostic imaging. 2nd ed. London: Saunders Ltd.; 2004. ISBN:0702026204
95. Hamilton WJ, Simon G, Hamilton I. From surface andradiological anatomy for students and general practitioners. In: Abdominal contents. 5th ed. Cambridge: W. Heffer & Sons Ltd; 1971. pp. 237 and 250.
96. Sargon M. Anatomi Akıl Notları, 2. Baskı. Guneş Tıp Kitabevleri: Ankara/Turkey; 2017.

97. Dietrich CS 3rd, Gehrich A, Bakaya S. Surgical exposure and anatomy of the female pelvis. Surg Clin North Am. 2008;88(2):223–43., v. https://doi.org/10.1016/j.suc.2008.01.003.
98. Precise Neurovascular Anatomy for Radical Hysterectomy Shingo Fujii. Kentaro Sekiyama ISBN 978-981-13-8097-6 ISBN 978-981-13-8098-3 (eBook). https://doi.org/10.1007/978-981-13-8098-3. Cham: Springer; 2020.
99. Yabuki Y, Asamoto A, Hoshiba T, et al. Radical hysterectomy: an anatomic evaluation of parametrial dissection. Gynecol Oncol. 2000;77:155–63.
100. Yabuki Y, Sasaki H, Hatakeyama N, et al. Discrepancies between classic anatomy and gynecologic surgery on pelvic connective tissue structure: harmonization of those concepts by collaborative cadaver dissection. Am J Obstet Gynecol. 2005;193:7–15.
101. Fujii S, Takakura K, Matsumura N, et al. Precise anatomy of the vesicouterine ligament for radical hysterectomy. Gynecol Oncol. 2007;104:186–91.
102. Raspagliesi F, Ditto A, Fontanelli R, et al. Nerve-sparing radical hysterectomy: a surgical technique for preserving the autonomic hypogastric nerve. Gynecol Oncol. 2004;93:307–14.
103. Niikura H, Katahira A, Utsunomiya H, et al. Surgical anatomy of intrapelvic fasciae and vesicouterine ligament in nerve-sparing radical hysterectomy with fresh cadaver dissections. Tohoku J Exp Med. 2007;212:403–13.
104. Yang X, Wang J, Wang Y, Fan Q, Li Y, Wang Y. Surgical technique based on space anatomy for laparoscopic radical trachelectomy with uterine artery preservation. J Laparoendosc Adv Surg Tech A. 2021;31(6):705–9. https://doi.org/10.1089/lap.2020.0461. Epub 2020 Oct 21
105. Dicker RC, Greenspan JR, Strauss LT, Cowart MR, Scally MJ, Peteson HB, et al. Complications of abdominal and vaginal hysterectomy among women of reproductive age in the United States. The collaborative review of sterilization. Am J Obstet Gynecol. 1982;144:841–8.
106. Goodno JA Jr, Powers TW, Harris VD. Ureteral injury in gynecologic surgery: a ten-year review in a community hospital. Am J Obstet Gynecol. 1995;172:1817–20.
107. Harkki-Siren P, Sjoberg J, Tiitinen A. Urinary tract injuries after hysterectomy. Obstet Gynecol. 1998;992:113–8.
108. Hurd WW, Chee SS, Gallagher KL, Ohl DA, Hurteau JA. Location of the ureters in relation to the uterine cervix by computed tomography. Am J Obstet Gynecol. 2001;184(3):336–9.
109. Ihse I, Arnesjo B, Jonsson G. Surgical injuries of the ureter. A review of 42 cases. Scand J Urol Nephrol. 1975;9(1):39–44.
110. Gangai MP, Agee RE, Spence CR. Surgical injury to the ureter. Urology. 1976;8(1):22–7.
111. Watterson JD, Mahoney JE, Futter NG, Gaffield J. Iatrogenic ureteric injuries: approaches to etiology and management. Can J Surg. 1998;41(5):379–82.
112. Thompson JD. Operative injuries to the ureter: prevention, recognition, and management. In: Rock JA, Thompson JD, editors. TeLinde's operative gynecology. 8th ed. Philadelphia, PA: Lippincott-Raven; 1997. p. 1135–73.
113. Motola JA, Shahon RS, Smith AD. Anatomy of the ureter. Urol Clin North Am. 1988;15(3):295–9.
114. Sorinola O, Begum R. Prevention and management of ureteric injuries. Hosp Med. 2005;66(6):329–34.
115. Dyson M. Urinary system. In: Williams PL, editor. Gray's anatomy. 38th ed. New York: Churchill Livingston; 1998. p. 1828–31.
116. Gemer O, Simonovsky A, Huerta M, Kapustian V, Anteby E, Linov L. A radiological study on the anatomical proximity of the ureters and the cervix. Int Urogynecol J Pelvic Floor Dysfunct. 2007;18(9):991–5. https://doi.org/10.1007/s00192-006-0269-5 Epub 2007 Jan 13

Chapter 4
Ureteropelvic Junction Obstruction

Bilge Turedi Sezer

Abstract Ureteropelvic junction obstruction (UPJO) is the most common obstructive uropathy in children with an incidence of 1/750–1000 live births. It can be diagnosed during the investigation of antenatal hydronephrosis or by symptoms in older children. The most common cause of UPJO is a congenital intrinsic narrowing of the proximal ureter at the ureteropelvic junction level. Ultrasonography and dynamic renal scan are used for diagnosis. In patients without a decrease in renal function, parenchymal thinning, increasing hydronephrosis non-surgical management with close monitoring are preferred. For patients needing surgical treatment, the gold standard method is still Anderson-Hynes dismembered pyeloplasty. With the increased use of minimally invasive surgical techniques, laparoscopic or robotic-assisted pyeloplasty techniques are used for surgical treatment. This chapter focuses on the description, etiology, and pathophysiology of ureteropelvic junction obstruction, clinical presentation, diagnosis, management, and long-term follow-up.

Keywords Ureteropelvic junction obstruction · UPJO · Congenital anomalies · Urinary tract · Pyeloplasty · Laparoscopic pyeloplasty · Robot-assisted pyeloplasty

Abbreviations

ALARA	As low as reasonably achievable
Alpha-GST	Alpha-glutathione S-transferase
ANH	Antenatal hydronephrosis
APRPD	Anteroposterior renal pelvis diameter
CAKUT	Congenital anomalies of the kidney and urinary tract
CHARGE Syndrome	Coloboma, heart disease, atresia chcanae, retarded growth, genital anomalies, ear anomalies

Test your learning and check your understanding of this book's contents: use the "Springer Nature Flashcards" app to access questions. To use the app, please follow the instructions in Chapter 1.

B. T. Sezer (✉)
Konya City Hospital, Konya, Turkey

M. Abdel-Gawad et al. (eds.), *The Ureter*,
https://doi.org/10.1007/978-3-031-36212-5_4

CT	computerized tomography
DMSA	Dimercaptosuccinic acid
DTPA	Diethyl-enetriaminepentacetate
GFR:	Glomerular filtration rate
KIM	Kidney injury molecule
MAG-3	Mercaptoacetyl triglycine
MRI	Magnetic resonance imaging
MRU	Magnetic resonance urography
NGAL	Neutrophil gelatinase-associated lipocalin
PUV	Posterior urethral valve
RALP	Robot-Assisted Laparoscopic Pyeloplasty
SFU	Society of Fetal Urology
VACTERL Association	Vertebral, anorectal, cardiac, tracheoesophageal, renal, limb
UPJO	Ureteropelvic junction obstruction
UTD	Urinary tract dilatation
UTI	Urinary tract infection
VCUG	Voiding cystourethrography
VUR	Vasicoureteral reflux

Learning Objectives

- To describe the causes of ureteropelvic junction obstruction
- To describe the evaluation and indications for treatment of ureteropelvic junction obstruction
- To describe the techniques for the repair of ureteropelvic junction obstruction
- To describe the diagnosis and management of complications following ureteropelvic junction repair

4.1 Introduction

The incidence of antenatal hydronephrosis (ANH) is increasing with the widespread use of antenatal ultrasonography today [1]. The most common cause of antenatal hydronephrosis is ureteropelvic junction obstruction, which is seen with a frequency of approximately 1/750–1/1000. It is seen more in boys than girls and it is also seen more on the left side than on the right side [2]. The incidence of bilaterality is around 10% [3]. Although it is generally seen sporadically, familial cases may also be seen [4]. It can be associated with some urological congenital anomalies such as multicystic dysplastic kidneys and horseshoe kidney [5].

4.2 Etiology and Pathophysiology

Some different theories have been proposed in the literature for the development of UPJO. Although there are different opinions, the etiology is still not clear. Some genetic markers in pathological specimens have been studied in recent years. Some genes with upregulated and downregulated expression have been identified [6]. But these studies have not yet been reflected in clinical practice. It is expected that targeted treatment options will come to the fore with the revealing of some genes and markers that can diagnose patients and identify patients who will go to surgery.

The etiological causes of UPJO can be classified as intrinsic or extrinsic. Intrinsic causes include valvular mucosal folds and fibroepithelial polyps [7]. In most cases, smooth muscle hypertrophy leading to intrinsic narrowing, increase in extracellular matrix elements, and an increase in proinflammatory cells and ureteral segment with decreased peristalsis seem to be responsible [8]. Extrinsic causes include kinks, fibrosis, and aberrant vascular compression [9].

Pelviureteric junction obstruction may lead to different clinical presentations. It can be diagnosed during the investigation of antenatal hydronephrosis in older children with different symptoms.

4.2.1 UPJO Causes

4.2.1.1 Congenital Causes

1. **Ureteral Adynamic Segment:** In most cases, there is a stenosis in the proximal ureteral segment and kinking at the level of entrance to the pelvis. Although the mechanism has not been fully elucidated, it is thought to be caused by the defect in the development of the circular muscle layer and collagen in the proximal ureter or the difference in their composition
2. **High Insertion of the Ureter into the Renal Pelvis**: It causes an impaired emptying of urine due to angulation of the ureteropelvic junction.
3. **Aberrant Crossing Vessel to Lower Pole**: In about 10% of UPJO, intermittent obstruction is seen due to compression of the aberrant vessel leading to the lower pole due. It causes intermittent compression on the ureter and obstruction of the pelvis which affects urine drainage. Patients with aberrant vascular compression may be presented with intermittent increasing hydronephrosis and pain. Increases and decreases in hydronephrosis may occur on repeated ultrasonography at follow-up. In older children, intermittent renal colic pain may develop. Diagnosis can be made preoperatively with cross-sectional imaging or can be made intraoperatively.

4. **Congenital Anomalies:** Malrotation of the kidney or anomalies like horseshoe kidney might cause impairment in urine emptying due to malposition of the pelviureteric junction.
5. **Other Rare Intrinsic Causes**: These rare causes include mucosal folds and ureteral polyps.

4.2.1.2 Acquired Causes

1. **Extrinsic Causes**: These include the compression effect of a retroperitoneal mass like a tumor or lymphadenopathy and fibrosis
2. **Intrinsic Causes**: Ureteral scarring due to impacted stones, inflammation, rarely radiation, and ureteral tumors may cause UPJO.
3. **Iatrogenic Causes**: Previous endoscopic interventions, after surgery of recurrent UPJO, or after previously failed pyeloplasty are among these iatrogenic causes.

4.3 Clinical Presentation

Although there are symptomatic patients, UPJO is mostly encountered as an asymptomatic disease in newborns with antenatal diagnosis [10]. Normal values of urinary tract dilatation measurements in the antenatal period for patients with antenatal hydronephrosis are shown in Table 4.1. Postnatal assessment schemes of the patients are determined due to these risk groups which were created according to the Urinary Tract Dilatation (UTD) classification. Risk stratification groups are shown in Table 4.2. Postnatal imaging and follow-up are decided according to these risk groups.

The absence of ureteral dilatation and isolated hydronephrosis in the postnatal evaluation of antenatal hydronephrosis might alert UPJO and should direct us to plan further investigations. It can be diagnosed with a palpable abdominal mass in a newborn with UPJO. Sometimes, this may be the only finding.

Table 4.1 Normal values of Urinary Tract Dilatation(UTD) classification

Ultrasound findings	Presentation time		
Anterior-posterior renal pelvis diameter (APD)	16–27 weeks	>28 weeks	Postnatal (>48 h)
	<4 mm	<7 mm	<10 mm
Calyceal dilatation			
Central	–	–	–
Peripheral	–	–	–
Parenchymal thickness	Normal	Normal	Normal
Parenchymal appearance	Normal	Normal	Normal
Ureter	Normal	Normal	Normal
Bladder	Normal	Normal	Normal
Unexplained oligohydramnios	–	–	

Table 4.2 Urinary Tract Dilatation (UTD) risk stratification

Prenatal presentation			
16–27 weeks APD 4–7 mm	≥ 28 weeks 7–10 mm	16–27 weeks ≥ 7 mm	≥ 28 weeks ≥ 10 mm
Central or no calyceal dilatation		Peripheral calyceal dilatation	
Parenchymal thickness normal		Abnormal	
Parenchymal appearance normal		Abnormal	
Ureters normal		Abnormal	
Bladder normal		Abnormal	
No unexplained oligohydramnios		Unexplained oligohydramnios	
UTD A1 -Low risk		UTD A2-A3 Increased risk	

Congenital anomalies of the kidney and urinary tract (CAKUT) are increasingly researched the topic and clinical presentation ranges from mild, asymptomatic anomalies like duplex system ureter or minimal UPJO to severe, life-threatening pathologies like bilateral renal agenesis or renal dysplasia. Renal anomalies may be a part of a syndrome or association [11]. Additional anomalies such as anorectal malformation, multicystic dysplastic kidney, VACTERL (vertebral, anorectal, cardiac, tracheoesophageal, renal, limb) association, CHARGE (coloboma, heart disease, atresia choanae, retarded growth, genital anomalies, ear anomalies) syndrome or congenital heart diseases, may be present [12]. Therefore, careful examination of all systems is important in these patients. In some asymptomatic patients with suspicious ultrasonographic findings, further investigation may be planned.

Patients with severe hydronephrosis in the high-risk group may develop pyonephrosis in the postnatal period, and high fever, poor general condition, decreased sucking, and decreased functions of the newborn may be seen. UPJO should be suspected in neonates with hydronephrosis and urinary tract infection (UTI) [13]. Urgent drainage is required when diagnosed with ultrasonography. Diagnosis can be clarified by examinations to be performed after nephrostomy drainage and parenteral antibiotic therapy. Older children may present with intermittent renal colic pain or may be detected incidentally in a radiological examination performed for another reason. UPJO is also a risk factor for stone formation and the patient may be presented with symptoms due to kidney stone formation. Due to the small number of patients and few studies in the literature, the evidence regarding the occurrence of hypertension is not clear. Rarely, it can be detected incidentally during the examination after abdominal trauma. Fluctuating hydronephrosis and intermittent symptoms are typical in patients with lower pole aberrant vascular compression as the cause of extrinsic UPJO.

4.4 Laboratory Tests

All patients should be evaluated with complete blood count, and biochemical parameters including kidney function tests (serum creatinine, glomerular filtration rate (GFR), and blood urea nitrogen (BUN). If a urinary tract infection is present, the patient may have leucocytosis and pyuria. Urinalysis and urine culture should be sent for evaluation.

There are no specific tests diagnostic for UPJO yet. Some studies discussing urinary and serum biomarkers, such as alpha-GST (alpha-glutathione S-transferase) and NGAL(neutrophil gelatinase-associated lipocalin) in obstructive uropathy, have not become a part of routine laboratory evaluation for these patients [14]. Sangeetha et al. found some urinary biomarkers that differentiate UPJO from nonobstructive dilatation in children. They offered a panel including Ca 19–9, NGAL, and KIM (kidney injury molecule) for diagnosis of UPJO in children [15]. Future studies focusing on the standardization of biomarkers may help clinicians for evaluating patients without serial imaging methods.

4.5 Imaging Methods

Different imaging methods can be used for diagnosis. Imaging studies are useful for both diagnosis and follow-up of patients with UPJO. Minimal invasive techniques are preferred by following the ALARA (as low as reasonably achievable) principle in children. Prenatal imaging is also important for the diagnosis of patients with antenatal hydronephrosis. Different grading systems are used for the evaluation of these patients like an anteroposterior renal pelvis diameter (APRPD), SFU (Society of Fetal Urology) grading system, and UTD (urinary tract dilatation) grading system. APRPD is thought to be dependent on variable factors and may not be standardized in clinical practice [16]. The Society of Fetal Urology (*SFU*) grading system has four main grades evaluating pelvicalyceal dilatation. Only fourth grade includes parenchymal thinning.

The UTD grading system was developed in 2014 by eight societies including the American College of Radiology, the American Institute of Ultrasound in Medicine, the American Society of Pediatric Nephrology, the Society for Fetal Urology, the Society for maternal–Fetal Medicine, the Society for Pediatric Urology, the Society for Pediatric Radiology and the Society of Radiologists in Ultrasound [17] and updated in 2021 [18]. UTD classification depends on both prenatal and postnatal findings and some related risk groups were determined for follow-up. Follow-up should be continued in the postoperative period and attention should be paid to both short-term and long-term complications.

4.5.1 *Ultrasonography*

Diagnosis can be made with antenatal ultrasonography. Patients are divided into risk groups according to the ultrasonographic findings in the antenatal period and control ultrasonographic. Evaluation should be planned in the postnatal period. If certain conditions are suspected, ultrasonography should be performed in the early postnatal period. Ultrasonography should be performed in the early postnatal period in patients with severe dilatation, suspicion of decreased kidney function, and suspected bladder outlet obstruction. Otherwise, control ultrasonography should be planned after the postnatal physiologic oliguria period which is between postnatal 5th–7th days. Anterior-posterior diameter in the transverse plane measured from the renal hilus level, the presence of extrarenal pelvis, parenchymal thickness, parenchymal echogenicity, degree of hydronephrosis, ureteral dilatation, and bladder wall thickness should be measured in postnatal ultrasonography.

Dilatation of the ureter can give information about the level of obstruction in the urinary system. The absence of a visible ureter increases the probability of a UPJO diagnosis. The presence and dilatation of the ureters behind the bladder can be considered primarily in favor of ureterovesical junction obstruction. In patients with AP diameter >5 cm and significant calyceal dilatation, renal function can be preserved with temporary nephrostomy drainage until the examinations are completed. If ultrasonographic findings are compatible with UPJO, further investigations can be planned to confirm the diagnosis.

4.5.2 *Scintigraphy*

In patients with suspected UPJO, dynamic MAG-3 (mercaptoacetyl triglycine) scintigraphy is used as a further functional examination, in which drainage can be evaluated and separate renal functions can be measured. DTPA (diethylenetriaminepentacetate) can also be used for the same purpose, but it is known that the excretion of MAG-3 gives clearer information. Today, MAG-3 scintigraphy is preferred primarily in children with suspected UPJO. This examination must be performed with optimal hydration. Changing the position during the procedure is also important for optimal measurement. Bladder fullness also affects the results, so bladder catheterization is recommended for optimal evaluation of drainage. The drainage curve of the kidneys is revealed using diuretics and urinary stasis is evaluated. The Renogram of a patient with right UPJO is shown in Fig. 4.1. It shows the deterioration in differential right kidney function and the curve with evidence of obstruction.

Ideally, it should be done after the third month. If the patient's kidney function is generally impaired, the result may be misleading. In such a case, DMSA (dimercaptosuccinic acid) scintigraphy may be preferred for treatment decisions. Today, in clinical practice, a decrease of <40% in separate renal function is accepted as an indication for surgery [19]. The decrease in renal function can be evaluated with repeated scintigraphic measurements in patients under close follow-up.

European Association of Urology (EAU) / European Society for Pediatric Urology (ESPU) guidelines recommend surgical intervention in case of an impaired split renal function due to obstruction or a decrease of split renal function in subsequent studies and increased anteroposterior diameter in the US, and grade IV dilatation as defined by the Society for Fetal Urology [20].

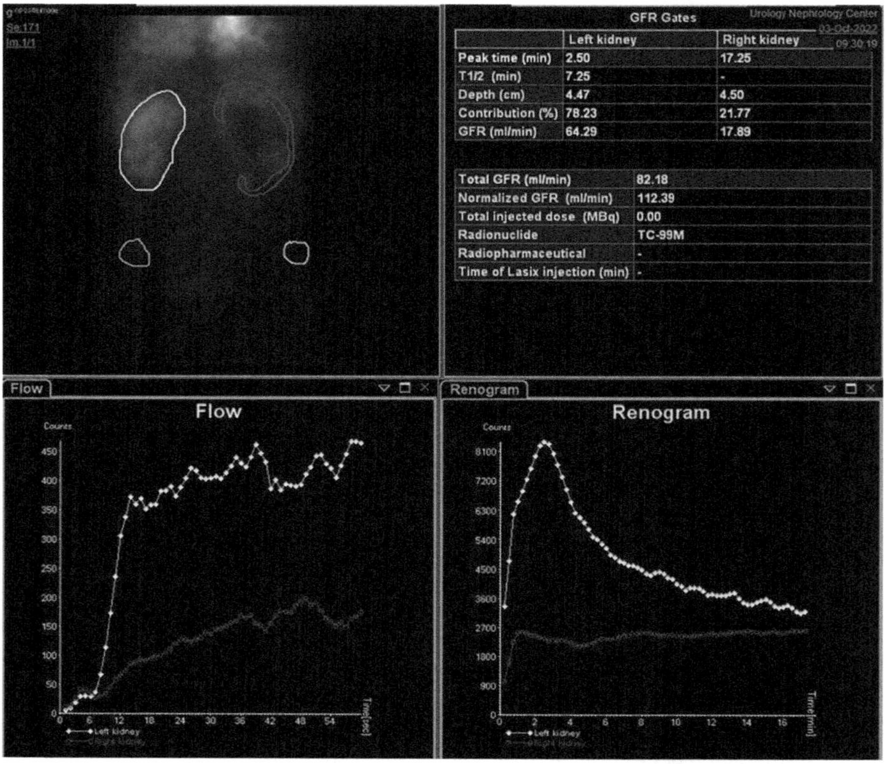

Fig. 4.1 Renogram of a patient with right UPJO. It shows that the differential right kidney function is 22% and with evidence of obstruction, as seen in the curve. From the courtesy of Dr. Bedeir Ali-El-Dein

4.5.3 Magnetic Resonance Imaging (MRI)/Magnetic Resonance Urography (MRU)

Another imaging method that is widely used today is MRU. It may be preferred because it provides detailed anatomical and functional information. Dilated renal pelvis without ureteral dilatation may be seen on MRI (Fig. 4.2) While it may be preferred in children because of not contain radiation, the need for anesthesia is restrictive in clinical practice. In anatomical disorders such as double collecting systems, MR urography can be an anatomical and functional guide. Combined MRU and magnetic resonance angiography can also be used for patients with suspected aberrant crossing lower pole vessels (Fig. 4.3).

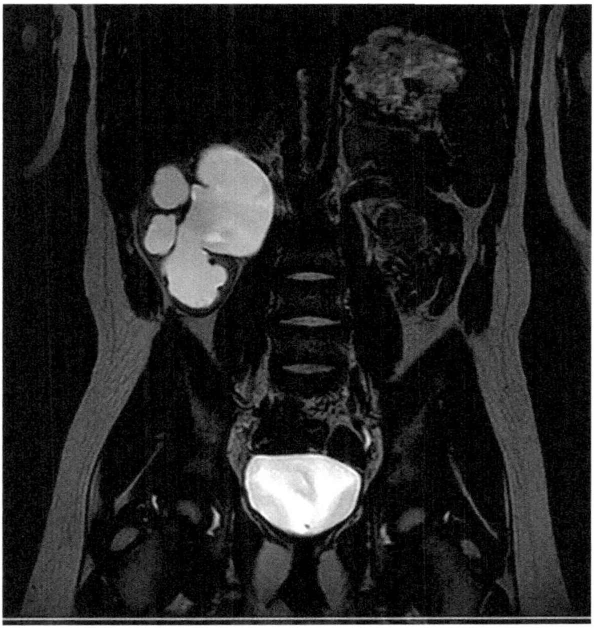

Fig. 4.2 Magnetic resonance urography (MRU) of the same patient showing right UPJO. From the courtesy of Dr. Bedeir Ali-El-Dein

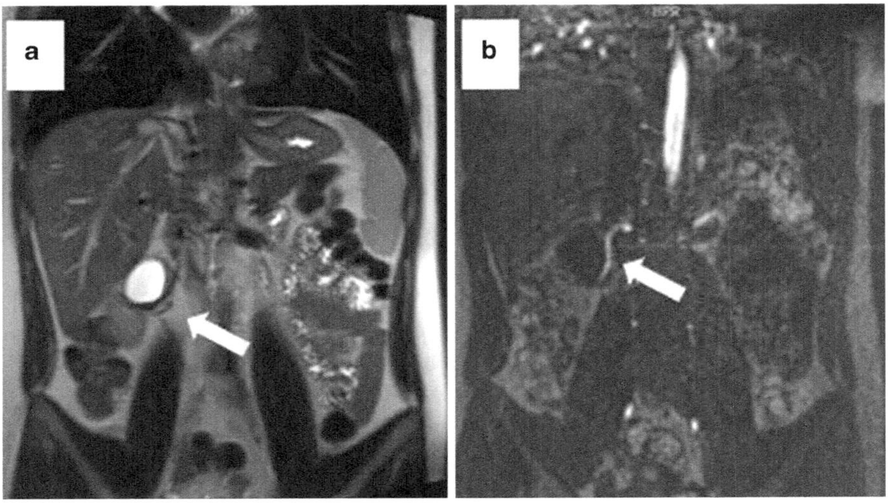

Fig. 4.3 Magnetic resonance urography (MRU) (**a**) and Magnetic resonance angiography (**b**) imaging of aberrant crossing lower pole vessel

4.5.4 Voiding Cystourethrography (VCUG)

If there is bilateral dilatation and posterior urethral valve (PUV) is suspected in a male newborn or especially if dilated ureters are seen, VCUG can be performed to reveal the accompanying vesicoureteral reflux (VUR). VCUG should also be performed in cases of suspected obstructive and refluxive megaureters. It can also help detect the presence of VUR while giving detailed anatomical information about the urethra and bladder.

4.5.5 Computerized Tomography (CT)

CT for UPJO is not the primary investigation in routine practice, but the disease can be diagnosed by CT in patients presenting with trauma or in suspected urinary tract stone disease.

4.5.6 Pressure-Flow Studies-Whitaker

This test has historical importance and is not routinely used in clinical practice. It is a pressure-flow study assessing the obstruction of the affected kidney. After placement of a nephrostomy tube under general anesthesia, saline is given with a constant perfusion rate. The pressure of the pelvis and ureter is measured through the same cannula with simultaneous bladder catheterization. Whitaker test is the first to determine the increased pelvic pressure while nearly normal flow rates and its effect on kidney function [21].

4.5.7 Antegrade Pyelogram

In patients with nephrostomy drainage, antegrade pyelography may be done to show obstructed system with no/minimal urine passage to the ureter from the renal pelvis. Late images may help to confirm the impaired drainage and pelvic urinary stasis.

4.6 Differential Diagnosis

The most commonly seen etiology of antenatal hydronephrosis is transient hydronephrosis. UPJO is the second most common etiological pathology of antenatal hydronephrosis [22]. In addition, the list of differential diagnoses includes vesicoureteral reflux, multicystic dysplastic kidney (MCDK), vesicoureteric junction obstruction (VUJO), duplex system, megaureter, and posterior urethral valves. Also, a stone obstructing the urine flow distal to the pelviureteric junction may present with UPJO-like symptoms. Extrinsic compression by fibrotic tissue, retroperitoneal tumor, or an aberrant lower pole crossing vessel may create the same clinical status and symptoms.

4.7 Tretament Options

4.7.1 Conservative Management

Today, with the widespread use of antenatal ultrasonography, it is diagnosed more frequently. Most of the patients have transient hydronephrosis and usually regress in postnatal follow-up. Conservative follow-up may be preferred if the differential renal function is preserved in the radiological and scintigraphic evaluations if parenchymal thinning or an increase in hydronephrosis is not detected in serial ultrasonography and the patient is asymptomatic. If there is a concern about worsening in serial ultrasonographic evaluation, dynamic scintigraphy can be repeated and checked for a decrease in renal function. If the patient is symptomatic during the follow-up, he/she should be re-evaluated in terms of the surgical decision. Surgical indications include a decrease in the differentiated renal function below 40%, a decrease in renal function of more than 10% in consecutive measurements, stasis unresponsive to diuretics in scintigraphy, increase in hydronephrosis, dilatation of SFU grade 3–4, and being symptomatic in follow-up [19]. In patients with severe hydronephrosis (Anterior-posterior pelvic diameter(APD) > 5 cm) at the time of diagnosis, nephrostomy drainage can save time in terms of performing the examinations and preserving kidney functions until the operation.

Overall, the indications for surgery in follow-up are:

- Less than 40% in the split function of the affected kidney on the diuretic renogram
- Increasing hydronephrosis
- Parenchymal thinning due to severe bilateral UPJO
- Decrease in renal function of more than 10% in consecutive measurements
- Being symptomatic in follow-up (pain, recurrent UTI despite using prophylactic antibiotics)

4.7.2 Surgical Treatment

4.7.2.1 Open Pyeloplasty

Today, the gold standard surgical method is Anderson Hynes's dismembered pyeloplasty [23]. An open approach can be performed through the flank incision or dorsal lumbotomy. It can be applied retroperitoneally by lumbotomy. Pyeloplasty with a mini-incision of approximately 2 cm is the frequently preferred method in infants [24]. The main steps of the method can be counted as separation of the ureter and pelvis, excision of the narrow UP junctional segment, spatulation of the healthy ureter, and completion of the ureteropelvic anastomosis without tension. Obstructed pelviureteric junction is seen before and after the dismembering of UPJ in Fig. 4.4. Impairment of ureteral vascularisation during a release may cause stricture development. It is important to make a tension-free anastomosis with the healthy part of the ureter. During this technique, different drainage catheters can be used to protect the anastomosis. Transanastomotic double-J (DJ) stent is commonly placed. However, catheters with external drainage can also be used. Today, stentless pyeloplasty is also a method used. Nagdeve et al. found that the length of hospital stay was shortened in pyeloplasty with stent placement but the difference had not been found statistically significant in their study [25]. While anastomotic leakage and clot formation are common in stentless patients, stent-related complications are common in stented patients. Liu et al. found no significant differences in operative time, success, hospital stay, improvement of renal functions, and overall complications for the external stented, DJ stented, and stent-less procedures in pediatric pyeloplasty in their meta-analysis [26].

4.7.2.2 Laparoscopic Pyeloplasty

Minimally invasive surgical methods have come to the forefront of urologic surgery in recent years [26]. Laparoscopic pyeloplasty was first performed in adult patients and a few years later, it started to be applied in pediatric patients as well [27, 28]. Laparoscopic intracorporeal suturing is a technique that requires experience. The importance of experience is increasing, especially with miniaturized instruments

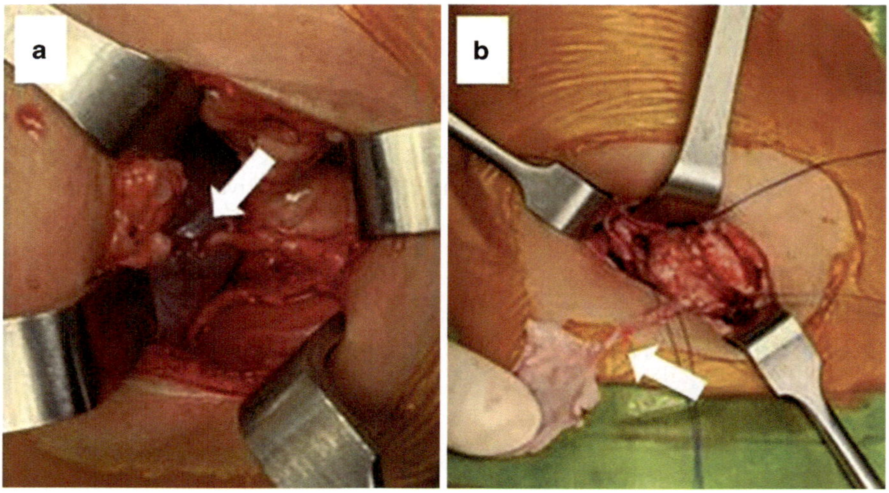

Fig. 4.4 (**a**) Obstructed ureteropelvic junction (white arrow) (**b**) view of the ureteropelvic junction after dismembering (white arrow)

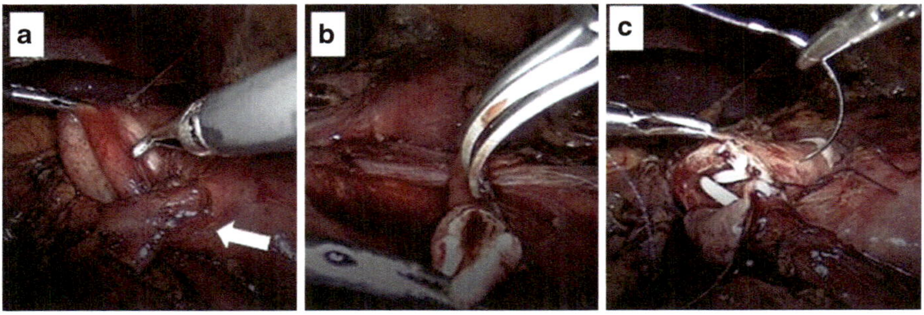

Fig. 4.5 (**a**) Laparoscopic view of crossing pole vessel causing extrinsic obstruction at the ureteropelvic junction (white arrow) (**b**) spatulation of the ureter and (**c**) completion of anastomosis after antegrade stent placement

used in children. Laparoscopic pyeloplasty can be performed transperitoneal or retroperitoneal. Transperitoneal laparoscopic pyeloplasty can be performed either transmesocolic or by standard approach by releasing the colon. The advantage of laparoscopic pyeloplasty is that it provides a wide field of view and allows visualization of the aberrant vein leading to the lower pole that compresses the ureteropelvic junction. A wide crossing lower pole vessel compressing the ureter at the level of the pelviureteric junction is seen in Fig. 4.5. In addition, the laparoscopic approach has all other advantages of laparoscopy such as rapid recovery, short hospital stay, less postoperative pain, and high patient comfort.

4.7.2.3 Robot-Assisted Laparoscopic Pyeloplasty (RALP)

Today, with the spread of minimally invasive techniques, RALP is increasingly used. Robotic pyeloplasty can be performed retroperitoneal or transperitoneal. Robotic surgery has advantages such as greater maneuverability, ease of suturing, shorter hospital stay, and fewer postoperative complications [29]. High cost and learning curve are among the disadvantages. Studies have found that all minimally invasive techniques in UPJO surgery are safe and effective. It is known that the laparoscopic technique is effective and less invasive than the open technique. Depending on the surgeon's experience, the laparoscopic or robotic-assisted laparoscopic method may be preferred.

4.7.2.4 Alternative Techniques

The Culp de Weerd pyeloplasty

In the Culp de Weerd pyeloplasty technique, a renal pelvic spiral flap is used to widen the pelviureteral junction. It does not include standard dismembering. It is usually suitable for patients having a strictured proximal ureter due to failed pyeloplasty or endopyeleotomy. If there is a large extrarenal pelvis, the spiral flap technique may be much more effective [30].

Foley Y-V plasty

It was developed for pelviureteric junction obstruction due to high ureteral insertion. If a pelvic reduction is needed, or proximal ureteric stenosis is present, this technique may not be effective.

Scardino Prince Vertical Flap

In this historical operative technique, a flap created from the medial part of the pelvis is used for proximal ureteric stenosis. It is less effective than a spiral flap regarding flap length when needed for long strictures.

Ureterocalicostomy

This technique starts with the mobilization of the kidney for easy access to the lower pole. Lower pole parenchyma is resected. After mobilization of the inferior calyx, the ureter is spatulated laterally and anastomosed with the calyx. It is usually preferred when there is an increased risk of failure for re-do cases, and also for rotational and fusion anomalies of the ureter. The technique has advantages in patients with horseshoe kidneys because it allows the reconstruction without touching the isthmus.

Endopyelotomy

It can be performed via an antegrade or retrograde approach. After an antegrade access to the calyx, a guidewire is sent to the bladder through the ureter. Retrograde manner should be preferred if the ureter can not be catheterized with a guidewire. With the retrograde approach, a ureteroscope is inserted with the guidance of wire, and endopyelotomy is performed with Holmium-YAG (Holmium yttrium-aluminum-garnet) laser. Balloon dilatation of the incision area is done and a ureteral stent is placed. If an endopyelotomy is planned, it should be ensured that there is no crossing aberrant lower pole vessel with preoperative imaging methods such as CT angiography or MR angiography. The success of endoscopic techniques is not as high as open pyeloplasty.

Transposition of Lower Pole Crossing Vessels: Vascular Hitch Procedure

The vascular hitch method is also among the surgical options in aberrant lower pole vessels. It aims to eliminate the pressure and provide drainage. There are various publications in the literature that give different results. There are also publications advocating that it should not be preferred because there may be accompanying intrinsic stenosis. Zahn et al. advocated that concomitant intrinsic stenosis is rare and it may be performed safely with the intraoperative diuretic test. At the same time, they argued that it is more advantageous compared to laparoscopic pyeloplasty because there is no risk of anastomotic stenosis or leak, no need for intraluminal stenting, and short operation time [31].

Overall, although re-do pyeloplasty includes the same technical details as primary surgery, ureterocalicostomy may be needed in patients who can not undergo dismembered pyeloplasty because of the limited length or mobility of the ureter. Lindgren et al. evaluated 16 patients who underwent re-do pyeloplasty and shared that robotic reoperation can be a safe and effective method in redo cases [32]. Endopyelotomy is an alternative method used in patients for primary or secondary procedures who are known to have no aberrant vascular compression [33].

In the presence of horseshoe kidneys and UPJO, the surgical technique is the same as in normal cases. Blanc et al. shared their experience of laparoscopic pyeloplasty in 10 children with horseshoe kidneys and found it effective for UPJO patients having horseshoe kidneys [34]. Ureterocalicostomy may be preferred in cases where the ureteropelvic anastomosis is not suitable due to the abnormal location of the kidney.

4.8 Postoperative Follow-Up and Long-Term Outcome

In cases of stent placement, follow-up for stent-related risks, such as irritative symptoms, UTI, migration, and flank pain during voiding due to high pressure reflecting the renal pelvis, should be conducted [35]. Stent removal should be performed under anesthesia in children. There is no consensus on the removal time in the literature. However, It mostly depends on the clinical practice of centers.

Although there are different clinical applications, control ultrasonography can be performed between 4 and 6 weeks after stent removal. If hydronephrosis has improved, follow-up can be continued by ultrasonography controls with widened intervals [36]. If there is no improvement in ultrasonographic findings, the diuretic renogram may need to be repeated and a re-decision regarding the need for surgical intervention may be required. In the literature, the success rate of the operation is stated as 85–90% ([37]).

Among the complications, anastomotic stenosis is seen at a rate of 2–5% [38]. Urinoma formation, fistula formation, the persistence of obstruction, or stent-related complications can also be seen. In a study with 49 postpubertal patients with antenatal hydronephrosis who underwent open pyeloplasty at an average of 4.7 months, an increase in renal function and a shortened drainage time were observed after puberty. Additional surgery was required in 4% of patients with increased hydronephrosis [39]. There is no study with a high level of evidence in the literature regarding the long-term results of conservatively followed patients. Polok et al. assessed the long-term outcome of 35 patients who had open pyeloplasty for UPJO and 4 patients (11.1%) required surgical interventions due to complications. Complications were seen at the earliest 16 months in their patients' postoperative follow-up and they reported that the two postoperative years are important for complication occurrence and follow-up should be done properly in this period [40]. Lee et al. evaluated the long-term results of 55 patients who underwent pyeloplasty and reported that a decrease in renal function usually developed after 10 years after pyeloplasty. They recommend evaluation every 5 years until 20 years postoperatively [41]. To evaluate the long-term outcomes of UPJO patients, randomized controlled clinical studies that include patients who have undergone surgery and are followed conservatively are needed.

Questions

1. Which one is the most common cause of antenatal hydronephrosis?
   (a) UVJO
   (b) MCDK
   (c) PUV
   (d) UPJO
   (e) Transient hydronephrosis

Answer: (d)

2. Which one is the most commonly seen clinical presentation of UPJO?
   (a) Antenatal hydronephrosis
   (b) Colicky pain
   (c) UTI
   (d) Incidental
   (e) Hematuria

Answer: (a)

3. Which is the most commonly used method for diagnosis and follow-up?
   (a) CT urography
   (b) Voiding cystourethrography (VCUG)
   (c) MR urography
   (d) MAG-3 scintigraphy
   (e) Ultrasonography

Answer: (e)

4. Which is the gold standard technique for surgical treatment of UPJO?
   (a) Culp de Weird pyeloplasty
   (b) Vascular hitch procedure
   (c) Endopyelotomy
   (d) Anderson-Hynes dismembered pyeloplasty
   (e) Ureterocalycostomy

Answer: (d)

5. Which is not an early complication of pyeloplasty?
   (a) Hypertension
   (b) Anastomotic leak
   (c) Urinoma
   (d) Fistula formation
   (e) Stent-related complications

Answer: (a)

References

1. Mallik M, Watson AR. Antenatally detected urinary tract abnormalities: more detection but less action. Pediatr Nephrol. 2008;23(6):897–904. https://doi.org/10.1007/s00467-008-0746-9.
2. Bauer SB. Anomalies of the kidney and ureteropelvic junction. In: Walsh PW, Retik AB, Vaughan Jr ED, Wein AJ, editors. Campbell's Urology. 7th ed. Philadelphia: WB Saunders Company; 1998. p. 1739–49.
3. Duong HP, Piepsz A, Collier F, Khelif K, Christophe C, Cassart M, Janssen F, Hall M, Ismaili K. Predicting the clinical outcome of antenatally detected unilateral pelviureteric junction stenosis. Urology. 2013;82(3):691–6. https://doi.org/10.1016/j.urology.2013.03.041. Epub 2013 May 29
4. Mackintosh P, Almarhoos G, Heath DA. HLA linkage with familial vesicoureteral reflux and familial pelvi-ureteric junction obstruction. Tissue Antigens. 1989;34(3):185–9. https://doi.org/10.1111/j.1399-0039.1989.tb01735.x.
5. Cascio S, Sweeney B, Granata C, Piaggio G, Jasonni V, Puri P. Vesicoureteral reflux and ureteropelvic junction obstruction in children with horseshoe kidney: treatment and outcome. J Urol. 2002;167(6):2566–8.
6. Isali I, McClellan P, Wong TR, Gupta S, Woo L. A systematic review of underlying genetic factors associated with ureteropelvic junction obstruction in stenotic human tissue. J Pediatr Urol. 2022:S1477-5131(22)00326-6. https://doi.org/10.1016/j.jpurol.2022.07.022. Epub ahead of print.
7. Shive ML, Baskin LS, Harris CR, Bonham M, JD MK. Ureteral fibroepithelial polyp causing urinary obstruction. J Radiol Case Rep. 2012;6(7):23–8. https://doi.org/10.3941/jrcr.v6i7.1076. Epub 2012 Jul 1
8. Yiee JH, Johnson-Welch S, Baker LA, Wilcox DT. Histologic differences between extrinsic and intrinsic ureteropelvic junction obstruction. Urology. 2010;76(1):181–4. https://doi.org/10.1016/j.urology.2010.02.007. Epub 2010 Apr 14
9. Stern JM, Park S, Anderson JK, Landman J, Pearle M, Cadeddu JA. Functional assessment of crossing vessels as etiology of ureteropelvic junction obstruction. J Endourol. 2007;69:1022–4.
10. Anthony Herndon CD. Antenatal hydronephrosis: differential diagnosis, evaluation, and treatment options. Sci World J. 2006;6:21. Article ID 379298. https://doi.org/10.1100/tsw.2006.366.
11. Avanoglu A, Tiryaki S. Embryology and morphological (Mal)Development of UPJ. Front Pediatr. 2020;8:137. https://doi.org/10.3389/fped.2020.00137.
12. Rodriguez MM. Congenital anomalies of the kidney and the urinary tract (CAKUT). Fetal Pediatr Pathol. 2014;33(5–6):293–320. doi: https://doi.org/10.3109/15513815.2014.959678. Epub 2014 Oct 14.
13. Lorenzo AJ, Csaicsich D, Aufricht C, Khoury AE. Obstructive genitourinary disorders. Amsterdam: Elsevier BV; 2008. https://doi.org/10.1016/B978-0-323-04883-5.50043-X.
14. Bieniaś B, Sikora P. Potential novel biomarkers of obstructive nephropathy in children with hydronephrosis. Dis Markers. 2018;2018:1015726. https://doi.org/10.1155/2018/1015726.

15. Pereira AK, Reis ZS, Bouzada MC, de Oliveira EA, Osanan G, Cabral AC. Antenatal ultrasonographic antero-posterior renal pelvis diameter measurement: is it a reliable way of defining fetal hydronephrosis? Obstet Gynecol Int. 2011;2011:861–5. https://doi.org/10.1155/2011/861865.
16. Sangeetha G, Babu R. Comparing accuracy of urinary biomarkers in differentiation of ureteropelvic junction obstruction from nonobstructive dilatation in children. Pediatr Nephrol. 2022;37(10):2277–87. https://doi.org/10.1007/s00467-022-05488-3. Epub 2022 Mar 3
17. Nguyen HT, Benson CB, Bromley B, et al. Multidisciplinary consensus on the classification of prenatal and postnatal urinary tract dilation (UTD classification system). J Pediatr Urol. 2014;10:982–98.
18. Nguyen HT, Phelps A, Coley B, Darge K, Rhee A, Chow JS. 2021 update on the urinary tract dilation (UTD) classification system: clarifications, review of the literature, and practical suggestions. Pediatr Radiol. 2022;52(4):740–51. https://doi.org/10.1007/s00247-021-05263-w. Epub 2022 Jan 4
19. Dhillon HK. Prenatally diagnosed hydronephrosis: the Great Ormond Street experience. Br J Urol. 1998;81(Suppl 2):39–44. https://doi.org/10.1046/j.1464-410x.1998.0810s2039.x.
20. Fernbach SK, Maizels M, Conway JJ. Ultrasound grading of hydronephrosis: introduction to the system used by the Society for Fetal Urology. Pediatr Radiol. 1993;23(6):478–80. https://doi.org/10.1007/BF02012459.
21. Whitaker RH. Methods of assessing obstruction in dilated ureters. Br J Urol. 1973;45(1):15–22.
22. Nguyen HT, Herndon CD, Cooper C, Gatti J, Kirsch A, Kokorowski P, Lee R, Perez-Brayfield M, Metcalfe P, Yerkes E, Cendron M, Campbell JB. The Society for Fetal Urology consensus statement on the evaluation and management of antenatal hydronephrosis. J Pediatr Urol. 2010;6(3):212–31. https://doi.org/10.1016/j.jpurol.2010.02.205. Epub 2010 Apr 15
23. Anderson JC, Hynes W. Retrocaval ureter; a case diagnosed pre-operatively and treated successfully by a plastic operation. Br J Urol. 1949;21(3):209–14. https://doi.org/10.1111/j.1464-410x.1949.tb10773.x.
24. Liu X, Wang X. Open surgery in the era of minimally invasive surgery: pyeloplasty via a mini flank incision in the treatment of infants with ureteropelvic junction obstruction. Urol J. 2020;17(2):169–72. https://doi.org/10.22037/uj.v0i0.5405.
25. Nagdeve NG, Bhingare PD, Sarawade P. A randomized control trial comparing outcome after stented and nonstented Anderson-Hynes dismembered pyeloplasty. J Indian Assoc Pediatr Surg. 2018;23(4):186–91. https://doi.org/10.4103/jiaps.JIAPS_58_17.
26. Liu X, Huang C, Guo Y, Yue Y, Hong J. Comparison of DJ stented, external stented and stentless procedures for pediatric pyeloplasty: a network meta-analysis. Int J Surg. 2019;68:126–33. https://doi.org/10.1016/j.ijsu.2019.07.001. Epub 2019 Jul 4
27. Schuessler WW, Grune MT, Tecuanhuey LV, Preminger GM. Laparoscopic dismembered pyeloplasty. J Urol. 1993;150(6):1795–9. https://doi.org/10.1016/s0022-5347(17)35898-6.
28. Peters CA, Schlussel RN, Retik AB. Pediatric laparoscopic dismembered pyeloplasty. J Urol. 1995;153(6):1962–5.
29. Silay MS, Spinoit AF, Undre S, Fiala V, Tandogdu Z, Garmanova T, Guttilla A, Sancaktutar AA, Haid B, Waldert M, Goyal A, Serefoglu EC, Baldassarre E, Manzoni G, Radford A, Subramaniam R, Cherian A, Hoebeke P, Jacobs M, Rocco B, Yuriy R, Zattoni F, Kocvara R, Koh CJ. Global minimally invasive pyeloplasty study in children: Results from the Pediatric Urology Expert Group of the European Association of Urology Young Academic Urologists working party. J Pediatr Urol. 2016;12(4):229–7. https://doi.org/10.1016/j.jpurol.2016.04.007. Epub 2016 May 12
30. Kausik S, Segura JW. Surgical management of ureteropelvic junction obstruction in adults. Int Braz J Urol. 2003;29(1):3–10. https://doi.org/10.1590/s1677-55382003000100002.
31. Zahn K, Younsi NF, Stein R. Subpelvine Stenose & kreuzende Gefäße – Pro "vascular hitch" [Pelviureteric junction obstruction and crossing vessels: pro "vascular hitch"]. Aktuelle Urol. 2020;51(2):116–20. https://doi.org/10.1055/a-1001-1948. Epub 2019 Nov 7. German

32. Lindgren BW, Hagerty J, Meyer T, Cheng EY. Robot-assisted laparoscopic reoperative repair for failed pyeloplasty in children: a safe and highly effective treatment option. J Urol. 2012;188(3):932–7. https://doi.org/10.1016/j.juro.2012.04.118. Epub 2012 Jul 20
33. Corbett HJ, Mullassery D. Outcomes of endopyelotomy for pelviureteric junction obstruction in the paediatric population: a systematic review. J Pediatr Urol. 2015;11(6):328–36. https://doi.org/10.1016/j.jpurol.2015.08.014. Epub 2015 Oct 22
34. Blanc T, Koulouris E, Botto N, Paye-Jaouen A, El-Ghoneimi A. Laparoscopic pyeloplasty in children with horseshoe kidney. J Urol. 2014;191(4):1097–103. https://doi.org/10.1016/j.juro.2013.10.059. Epub 2013 Oct 17
35. Abdelwahab M, Abdelaziz A, Aboulela W, Shouman AM, Ghoneima W, Shoukry A, Kassem A, Abdelhamid M, Abdelhakim M, ElGhoneimy M, Morsi H, Badawy H, Elkady A. One week stenting after pediatric laparoscopic pyeloplasty; is it enough? J Pediatr Urol. 2020;16(1):98.e1–6. https://doi.org/10.1016/j.jpurol.2019.10.016. Epub 2019 Oct 25
36. Almodhen F, Jednak R, Capolicchio JP, Eassa W, Brzezinski A, El-Sherbiny M. Is routine renography required after pyeloplasty? J Urol. 2010;184(3):1128–33. https://doi.org/10.1016/j.juro.2010.05.017. Epub 2010 Jul 21
37. Tubre RW, Gatti JM. Surgical approaches to pediatric ureteropelvic junction obstruction. Curr Urol Rep. 2015;16(10):72. https://doi.org/10.1007/s11934-015-0539-1.
38. Lim DJ, Walker RD 3rd. Management of the failed pyeloplasty. J Urol. 1996;156(2 Pt 2):738–40. https://doi.org/10.1097/00005392-199608001-00048.
39. Chertin B, Pollack A, Koulikov D, Rabinowitz R, Shen O, Hain D, Hadas-Halpren I, Farkas A. Does renal function remain stable after puberty in children with prenatal hydronephrosis and improved renal function after pyeloplasty? J Urol. 2009;182(4 Suppl):1845–8. https://doi.org/10.1016/j.juro.2009.03.008. Epub 2009 Aug 18
40. Polok M, Apoznański W. Anderson-Hynes pyeloplasty in children - long-term outcomes, how long follow up is necessary? Cent European J Urol. 2017;70(4):434–8. https://doi.org/10.5173/ceju.2017.1431. Epub 2017 Sep 9
41. Lee HE, Park K, Choi H. An analysis of long-term occurrence of renal complications following pediatric pyeloplasty. J Pediatr Urol. 2014;10(6):1083–8. https://doi.org/10.1016/j.jpurol.2014.03.015. Epub 2014 May 6

Chapter 5
Ureterocele

Mohamed A. Baky Fahmy

Abstract Almost 1% of human infants are born with urogenital abnormalities, many of which are linked to irregular connections between the distal ureters and the bladder. Ureterocele is an abnormal intravesical dilatation of the terminal ureter. In the past, most cases were detected postnatally when the child presented with urinary tract infections or urine dribbling. Ureteroceles may present both diagnostic and treatment challenges among urologists and pediatric surgeons. The diagnosis of ureterocele may be obvious in some cases, but at times, it is less clear and is then only diagnosed with a high index of suspicion and contingent on special investigations. The management of ureterocele varies according to its effects on obstruction, reflux, continence, and renal function. Therefore, it is imperative for the urologists to be aware of the variable clinical and radiological presentations and treatment options to yield the best possible results. Recently; with availability of ultrasound facilities allover the world, most cases of ureteroceles are diagnosed antenatally, but only limited centers can afford antenatal or early postnatal management. The treatment needs to be tailored for each case; depending on other factors such as the location of ureterocele, the age of the child, presence of a duplex or single system, the function of the kidney or the moiety, and the status of vesicoureteral reflux.

Keywords Ureterocele · Congenital urinary anomalies · Moiety · Duplex · Vesicoureteric reflux

Abbreviations

AHN	Antenatal hydronephrosis
BOO	Bladder Outlet Obstruction
CAP	Continuous Antibiotic Prophylaxis

Test your learning and check your understanding of this book's contents: use the "Springer Nature Flashcards" app to access questions. To use the app, please follow the instructions in Chapter 1.

M. A. Baky Fahmy (✉)
Pediatric Surgery, Al-Azhar University, Cairo, Egypt

M. Abdel-Gawad et al. (eds.), *The Ureter*,
https://doi.org/10.1007/978-3-031-36212-5_5

CECT	Contrast-enhanced computed tomography
CND	Common Nephric Duct
CT	Computerized tomography
IVP	Intravenous pyelogram
PUJ	Pelviureteric junction
URL	Ureteroscope lithotripsy
USS	Ultrasound
UTIs	Urinary tract infections
VCUG	voiding cystourethrography
VUR	Vesicoureteric Reflux

5.1 Embryological and Anatomical Background

Developmental and anatomical configuration of the vesicoureteric junction is one of the most complex area in the body and its development is not completely understood. The bladder develops through mesenchymal-epithelial interactions between the endoderm of the urogenital sinus and mesodermal mesenchyme, with many key signaling factors include shh, TGF-β, Bmp4, and Fgfr2 genes [1].

The ureteric bud starts as an epithelial outgrowth that sprouts from the base of the Wolffian ducts. The initial integration site between urogenital sinus and the paired Wolffian ducts at early embryonic life was poorly understood, but recent embryonic studies provided new insights into the normal process of ureter maturation, and shed some light on possible causes of obstruction, reflux and ureteral abnormalities which affect 1–2% of the human population.

During early stages of development, the Wolffian ducts open into the cloaca, which later divided into the hindgut and the urogenital sinus. The proximal ureteric bud differentiates into the ureter, which initially join the bladder indirectly, via the primitive Common Nephric Duct (CND). However, to establish direct connections with the bladder, the ureters disassociate from the Wolffian ducts and merge with the bladder epithelium in the trigone, as sequence of perforation of the Chwalla's membrane, allowing the formation of a normal ureteral orifice. If this membrane does not completely perforate, a ureterocele results. The Chwalla's membrane is a doubled layered ureterovesical membrane that temporarily obstruct this region between the 37th and 43th days after conception, this membrane divided the Wolffian duct from the urogenital sinus at the time of formation of the ureteral sac during early embryonic development [2].

Precise positioning of the ureter orifice in the trigone depends on the ureteric bud sprouting at a stereotypical position on the Wolffian duct; abnormalities in this process can result in reflux and obstruction [3]. Expansion of the CND would enable the ureter to move away from the Wolffian duct, while insertion of the CND into the bladder and its differentiation into the trigone would reposition the ureter orifice at the proper site [4]. Mature connections are established during ureteric maturation, and the distal ureter maturate later on to form a continent vesicoureteric junction and a separate vas duct. This complex area became the scene of many congenital anomalies; mainly an ureterocele, ectopic ureter and vesicoureteric reflux [5]. It was previously thought that the trigonal musculature developed primarily from the Wolffian duct, but it has been shown to develop primarily from bladder mesenchyme. Following emergence of the ureters from the Wolffian ducts, extensive epithelial remodeling brings the ureters to their final trigonal positions via vitamin A-induced apoptosis as suggested by Batourina et al. [6] Ureterocele is a congenital pathology that has been attributed to the delayed rupture or persistence of the Chwalla's membrane. The most other common anomalies include partial and total duplication, ectopic orifices, ureterocele, ureterovesical junction incompetence causing ureteral reflux, and intrinsic obstruction of ureter [7]. Embryologically the congenital ureteric obstructions may be divided in two major groups: intrinsic ureteral obstructions and obstructions of the ureterovesical junction; which subsequently divided into three sections:

- Terminal portion (juxtavesical ureter)
- Intramural portion
- Submucosal portion (lying under the mucosa of the bladder)

Anatomically the ureter is most narrow at the ureterovesical junction, followed by the ureteropelvic junction, and then at the crossing of the iliac vessels [8].

The intramural segment of the ureter runs obliquely through the bladder wall. Near the bladder the terminal ureter is enveloped by the muscular layer of Waldeyer. It coalesces with bundles of the detrusor muscle in the bladder wall and consists of coarser longitudinally muscle bundles (Fig. 5.1).

Reflux of urine is prevented because the ureter passes diagonally through the bladder wall musculature for a short distance before entering the bladder lumen. The length of this intramural part of the ureter in adults is 1.2–2.5 cm (in neonates 0.5–0.8 cm) [9].

Definition: Since 1984 the nomenclature and classification of the ureterocele were standardized by the Committee on Terminology, Nomenclature, and Classification, Section on Urology, American Academy of Pediatrics [10].

In ICD-10 version the ureterocele considered as the last item of the other specified disorders of kidney and ureter under the code of (N28.8).

The term "cele" denoting a swelling or hernia in a specified part, its origin from Greek kēlē which means 'tumour'.

Ureterocele is a cystic dilatation of the terminal lower ureter at its entry into the mucosa of urinary bladder, it is located inside the bladder or the urethra, or both.

Sometimes ureterocele represented shortly as "Uceles".

Incidence: The incidence of ureterocele is variable; at autopsy it is 1:500; and generally, it affects women more than men, with a 6:1 ratio. It predominantly affecting Caucasians than other ethnic groups [11].

The incidence shows a wide range in the literature, and it is range from 1/500 to 1/12000 [12].

Alvarado et al. [13] reported a lower incidence in children of 7 out of every 10 million children under the age of 6 years in some localities. According to Schultz

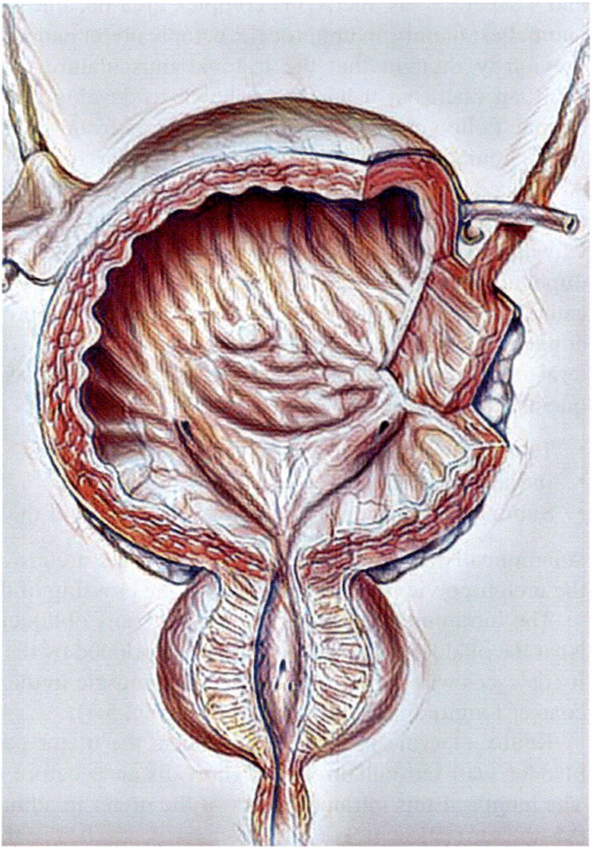

Fig. 5.1 The intramural segment of the ureter which runs obliquely through the bladder wall. The terminal ureter is enveloped by the muscular layer of Waldeyer. (This photo designed by Prof S A Salam, professor of surgery, Al-Azhar university

et al. [14] ureteroceles are known to happen roughly in 1 in 4000 children. Duplicate ureters with bifid ureters being five times more common than completely duplicated ones. Bilateral duplications are found in 39% of cases [15].

Eighty percent of ureteroceles occur in duplex systems, and 10% of ureteroceles are bilateral.

If a ureterocele occurs in a duplex system, the upper pole moiety is always affected. Single-system ureteroceles are relatively rare but are more common in males. Ureteroceles in the upper pole moiety of a duplex system are more common in females, occurring four to seven times more frequently than in males. In 70% of upper pole ureteroceles, the ureteric orifice is in an ectopic position at the bladder neck or in the proximal urethra.

Most cases are congenital, but acquired type of ureterocele is rare, and it seen in adults and associated with other lower ureteric pathologies. At the meantime the true prevalence of vesicoureteric reflux (VUR) in healthy infants and children is not well known. Bailey [16] reviewed 15 articles on the subject and concluded that

VUR may be present in 0.4–1.8% of normal healthy children, but a lower figure probably being more accurate.

Etiology: The precise embryologic etiology of the ureterocele remains unknown, but theorised causes include the following:

Ureteroceles may be caused by obstruction due to incomplete breakdown of Chwalla's membrane, a two-cell layer between the ureteral bud and the Wolffian duct. Alternatively, ureterocele formation may result from delayed arrival of the ureteral bud into the bladder, with expansion occurring as part of the flaring of the common excretory duct [17].

A third theory suggests that ureterocele formation is due to an intrinsic muscular deficiency of the distal ureter and bladder trigone [18].

The most commonly accepted theory behind ureterocele formation is obstruction of the ureteral orifice during embryogenesis, with incomplete dissolution of the Chwalla membrane. Failure of this membrane to completely perforate during development of the ureteral orifice is thought to explain the occurrence of a ureterocele [1].

Classification of Ureterocele: It is classified into the single or duplex system and acquired or congenital; acquired type is rare and seen in adults.

Ureterocele is also classified simply as orthotopic or ectopic one. In the orthotopic variety, the ureterocele is located on the trigone at the normal usual location of the ureteral orifice, but in ectopic type, the ureterocele is located distal to the trigone and may project well from the urethral orifice. The ectopic orifice is located at the bladder neck or more distal.

So ureteroceles are classified into intravesical or extravesical [19].

- ***Intravesical represent about 20% of the cases:*** the ureterocele is completely confined within the bladder, these tend to be associated with single systems and are more common in males, subtypes include:
  - **Stenotic**: small, stenotic ureteric orifice associated with obstruction of the upper tract.
  - **Non-obstructed**: large ureteric orifice that tends to balloon frequently.
- ***Extravesical (or ectopic) (80%):*** when the ureterocele extends to the bladder neck or urethra and tend to occur with duplex systems; most commonly in females, with many subtypes which include:
  - **Sphincteric**: ureterocele extends into bladder neck and urethra. The orifice is wide and usually opens proximal to the external sphincter, in males this subtype presented with urinary retention.
  - **Sphincterostenotic**: similar to sphincteric ureterocele, but the ureteric orifice is stenosed.
  - **Cecoureterocele**: ureterocele prolapses posterior to the urethra and anterior to the vagina, but the orifice is within the bladder (affects girls only). This type can cause urethral obstruction.
  - **Blind ectopic**: similar to sphincteric, but there is no detectable ureteric orifice.

Pseudoureterocoeles are acquired dilatations of the submucosal portion of the distal ureter that mimic simple ureterocele. The appearance of the radiolucent wall surrounding the dilated distal ureteral segment is an important differentiating point (cobra head sign), which is characterising ureterocele (Fig. 5.2).

The distinction between real and pseudo types is important, since most pseudoureterocoeles are seen in elders, and were related to malignancy involving the bladder, in the later situation the lucency or halo around the ureteric orifice is thicker than that of a ureterocele and is poorly defined; and in cases of tumors, it may be irregular and may show a filling defect within the ureterocele, with asymmetry of the dilated ureteral lumen [20].

In most cases of acquired pseudourteroceles there is evidence of an acquired cause, such as a calculus or abnormal vesical mucosal pattern. Rarely, thickening of this lucency is seen in a patient with a known congenital ureterocele, and it is usually associated with a complicating process, such as oedema with a calculus [20].

A simple classification is applicable; which based on the location of the orifice (intravesical vs ectopic), it is more commonly used because it has therapeutic implications, especially with respect to the likelihood of the presence of vesicoureteral reflux following transurethral puncture of the ureterocele.

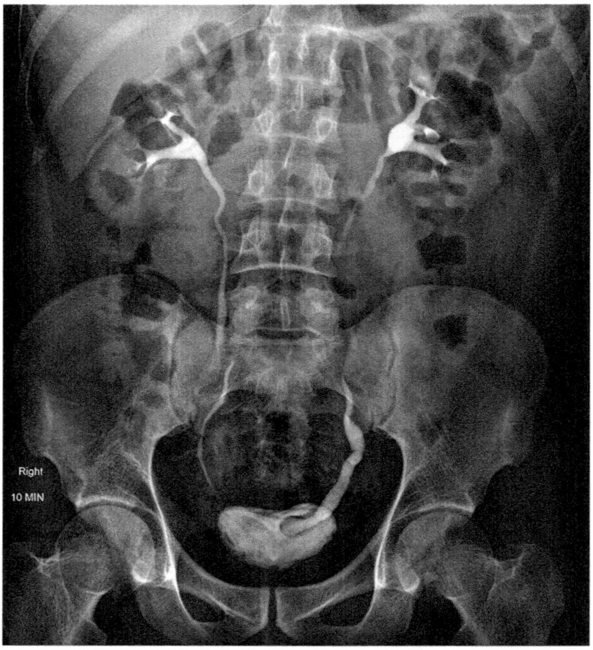

Fig. 5.2 IVP fluoroscopy showing the cobra head sign, dilatation of the distal left ureter, surrounded by a thin lucent line; which is consistent with ureterocele [50]. Under a modified Creative Commons Attribution-Non-commercial-Share Alike 3.0 Unported License, (Radiopaedia)

5.1.1 Associated Anomalies

Duplex kidneys: Eighty percent of ureteroceles occur in duplex systems; which are a common congenital malformations of urogenital system, with an overall incidence of approximately 1–3% [21].

This anomaly was classified as complete or incomplete according to ureteral morphology, in which the renal unit is made up of two separate pelvicalyceal systems. The renal vessels, collecting system and ureter of duplex kidneys are respectively separated (Fig. 5.3).

Most patients with duplex kidneys have no significant clinical symptoms. But some complications like urolithiasis and vesicoureteral reflux (VUR) are relevant to duplex kidneys (Fig. 5.4).

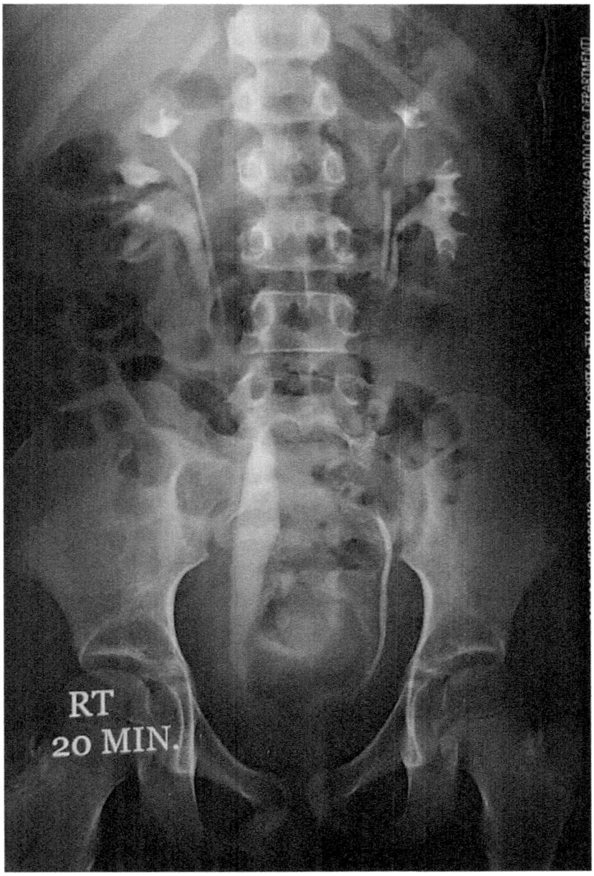

Fig. 5.3 IVP showing after 20 min a bilateral duplication of the kidneys and ureters

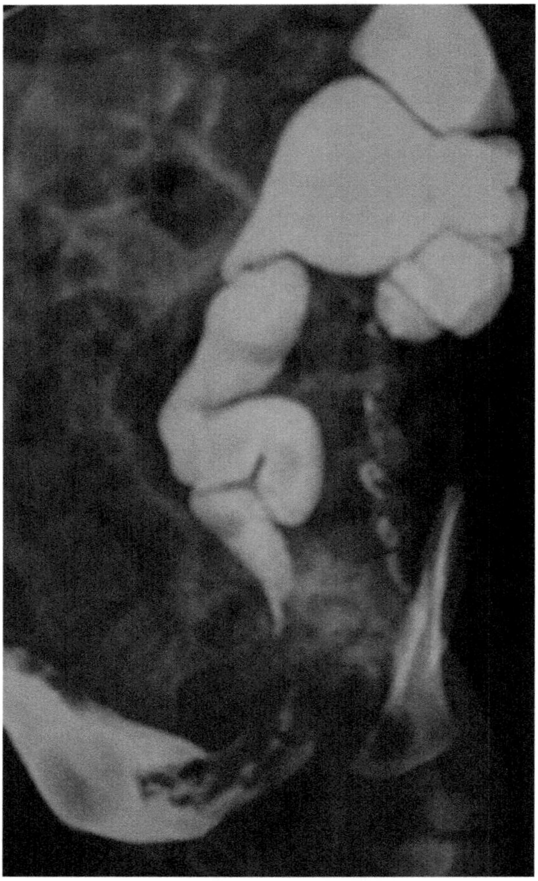

Fig. 5.4 A Left sided ureterocele with a marked reflux and hydronephrosis in one moiety of a left duplex in IVP study

Upper moiety complications are related to the ureteral ectopic insertion, usually complicated with a ureterocele or multi-cystic dysplastic moiety kidney [22]. The most common upper moiety complication is urinary tract obstruction due to a ureterocele.

A prolapsing ureterocele is almost always associated with a duplex kidney ipsilaterally. The ureter from the upper moiety of a duplex kidney is inserted more caudally than normal and is prone to obstruction at the level of the VUJ. The lower moiety ureter is often inserted more laterally and is prone to vesicoureteric reflux. As either of the moieties can be functioning poorly in a duplex system [23].

Kidney triplication with ectopic ureterocele: In 1870 Wrany [24] first described a triplex kidney with ureterocele which was diagnosed in a 3-year-old girl autopsy. Until 2020; about 100 cases of renal triplication are described in scientific literature. A little over than 20 cases is associated with ureterocele. Successful outcome of endoscopic treatment of ectopic ureterocele was reported [25].

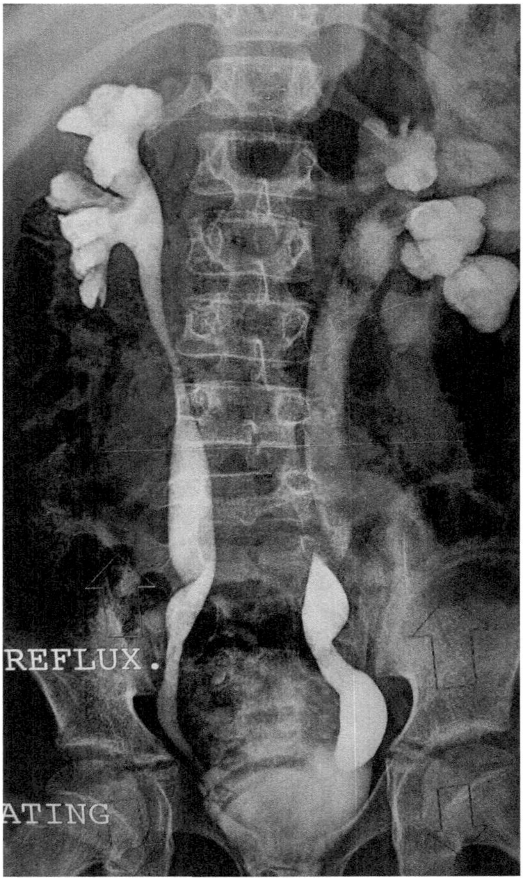

Fig. 5.5 An IVP with bilateral marked hydroureter and hydronephrosis with a left sided large ureterocele, and a marked right sided reflex

Hydronephrosis: Different grades of hydroureter with or without hydronephrosis, uni or bilateral are detectable with ureteroceles; which may be duet or reflux or ureteric obstruction (Fig. 5.5).

Multicystic dysplastic kidney: Ureterocele is occasionally seen in association with a multicystic dysplastic kidney; which is usually nonfunctioning (Fig. 5.6).

Renal agenesis: Ureterocele may be diagnosed with a single urinary collecting system with or without hydronephrosis. Unilateral renal agenesis with ureterocele is uncommon. The coexistence of unilateral renal agenesis, ureterocele, and a blind ended proximal ureter is also very rare [26].

It is generally thought that renal agenesis occurs due to a lack of any induction effect between mesonephric blastema and ureteric buds, caused by a developmental problem of the mesonephric duct during early embryonic development.

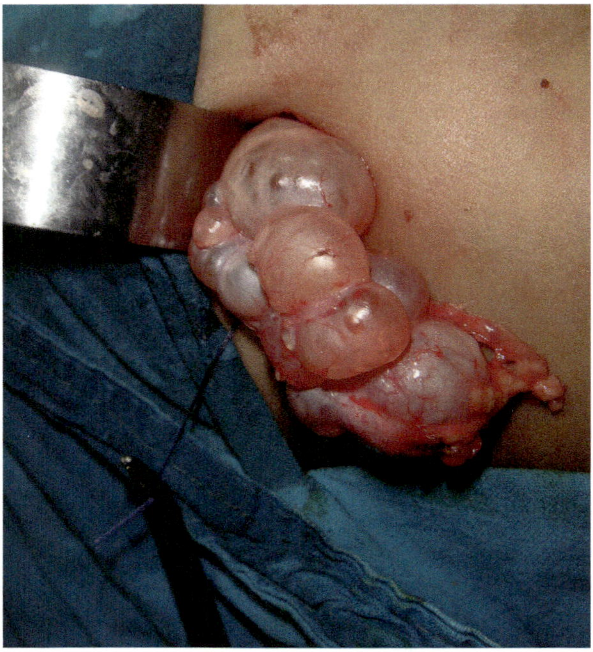

Fig. 5.6 Polycystic dysplastic nonfunctioning left kidney associating ureterocele seen in an operative photograph

5.1.2 Diagnosis

Antenatal: The majority of babies with a ureterocele and duplex kidneys present antenatally. Widespread prenatal screening has resulted in a recently increased detection of the congenital anomalies of the kidneys and urinary tract. Antenatal hydronephrosis (AHN) is one of the most common anomalies detected on routine prenatal ultrasounds, it affects 1–4.5% of all pregnancies [27]. At the meantime vesicoureteral reflux (VUR) and ureteroceles are among the most common congenital anomalies diagnosed in utero or after birth; ureterocele represents 5% of cases of AHN [28]. Ureteroceles are often identified on antenatal ultrasound, presenting as hydroureteronephrosis, or as hydronephrosis in the upper or lower part of the kidney with duplex system and in some occasions the ureterocele itself could be identified as a cystic swelling within the bladder in the transsexual view [29].

Postnatal diagnosis: Postnatal diagnosis is confirmed with renal ultrasound, though, historically, ureterocele has been mainly identified with voiding cystourethrography (VCUG), with a swelling displacing the intravesical contrast. Although patients with ureteroceles are often clinically asymptomatic, the ureteral obstruction can lead to severe hydroureteronephrosis, with associated parenchymal thinning and potential functional loss of the upper moiety. UTIs can ascend to the upper tract and present with pyelonephritis and/or sepsis [30]. Ureteroceles in adults are usually less obstructive, intravesical, and associated with a single system. A prolapsing

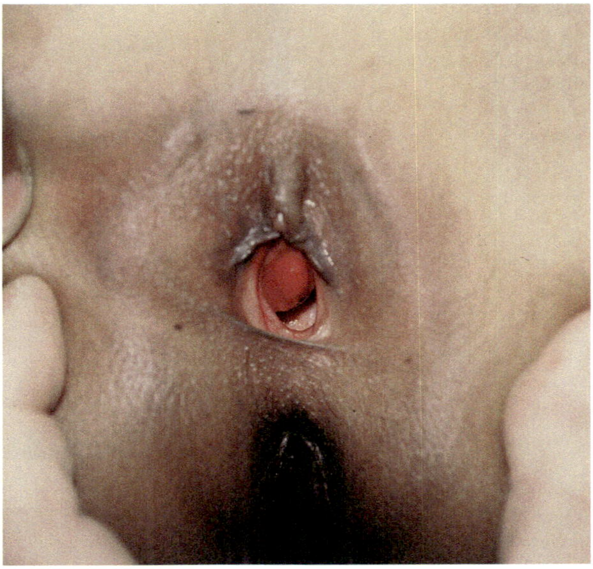

Fig. 5.7 Three years old girl with a ureterocele protruding from the urinary meatus; as an inter-labial red cystic swelling which should be differentiated from ureteral prolapse

ectopic ureterocele may be presented in the form of labial or/and inter-labial swelling as a red or purple in color cystic swelling protrudes from the urethral meatus, without surrounding it (Fig. 5.7).

5.1.3 Investigation

- Antenatally the ultrasound of the renal tract shows a thin-walled cyst in the bladder often associated with a duplex system and a usually ectopic, and rarely orthotopic dilated ureter. If there are concerns about obstruction; USS should be performed immediately after birth with a view to urgent surgical treatment. Small lower positioned ureteroceles may remain unrecognized with this US [31] (Fig. 5.8).
- VCUG: can identify ureterocele location, size, and associated VUR (reflux into the lower moiety of an associated duplex kidney is seen in 50% of the cases). This should be performed early in the post-natal period if there is evidence of BOO, otherwise defer 3–6 months (Fig. 5.9).
- MAG3 renogram: is useful to exclude obstruction, because it is a the favorable imaging and the more efficient for detection of renal extraction.
- DMSA renogram: is used also to assess renal moiety function and demonstrate renal cortical abnormalities in the presence of reflux.
- Contrast-enhanced computed tomography (CECT): scanning of the abdomen and pelvis provides additional clues for diagnosing simple or ectopic ureterocele

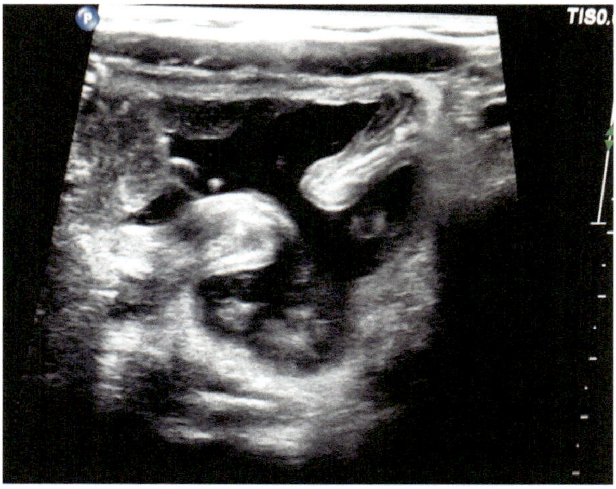

Fig. 5.8 An USS showing an unusual thick walled ureterocele opening into the bladder

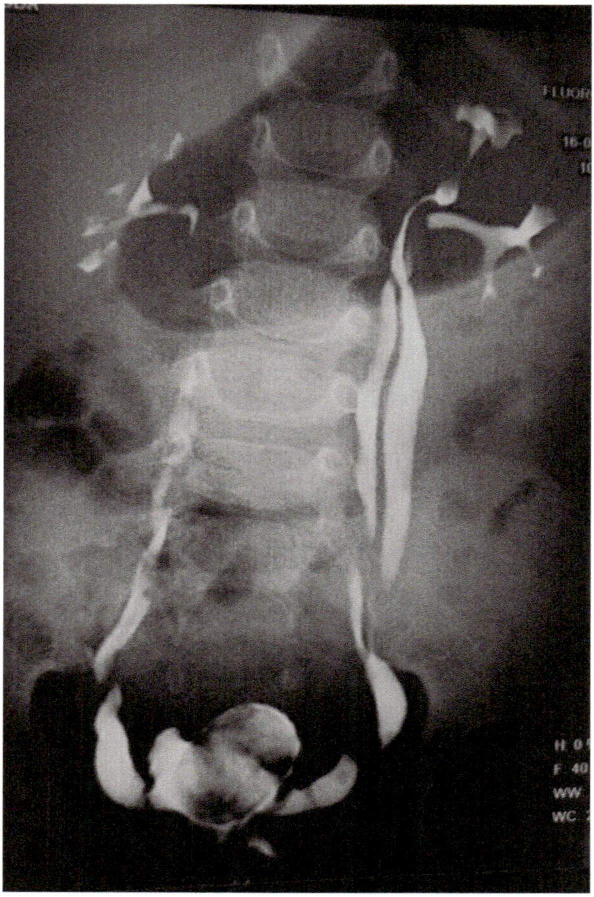

Fig. 5.9 VCUG showing ureterocele, bilateral reflux and a left sided duplex

in adults when kidney ultrasonography findings are equivocal. CT can reveal the presence of a duplicated collecting system, hydronephrotic upper pole segment, and dysplastic upper pole moiety. It is also an excellent tool to detect ureteral calculi; however, abnormal ureteral anatomy and ureteral dilatation are better imaged with MRI (Fig. 5.10).

- MRI is an excellent anatomical study for evaluating rare cases with suspected dysplastic, nonfunctioning, ectopic renal moieties and ectopic ureteral insertion.
- Dynamic MRI allows reliable assessment of individual renal function and urinary excretion. A combination of static and dynamic sequences appears to have particular value in the diagnostic work-up of congenital urinary tract anomalies including evaluation of duplex kidneys in children, permitting exact morphologic-functional correlation [32].
- Cystoscopy: can be used for diagnosis and as well for endoscopic treatment [33].

Presentation: Depending on the size and location of the ureterocele, it ranges from a non symptomatic quiescent lesion to a prolapsed mass through the bladder neck causing bladder outlet obstruction, or even protruded outside the introitus. However, the most common presentation in young as well as older pediatric populations is a UTI. Most cases of ureterocele are associated with hydroureteronephrosis, VUR, and complete ureteral and renal duplication (duplex kidney) [34].

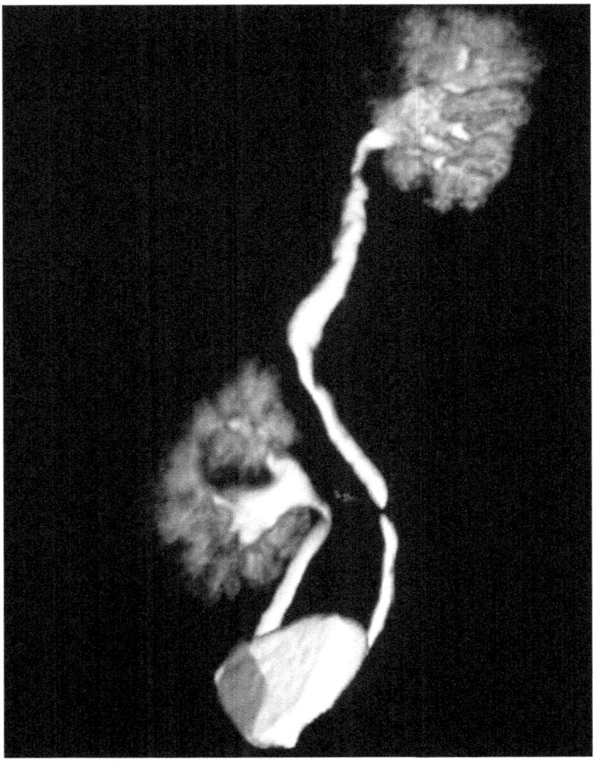

Fig. 5.10 Contrast-enhanced computed tomography showing a Rt sided ectopic kidney with an obvious intravesical ureterocele

VUR may be the result and can be present in the upper moiety or both of the moieties. Patients with bifid ureters usually have no symptoms. In three situations, however, symptoms may occur if there is vesicoureteral reflux (VUR), if a uretero-pelvic junction obstruction exists in the inferior branch of the bifid ureter, or (less commonly) if ureteroureteric reflux occurs because of a functional obstruction distal to the branch point in the ureter.

The voiding cystourethrogram sometimes shows reflux into a "drooping lily," the indirect sign of a duplex kidney. The "drooping lily" refers to the renal pelvis of the refluxing lower pole system: the pelvis is in a lower than normal position and is frequently laterally displaced, resulting in the appearance of the drooping petals of a lily. Ureteroceles containing stones present as a unique challenge, urinary stones are a common urologic condition and are detected in 5%–40% of cases of ureterocele [34]. However, stone formation in the ureterocele is rare in children, with only a few previously reported [35].

Iincontinente is a rare presentation in older children, and urinary drippling is not rare. Other variable clinical presentation may include loin pain, lower abdominal pain, urinary tract infection, hematuria, or retention [36].

Incidentally detected ureterocele: In adults and on some occasions a ureterocele may be discovered incidentally during pelvic or prostatic surgeries. Treatment of such ureteroceles should be determined according to the ureterocele's size, anatomic configuration, and location and by the degree of obstruction of the affected renal unit. Surgical excision of the ureterocele at the time of radical prostatectomy may be the best approach for patients requiring treatment [37].

5.1.4 Differential diagnosis

- Bladder diverticula which are hernias of the bladder mucosa through muscular fibers of the bladder wall resulting in a thin-walled structure that poorly empties during micturition. Bladder diverticula are either congenital or acquired. Such cases my be confused with ureterocele, specially at younger ages. The mainstay difference of diverticula that it is essential an extravesical extension (Fig. 5.11). The incidence of congenital bladder diverticula is reported to be 1.7% [38].
- Differential diagnosis of ureteroceles on US include; Gartner duct cyst or the wolffian duct cyst, which are seen extravesical and may be associated with genital or renal anomalies.
- On contrast studies like MCUG; ureterocele should be differentiated from air bubble, blood clot, lithiasis, tumor, or balloon catheter [39].
- Ureteroceles should be also differentiated from the rare cases of pipestem megaureter; which is a dilated ureter without an overt obstructing lesion. Two basic types exist, these are the refluxing and non-refluxing types.

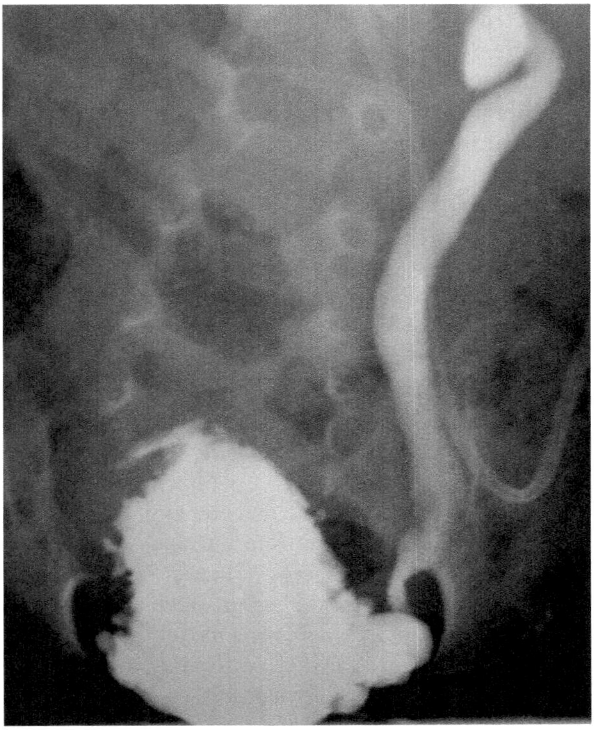

Fig. 5.11 A child with left sided bladder diverticulum with marked reflux seen during VCUG, which should be differentiated from ureterocele

5.1.5 Management

Literature is still struggling to find the best practical guidelines in managing ureteroceles. Broadly speaking, management aims frequently sought for include persevering the renal function up to the maximum possible extent, preventing and treating VUR in a timely manner if it arises or if it is already present, keeping the kidney drainage intact in order to preserve renal parenchymal tissue, preventing bladder outlet obstruction and maintaining child's continence [40].

The lack of standardisation of treatment of ureterocele was highlighted in a study by Merguerian et al. [41] in 2010, they reported that most pediatric urologists saw fewer than 10 cases per year, and there was significant variation in their managements, especially in cases of intravesical ureterocele with duplicated system.

Contemporary trends in treatment of children with ureterocele means conservative or minimally invasive surgical tactics with high possibility of getting good results. It is important to diagnose uretroceles early; as surgical decompression soon after diagnosis and further investigations are important to prevent renal complications. Initial management is based on relieving the obstruction with an endoscopic puncture of the ureterocele, utilizing cautery or laser, although endoscopic puncture can potentially introduce secondary VUR into the punctured ureter and collecting system.

Antibiotic prophylaxis: Pediatric urologists frequently rely on continuous antibiotic prophylaxis (CAP) for managing cases of VUR, and ureterocele, unless a definitive treatment is applied. The main aim of CAP is to prevent urinary tract infection and long-term complications. Nevertheless, its efficacy has been a source of considerable debate, and pediatricians have varied opinions on who would benefit from it.

Early endoscopic unroofing of the urtelocele: Transurethral endoscopic incision is an established treatment option for management of obstructing ureterocele. The advantage of this simple technique is that it helps to drain the obstructed urinary tract, providing hope of improving function and rendering the frequency of doing unnecessary heminephrectomy. The disadvantage of this method is that secondary VUR into the upper pole may supervene, making reimplantation necessary [41]. After incision, the ureterocele collapses and appears as a pseudomass within the bladder.

Transurethral endoscopic incision could be achieved by using monopolar electrocautery or holmium laser A recent study was carried out to evaluate the outcomes of those two different energy sources, i.e., monopolar electrocautery versus holmium laser in 44 patients, and it proved that both laser and monopolar incision have similar efficacy in decompressing the ureterocele in long-term follow-up. However, laser has added advantage of performing a stone lithotripsy with the same instruments with lesser morbidity and lower incidence of persistent reflux [42].

Definitive management is similar to that for ectopic ureter, with upper pole heminephrectomy in symptomatic, poorly functioning systems, or vesicoureteral reimplantation with the goal of renal preservation. Excision of the ureterocele and bladder neck reconstruction are often required to remove the residual ureterocele. If surgical intervention is performed prior to endoscopic puncture, the ureterocele may be left in place and the upper ureter anastomosed to the lower ureter (ureteroureterostomy) to divert the obstructed upper ureter.

Henry Morris at 1904 [43] reported that grafting into the bladder—cystoureterostresis or uretero-cysto-neostomy ought to be the operation of choice when it can.

Today, ureteral reimplantation remains the management of choice for distal ureteral reconstruction. In situations where the remnant ureter is not long enough for ureteroneocystostomy, alternative procedures including psoas hitch, Boari flap, ureteroureterostomy, transureteroureterostomy, substitution ureteral reconstruction, or autotransplantation are used. These procedures for distal ureteral reconstruction have traditionally been performed using an open approach (Fig. 5.12).

But in 2001, laparoscopic Boari flap was described in three patients for distal ureteral obstruction due to stricture disease [44].

A few years later, Allaparthi et al. [45] reported successful robot-assisted laparoscopic Boari flap/ureteral reimplant, establishing its feasibility and safety.

Ureteroceles containing stones present as a unique challenge: When a calculus has to be removed from within the ureterocele, a large opening lead to de novo

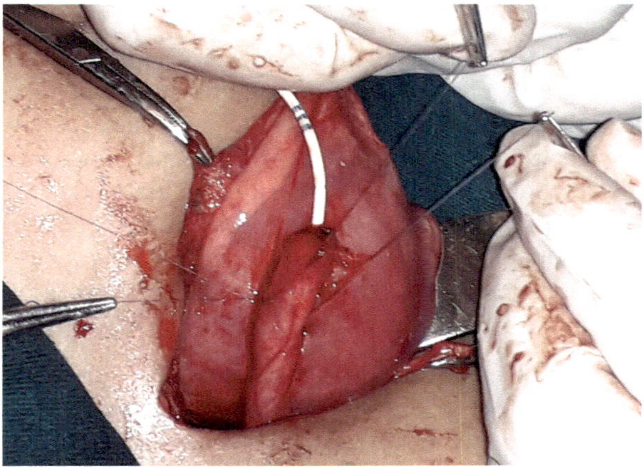

Fig. 5.12 Operative photograph showing the extra-vesical ureteral reimplantation following Lich-Gregoir (LG) technique

vesicoureteral reflux (VUR), which may result in recurrent infections and renal parenchymal damage.

Transvesical laparoscopic ureterolithotomy with partial suturing of the incision at the roof of the.

ureterocele is another good treatment option, particularly for asymptomatic patients [36].

So surgical options for ureteroceles include simple aspiration for prolapse of the ectopic ureterocele, distal enlargement of the meatus, upper pole or total nephrectomy, ureteropelvic or uretero-ureteral anastomosis with segmental ureterectomy, ipsilateral ureterovesical reimplantation with total resection of the ureterocele, and total resection of the pathologic tract with parietal reconstruction/reimplantation [46].

5.1.6 New Advances in Management of Ureteroceles

- Transvesical laparoscopic surgery has been recently tried through a cross trigonal ureteral reimplantation for correction of VUR. It carries the advantages of diminished postoperative surgical pain, shortened hospital stay and acceptable cosmesis [47].
- Laparoscopic selective clipping of upper moiety vasculature and ureter has been recently tried to deal with ectopic ureter associated with poor functioning renal moiety [48].

Follow up: Follow-up care for all cases includes serial monitoring of renal function, periodic evaluation of voiding symptoms and bladder function, and interval radiologic studies to assess renal growth, hydroureteronephrosis, and vesicoureteral reflux.

Complications:

- Endoscopic incision of ureterocele: This is infrequently definitive therapy, except in cases of a single-system intravesical ureterocele. Iatrogenic vesicoureteral reflux, especially in extravesical ureteroceles, can occur.
- Upper pole heminephrectomy: This technique has the highest risk of vascular compromise of lower pole with potential loss of kidney function can occur. The need for further lower tract reconstruction due to persistent reflux, infection, or failure to decompress the ureterocele is a possible complication.
- Excision of ureterocele and ureteral reimplantation [49]: Postoperative complications include the following:
  - Problematic hematuria and/or bladder spasms
  - Damage to bladder neck and subsequent innocence
  - Injury to the contralateral ureteral orifice
  - Compromise of blood supply to the lower pole ureter

Questions

1. The Chwalla's membrane:
   (a) Is a doubled layered ureterovesical membrane
   (b) Temporarily obstruct the ureterovesical region
   (c) Appear between the 37th and 43th days after conception
   (d) Divided the Wolffian duct from the urogenital sinus
   (e) All of the above

Answer: (e)

2. The length of this intramural part of the ureter is:
   (a) In adults it is 3–5 cm
   (b) In neonates it is 0.5–0.8 cm
   (c) In adults it is 7 cm
   (d) In children it is about 4 cm
   (e) It is always variable

Answer: (b)

3. The incidence of ureterocele:
   (a) At autopsy it is 1:500
   (b) Affecting Africans than other ethnic groups
   (c) Affecting man than women
   (d) Most cases reported at older age
   (e) All of the above

Answer: (a)

4. The management of ureterocele varies according to:

    (a) The location of ureterocele
    (b) Presence of a duplex or single system
    (c) The function of the kidney
    (d) The function of the moiety
    (e) All of the above

Answer: (e)

5. Ureterocele subtypes:

    (a) Intravesical cases represent about 80% of the cases.
    (b) Extravesical (or ectopic) represent 20% of the cases.
    (c) When it extends to the bladder neck or urethra it tends to occur with duplex systems.
    (d) Sphincteric: ureterocele extends into bladder neck, but it will not never extend to the urethra.
    (e) The orifice is usually wide and usually opens distal to the external sphincter.

Answer: (c)

6. Ureterocele subtypes:

    (a) In males the sphincteric subtype usually presented with urinary retention.
    (b) In cecoureterocele subtype the ureterocele prolapses anterior to the urethra in male
    (c) Cecoureterocele is usually posterior to the vagina
    (d) The orifice of cecoureterocele is outside the bladder.
    (e) This type can cause urethral obstruction.

Answer: (a)

7. Associated anomalies:

    (a) Thirty percent of ureteroceles occur in duplex system
    (b) Duplex system is not a common congenital malformations of urogenital system
    (c) Duplex system had an overall incidence of approximately 1–3%.
    (d) Duplex system was classified as complete or incomplete according to its relation with the kidney.
    (e) In Duplex anomaly the renal vessels, collecting system and ureter of duplex kidneys are not separated.

Answer: (c)

References

1. Domenech G, Tejedo A, Vilanova J. Contribuition al estudio de la membrana ureteral de Chwalla. Su importancia clinica. Arch Esp Urol. 1973;26:355–9.
2. Mendelsohn C. Using mouse models to understand normal and abnormal urogenital tract development. Organogenesis. 2009;5(1):32–40.
3. Mackie GG, Stephens FD. Duplex kidneys: a correlation of renal dysplasia with position of the ureteral orifice. J Urol. 1975;114:274–80.
4. Batourina E, Choi C, Paragas N, Bello N, Hensle T, Costantini FD, Mendelsohn CL. Distal ureter morphogenesis depends on epithelial cell remodeling mediated by vitamin A and Ret. Nat Genet. 2002;32(1):109–15.
5. Batourina E, Tsai S, Lambert S, Sprenkle P, Viana R, Dutta S, Mendelsohn CL. Apoptosis induced by vitamin A signaling is crucial for connecting the ureters to the bladder. Nat Genet. 2005;37(10):1082–9.
6. Fröber R. Surgical atlas surgical anatomy of the ureter. BJU Int (Papier). 2007;100(4):949–65.
7. Lierse W. Becken. In: von Lanz T, Wachsmuth W, editors. Praktische Anatomie, Bd 2, Teil 8A. Berlin: Springer; 1984.
8. Liaw A, Cunha GR, Shen J, Cao M, Liu G, Sinclair A, Baskin L. Development of the human bladder and ureterovesical junction. Differentiation. 2018; https://doi.org/10.1016/j.diff.2018.08.004.
9. Lierse W. Ureter. In: Applied anatomy of the pelvis. Springer: Berlin; 1987. p. 136–45.
10. Glassberg KI, Braren V, Duckett JW, Jacobs EC, King LR, Lebowitz RL, Perlmutter AD, Stephens FD. Suggested terminology for duplex systems, ectopic ureters and ureteroceles. J Urol. 1984;132(6):1153–4.
11. Kumar GA, Babu BP, Lavakumar A, Sindhuri A. Giant ureterocele management in an adult male: a rare case report. J Sci Soc. 2020;47(3):185.
12. Shah H, Tiwari C, Shenoy NS, Dwivedi P, Gandhi S. Transurethral incision of ureteroceles in paediatric age group. Turk J Urol. 2017;43(4):530–5.
13. Alvarado-García R, Gallego-Grijalva J, García-Arano G. Ureterocele en niños. Cirugía y Cirujanos. 2004;72(2):117–20.
14. Schultz K, Yoneka Toda L. Genetic basis of ureterocele. Curr Genomics. 2016;17(1):62–9.
15. Timothy RP, Deeter A, Perlmutter AD. Ureteral duplication: clinical findings and therapy in 46 children. J Urol. 1971;105:445–51.
16. Bailey R. Vesicoureteric reflux in healthy infants and children. In: Hodson J, Kincaid-Smith P, editors. Reflux nephropathy. New York: Masson Publishing; 1979. p. 59–61.
17. Tanagho EA. Embryologic basis for lower ureteral anomalies: a hypothesis. Urology. 1976;8:451–64.
18. Stephens FD. Aetiology of ureteroceles and effects of ureteroceles on the urethra. Br J Urol. 1968;40:483.
19. Stephens D. Caecoureterocele and concepts on the embryology and aetiology of ureteroceles. Aust N Z J Surg. 1971;40:239.
20. Thornbury J, Silver T, Vinson R. Ureterocelesvs. Pseudoureuteroceles in adults. Radiology. 1977;122(1):81–4. https://doi.org/10.1148/122.1.81.
21. Hunziker M, Kutasy B, D'Asta F, Puri P. Urinary tract anomalies associated with high grade primary vesicoureteral reflux. Pediatr Surg Int. 2012;28(2):201–4.
22. Pan Y, Chen G, Chen H, Zhu Y, Chen H. The left ureterocele and stone of calyceal diverticulum in the patient with bilateral incomplete duplex kidneys managed by flexible ureteroscopy: a case report and literature review. BMC Urol. 2020;20(1):1–6.
23. Privett JT, Jeans WD, Roylance J. The incidence and importance of renal duplication. Clin Radiol. 1976;27(4):521–30.
24. Smith I. Triplicate ureter. Br J Surg. 1946;34(134):182–5. https://doi.org/10.1002/bjs.18003413409.

25. Osipov IB, Lebedev DA, Lifanova MV. Kidney triplication with ectopic ureterocele: a case report. BMC Urol. 2020;20:54. https://doi.org/10.1186/s12894-020-00625-2.
26. Park JJ, Kim WB, Kim WK, et al. Renal agenesis with ureterocele, duplicated megaureter and translocation of seminal vesicle: a case report and review of the literature. J Mens Health. 2021:1–5. https://doi.org/10.31083/jomh.2021.088.
27. Liu DB, Armstrong WR 3rd, Maizels M. Hydronephrosis: prenatal and postnatal evaluation and management. Clin Perinatol. 2014;41(3):661–78.
28. Castagnetti M, Cimador M, Esposito C, Rigamonti W. Antibiotic prophylaxis in antenatal nonrefluxing hydronephrosis, megaureter and ureterocele. Nat Rev Urol. 2012;9(6):321–9.
29. Whitten SM, McHoney M, Wilcox DT, New S, Chitty LS. Accuracy of antenatal fetal ultrasound in the diagnosis of duplex kidneys. Ultrasound Obstet Gynecol. 2003;21:342–6. https://doi.org/10.1002/uog.40.
30. Tangal S, Boga MS, Kutsal O, Haliloglu AH. Adult unilateral duplex system ureterocele with multiple calculi. Eur Res J. 2015;1:71–3.
31. Dacher JN. Abnormalities of the lower urinary tract and urachus. In: Fotter R, editor. Pediatric uroradiology. Medical radiology (diagnostic imaging). Berlin: Springer; 2001. https://doi.org/10.1007/978-3-642-56484-0_8.
32. Rohrschneider WK, Stegen P. Magnetic resonance imaging. In: Fotter R, editor. Pediatric uroradiology. Medical radiology (diagnostic imaging). Berlin: Springer; 2001. https://doi.org/10.1007/978-3-642-56484-0_2.
33. John R, Brewster SF, Biers S, Neal NL. Chapter 16: Pediatric urology. In: Oxford handbook of urology. Oxford: Oxford University Press; 2019.
34. Shokeir AA, Nijman RJ. Ureterocele: an ongoing challenge in infancy and childhood. BJU Int. 2002;90(8):777–83.
35. Dominichi A, Travaglini F, Maleci M, et al. Giant stone in a complete duplex ureter with ureterocele. A case report. Urol Int. 2003;71:336–7.
36. Satoji Y, Tobu S, Udo K, Noguchi M. Transvesical laparoscopic surgery for a Stone in the ureterocele. J Endourol Case Rep. 2020;6(4):283–6.
37. Leventis A, Miles B, Gonzales E, et al. Diagnosis and management of incidental ureterocele during the treatment of clinically localized prostate cancer. World J Urol. 2000;18:444–8. https://doi.org/10.1007/s003459900080.
38. Abou Zahr R, Chalhoub K, Ollaik F, Nohra L. Congenital bladder diverticulum in adults: a case report and review of the literature. Case Rep Urol. 2018: 9748926. https://doi.org/10.1155/2018/9748926.
39. Bellah RD, Long FR, Canning DA. Ureterocele eversion with vesicoureteral reflux in duplex kidneys: findings at voiding cystourethrography. AJR. 1995;165:409–13
40. Ali SI, et al. Management of ureteroceles: review article. J Biol Today's World. 2020;9(10):001–4.
41. Avni EF, Gallety E, Rypens F, et al. A hypothesis for the higher incidence of vesico-ureteral reflux and primary megaureters in male babies. Pediatr Radiol. 1992;22:1–4.
42. Sharma A, Garg G, Sharma A, Kumar M, Sankhwar SN. Comparison of electrocautery versus holmium laser energy source for transurethral ureterocele incision: an outcome analysis from a tertiary care institute. Lasers Med Sci. 2021;36:521–8.
43. Morris H. Surgical diseases of the kidney and ureter including injuries, malformations and misplacements (Vol. 2). Cassell and Company; 1904.
44. Fugita OE, Dinlenc C, Kavoussi L. The laparoscopic Boari flap. J Urol. 2001;166(1):51–3.
45. Allaparthi S, Ramanathan R, Balaji KC. Robotic distal ureterectomy with boari flap reconstruction for distal ureteral urothelial cancers: a single institutional pilot experience. J Laparoendosc Adv Surg Tech. 2010;20(2):165–71.
46. Caione P, Nappo SG, Collura G, et al. Minimally invasive laser treatment of ureterocele. Front Pediatr. 2019;7:106.
47. Kawauchi A, et al. Transvesical laparoscopic cross-trigonal ureteral reimplantation for correction of vesicoureteral reflux: initial experience and comparisons between adult and pediatric cases. J Endourol. 2009;23:1875–8.

48. Romao RL, et al. Laparoscopic ureteral ligation (clipping): a novel, simple procedure for pediatric urinary incontinence due to ectopic ureters associated with non-functioning upper pole renal moieties. J Pediatr Urol. 2014;10:1089–94.
49. Sander JC, Bilgutay AN, Stanasel I, Koh CJ, Janzen N, Gonzales ET, et al. Outcomes of endoscopic incision for the treatment of ureterocele in children at a single institution. J Urol. 2015;193(2):662–6.
50. Niknejad M. Ureterocele (cobra head sign). Case study, Radiopaedia.org. (Accessed on 15 Nov 2021). https://doi.org/10.53347/rID-61541

Chapter 6
Vesicoureteral Reflux

Fahad Alyami and Ziad M. Nakshabandi

Abstract Vesicoureteral reflex (VUR), which predisposes patients to recurrent pyelonephritis by permitting bacteria to reach the kidney, may lead to renal scarring and eventual renal impairment, hypertension, and chronic kidney disease. However, we now have a better understanding of the disease, thereby enabling less aggressive treatment of VUR. After proper diagnosis and exclusion of secondary VUR, we manage VUR conservatively, and reserve surgical intervention only for specific cases.

Keywords Vesicoureteral reflux · UTI · Hydronephrosis · Children

Learning Objectives
- This chapter discusses the overall incidence, natural history, types, presentation, and diagnosis of vesicoureteral reflex (VUR). After reading this chapter, the reader will be able to describe the predictors of spontaneous resolution, management goals, and different treatment options for VUR, especially in children.

Test your learning and check your understanding of this book's contents: use the "Springer Nature Flashcards" app to access questions. To use the app, please follow the instructions in Chapter 1.

F. Alyami (✉)
King Saud University, College of Medicine, King Faisal Specialist Hospital and Research Centre, Riyadh, Saudi Arabia
e-mail: faalyami@ksu.edu.sa

Z. M. Nakshabandi
National Center for Health Workforce Planning, SCFHS, Riyadh, Saudi Arabia
e-mail: z.nakshabandi@scfhs.org.sa

M. Abdel-Gawad et al. (eds.), *The Ureter*,
https://doi.org/10.1007/978-3-031-36212-5_6

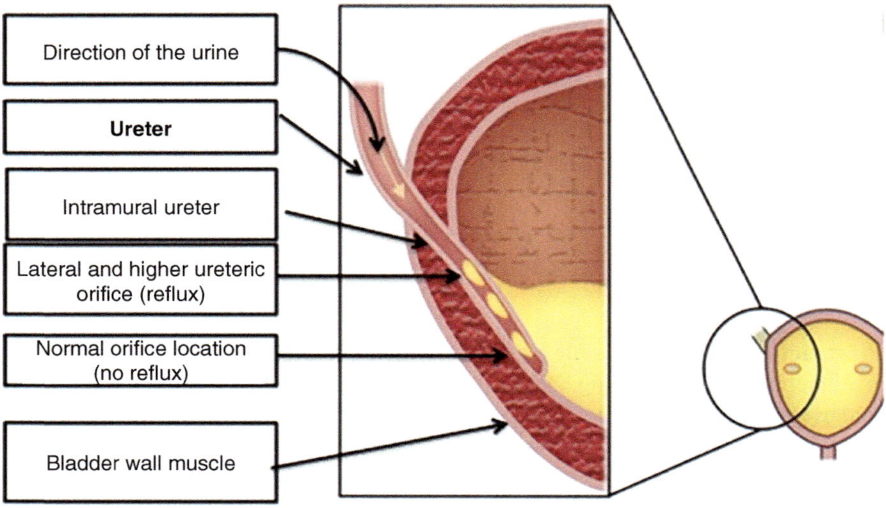

Fig. 6.1 anatomy of the ureterovesical junction

6.1 Introduction

Vesicoureteral reflux (VUR) is defined as the retrograde flow of urine from the bladder to the ureter and kidneys secondary to an incompetent ureterovesicoureteral junction (UVJ), which works as a one-way valve. Different factors play a role in creating this physiological valve, including the length of the submucosal tunnel, width of the ureteric orifice, presence of supporting bladder muscle at the trigone, and ureteral peristalsis [1, 2] (Fig. 6.1). VUR usually occurs during voiding due to an increase in bladder (intravesical) pressure, but it can also occur passively during filling. When assessing a patient with VUR, it is important to know if the reflux is caused by a deficient UVJ (primary VUR) or secondary to factors that compromise UVJ function, such as high intravesical pressures or other functional factors (secondary VUR). The management of secondary VUR should be directed at the underlying cause.

6.1.1 Prevalence

Although VUR is commonly seen in children, accurate assessment can be difficult owing to the tendency of spontaneous resolution and under-detection, especially in asymptomatic children. The overall incidence of VUR in the pediatric population was found to be 0.4–1.8% [3]. In contrast, the incidence of VUR is within 30–50% in children with urinary tract infection (UTI) and 15%–30% in children with antenatal hydronephrosis [4–6]. The rate of VUR is higher in males than in females in the first year of life, with prevalence rates shifting to 1:1 by 2 years of age. The diagnosis of VUR in infants was more predominant in males for antenatal screening than in females, who were predominantly diagnosed with after febrile UTI.

The incidence of VUR in siblings of children with VUR reaches 27% and decreases with age. Additionally, the incidence of VUR in the offspring of patients who were diagnosed with VUR was approximately 36%. As our understanding of the natural history and pathophysiology of VUR has improved, unnecessary invasive testing to diagnose it (in the absence of febrile UTI) is unwarranted. The AUA does not recommend VUR screening in siblings and offspring because the health benefits of identifying VUR in these patients has not been proven. It is recommended that this information be shared with the family to permit an informed decision recognizing that identifying and managing VUR may or may not be beneficial to the child [7].

Race also plays a role in the incidence of VUR. Children of African descent have a lower incidence of VUR than those of Caucasian descent. Girls of Asian descent are less likely to have scarring associated with reflux than Caucasian girls [8, 9].

6.1.2 *Grading of Reflux*

The International Reflux Grading System classifies VUR into five grades based on a voiding cystourethrogram (VCUG), which is commonly used for diagnosis (Fig. 6.2). Radionuclide cystogram (RNC) is another popular option to evaluate

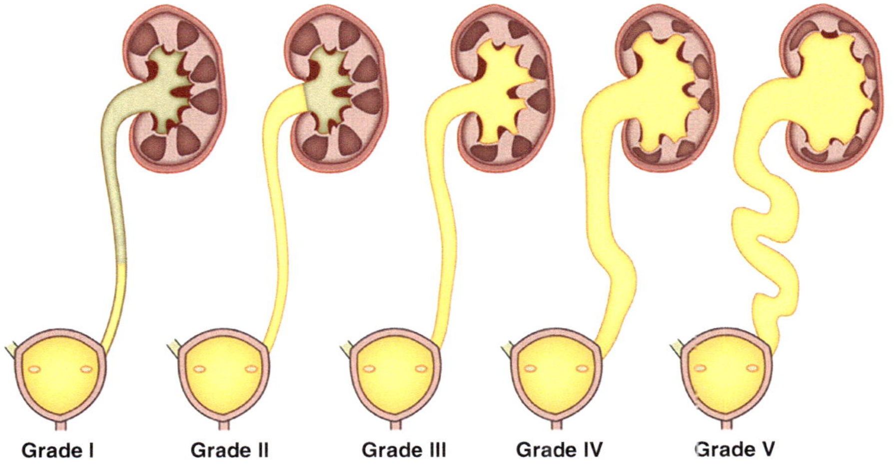

Fig. 6.2 Grading system for VUR. Grade 1: reflux in to non-dilated ureter. Grade 2: reflux in the pelvic and calyces without dilation. Grade 3: mild to moderate dilation of the ureter and pelvic. Grade4: moderate dilation and/or tortuosity of the ureter with some blunting of the calyces. Grade 5: sever dilation and tortuosity of the ureter, renal pelvic and calyces with blunting of the calyces

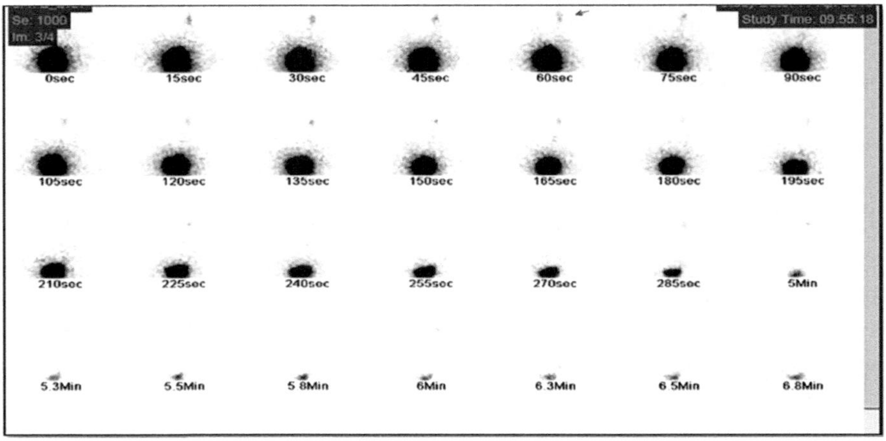

Fig. 6.3 Nuclear voiding cystography shows right VUR

VUR and it has a different grading system. Some pediatric urologists use it for follow-up only (Fig. 6.3) [10].

The use of a grading system helps us understand the natural history of the disease, predict the possible resolution rate, and individualize our management of children with VUR based on risk stratification and evidence-based data.

6.1.3 Natural History of Primary VUR

Spontaneous resolution is one of the main hallmarks of primary VUR in children, and we rely on it mostly when embarking on a conservative management approach. Different factors play a role in predicting the resolution of VUR, including sex, age at presentation, grade, laterality, and mode of clinical presentation [11]. Remodeling of the UVJ in a stable bladder dynamic helps the body overcome VUR as children grow. Boys with VUR have a greater likelihood of spontaneous resolution within the first year of life than do girls. A resolution rate of 29% was reported in boys aged <1 year with VUR grades IV and V. The same study reported that, in both girls and boys after their first year of life, the annual reported resolution rate was only 9% [12].

The chance of spontaneous resolution is higher when patients are younger than one year at presentation, have a lower grade of reflux (grade I–III), and are asymptomatic (antenatal hydronephrosis) [11]. A meta-analysis performed by the AUA in 2010 revealed an overall VUR resolution rate in infants less than one year of 49.9 per 100 patients and 52.0 per 100 renal units, with a range of follow-up times between 12 and 48 months. In children over one year, the overall resolution rate was 53.2 per 100 children, with the highest rates occurring between 24 and 36 months (range, 2–71 months) [13]. The AUA Vesicoureteral Reflux Practice Guidelines Committee analyzed raw data from multiple published series (Fig. 6.4). Persistence

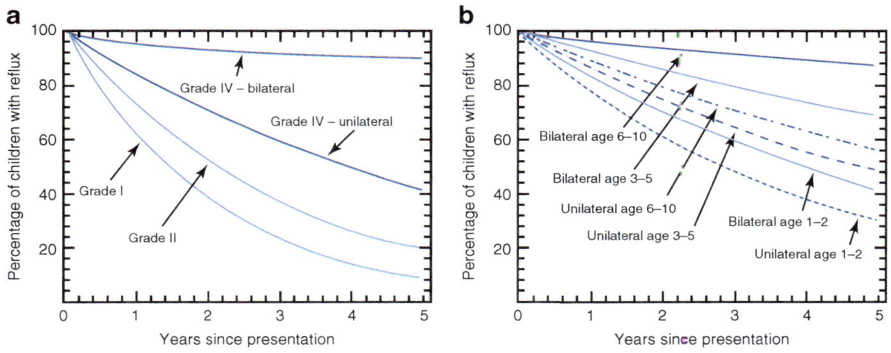

Fig. 6.4 The likelihood of spontaneous VUR resolution in percentages of patients with VUR followed up to 1–5 years: (**a**) for VUR grades I, II, and IV and (**b**) for VUR grade III by patient age at presentation. Reproduced with permission from "Pediatric Vesicoureteral Reflux Guidelines Panel Summary Report on the Management of Primary Vesicoureteral Reflux in Children, J S Elder, C A Peters, B S Arant Jr et al., Journal of urology Urol, 1997 May;157(5):1846–51"

of VUR is more common in patients with higher grades (IV–V), bilateral VUR, ureteral dilation, and in those with prior evidence of renal scarring. Spontaneous resolution of the reflux occurs in a proportion of children with duplicated collecting systems and reflux into the lower pole moiety, similar to that seen in single-system reflux, but it might take a longer time to resolve. The presence of renal cortical abnormalities, bladder dysfunction, and breakthrough febrile UTI are negative predictive factors for reflux resolution [14–16].

Few tools were published to help us predict the rate of VUR resolution. Estrada et al. 2009 developed a nomogram to predict spontaneous resolution rates, taking in consideration VUR grade and 2 years follow-up (the resolution rates for grades I, II, III, and IV/V were 72%, 61%, 49%, and 32%, respectively) [17]. The Vesicoureteral Reflux Index (VURI) developed by Kirsch et al. is a novel and validated prediction tool that incorporates timing of reflux, presence of associated anomalies, sex, and VUR grade to predict complete or partial resolution of reflux by at least two grades. It has been validated for children younger than and older than 24 months of age, and they reported that female sex, high-grade VUR, ureteral anomalies, and filling reflux are associated with a longer time to improvement and non-resolution.

6.2 Diagnosis and Presentation

6.2.1 Antenatal presentation

With the widespread use of prenatal US, antenatal hydronephrosis (ANH) has become a common finding [18, 19]. The need for routine postnatal VCUG for all newborns with ANH has decreased, as we have a better understanding of VUR and reflux is found to be a benign disease in the absence of febrile UTI. Studies found VUR to be present in 17% (range, 1–40%) of children with history of antenatal US and postnatal US confirmation. VCUG is performed in children with high-grade Society of Fetal Urology grade 3–4 hydronephrosis, bilateral hydronephrosis in boys, ureteral dilation, or other anatomical abnormalities, such as ureterocele, duplication anomalies, or neurogenic bladder. This cultural shift in evaluation and the decrease in the routine use of VCUG, might lead to a change in the reported prevalence of VUR in children with ANH. Additionally, studies have found that boys are more affected by VUR during workup for ANH [20].

6.2.2 Urinary Tract Infections (UTIs)

Febrile UTI is a common and important clinical pediatric diagnosis. We treat it aggressively and try to avoid recurrence to preserve the upper tract and prevent long-term complications, including renal scarring, hypertension, and end-stage renal disease. Imaging plays an important role in the assessment of children with a history of febrile UTI to identify any abnormalities of the urinary tract that require additional evaluation or management. A consensus regarding the optimal imaging strategy for children after the first febrile UTI is lacking; however, there is agreement on the need for US as it is a non-invasive test that can help stratify patients and assess the upper and lower urinary tracts. The American Academy of Pediatrics recommends US for all infants and children aged 2–24 months after their first febrile UTI [21].

Voiding cystourethrography (VCUG) is the test of choice for assessing the presence and grade of VUR (Fig. 6.5). It is an expensive and invasive diagnostic tool that poses a risk of radiation exposure in children. The decision to perform VCUG for infants and children should consider the likelihood of VUR, severity, and recurrence of UTI. We perform VCUG for children with (1) recurrent febrile UTI, (2) febrile UTI with abnormal anatomical findings on US, (3) febrile UTI with high-grade fever >39 °C with an atypical organism other than *E. coli*, (4) febrile UTI with a family history of VUR, and 5) family preference after febrile UTI.

The RIVUR trail (randomized intervention for vesicoureteral reflux) reported that 81% of the 607 children with VUR diagnosed after febrile or symptomatic UTI reached 92% female [22]. Radionuclide cystogram (RNC) is an alternative modality for diagnosis but it is not popular due to poor anatomical details and chance of missing low grade VUR (Fig. 6.3). RNC can be used to monitor reflux resolution during follow-up. Dimercaptosuccinic acid (DMSA) is another imaging modality used to assess children with VUR or recurrent febrile UTI (Fig. 6.6). It is mainly used to detect acute pyelonephritis in the acute setting and renal scarring during follow-up. It is beyond the scope of this chapter to elaborate on the indication for DMSA in children with febrile UTI in general. There is no consensus about the proper use of DMSA in VUR assessment; in our practice, we tend to perform DMSA for the following: 1) children with a history of recurrent febrile UTI with any grade of VUR, 2) high-grade VUR as a baseline in case of developing UTI, and 3) VUR in a single functioning kidney.

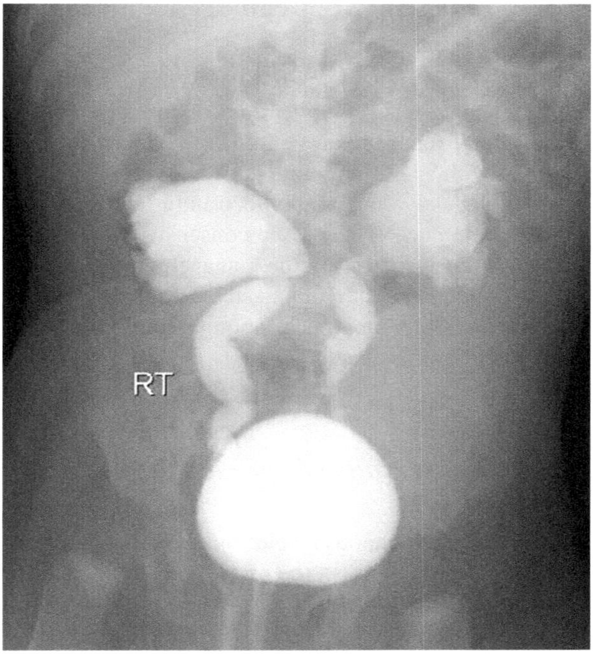

Fig. 6.5 The figure shows voiding cystourethrogram (VCUG) of one-year old boy with bilateral grade V vesicoureteral reflux. From the courtesy of Dr. Bedeir Ali-El-Dein

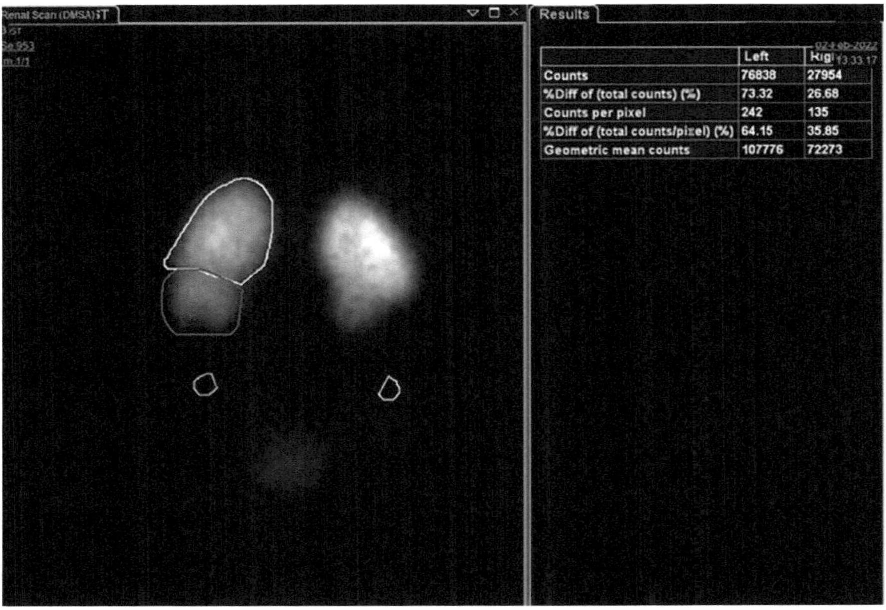

Fig. 6.6 This is 99 mTC-DMSA scan. It shows Multiple photopenic areas o: patches of pyelonephritis and scarring in both kidneys secondary to vesicoureteral reflux. From the courtesy of Dr. Bedeir Ali-El-Dein

6.3 Management of Children with Primary VUR

The goals of management are to prevent UTI, preserve the upper urinary tract; and avoid any long-term complications of untreated VUR, such as renal scarring, hypertension, and renal impairment. Many factors must be considered when managing children with VUR, including the VUR grade, laterality, history of UTI, presence of bladder bowel dysfunction, toilet training status, patient and family compliance, and family preference. There is no consensus on the optimal management in children, and there are variations in the management approach among guidelines and practitioners. The use of individualized care and risk stratification is becoming a popular and well-accepted approach among pediatric urologists, and will be discussed in more detail in this chapter.

6.3.1 Conservative Approach

The overall spontaneous resolution rate of VUR in infants aged 1–4 years can reach up to 50% (girls > boys); the resolution rate is high in infants, and VUR resolves at a yearly rate of 9% after infancy. During follow-up, the spontaneous resolution rate (72% for grade I, 61% for grade II, 49% for grade III, and 32% for grade IV–V) and the resolution rate were higher when the VUR grade was lower, VUR was bilateral, patients were younger, and VUR was detected on screening for patients with fetal hydronephrosis or suspected familial VUR [23]. The spontaneous resolution rate for high-grade (grades IV and V) congenital VUR was high in boys during the infant year (29%), whereas in girls and boys, the infant year the resolution rate was 9% yearly during follow-up. The negative prognostic factors for resolution were recurrent UTI and bladder dysfunction [24].

As pediatric urologists, we rely on spontaneous resolution of VUR and consider it a benign disease. Spontaneous resolution can take time, and we aimed to optimize the bladder and the remainder of the urinary tract condition to prevent UTI.

For children who are not toilet-trained and have VUR diagnosed as part of hydronephrosis work-up, follow-up observation with optional continuous antibiotic prophylaxis (CAP) is recommended for grades I–II; whereas, CAP is recommended for grade III or higher, and should also be considered in patients with a history of febrile UTI. Trimethoprim and sulfamethoxazole have been used in combination in many clinical studies and are considered standard medications. However, they should not be administered to infants aged <2 months. Thrombotic thrombocytopenic purpura and hemolytic-uremic syndrome are listed as serious adverse reactions on the package insert, and adequate observation by blood tests is necessary. Instead, ampicillin, amoxicillin, and cephalexin are appropriate prophylactic drugs for children aged <3 months [25].

For toilet-trained children, follow-up observation is recommended for grades I–II VUR without renal scarring, whereas CAP is recommended for those with grades III–V VUR with renal scarring. In the RIVUR trial, children with grade III or IV VUR were more likely to have febrile or symptomatic UTI than those with grade I or II (23% vs. 14 percent) [22]. CAP is also recommended if they have bowel bladder dysfunction (BBD) as they are at a higher risk of developing UTI, and it can be stopped if the BBD is rehabilitated.

CAP is a widely accepted option and the cornerstone for a conservative approach for VUR, as it prevents recurrent episodes of febrile UTI and consequent new renal scars. The RIVUR trial showed that using a combination of trimethoprim and sulfamethoxazole reduced the occurrence of UTI by approximately 50% (from 27.4% to 14.8%) in patients aged 2–71 months with VUR diagnosed after the first UTI but did not prevent new renal scarring. Additionally, there was a higher risk of UTI due to antibiotic-resistant bacteria in the CAP group (68.4% vs 24.6%), which is a well-documented side-effect of antibiotic prophylaxis [22].

Boys with urinary tract abnormalities, specifically VUR, benefit greatly from newborn circumcision in the prevention of UTIs. Early circumcision may be considered as part of the conservative approach because it is effective in reducing the risk of infection in children without abnormalities as the risk of UTI is approximately 1% and the number-needed-to-treat to prevent one UTI is 111 [26]. In boys with recurrent UTI or high-grade VUR, the risk of UTI recurrence was 10% and 30%, respectively; and the numbers-needed-to-treat are 11 and 4, respectively [26].

The choice between CAP and follow-up observation should be based on different patient characteristics, including age, history of febrile UTI, presence of voiding dysfunction or BBD, and the presence of dilating hydronephrosis or high-grade VUR (grade III to IV). In our practice, the Indications for CAP are (1) patients with a history of febrile UTI awaiting work-up, (2) all patients who are not toilet-trained with any grade of VUR regardless of the severity of grade, (3) all toilet trained patients with BBD regardless of the severity of VUR, and (4) all patients with high-grade reflux (grade III to IV). As BBD becomes apparent after toilet training, we will discuss the indications for CAP before and after toilet training.

6.3.1.1 Before Toilet Training

If VUR is diagnosed as part of the ANH work-up or is an incidental finding of hydronephrosis with no history of UTI; it is recommended that CAP should be started for grade III or higher VUR and it is optional for grades I–II VUR.

CAP is recommended irrespective of the severity of VUR if the patient has a history of febrile UTI, especially in patients aged <1 year. It is optional to stop CAP for patients aged 1 year old with grades I–II VUR, and if this option is taken, proper family counseling, which includes discussing the risks and benefits of management, should be taken into consideration.

6.3.1.2 After Toilet-training

As the chances of having a UTI decrease significantly in children with VUR after toilet training, CAP is stopped at that age. CAP is recommended for patients with any VUR grade in the presence of renal cortical abnormalities or scarring, even after toilet training.

In the presence of BBD, given that the risk of febrile UTI is high, it is recommended that CAP should be continued for all grades of VUR and focus placed on addressing the BBD before we stop CAP. If the child develops febrile UTI and fails medical treatment, it is recommended to treat the BBD before any surgical options, to increase the success rate and prevent VUR recurrence.

6.3.2 *Timing of Discontinuation of CAP*

Currently, there is no clear consensus on the proper timing of CAP discontinuation. The classic and well-supported approach in the literature is to continue up to the age of toilet training [27–32]. Some advocate stopping at 1–2 years of age, especially for low-grade reflux (grade I–II) [33]. Re-initiation of CAP is recommended for any new-onset or recurrence of breakthrough UTI.

6.3.3 *Treatment of BBD*

Behavioral therapy is the cornerstone in managing BBD in toilet-trained children with VUR. Patients are encouraged to empty the bladder and bowel regularly, and a voiding diary can be a good monitoring tool in the clinic.

Treatment of constipation by increasing fluid and fiber intake, dietary modification, and the use of laxatives, if indicated, is also an important aspect in the management of children with VUR and BBD.

Biofeedback therapy can be an option in children aged ≥5 years, especially if they have voiding dysfunction with or without detrusor sphincter dyssynergia on uroflowmetry and electromyography (EMG) [34]. This approach helps patients understand the contraction of the pelvic floor muscles, and this understanding will be used to improve lower urinary tract function.

6.3.4 *Surgical Options and Indication*

The indications for surgical intervention are controversial and include the following (1) breakthrough UTI and failed medical management; (2) girls older than 6 years with persistent VUR (especially grade III or higher); and (3) presence of renal scarring and no resolution of VUR after the age of toilet training.

Some indications are controversial and are considered as relative inductions: (1) high-grade VUR, especially bilateral to avoid poor bladder emptying and cycling; (2) the presence of renal impairment (at detection or during follow-up); (3) recurrent UTI in children who are toilet-trained and are not candidates for a prolonged course of CAP; (4) high-grade VUR with lower urinary tract dysfunction; and (5) poor compliance to CAP with recurrent UTI or the presence of renal scarring.

6.3.5 *Endoscopic Injection*

The reflux resolution rate after endoscopic injection was lower than that after ureteric reimplantation surgery, which is one of the most widely used minimally invasive options with better results for low-grade VUR. Metanalysis showed that the reflux resolution rate after the first endoscopic injection was 74%. The resolution rates of grade II, grade III, and grade IV VUR were 79%, 72%, and 63%, respectively [35]. The incidence of UTI was lower after endoscopic injection than after open surgery (15% vs. 38%), and the incidence of febrile UTI was also lower after endoscopic injection than after open surgery (5% vs. 24%) [36]. The VUR resolution rate after open surgery was unaffected by the presence of BBD, whereas it was significantly lower after the endoscopic approach [13]. The success rate of endoscopic therapy is even lower in children with anatomical abnormalities, such as duplication anomalies, BBD, or neurogenic bladder. Possible complications of the endoscopic approach include new-onset contralateral VUR, ureteral obstruction, or persistence of VUR.

6.3.6 *Open Surgery for VUR*

Open surgical reimplantation of the ureters is a highly successful procedure, with reported success rates of 95–99%, regardless of the severity of VUR [13]. Open reimplantation procedures are based on the basic technique described by Politano and Leadbetter, and include the following approaches:

- Intravesical approach:
- The bladder is opened, and the ureters are reimplanted by tunneling a ureteral segment through the detrusor muscle to create a submucosal tunnel with a length-to-diameter ratio of 5: 1, by applying Paquin's rule. Modifications of the basic technique, described by Politano and Leadbetter, are named after surgeons who developed each of the variants (e.g., Cohen and Glenn-Anderson). The Cohen cross-trigonal reimplantation is the most common open surgical procedure used to treat pediatric VUR.
- Extravesical approach
- In this approach, reimplantation is performed without opening the bladder, by creating a tunnel through opening the bladder muscle, tunneling the ureter between the muscle and mucosa and closing the muscles on it (Lich-Gregoir

reimplantation procedure). The Lich-Gregoir procedure is a commonly performed procedure for VUR in the pediatric population especially for children with unilateral VUR. Studies showed some children who underwent bilateral extravesical ureteral reimplantation might experience a transient voiding dysfunction and it tends to resolve after few weeks of clean intermittent catheterization.

The success rate of open surgery has been proven to be high, irrespective of the technique used, and it is indicated for patients with anatomical or functional abnormalities of the urinary tract (e.g., BBD and duplicated ureter). The success rates of open surgery for primary VUR were reported to be as high as 95–99%, irrespective of the severity [13]. Studies also show that in open surgery, the success rate between groups with BBD and those without BBD were 88.4–100% vs. 92–100%, respectively [37, 38].

6.3.7 Laparoscopic and Robotic Surgery for VUR

1. Intravesical approach

   The laparoscopic transvesical Cohen's technique has a success rate (91–96%) close to that of open surgery [39–46]. However, the learning curve and difficulty of the procedure are the two limiting factors affecting the adoption of this technique among pediatric urologists. Possible complications include intraperitoneal urine leakage and anastomotic strictures. The incidence of complications was higher with a smaller bladder capacity; younger patients and proper patient selection helped decrease the complication rate. Laparoscopic Politano–Leadbetter technique has high reported success rate of up to 94% [47].
2. Extravesical approach

   This approach has an advantage over the intravesical laparoscopic approach, because it has a larger working space. The reported success rate is similar to that of open surgery (93.5–100%) [48]. Bladder dysfunction, including urinary retention, is a potential complication after any type of extravesical ureteric reimplantation; with incidences of 6.5% after laparoscopic surgery [49] and was approximately 3–20% after open surgery [50, 51].
3. Robot-assisted surgery.

   Robot-assisted ureteric reimplantation using the extravesical approach is commonly adopted by pediatric urologists. Two case series reported comparable outcomes between robot-assisted reimplantation and the open approach in children with VUR [52, 53]. Multicenter reviews from different tertiary centers showed lower success rates and higher complication rates associated with robot-assisted reimplantation than with open reimplantation.

Robot-assisted ureteric reimplantation is widely utilized over the laparoscopic approach, and it overcomes the technical difficulties surgeons face in performing pelvic surgery laparoscopically owing to the limited working space. Comparatively, robot-assisted surgery and the laparoscopic approach had similar success rates

(92–93%), with no reported serious complications. Unsurprisingly, the cost of robot-assisted ureteric reimplantation was reported to be significantly higher than that of laparoscopic surgery, and the learning curve is shorter and easier to adopt.

6.4 Summary

In managing VUR, secondary VUR should be ruled out, as it requires a different management approach than that for primary VUR. Spontaneous resolution is one hallmark of primary VUR in children and we rely on it when we embark on conservative management approach. In our practice, we moved toward individualized care, risk stratification, and predictive models to guide our management approach and provide our patients with the best care needed with minimal morbidity.

Questions

1. 1-month-old baby boy with history of left antenatal hydronephrosis and developed an attack of febrile UTI, which was treated with intravenous antibiotics. His US showed an SFU grade 3 Lt hydronephrosis. The most appropriate next step is:
   (a) Follow up US after 3 months.
   (b) Voiding cystourethrogram.
   (c) Nuclear cystogram
   (d) Cystoscopy

Answer: (b)

2. The best modality to diagnose VUR is:
   (a) Voiding cystourethrogram (VCUG).
   (b) Nuclear cystogram.
   (c) Magnetic resonance urography (MRU)
   (d) Cystoscopy

Answer: (a)

3. Two weeks old girl diagnosed with left SFU grade IV VUR as part of her antenatal hydronephrosis work up. If a decision was taken to start her on antibiotic prophylaxis. What is the most appropriate antibiotic for her?
   (a) Cefuroxime
   (b) Nitrofurantoin
   (c) Amoxicillin
   (d) Sulfamethoxazole and trimethoprim

Answer: (c)

4. Which of the following is an absolute indication for surgery for a child with VUR?
   (a) 4 Years old boy with recurrent febrile UTI despite CAP and no BBD.
   (b) 2 years old boy with bilateral VUR and bilateral renal scarring.
   (c) 2 years old boy with left grade V VUR and reduced left kidney function (35%).
   (d) 6 years old boy with bilateral grade 3 VUR.

Answer: (a)

5. In open ureteric reimplantion the length-to-diameter ratio needed is:
   (a) 4:1
   (b) 5:1
   (c) 3:1
   (d) 2:1

Answer: (b)

References

1. Paquin AJJ. Ureterovesical anastomosis: the description and evaluation of a technique. J Urol. 1959;82:573–83.
2. Cussen LJ. Dimensions of the normal ureter in infancy and childhood. Investig Urol. 1967;5:164–78.
3. Bailey RR. Vesicoureteral reflux in healthy infants and children. In: Hodson CJ, Kincaid-Smith P, editors. Reflux nephropathy. New York: Masson; 1979. p. 59–61.
4. Smellie JM, Normand IC. Clinical features and significance of urinary tract infection in children. Proc R Soc Med. 1966;59:415–6.
5. Berrocal T, Pinilla I, Gutiérrez J, et al. Mild hydronephrosis in newborns and infants: can ultrasound predict the presence of vesicoureteral reflux. Pediatr Nephrol. 2007;22(1):91–6.
6. Garne E, Loane M, Wellesley D, et al. Eurocat Working Group: congenital hydronephrosis: prenatal diagnosis and epidemiology in Europe. J Pediatr Urol. 2009;5(1):47–52.
7. https://www.auanet.org/guidelines/guidelines/vesicoureteral-reflux-guideline#x3317
8. Chand DH, Rhoades T, Poe SA, et al. Incidence and severity of vesicoureteral reflux in children related to age, gender, race and diagnosis. J Urol. 2003;170(4):1548–50.
9. Howard RG, Roebuck DJ, Yeung PA, Chan KW, Metreweli C. Vesicoureteric reflux and renal scarring in Chinese children. Br J Radiol. 2001;74:331–4.
10. Willi U, Treves S. Radionuclide voiding cystography. Urol Radiol. 1983;5:161–73.
11. Estrada CR Jr, Passerotti CC, Graham DA, et al. Nomograms for predicting annual resolution rate of primary vesicoureteral reflux: results from 2,462 children. J Urol. 2009;182:1535–41.
12. Sjöström S, Sillén U, Bachelard M, Hansson S, Stokland E. Spontaneous resolution of high grade infantile vesicoureteral reflux. J Urol. 2004;172:694–8.
13. Peters CA, Skoog SJ, Arant BS Jr, et al. Summary of the AUA guideline on management of primary vesicoureteral reflux in children. J Urol. 2010;184:1134–44.
14. Knudson MJ, Austin JC, McMillan ZM, et al. Predictive factors of early spontaneous resolution in children with primary vesicoureteral reflux. J Urol. 2007;178:1684–8.
15. Yeung CK, Sreedhar B, Sihoe JD, et al. Renal and bladder functional status at diagnosis as predictive factors for the outcome of primary vesicoureteral reflux in children. J Urol. 2006;176:1152–6. discussion 1156–7

16. Sjöström S, Sillén U, Jodal U, Sameby L, Sixt R, Stokland E. Predictive factors for resolution of congenital high grade vesicoureteral reflux in infants: results of univariate and multivariate analyses. J Urol. 2010;183:1177–84.
17. Kirsch AJ, Arlen AM, Leong T, Merriman LS, Herrel LA, Scherz HC, Smith EA, Srinivasan AK. Vesicoureteral reflux index (VURx): a novel tool to predict primary reflux improvement and resolution in children less than 2 years of age. J Pediatr Urol. 2014;10(6):1249–54.
18. Blyth B, Snyder HM, Duckett JW. Antenatal diagnosis and subsequent management of hydronephrosis. J Urol. 1993;149:693.
19. Robyr R, Benachi A, Daikha-Dahmane F, et al. Correlation between ultrasound and anatomical findings in fetuses with lower urinary tract obstruction in the first half of pregnancy. Ultrasound Obstet Gynecol. 2005;25:478.
20. Yeung CK, Godley ML, Dhillon HK, et al. The characteristics of primary vesico-ureteric reflux in male and female infants with pre-natal hydronephrosis. Br J Urol. 1997;80:319.
21. SUBCOMMITTEE ON URINARY TRACT INFECTION. Reaffirmation of AAP Clinical Practice Guideline: the diagnosis and management of the initial urinary tract infection in febrile infants and young children 2-24 months of age. Pediatrics. 2016;138:e20163026.
22. Hoberman A, Greenfield SP, Mattoo TK, et al. Antimicrobial prophylaxis for children with vesicoureteral reflux. N Engl J Med. 2014;370:2367–76.
23. Hollowell JG. Outcome of pregnancy in women with a history of vesico-ureteric reflux. BJU Int. 2008;102:780–4.
24. Sjöström S, Sillén U, Bachelard M, Hansson S, Stokland E. Spontaneous resolution of high grade infantile vesicoureteral reflux. J Urol. 2004;172(2):694–8. discussion 699
25. Nickavar A, Sotoudeh K. Treatment and prophylaxis in pediatric urinary tract infection. Int J Prev Med. 2011;2(1):4–9.
26. Singh-Grewal D, Macdessi J, Craig J. Circumcision for the prevention of urinary tract infection in boys: a systematic review of randomised trials and observational studies. Arch Dis Child. 2005;90:853.
27. Thompson RH, Chen JJ, Pugach J, Naseer S, Steinhardt GF. Cessation of prophylactic antibiotics for managing persistent vesicoureteral reflux. J Urol. 2001;166:1465–9.
28. Al-Sayyad AJ, Pike JG, Leonard MP. Can prophylactic antibiotics safely be discontinued in children with vesicoureteral reflux? J Urol. 2005;174(4 Pt 2):1587–9.
29. Alconcher LF, Meneguzzi MB, Buschiazzo R, Piaggio LA. Could prophylactic antibiotics be stopped in patients with history of vesicoureteral reflux? J Pediatr Urol. 2009;5:383–8.
30. Kitchens DM, Herndon A, Joseph DB. Outcome after discontinuing prophylactic antibiotics in children with persistent vesicoureteral reflux. J Urol. 2010;184(4 Suppl):1594–7.
31. Leslie B, Moore K, Salle JL, et al. Outcome of antibiotic prophylaxis discontinuation in patients with persistent vesicoureteral reflux initially presenting with febrile urinary tract infection: time to event analysis. J Urol. 2010;184:1093–8.
32. Drzewiecki BA, Thomas JC, Pope JC 4th, Adams MC, Brock JW 3rd, Tanaka ST. Observation of patients with vesicoureteral reflux off antibiotic prophylaxis: physician bias on patient selection and risk factors for recurrent febrile urinary tract infection. J Urol. 2012;188(4 Suppl):1480–4.
33. Moriya K, Mitsui T, Kitta T, et al. Early discontinuation of antibiotic prophylaxis in patients with persistent primary vesicoureteral reflux initially detected during infancy: Outcome analysis and risk factors for febrile urinary tract infection. J Urol. 2015;193:637–42.
34. Alyami F, Ewida T, Alhazmi H, Trbay M, Arafa M, Tahir M, Neel KF. Biofeedback as single first-line treatment for non-neuropathic dysfunctional voiding children with diurnal enuresis. Can Urol Assoc J. 2018;13(1):E7–9.
35. Elder JS, Diaz M, Caldamone AA, et al. Endoscopic therapy for vesicoureteral reflux: a meta-analysis. I. Reflux resolution and urinary tract infection. J Urol. 2006;175:716–22.
36. Lmore JM, Kirsch AJ, Heiss EA, Gilchrist A, Scherz HC. Incidence of urinary tract infections in children after successful ureteral reimplantation versus endoscopic dextranomer/hyaluronic acid implantation. J Urol. 2008;179:2364–7.

37. Aboutaleb H, Bolduc S, Bagli DJ, Khoury AE. Correlataion of vesicoureteral reflux with degree of hydronephrosis and the impact of antireflux surgery. J Urol. 2003;170:1560–2.
38. Lavine MA, Siddig FM, Cahn DJ, Caesar RE, Koyle MA, Caldamone AA. Vesicoureteral reflux after ureteroneocystostomy: indications for postoperative voiding cystography. Tech Urol. 2001;7:50–4.
39. Yeung CK, Sihoe JD, Borzi PA. Endoscopic cross-trigonal ureteral reimplantation under carbon dioxide bladder insufflation: a novel technique. J Endourol. 2005;19:295–9.
40. Kutikov A, Guzzo TJ, Canter DJ, Casale P. Initial experience with laparoscopic transvesical ureteral reimplantation at the Children's Hospital of Philadelphia. J Urol. 2006;176:2222–5.
41. Kawauchi A, Naitoh Y, Soh J, Hirahara N, Okihara K, Miki T. Transvesical laparoscopic cross-trigonal ureteral reimplantation for correction of vesicoureteral reflux: initial experience and comparisons between adult and pediatric cases. J Endourol. 2009;23:1875–8.
42. Canon SJ, Jayanthi VR, Patel AS. Vesicoscopic cross-trigonal ureteral reimplantation: a minimally invasive option for repair of vesicoureteral reflux. J Urol. 2007;178:269–73.
43. Chung MS, Han SW, Jung HJ, et al. Transvesicoscopic ureteral reimplantation in children with bilateral vesicoureteral reflux: surgical technique and results. J Laparoendosc Adv Surg Tech A. 2012;22:295–300.
44. Hong CH, Kim JH, Jung HJ, Im YJ, Han SW. Single-surgeon experience with transvesicoscopic ureteral reimplantation in children with vesicoureteral reflux. Urology. 2011;77:1465–9.
45. Emir H, Mammadov E, Elicevik M, Buyukunal C, Soylet Y. Transvesicoscopic cross-trigonal ureteroneocystostomy in children: a single-center experience. J Pediatr Urol. 2012;8:83–6.
46. Valla JS, Steyaert H, Griffin SJ, et al. Transvesicoscopic Cohen ureteric reimplantation for vesicoureteral reflux in children: a single-centre 5-year experience. J Pediatr Urol. 2009;5:466–71.
47. Soh S, Kobori Y, Shin T, et al. Transvesicoscopic ureteral reimplantation: Politano-Leadbetter versus Cohen technique. Int J Urol. 2015;22:394–9.
48. Riquelme M, Aranda A, Rodriguez C. Laparoscopic extravesical transperitoneal approach for vesicoureteral reflux. J Laparoendosc Adv Surg Tech A. 2006;16:312–6.
49. Bayne AP, Shoss JM, Starke NR, Cisek LJ. Single-center experience with pediatric laparoscopic extravesical reimplantation: safe and effective in simple and complex anatomy. J Laparoendosc Adv Surg Tech A. 2012;22:102–6.
50. David S, Kelly C, Poppas DP. Nerve sparing extravesical repair of bilateral vesicoureteral reflux: description of technique and evaluation of urinary retention. J Urol. 2004;172(4 Pt 2):1617–20.
51. Heidenreich A, Ozgur E, Becker T, Haupt G. Surgical management of vesicoureteral reflux in pediatric patients. World J Urol. 2004;22:96–106.
52. Hayashi Y, Mizuno K, Kurokawa S, et al. Extravesical robot-assisted laparoscopic ureteral reimplantation for vesicoureteral reflux: initial experience in Japan with the ureteral advancement technique. Int J Urol. 2014;21:1016–21.
53. Schober MS, Jayanthi VR. Vesicoscopic ureteral reimplant: is there a role in the age of robotics? Urol Clin North Am. 2015;42:53–9.

Chapter 7
Radiology and Imaging of the Ureter

Mostafa El-Ksas, Hashim Farg, and Tarek A. El-Diasty

Abstract The ureter is responsible for a significant share of urinary tract problems, such as renal colic, flank pain, hematuria and impaired renal function.

There are multiple, different imaging modalities to examine the ureters and identify ureteric lesions. Proper choice of imaging technique provides an opportunity for accurate diagnosis and proper treatment; however, a definite diagnosis sometimes requires endoscopic techniques, biopsy and/or surgical excision and histopathological examination.

In this chapter, we will explore the different radiological modalities used in the evaluation of ureter. The radiological techniques of different imaging studies will be highlighted.

Keywords Ureter · Urinary tract · Imaging · X-Ray · IVU · US · CT · MRI · Calculus · UC

Test your learning and check your understanding of this book's contents: use the "Springer Nature Flashcards" app to access questions. To use the app, please follow the instructions in Chapter 1.

M. El-Ksas
Specialist of diagnostic radiology, medical imaging and interventional radiology, Radiology Department, Urology and Nephrology Center, Mansoura University, Mansoura, Egypt

H. Farg
Fellow of diagnostic radiology, medical imaging and interventional radiology, Radiology Department, Urology and Nephrology Center, Mansoura University, Mansoura, Egypt

T. A. El-Diasty (✉)
Consultant of diagnostic radiology, medical imaging and interventional radiology, Radiology Department, Urology and Nephrology Center, Mansoura University, Mansoura, Egypt

M. Abdel-Gawad et al. (eds.), *The Ureter*,
https://doi.org/10.1007/978-3-031-36212-5_7

7.1 Introduction

Until the 1970s, the main radiologic evaluation required ureteric opacification during excretory urography, retrograde pyelography or antegrade nephroureterography. Ultrasonography (US), computerized tomography (CT), magnetic resonance imaging (MRI) have come to replace those earlier techniques.

The ureter is a muscular conduit that carries urine from the renal pelvis to the urinary bladder. It arises proximally from the renal pelvis at the ureteropelvic junction (UPJ) and empties distally into the urinary bladder at the ureterovesical junction (UVJ). It remains retroperitoneal throughout its course, has an approximate length of 25 cm, and has a normal diameter of less than 3 mm. Histologically, it has an inner cell layer of watertight urothelium surrounded by an outer smooth muscle layer with coordinated contractions [1].

The ureter is responsible for a significant share of urinary tract problems such as renal colic, flank pain, hematuria and impaired renal function. Because of its retroperitoneal position, thin caliber and long course it is often difficult to diagnose ureteric lesions by conventional imaging methods such as plain X-Ray, US or intravenous urography (IVU). Because of its small caliber, small ureteric lesions may completely obstruct its lumen and cause obstructive nephropathy [2].

Close association of the abdomino-pelvic viscera and blood vessels places the ureter at risk for inflammatory, infectious, or malignant processes of the intestines, appendix, prostate, oviducts, uterus, ovaries, aorta, iliac vessels and for complications of surgery on these structures [3].

The ureter has 3 physiologic narrowings: (a) the UPJ, (b) the crossing over the iliac vessels (c) the UVJ. These narrowings may result in ureteric stones becoming trapped and obstructing at these specific levels. These narrowings may also limit retrograde instrumentation performed for diagnostic or therapeutic purposes. The close association of the ovarian vessels at the level of the pelvic brim and the uterine artery in the rectouterine fold render the ureters subject to injury during oophorectomy or hysterectomy, as they are just deep to the crucial vasculature [3].

The diagnosis, screening and evaluation of ureteric lesions is usually by imaging studies however, a definite diagnosis is only obtained, in certain cases, by endoscopy, biopsy and sometimes surgical excision and histopathological examination.

Cross-sectional imaging with CT and/or MRI has become the diagnostic routine for the study of patients with ureteric lesions. CT is more widely available than MRI, however both modalities allow comprehensive evaluation of the ureter and surrounding structures. Other CT advantages include the use of curved planar reformatted images, multiplanar reconstruction (MPR), maximum intensity projection (MIP) and three-dimensional (3D) reconstruction. The detectability of air and calcifications is usually better using CT scan than MRI, although these conditions can also be detected on MRI. MRI is currently considered as a problem-solving imaging technique if CT is not diagnostic. MRI is also recommended when CT cannot be performed, such as in pregnant women and in patients with a contrast medium contraindication. MRI has also the advantage of high soft-tissue resolution without radiation exposure. Better tissue characterization can be obtained using dynamic contrast enhanced MRI and diffusion weighted MRI. CT carries the risk of radiation exposure and side effects of iodinated contrast medium. On the other hand, MRI is not routinely used in the evaluation of ureteric lesions and is reserved for problematic cases due to high cost, limited availability, and scanning duration [4].

7.2 Different Modalities of Ureteric Imaging

7.2.1 Plain X-Ray of the Kidneys, Ureters and Bladder (KUB)

The plain abdominal X-Ray film (kidney, ureter, bladder; KUB) can be considered the initial and widely available imaging technique for the ureter exploration. The plain X-Ray film must be of good quality and carefully examined: low kilovoltage for higher contrast and lower diffuse radiation, local compression to push away the superposition of the interfering gas, lateral and oblique views to specify the topography of an abnormal radio-opaque shadows. Some ureteric or periureteric abnormalities can be seen on plain X-Ray abdominal film such as stones, mass effect, abnormal gas shadows, fatty radiolucency, and calcifications. Some abnormal findings such as calcifications may be concealed after the opacification of the urinary tract [5].

Plain pelvi-abdominal films are usually indicated for the evaluation of radiopaque urinary tract stones (calcium-containing stones, struvite, cystine) (Figs. 7.1a and 7.2a). An advantage of the plain film is that it can be performed in pregnant and pediatric patients, since the amount of radiation exposure is limited [5].

7.2.2 Intravenous Urography (IVU)

Intravenous urography (IVU); also known as antegrade ureteropyelography was the most recommended radiologic examination for the diagnosis of urinary tract abnormalities until the end of the twentieth century. However, IVU is still being requested by clinicians, particularly urologists, and is still being performed by radiologists, especially in the developing countries [6]. IVU is still used excessively in Egypt. The presence of urinary tract calculi is the most frequent IVU finding, which reveals that urolithiasis could be the main indication for IVU (Figs. 7.1b and 7.2b).

Three-minute IVU film can be used to assess a functional abnormality. The optimal ureteric opacification is usually obtained 10–15 min after injection of the contrast agent. The ureteric opacification is improved with the ureteric compression that allows a better filling of the upper portion of the ureter and total ureteric

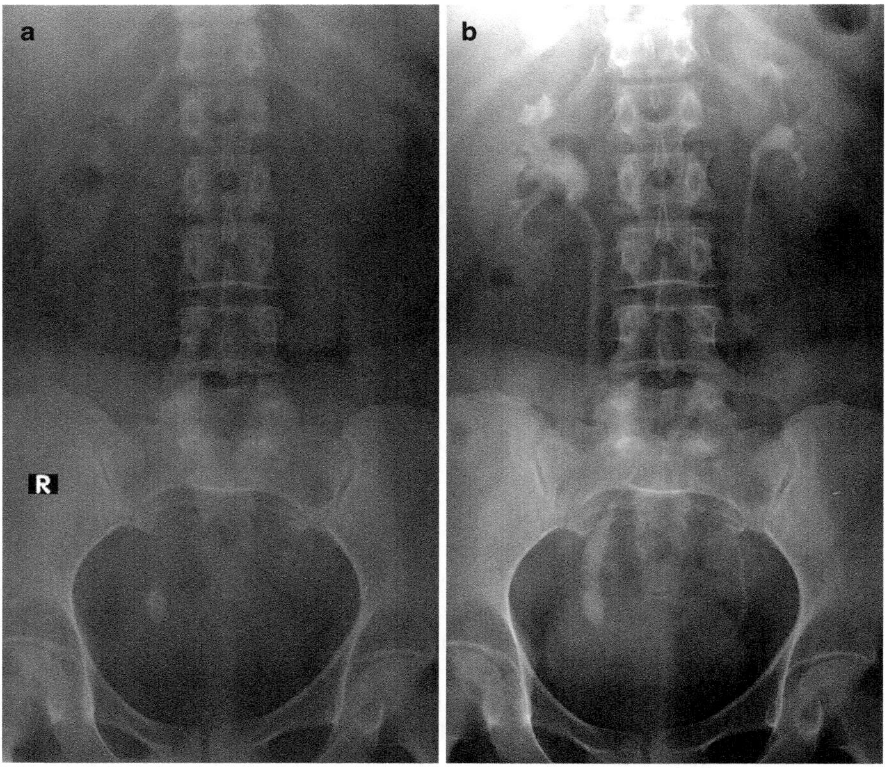

Fig. 7.1 (**a**) KUB reveals a radio-opaque shadow at the right aspect of the pelvic region. (**b**) IVU (excretory phase) reveals mild right hydroureteronephrosis down to a stone at the lower end of the right pelvic ureter

opacification. Localized compression of the ureter with a pad is used to improve visualization of some hidden segments. Compression can be performed with a device attached to the patient or to the table, consisting in a belt placed around the anterior abdominal wall, which maintains a foam pads or balloon upon the abdomen. Abdominal compression is contraindicated in the following: renal colic, recent abdominal surgery, those with a painful or tender abdomen, suspicious aortic aneurysm, or abdominal mass. Its usefulness remains unquestionable when a precise analysis of the ureteric lumen is needed. Other technical variants are needed in some circumstances [5].

Delayed IVU films are obtained in case of slow opacification of the ureter. Positioning IVU films may be used to facilitate the progression of the contrast media when the urinary tract is dilated. Slow ureteric opacification may result from absence of peristalsis and sedimentation of the contrast media. Tomographic views of the ureter and videotape recording of the ureteric peristalsis are rarely used. Oblique views are necessary when a ureter displacement is suspected or to suppress

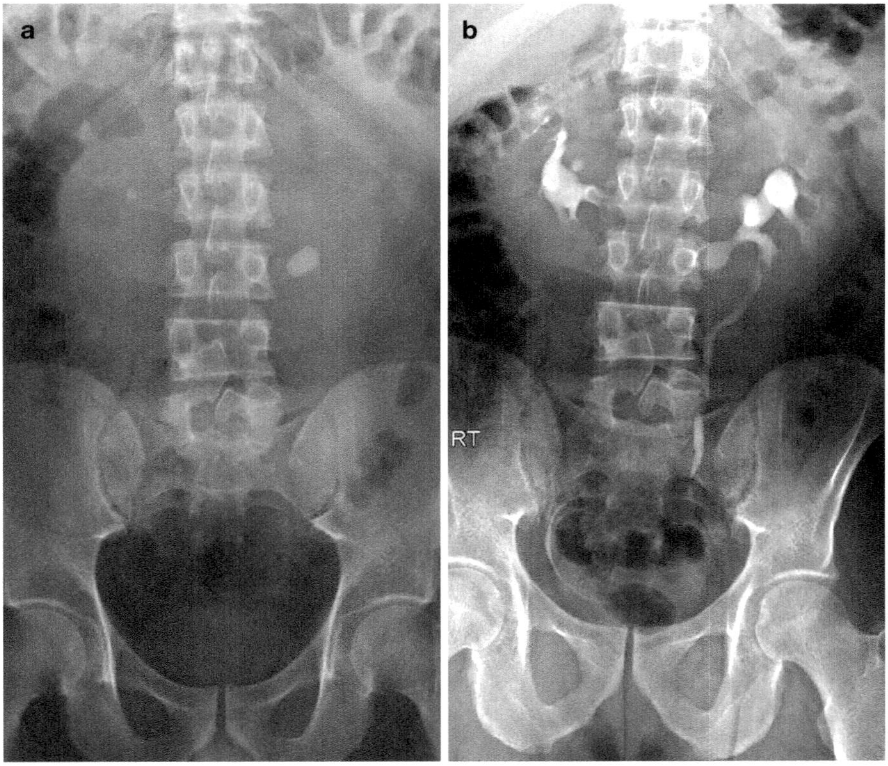

Fig. 7.2 (**a**) KUB reveals two radio-opaque shadows at both upper lumbar regions. (**b**) IVU (excretory phase) reveals malrotated both pelvi-calyceal systems with abnormal medialization of both renal lower poles suggestive of horse-shoe kidney. Two right middle and left lower calyceal stones. No hydronephrosis at both renal compartments with non-dilated opacified both ureters

superimposition. The IVU films in the prone and vertical positions are very useful as well as post-voiding films to study the ending ureter.

The IVU technique of the intermittent ureteric obstruction requires special protocols such as higher doses of contrast media, hyperdiuresis with injection of 0.5 mg/kg of furosemide intravenously or a quick perfusion of an isotonic saline solution.

7.2.3 *Retrograde Ureteropyelography (RUP)*

Retrograde ureteropyelography (RUP) was the first method devised for imaging the urinary collecting system, and until the development of early IVU agents in the 1930s, it was the only way of imaging the collecting system.

RUP is a radioendoscopic technique requiring special equipment (a uroradiological room with facilities for radiological and endoscopic procedures) as well as hygiene and radio protection conditions. The image quality is a very important matter and digital imaging from the X-ray intensifier is very useful. A catheter is placed in the ureter of interest, with its tip positioned at the distal ureter. Water-soluble contrast appropriate for the urinary system is instilled slowly to gently distend the upper collecting system (Pollack et al.). The exam is always preceded by a plain abdominal X-Ray film and performed by cystoscopic catheterization of the ureteric orifice with a Chevassu bulb-tipped probe, which reduces contrast leakage, followed by injection of 5–8 cc of contrast under fluoroscopically guidance. Sometimes more contrast must be injected if the urinary tract is dilated. Low-concentration HOCM with (250 mg of iodine per 100 ml) diluted to 30% is used so that small filling defect images are not concealed. LOCM do not provide additional advantages. Injection of air as CM to find a radiotransparent calculus is no longer used. The injection of CM must be stopped when a totally and satisfactory opacification of the urinary tract is obtained. If the patient is experiencing pain, or if a lymphatic or pyelotubular reflux is visualized, the injection must be stopped. The films are obtained with a total filling of the ureter in antero-posterior and oblique positions and also at the level of the obstacle with magnification. A later film, 5 min after the withdrawal of the catheter, is obtained to be sure of the drainage of the urinary tract. The procedure could be done under local anesthesia of the urethra, in particular in women [5].

Spot images are obtained of areas of interest. Distention of the upper collecting system is painful, so overdistention is avoided. Overdistention also results in pyelosinus and pyelovenous backflow, degrading the image. The patient may need to be rolled into decubitus positions to fill out the lower pole calyces. Post void images are obtained.

A general anesthesia could be necessary in men and if a therapeutic approach is planned. The RUP must be interpreted in relation to the retrograde injection of the contrast agent that reduces peristalsis. The films obtained after the with draw al of the catheter give some physiological information. Using this technique depends on the success of the catheterization of the ureteric meatus. The meatus is inaccessible in case of invasion of the bladder trigone by a tumor, deformation of the bladder by prostatic hypertrophy or meatus stenosis after surgery or radiotherapy. RUP is obviously impossible in case of ureterointestinal anastomosis [5].

7.2.4 Anterograde Pyelography (AP)

Anterograde pyelography (AP) is performed by injecting a contrast media using a nephrostomy catheter or by direct puncture of the pelvis, complementing or substituting RUP (Fig. 7.3). AP also allows the urodynamic study of the urinary tract. Today, it is for the most part the first-step procedure in all percutaneous interventions. The technique depends on whether it is used as a diagnostic or therapeutic

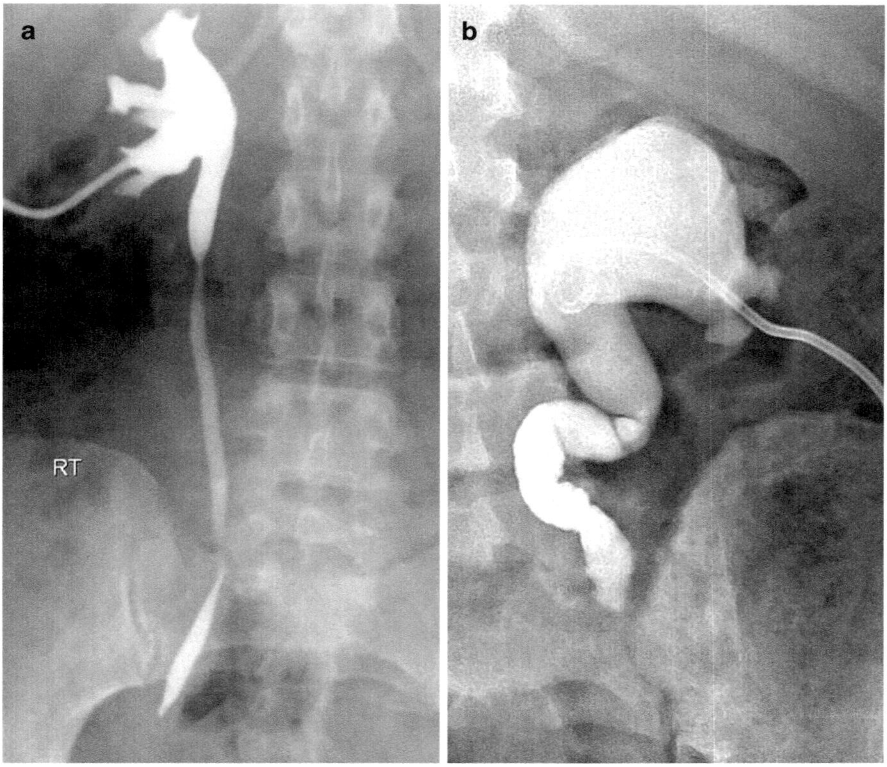

Fig. 7.3 Antegrade pyelography. (**a**) Mild right hydroureteronephrosis with arrest of the contrast at the pelvic ureter denoting ureteric stricture. (**b**) Moderate left hydroureteronephrosis with abrupt arrest of the contrast at the iliac ureter denoting ureteric stricture

approach and also on whether the renal pelvis is dilated. The exam is performed with local anesthesia in the prone position. The puncture could be guided with fluoroscopic or US guidance.

Fluoroscopic guided puncture is done vertically in a posterior approach after the localization of the kidney, 1 cm inside the middle of the bipolar line. The needle is advanced until a reflux of urine is obtained. This technique is used when the renal pelvis is not dilated and allows the opacification of the urinary tract. Intravenous injection of the contrast media can also be used for defining anatomy and position of the kidneys and to directly guide the puncture to a postero-inferior calyx. More recently, CT technical improvements allow real-time fluoroscopy. CT fluoroscopy provides a precise guidance and an optimal selection of the adequate calyx for antegrade pyelography and further therapeutic intervention on the upper urinary tract via an antegrade route [5].

US guided puncture is the easiest method when the pelvis is dilated. US guidance makes it possible to determine the axis of the puncture to the targeted calyx and follows the progression of the needle, avoiding colon, liver and spleen, and confirms its correct position. The puncture, posterior or postero-lateral, must be done with a fi ne CHIBA-type needle. A good position is confirmed with urine aspiration. Three things must be done when the needle is in a correct position: a bacteriological study of a sample of the urine, pressure measurement (less than 10 cm H_2O) and verification of the needle position after injection of a small quantity of contrast media. Opacification of the urinary tract is made by the injection of the iodine-diluted CM under fluoroscopic guidance. The quantity of the contrast media that must be administrated depends on the volume of the urinary tract. If the urinary tract is pressurized, it must be drained before opacification. Opacification makes it possible to completely visualize the ureter or just up to the obstacle if it is too tight. The films are made in different incidences. The urinary tract must be emptied before the withdrawal of the needle. AP is particularly useful for the opacification of the ureter in the transplanted kidney, where the retrograde approach is very difficult and sometimes impossible. The kidney is generally localized and punctured under US guidance [5].

7.2.5 *Ultrasonography (US)*

If the kidneys can easily and reliably be evaluated by ultrasonography (US), the ureteric US evaluation is more often limited to the proximal part of the lumbar ureter and the distal portion through the bladder.

It is difficult to visualize the normal ureters by US; however, diagnosis of various abnormalities associated with ureteric dilatation is possible in many instances. US examination almost exclusively concerns hydronephrotic kidneys, mostly searching for ureteric stones. To improve analysis of the ureter in these conditions, special US techniques are used. The proximal portion of ureter can be visualized (in case of dilatation) through the lower pole of the kidney using a postero-lateral approach with the patients in supine or oblique position, preferably with a well-distended bladder. Scanning is performed longitudinally and transversally, generally with 3.5 MHz transducer. It is important to use real-time scanning to search for the landmarks of the psoas to explore the retroperitoneum. [5].

The lower lumbar ureter can be explored when it crosses the common iliac vessels, particularly in thin patients. The patient should be positioned in a contra-lateral oblique position and the transducer has to be positioned longitudinally in the iliac fossa. Color Doppler is very helpful in this setting to identify the ureter and differentiate it from the iliac vessels. Visualization of the lower pelvic ureter requires bladder distension.

Endorectal approaches have been proposed to improve sensitivity of distal ureter examination. A transperineal route could improve US reliability in detecting abnormalities of this ureteric section. Suprapubic scanning is performed longitudinally and transversely. A post-voiding scan of the bladder can be useful in some circumstances. Water intake before examination is very useful in creating a diuretic situation with frequent ureteric jets. In certain cases, such as renal colic, very important diagnostic tool is the demonstration of ureteric jets on color Doppler US. It is important to know the limitations of detecting ureteric jets, which depends on diuresis and urine density differences between the ureter and bladder. The technique requires an incompletely emptied bladder and is very time consuming (5–20 min). Demonstration of twinkling artifacts using color Doppler has been described as a good echographic tool to identify some ureteric stones [5].

US is a practical method for diagnosis of ectopic ureter, ureterocele, and certain causes of ureteric obstruction that compares favorably with contrast radiography because it is quicker, does not involve use of contrast media or ionizing radiation, and usually requires no sedation or anesthesia. US is a convenient method for examining adjacent organs, principally the kidneys and bladder, that may be affected with ureteric abnormalities. Also, US guidance facilitates certain interventional diagnostic procedures for the ureters.

Endoluminal US was used to evaluate different causes of ureteric obstruction. It allows depiction of the ureteric wall and periureteric structures, however this technique is limited by the cost of the probe. It is performed at the same time as ureteroscopy, but the probe can be also introduced along the anterograde route. A 12.5- or 20-MHz frequency 6.2-F catheter-based transducer gives cross-sectional imaging of the ureter. Depending on the frequency used, a 3-cm-deep cross-sectional image showing the ureteric wall and periureteric tissue is provided and reconstructed 3D image also can be obtained [5].

7.2.6 Computerized Tomography (CT)

Over the past decade, computerized tomography urography (CTU) has emerged as the primary imaging modality for evaluating the urinary tract in various clinical settings. CT urography not only allows detailed assessment of the urinary tract but also enables direct visualization of adjacent structures and comprehensive evaluation of the abdomen and pelvis. CT urography is currently the first-line imaging modality for several indications, including hematuria, initial staging of urothelial tumors, and follow-up surveillance in patients with prior urothelial tumors. CT urography has essentially replaced intravenous urography as the first-line imaging modality in most of these settings and has been shown to have increased overall accuracy and sensitivity, particularly for evaluation of hematuria. Additional indications for CT urography include evaluation of urinary tract obstruction, depiction of complex congenital or postsurgical urinary tract anatomy, and any clinical scenarios where comprehensive evaluation of the urinary tract is needed. In this review, we focus specifically on ureteric abnormalities that can be identified at CT urography [7].

Nowadays, CT scanning is the "gold standard" of urologic imaging [8]. Multiphasic CT urography (CTU) has become the most suitable tool for the diagnosis of different urinary tract abnormalities, including congenital anomalies, infections, traumas, and tumors. In addition, its "one-stop-shop" use in the evaluation of vascular, parenchymal, and urothelial problems has a great impact on their management [9].

CTU not only allows detailed estimation of the urinary tract but also enables direct visualization of adjacent structures and overall evaluation of the abdomen and pelvis. Pathologic findings at CTU include congenital abnormalities, filling defects, dilatation, narrowing, and deviations in course.

With few exceptions, most observed that of the unenhanced CT performed for acute flank pain and stone disease. Continuing improvements in the spatial resolution and speed of newer CT scanners, combined with advanced MPR and volume rendering (VR) image reconstruction, have made CTU a comprehensive examination by which the kidneys and upper collecting system, ureters, and urinary bladder can be evaluated in one setting [10].

Various scanning techniques for CT urography have been described, but there is no universally accepted imaging protocol. In the most general sense, complete CT urography includes a non-enhanced phase, a contrast-enhanced phase, and an excretory phase. Several imaging protocols are currently used in clinical practice, some of which allow a decreased radiation dose [7].

Most CTU protocols are triphasic examinations that include non-contrast, enhanced, and delayed images. Non-contrast images extending from the top of the kidneys through the bladder are obtained to evaluate for calculi, fat containing lesions and parenchymal calcifications and to provide baseline attenuation for assessment of lesion enhancement [11].

Intravenous contrast is administered and following a 90–100 s delay, scanning of the abdomen and pelvis is performed during the nephrographic phase [10]. Homogeneous enhancement of the kidneys optimizes small renal mass detection. The final acquisition is during the excretory phase after a 12–15 min delay, when there is opacification and distention of the collecting systems, ureters, and bladder [10].

Most of the CT explorations of the ureter rely on the intravenous administration of contrast medium (CM). The main exception concerns the detection or evaluation of ureteric stone, which has gained wide acceptance among radiologists and referring clinicians in the last few years because of its excellent performance and because there is no need for CM injection. The iodine load is approximately 400 mg iodine per kg of body weight. When a multiphasic analysis of the renal parenchyma is not indicated on the basis of other radiological or clinical data, an ionic HOCM could be chosen because it results in increased diuresis and subsequently better filling of the excretory system. As helical acquisition is delayed after the injection, a possible intolerance to CM will not interfere with the quality of the breath-hold. Inversely, if the renal parenchyma has to be explored at the cortical and nephrographic phases, nonionic CM is often preferred due to better tolerance. In this case, the CM is administered using a power injector and three or four acquisitions are usually obtained: native, cortical phase, nephrographic phase and excretory time [12].

Excretory images allow for evaluation of the urothelium. While diagnostic unenhanced and nephrographic acquisitions are relatively easy to obtain, optimal opacification and distention of the ureters during the excretory phase can be more problematic [13].

The large number of very thin section images allows for isotropic presentation of the axially acquired data set in any chosen plane. Often on a workstation, CTU are frequently reviewed utilizing MPR, MIP, and 3D VR images. Curved planar reformations along the length of the ureters are also often helpful.

The emergence of volumetric imaging tools such as helical CT has resulted in the development of 3D reconstruction techniques. Some of the multidimensional algorithms were available at the time of sequential CT and were applied to immobile structures such as bone. Nevertheless, the emergence of helical CT has made it possible to use them in imaging the retroperitoneum, in particular kidneys and ureters, since acquisition of the entire volume in a single breath-hold is mandatory to avoid respiratory misregistration. Despite wide availability on most workstations, the application of 3D algorithms to the urinary tract have been the topic of few publications, most of them concerning the anatomy of the lower urinary tract after surgery.

The parameters of reconstruction may be adapted to 3D representation by increasing in-plane and longitudinal resolutions (reducing the field-of-view size and increasing the overlapping reconstruction ratio, respectively). When 5-mm-thick slices have been obtained, the volume should be reconstructed at least every 3 mm in order to reduce the step artifact. The number of slices to be manipulated may become substantial, but recent workstations are more efficient in handling large amounts of data. The different types of multidimensional reconstructions differ in the rendered effect and the process complexity. In particular, preprocessing of native data such as spatial segmentation may be an important time-consuming factor. Nevertheless, whatever representation mode is chosen, the preliminary analysis of native slices is essential: in the vast majority of cases, multidimensional representation does not add information to native slices. The main interest of 3D reconstructions is to provide clinicians a coronal representation of the whole urinary tract with which they have become familiar after years of prescribing EU. Shaded surface display (SSD) offers a real 3D representation, even in cases of complex anatomy. The gray scale encodes surface reflection from an imaginary source of illumination. The selection of the voxels participating in the reconstructed image is based on the choice of a density threshold: the pixels integrated into the image are those with densities over the selected threshold. A value in the range of 140–160 Hounsfield units (HU) allows the selection of opacified urine and the elimination of soft tissues. The bony structures are also included in the 3D dis- play; nevertheless, the interactive rotation of the 3D volume makes it possible to limit undesirable superimposition. Otherwise, pre-rendering editing may be applied in order to remove overlying anatomy that obscures the structures of interest. The anatomic segmentation is based on a region-of-interest drawing or connectivity-based algorithms, depending on the different workstation prototypes. In fact, the main drawback of SSD consists in the influence of the threshold selection on the final image: as observed in CT angiography, the selection of a thresh old higher than the density of pixels representing opacified urine results in pseudo-stenoses or even pseudo-interruption of the opaque column. Inversely, an excessively low level may result in the selection of extra-urinary pixels, yielding, for example, increased noise. Another limiting factor of SSD is the loss of density information: the gray scale is not allocated to Hounsfield units as on native scans, but to the 3D rendering mode using a shadowing technique. In this condition, opacified urine and ureteric stone may remain undifferentiated with this particular type of 3D display while careful analysis of native scans with interactive windowing is more prone to a correct diagnosis [5].

MIP is probably a more useful tool than SSD, particularly because the gray scale reflects CT attenuation and does not simulate light reflections as does SSD. Consequently, a ureteric stone will be distinguished from the urine as far as its density differs from that of urine and it is not completely surrounded by contrast medium. The MIP image is produced by casting rays through the data volume and displaying the maximum pixel value along each path. As the MIP algorithm projects the volume on a plane, the resulting image, even if containing information about the whole volume, is two-dimensional (Fig. 7.4). Therefore, the projection incidences have to be multiplied through a rotational axis. The main limiting factor of this mode of display is the initial essential phase of the prerendering editing mode aiming at the removal of all structures other than the urinary tract, which may turn out to be time-consuming if automated tools are not available on the workstation. When available, the multiplanar volume rendering (MPVR) algorithm may be useful, since it allows an MIP reconstruction of a selected volume with no need for

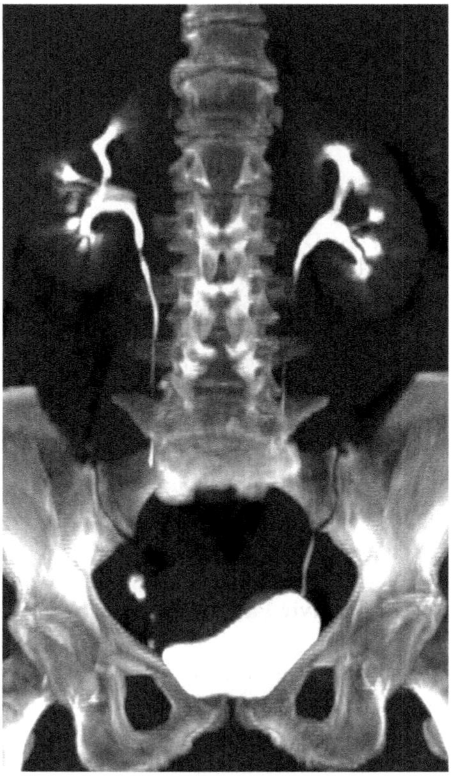

Fig. 7.4 CTU (MIP reformatted coronal image) reveals no hydroureteronephrosis with no pelvicalyceal or ureteric stones bilaterally as well as right pelvic phleboli

preliminary editing of data. It simply applies the MIP to a volume limited in thickness. The volume is adapted in such a way that it contains as much ureter as possible and avoids inclusion of undesirable structures. Thus, ureters are generally dis played separately, segment by segment. A volumetric data set with near-isotropic voxels is adapted to the application of virtual endoscopy. This technique is based on threshold image segmentation and surface-rendering algorithms. While the method has been widely applied to colon, trachea-bronchial tree and vessels, few data are available on the urinary tract. It is unlikely to detect lesions that are not visible on native scans, but can provide a better image of the lesion.

The VR technique is currently the most sophisticated 3D rendering technique and requires high-performance hardware. This technique does not result in information loss since all voxels participate to the calculation. Consequently, no preliminary editing of the data is required. Each voxel is assigned a color and opacity based on the CT attenuation, making it possible to evaluate the full range of tissue densities and their 3D spatial relationships (Fig. 7.5).

Finally, the most useful tool among the available multidimensional algorithms is probably curved MPR. It can be obtained either without opacification in case of ureteric dilatation or after CM opacification. Simple MPR reconstruction can be

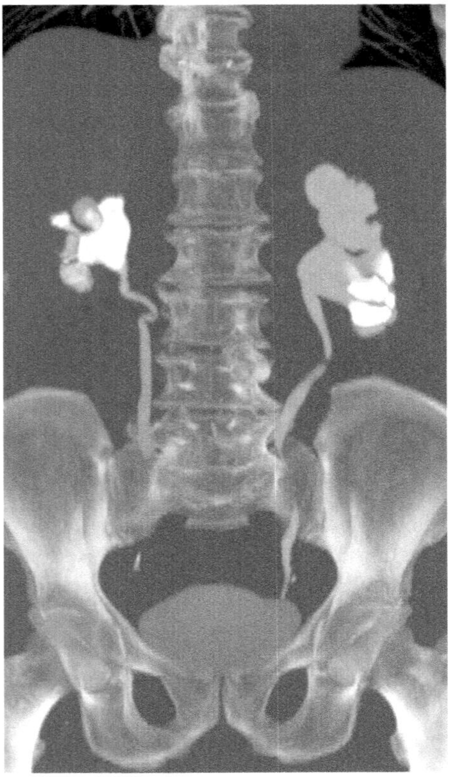

Fig. 7.5 CTU (MIP reformatted coronal image with 3D rendering technique) reveals mild right hydroureteronephrosis down to the iliac ureter with non-opacified distal ureter pelvicalyceal and moderate left hydroureteronephrosis down to the lower end of the pelvic ureter denoting bilateral ureteric strictures

used to improve the diagnosis of ureteric stone. It consists in the coronal oblique representation displaying the entire length of the ureter, obtained from the combination of segments of the ureter seen in adjacent CT images, thus depicting the whole ureter and its anatomic relationships on a single image. The delineation of the course of the curved reformation may be obtained from the lateral SSD representation. In the vast majority of cases, both ureters cannot be displayed simultaneously [5].

7.2.7 Magnetic Resonance Imaging (MRI)

In the past 20 years, MRI emerged as a promising, noninvasive imaging method in urology, and more recently, MR urography has been used as an effective imaging method for evaluating abnormalities of the urinary tract. Since the first description of MRU made by Henning in 1986, its diagnostic capability has been improving with increasingly sophisticated imaging sequences and very short acquisition times. Because of the long T2 of fluid in the collecting system, the first clinical studies were conducted using heavily T2-weighted sequences for visualization of the urine-filled urinary tract. Excretory MR is a more recent imaging method, similar to that of EU. Based on T1-weighted sequences taken after IV administration of gadolinium chelate, excretory MR provides both morphological and quantitative information about the urinary tract. The addition of fast 3D MR angiography provides even more valuable information on renal vasculature in patients in whom abnormal vascular anatomy or vascular diseases affect the urinary tract. Most studies have been performed on a unit with a 1.5-Tesla magnet, but good-quality images have also been obtained at 0.5 Tesla, although longer acquisition times or higher numbers of excitations are required [14].

CTU in most clinical practices throughout the world due to shorter examination times, improved efficiency and patient throughput, better availability and decreased technical and interpretative complexity compared to MR Urography (MRU) [15]. Nevertheless, MRU (when technically optimized) offers similar visualization of the ureters compared to CTU and for detection of non-calculous diseases of the collecting system has been shown to be as specific as CTU albeit with lower sensitivity [16]. MRU is non-ionizing and presents an ability to image the collecting systems, as well as, the kidneys and urinary bladder simultaneously as a comprehensive "one-stop-shop" examination [17]. Advances in MR imaging techniques including: parallel imaging, motion compensation and compressed sensing may dramatically shorten examination times improving image quality and patient tolerance for the MRU examination.

A comprehensive MRU requires anatomic coverage of the kidneys, urinary bladder and the collecting system in its' entirety including the pyelocaliceal system and ureters. The craniocaudal distance required to cover all of the anatomy of the urinary tract poses a technical challenge for many MRI systems [17].

A basic MRU examination typically includes T2-weighted (T2W) imaging obtained at standard and very long echo times (TE ~ 90 and >500 ms, respectively), T1-weighted (T1W) images acquired with dual-echo chemical shift imaging (CSI) and with fat suppression (FS) before and after gadolinium administration. When gadolinium enhanced images are acquired through DCE-MRI and when diffusion weighted imaging (DWI) is added to a basic MRU protocol, a "multi-parametric" MRU is achieved [17]. Delayed T1W gadolinium enhanced urographic phase images complete the protocol.

With heavily T2-weighted sequences, the urine is used as the intrinsic contrast agent, and so IV gadolinium chelate is not needed. Adequate distension of a renal collecting system and ureter is an important condition for complete assessment. Good oral hydration prior to the study is not indicated, because this may increase the fluid filled bowel loops. Intravenous infusion of saline allows for better distension of non-dilated ureters. Intravenous injection of furosemide a few minutes before the start of the examination is very effective, with maximal efficacy 10 min after injection. Compression devices, similar to those used in excretory urography, are not used. Voiding before the study is recommended.

Dynamic contrast-enhanced (DCE)-MRI can only be performed once using this set-up and can cover either the upper abdomen or the pelvis but not both. Vendors have proposed various solutions to overcome this challenge, and include: larger surface coils with wider useable FOV, integrated surface coils which enable linking of adjacent coils expanding the useable FOV and continuously moving table (CMT) MRI [18]. Dynamic MRU is based on glomerular filtration of gadolinium chelate. Intravenous administration of a low dose of gadolinium chelate (0.1 mmol/kg) is sufficient for evaluation of the urinary tract and is characterized by very low nephrotoxicity and also good dialyzability. In excretory MRU, there is a general gadolinium-related problem, which results from paramagnetic contrast agents leading to a shortening of both the T1 and T2 relaxation times of fluids and tissues. The most effective way to solve this problem is to inject furosemide few minutes before the injection of the contrast agent. A fast T1-weighted gradient sequence with very short repetition and echo times, demonstrates contrast enhanced urine, so that normal and abnormal renal cavities such as the renal pelvis and the ureters can be evaluated at different times and from various views, similarly to excretory urography. Acquisition time is 12 s for the multislice 2D turbo gradient echo sequence, but is significantly reduced by using the single-slice technique. The repetition of the sequence after the IV administration of gadolinium chelates up to 40–60 min, in an oblique coronal plan adjusted on the long axis of kidneys, provides both morphological and at least gross functional information about the urinary tract. Time-intensity curves obtained from parenchymal ROI are similar to those obtained during renal scintigraphy and may permit assessment of excretory function. An additional dose of furosemide can be administrated intravenously 20 min after IV injection of gadolinium chelate, as is usually done with renal scintigraphy. Comparative analysis may reveal asymmetry in the kinetics of enhancement of the kidneys. However, precise quantification is limited since there is no simple linear relationship between measured signal intensity and renal perfusion. The practicality of gadolinium-enhanced T1- weighted MR urography depends on renal excretory function. Good urographic effect is regularly obtained up to a serum creatinine concentration of 2 mg/dl. Due to longer acquisition times compared with T2-weighted sequences, image quality can be degraded by patient motion, especially in children. Finally, the most recent studies show the superiority of the gadolinium-enhanced MR urography over static fluid imaging in evaluation of acute flank pain.

Most abdominal and pelvic MRI surface coils offer an imaging field of view (FOV) of up to 40 cm which may be too small to cover the entire urinary tract simultaneously. A simple solution, though time consuming and somewhat impractical, is to cover the upper abdomen and pelvis separately. This requires moving the surface coil in between acquisitions and necessitates re-localization between stations [18]. Coil placement needs to be adjusted so that the field of view (FOV) covers the entire urinary tract from the top of the kidneys to the base of the bladder. Smaller FOV may be useful for complementary, focused examination. Asking patients to keep upper limbs above the head during the examination eliminates phase wrap artifacts. The use of respiratory compensation or breath gating, should reduce artifacts from breathing, which can significantly degrade images. However, single-breath-hold acquisition seems better than respiratory triggering, as long as the patient is able to suspend breathing during the acquisition time. The use of prospective or retrospective navigator gating may also improve image quality.

For T1-weighted sequences or short TE effective T2-weighted sequences, the adjunct of fat saturation, using STIR technique or presaturation bands, can be useful in order to eliminate signal from fatty tissues surrounding ureters. However, this increases the acquisition time and decreases the signal-to-noise ratio. Two acquisition protocols may be used to cover the entire volume of the urinary tract. The first protocol uses multiple one-slice, interleaved acquisitions obtained in various scanning planes, rotating in a stepwise manner from the coronal to the lateral view. The slice thickness usually ranges from 30 to 60 mm, and makes it possible to evaluate the entire ureter in different views. The main limitation of this thick-slice technique is a potential lack of spatial resolution due to partial volume effect. The second approach is to obtain multiple, 2D, thin slices and to subsequently acquire MIP reconstruction images of the entire urinary tract. The in-slice spatial resolution is optimal, but details such as small filling defects can also be removed on MIP images, although they are clearly visible on the individual source slices. This technique is also more sensitive to artifacts from breathing.

Even when coverage is possible, acquisition times can be prohibitive if modifications to existing protocols are not performed. One simple strategy to reduce acquisition time is to image in the coronal (as opposed to the axial) plane to reduce the number of slices required to achieve adequate coverage. Increasing slice thickness or reducing resolution through reductions in the number of phase-encoding steps can also shorten acquisition times to improve coverage.

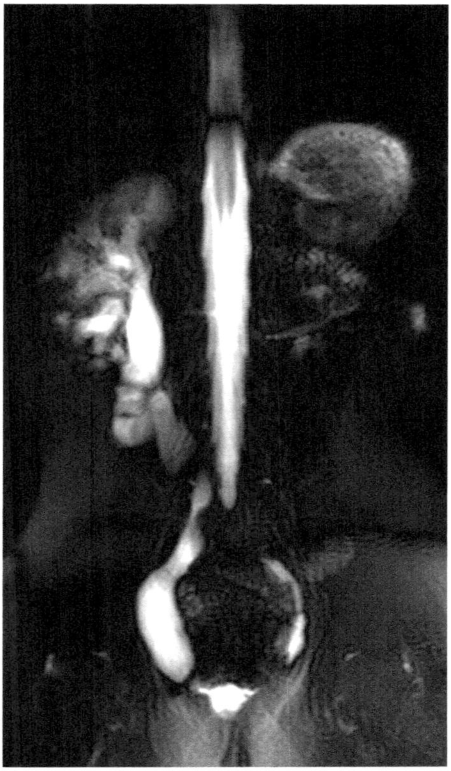

Fig. 7.6 MRU (coronal T2 weighted image "T2-WI") reveals moderate right hydroureteronephrosis with dilated ipsilateral tortuous ureter down the urinary bladder suggestive of congenital megaureter and nephrectomized left kidney with dilated left pelvic ureteric stump

Unenhanced MRU can be associated with virtual endoscopy of the upper urinary tract. Feasibility was demonstrated in all cases with dilatation but less than 50% of cases without dilatation. Lumen abnormalities (masses and stenosis) can be easily visualized with high diagnostic accuracy. MRU is now available alternative to excretory urography and contrast-enhanced CT in selected patients such as those allergic to iodinated contrast agents, pregnant women, or patients for whom radiation exposure is contraindicated. Recent technical improvements show that this technique is able to offer a highly accurate morphological and comprehensive functional diagnostic evaluation of the ureter in most conditions. It has the potential to become the preferred imaging modality for the diagnosis of suspected ureteric disease, significantly decreasing the need for excretory urography and retrograde pyelography (Figs. 7.6 and 7.7).

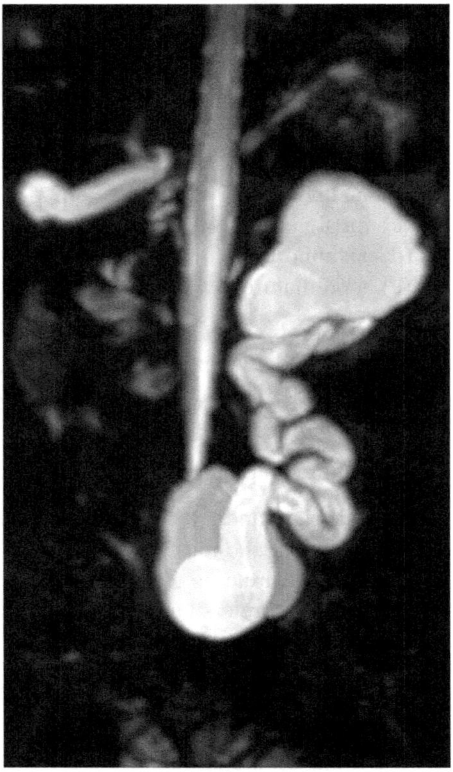

Fig. 7.7 MRU (coronal T2-WI) reveals dysplastic right kidney and marked left hydroureteronephrosis with dilated ipsilateral tortuous ureter down an extravesical ureterocele

7.2.8 Nuclear Renal Scan

Nuclear renal scan, also known as renal scintigraphy, is an imaging method that uses radiopharmaceuticals/radiotracers to evaluate urinary tract anatomy, physiology, and pathology. The various injected radiotracers are extracted from the blood by the kidneys and emit radiation, particularly gamma radiation, that is detected by gamma cameras. These studies are easy to perform and typically do not require sedation [5].

Diuretic renography is used for the assessment of urinary tract obstruction. It can distinguish between genuine obstruction and non-obstructive atonicity of the ureter that occurs with vesico-ureteric reflux (VUR), congenital malformations, or a non-compliant urinary bladder. Also, it has a role in the diagnosis of post-surgical or post-traumatic complications including urine leakage and urinoma development. Urinomas are seen as accumulations of radiotracer adjacent to the point of leakage [5].

7.3 Differential Diagnosis of Ureteric Filling Defects

7.3.1 Benign Causes

7.3.1.1 Calculus

Ureteric calculi are the most common cause of ureteric filling defects. Historically, the description of calculi as "filling defects" has applied to intravenous urography, where a calculus is seen as a defect in the contrast column. However, at CT, all urinary tract calculi have high attenuation and measure more than 200 HU (with the rare exception of indinavir calculi, which have soft-tissue attenuation). As a result, calculi are often obscured by the high attenuation of excreted contrast agent at CT urography and may not be identified as filling defects. Non enhanced CT is therefore the preferred modality for diagnosing ureteric calculi, and CT urography is not generally indicated. Nonetheless, calculi are occasionally seen at CT urography [7] (Fig. 7.8).

Calculi are often located at the normal anatomic sites of ureteric narrowing: the UPJ, pelvic brim, and UVJ. In some cases, the wall of the surrounding ureter may be thickened and edematous, resulting in the "soft-tissue rim" sign. Hydronephrosis is often

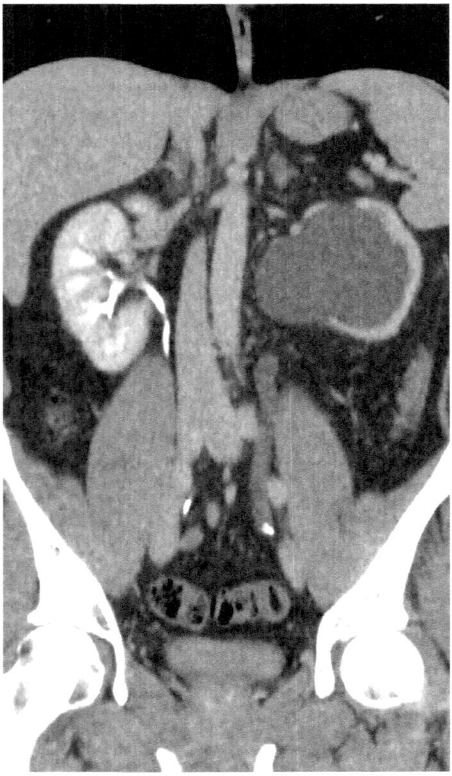

Fig. 7.8 CTU (MIP reformatted coronal image) reveals marked left hydroureteronephrosis down to two adjacent small stones at the iliac ureter

minimal in the setting of acute obstruction. Large stones (>5 mm) are less likely to pass and may require urologic intervention, such as ureteroscopic removal, shock wave lithotripsy, or stent placement. It is also important to identify duplicated ureters and to fully evaluate each for the presence of calculi, especially on non-enhanced images [7].

7.3.1.2 Ureterocele

Ureteroceles represent abnormal congenital dilatation of the distal-most portion of the ureter. The dilated portion of the ureter may herniate into the bladder secondary to the abnormal structure of uretrovesical junction (UVJ).

Most ureteroceles are congenital, usually associated with the ectopic insertion of the ureter with associated duplicated collecting system. In a minority of cases, ureteroceles are an isolated abnormality, and these are usually seen in adults.

The cobra head sign, also known as the spring onion sign, refers to dilatation of the distal ureter, surrounded by a thin lucent line, which is seen in patients with an adult-type ureterocele (Fig. 7.9).

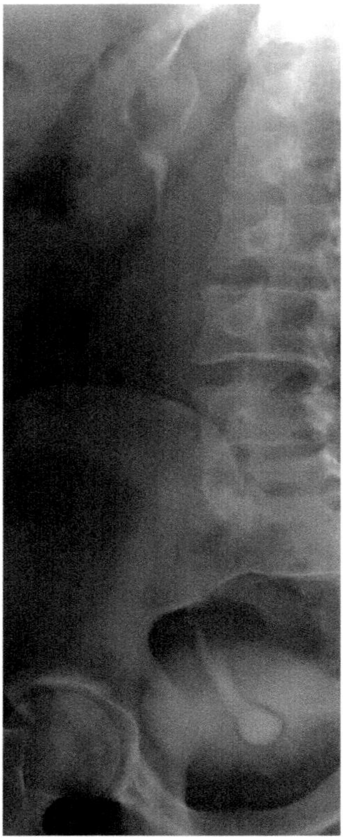

Fig. 7.9 IVU (excretory phase) (RAO) reveals complete right renal duplex with cobra head sign of the lower end of the pelvic ureter suggestive of ureterocele

7.3.1.3 Blood Clot

A ureteric clot can form after an intraureteric hemorrhage due to trauma, calculi, underlying malignancy, or anticoagulation. At imaging, clot material can appear as a small rounded filling defect or as a vermiform defect that fills the ureter. A clot does not enhance and can be identified on a non-enhanced image as hyperattenuating (>50 HU) relative both to urine and the surrounding soft tissues, occasionally with a urine-clot interface [18].

A clot also resolves at follow-up imaging studies. However, a small clot may be difficult to distinguish from UCC at initial identification at CT urography, and ureteroscopy and/or short-interval follow-up imaging may be necessary. A urologic consultation should also be considered to rule out the possibility of underlying malignancy [7].

7.3.1.4 Inflammation and Hyperplastic Lesions

Inflammatory and hyperplastic lesions of the ureter are uncommon and can manifest as solitary or multiple filling defects. These benign lesions cannot be reliably distinguished from tumors at CT urography, and ureteroscopic evaluation is often necessary [19]. Multiple filling defects can be due to benign entities such as:

1. ***Ureteritis cystica***

   Ureteritis Cystica is a rare benign entity of the urinary tract that is thought to occur due to chronic inflammation of the urothelium from recurrent urinary tract infection or nephrolithiasis and manifests as areas of glandular metaplasia at histopathology. These lesions are typically incidentally discovered during evaluation of the urinary tract for other causes and appear as numerous small uniform filling defects. Ureteric obstruction is rare. Treatment is usually conservative unless there are signs of obstruction or infection [20].
2. ***Malacoplakia***

   Malacoplakia is a rare form of granulomatous disease that can affect various organ systems but most commonly affects the genitourinary tract and is typically seen as soft yellowish plaques appearing on the mucosa. While the urinary bladder is the most common site of urinary tract involvement, ureters may be affected in up to 20% of cases [21].

   When the ureters are involved, patients can present with flank pain, hematuria, and fever. On CT, the lesions can appear as segmental ureteric thickening with or without proximal dilatation; hydronephrosis is rare but can occur. diagnosis is typically established by biopsy. Treatment involves antibiotic therapy and surgical resection of the plaques with or without ureteric stenting.
3. ***Leukoplakia (squamous metaplasia)***

   Benign lesion but high possibly turn premalignant [7].
4. ***Others***

   Fibroepithelial polyp, papilloma and nephrogenic adenomas; Benign lesions but radiologically not distinguishable from UCC [7].

7.3.1.5 Infection

1. ***Tuberculosis***

   Genitourinary tuberculosis may occur following hematogenous dissemination from the lungs. The ureters are involved in 50% of cases. In the early stages of disease, CT urography demonstrates dilatation and a ragged appearance of the ureter with wall thickening and inflammatory changes in the surrounding tissues. Occasionally, mucosal granulomas can be seen as filling defects at urography. as the disease progresses, short or long segment ulcerations form, which eventually lead to fibrosis and stricture formation resulting in a beaded or cork screw appearance of the ureter. Chronic thickening of the ureter may result in foreshortening and distortion of the architecture, referred to as "pipe-stem" ureter. The changes in the ureter are typically associated with ipsilateral renal cortical scarring, dilatation and distortion of the calyces, and renal parenchymal calcifications [21].
2. ***Fungus ball***

   Immunosuppressed patients are susceptible to opportunistic fungal infections. Candida and Aspergillus species can form fungus balls in the urinary tract. These mycetomas may contain air or calcifications. Rarely, a fungus ball can extend into the ureter and form a urobezoar, which can be obstructive [22].
3. ***Schistosomiasis***

   Schistosoma haematobium is a parasite that lays its eggs in the wall of the urinary tract and is endemic in Africa and the Middle East [23]. Reactive inflammation and edema surrounding the eggs can create a nodular filling defect. The eggs calcify over time, resulting in mural calcifications that may be visible at CT.

7.3.1.6 Ischemic or Vascular Origin

Renal papillary necrosis is the predominant cause of an ischemic filling defect, and its etiology includes analgesic abuse or overuse, sickle cell disease, pyelonephritis, renal vein thrombosis, tuberculosis, obstructive uropathy, and diabetes. Necrotic papillae can become dislodged and fall into the ureter, potentially resulting in hydronephrosis. If a ureteric filling defect is identified at CT urography, it is important to look for signs of papillary necrosis as a potential cause. Associated findings include caliceal cavities and blunting [7].

Vessels that cross over the ureter can occasionally cause vascular impressions that result in an apparent filling defect. For example, the ovarian vein crosses over the ureter near the L3 vertebral body. Rarely, thrombosis or dilatation of the ovarian vein may result in an obstructive uropathy known as ovarian vein syndrome [13].

7.3.1.7 Ureter Intussusception

Ureter intussusception is rare and usually occurs in an antegrade fashion as a result of a polyp, malignant tumors, or ureteric stone acting as a lead point; however, cases of iatrogenic intussusception following ureteroscopic procedures have also been reported [24]. In the absence of a lead point, ureter intussusception likely occurs as a result of weakening of the ureteric wall or mucosa, which can lead to telescoping of the weakened segment into the distal segment or very rarely the proximal segment [25].

On CT, the filling defect can be more clearly visualized, and a concentric ring of contrast may be seen around the invaginated intussuscepted segment. Retrograde ureteroscopic reduction can be attempted in cases that occur as a result of a surgical procedure, although the appropriate treatment is likely to be surgical excision with reconstruction [24].

7.3.2 Malignant Causes

7.3.2.1 Urothelial Carcinoma (UC)

Urothelial carcinoma (UC) frequently occurs in the urinary bladder; however, approximately 5% arise from the upper urinary tract. 25% of the upper tract tumors occur in the ureter, predominantly within the lower third. Patients usually present clinically with gross or microscopic hematuria, and up to one third of patients may experience flank pain or acute renal colic [26].

Increasing age, male gender, and smoking are among the most important risk factors for disease development. Synchronous bilateral lesion can be seen in 2–9% of patients with ureteric UC and 11–13%develops metachronous upper tract tumors within a mean period of 28 months [27]. Up to 50% of patients with upper tract UC, especially ureteric tumors, will develop metachronous tumors in the bladder within 2 years of surgical treatment [28].

This is related to the direction of flow of urine facilitating transfer of malignant cells from the upper to the lower urinary tract with subsequent malignant implants. Therefore, diligent assessment of the urinary tract is required at both initial and follow-up imaging for high-risk patients [26].

Upper tract UC typically manifest as single or multiple filling defects within the contrast enhanced ureter at IVU with or without proximal ureteric dilatation or hydronephrosis. Tracking of contrast into the interstices of the tumor is a characteristic feature and has been termed the “Stipple” sign, Long-standing obstruction may lead to poor renal excretion, which is the major limitation of IVU in detecting ureteric lesions [26].

RUP is usually performed to further investigate abnormalities detected at IVU, especially in inadequately excreting kidneys or cases of contrast allergy. As with

IVU, ureteric UC appears as a filling defect with proximal ureteric dilatation [26]. An "apple core" appearance may be seen with circumferential or eccentric lesions that infiltrate the ureter, giving the appearance of ureteric fixation and non-tapering margins [27].

The "goblet" sign is a classic imaging finding at RUP resulting from gradual localized ureteric dilatation around and distal to the filling defect, which is not typically seen with more acute causes of obstruction. Furthermore, the ureteric catheter may coil below the lesion at the time of the study, another characteristic feature that has been referred to as the Bergman sign on non-contrast CT images, UC is typically iso-hyperattenuating (5–30 HU) to urine but less attenuating than clot (40–80 HU) or calculus (N100 HU), although 2–7% may contain calcifications [26].

At CT urography, fully opacified urinary tract segments are essential for detection of upper tract carcinoma. Ureteric UC often results in dilatation of proximal ureteric segments and hydronephrosis [26]. Three distinct appearances have been described at CT, which include circumferential wall thickening, small masses (<5 mm in maximal diameter) and large infiltrating masses (>5 mm in maximal diameter) [29]. Viewing the opacified ureters at wider window settings such as bone windows aids in identifying subtle filling defects. Coronal reconstruction of the ureters provides anatomic views of the urinary tract similar to IVU, enabling evaluation of the longitudinal extension of a lesion and presence of multicentric disease [30]. The presence of a thickened enhancing ureteric wall and soft-tissue stranding in the periureteric fat is suggestive of extramural extension [26].

Recently, MRI plays a great role in the diagnosis of the upper urinary tract UC with valuable information about its size and extension. DWI may replace invasive retrograde urography or conventional imaging using intravenous injection of contrast medium in detecting the upper urinary tract UC (Fig. 7.10).

7.3.2.2 Metastasis

Metastatic disease to the ureter is extremely rare. The most common primary cancers that have been reported to metastasize to the ureters include colorectal, breast, stomach, prostate and cervical cancers as well as melanoma [31]. Primary malignancies of the lung and pancreas as well as acute myelogenous leukemia have also been implicated in previous reports [32]. Clinically, patients are often asymptomatic but may present with nonspecific symptoms such as flank pain and dysuria; hematuria is present in 20–30% of cases. Ureteric obstruction may develop gradually but can remain undetected. Recurrent urinary tract infections, unexplained proteinuria or progressive decline in renal function in the setting of a known primary malignancy should raise suspicion for ureteric involvement [31].

Three patterns of ureteric involvement have been described either transmural involvement of the ureteric wall, infiltration of the periureteric soft tissues or submucosal nodules [33].

The ureteric adventitia is the most common portion of the wall affected by metastases while mucosal involvement is uncommon. On CT imaging ureteric metastases

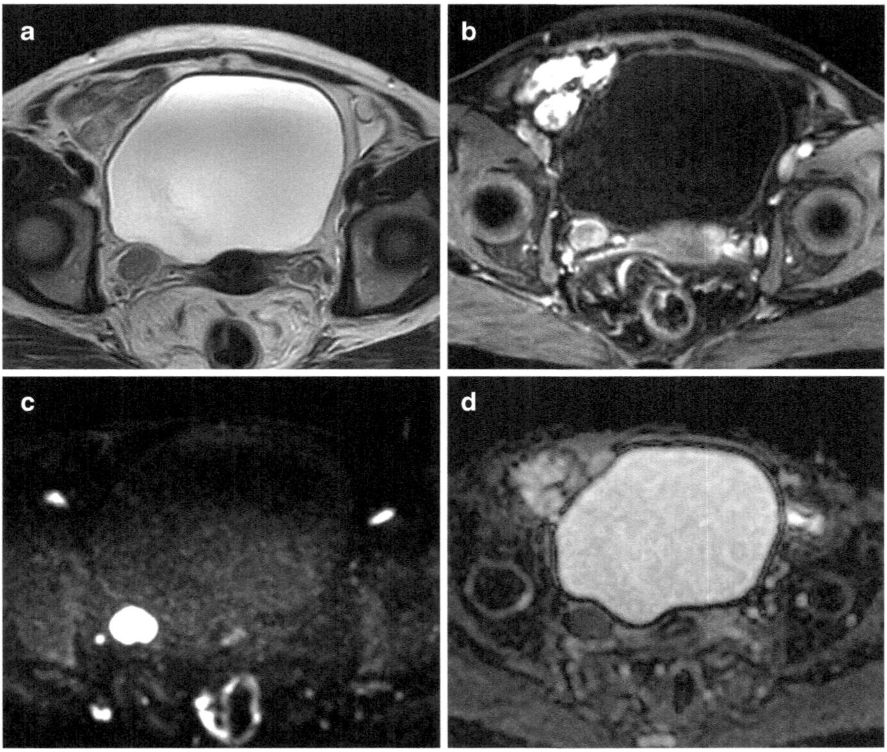

Fig. 7.10 Multiparametric MRI (axial images); (**a**) T2-WI, (**b**) post-contrast image, (**c**) DWI and (**d**) ADC map reveal an isointense soft tissue lesion at the lower end of the right pelvic ureter with restricted diffusion (high SI at DWI and low SI at ADC map) showing intense heterogenous enhancement after IV contrast administration with no extramural extension

typically appear as focal thickening and stricture formation with or without an associated mass with contrast enhancement.

It is prudent to visualize the enhancing lesion separate from any nodules or mass in the adjacent structures in order to confirm a ureteric metastasis rather than primary neoplasm or contiguous infiltration. Submucosal nodules manifest as one or more filling defects within the lumen at urography and are difficult to distinguish from primary ureteric malignancy. In patients with history of radiotherapy to the abdomen, retroperitoneal fibrosis (RPF) presents an additional diagnostic challenge, as it can occasionally mimic ureteric metastases [31].

Although fluoroscopy-guided retrograde brush biopsy has high accuracy in detecting primary ureteric malignancies, its use in detecting metastatic lesions is limited given that most metastases, including submucosal nodules, typically do not invade the mucosa. In addition, brush biopsy has limited value in differentiating metastases from RPF due to the predominantly extra-mucosal involvement with both entities [31]. Diagnosis of ureteric metastases may be confirmed by biopsy, which can be performed percutaneously using CT guidance if impact on management is anticipated [21].

7.3.2.3 Lymphoma

Primary lymphoma arising from the genitourinary tract is rare and accounts for less than 5% of extra-nodal lymphomas [34]. Non-Hodgkin's lymphoma (NHL) is the most common subtype of lymphoma that presents with extra-nodal disease. Most previous case reports of primary ureteric lymphoma are of the NHL subtype. While the most common genitourinary site for extra-nodal involvement is the kidney, isolated ureteric involvement has also been reported. The majority of patients are asymptomatic, but some present with non-specific symptoms of flank pain, renal colic, or hematuria. Hydroureter/Hydronephrosis is usually present on initial imaging evaluation although functional obstruction likely precedes radiologic evidence of ureteric/collecting system dilatation [35].

CT urography demonstrates diffuse, irregular, and concentric thickening of the affected ureteric walls with irregular narrowing of the ureteric lumen and proximal dilatation [36]. The tumor can involve the adventitia and grow away from the wall, which manifests as an area of nodular soft-tissue density on CT [35]. Post-contrast enhancement is typically present and is best evaluated on subtraction images [37]. Coronal images can be used to assess the longitudinal extent of the disease and evaluate response to therapy on follow up [38].

While ureteric mucosal biopsy with ureteroscopy has been shown to be useful in some cases, it may not yield adequate tissue especially when the outer wall is predominantly involved, therefore requiring CT guided percutaneous biopsy or surgery to confirm the diagnosis [35].

Secondary lymphomatous involvement of the ureters by retroperitoneal disease is more commonly encountered in clinical practice. It typically results in encasement or displacement of the ureter by retroperitoneal lymph nodes or lymphomatous masses. When displacement is present, it typically results in lateral deviation at the UPJ by para-aortic lymphadenopathy (LN) and medial displacement at the pelvic brim by iliac nodes. Ureteric obstruction is seen in only 14% of patients, although ureteric encasement may cause functional obstruction without radiographic dilatation [34].

On CT, secondary involvement of the ureter is suspected when there is concomitant retroperitoneal or pelvic lymph node enlargement and loss of tissue planes between the ureter and juxtaposed lymph nodes [39].

References

1. Lye CM, Fasano L, Woolf AS. Ureter myogenesis: putting Teashirt into context. J Am Soc Nephrol. 2010;21(1):24–30.

2. Masarani M, Dinneen M. Ureteric colic: new trends in diagnosis and treatment. Postgrad Med J. 2007;83(981):469–72.
3. Brooks JD. Anatomy of the lower urinary tract and male genitalia. In: Campbell-Walsh Urology. Philadelphia: W.B. Saunders; 2007.
4. El-Ghar MA, et al. CT and MRI in urinary tract infections: a spectrum of different imaging findings. Medicina. 2021;57(1):32.
5. Joffre F, Otal P, Soulie M, editors. Radiological imaging of the ureter. Cham: Springer; 2012.
6. Türk C, Knoll T, Petrik A, et al. Guidelines on urolithiasis. Eur Urol. 2012. Available from: https://uroweb.org/wp-content/uploads/20_Urolithiasis_LR-March-13-2012.pdf (Accessed 23 April 2014).
7. Potenta SE, et al. CT urography for evaluation of the ureter. Radiographics. 2015;35(3):709–26.
8. Hale Z, et al. Imaging the urologic patient: the utility of intravenous pyelogram in the CT scan era. World J Urol. 2014;32(1):137–42.
9. Abou-El-Ghar M, et al. Diagnosing urinary tract abnormalities: intravenous urography or CT urography. Rep Med Imaging. 2014;7:55–63.
10. Alderson SM, Hilton S, Papanicolaou N. CT urography: Review of technique and spectrum of diseases. Appl Radiol. 2011;40(7):6.
11. Sahni VA, Shinagare AB, Silverman SG. Virtual unenhanced CT images acquired from dual-energy CT urography: accuracy of attenuation values and variation with contrast material phase. Clin Radiol. 2013;68(3):264–71.
12. Lemaitre L, et al. Retroperitoneum and ureters. In: Spiral CT of the abdomen. Berlin: Springer; 2000. p. 277–317.
13. Lamba R, et al. Multidetector CT of vascular compression syndromes in the abdomen and pelvis. Radiographics. 2014;34(1):93–115.
14. Catalano C, et al. MR pyelography and conventional MR imaging in urinary tract obstruction. Acta Radiol. 1999;40(2):198–202.
15. Raman SP, Fishman EK. Upper and lower tract urothelial imaging using computed tomography urography. Urol Clin. 2018;45(3):389–405.
16. Sudah M, et al. Comprehensive MR urography protocol: equally good diagnostic performance and enhanced visibility of the upper urinary tract compared to triple-phase CT urography. PLoS One. 2016;11(7):e0158673.
17. Chung AD, et al. MRI evaluation of the urothelial tract: pitfalls and solutions. Am J Roentgenol. 2016;207(6):W108–16.
18. Hamilton J, Franson D, Seiberlich N. Recent advances in parallel imaging for MRI. Prog Nucl Magn Reson Spectrosc. 2017;101:71–95.
19. Ordon M, Andrew Ray A, John D'A R, Honey. Ureteritis cystica: a rare cause of ureteral obstruction. J Endourol. 2010;24(9):1391–3.
20. Poturalski MJ, Purysko AS, Herts BR. Ureteritis cystica. J Urol. 2015;193(4):1379–80.
21. Moosavi B, et al. Beyond ureterolithiasis: gamut of abnormalities affecting the ureter. Clin Imaging. 2016;40(4):678–90.
22. Paola D, Giuseppe, et al. Candida bezoars with urinary tract obstruction in two women without immunocompromising conditions. ScientificWorldJournal. 2011;11:1168–72.
23. Colley DG, et al. Human schistosomiasis. Lancet. 2014;383:2253–64.
24. Xu W, et al. Ureteral intussusception due to a polyp. Abdom Imaging. 2007;32(5):675–7.
25. Chiong E, Consigliere D. Antegrade ureteral intussusception: a rare complication of percutaneous endopyelotomy. Urology. 2004;64(6):1231.
26. Browne RFJ, et al. Transitional cell carcinoma of the upper urinary tract: spectrum of imaging findings. Radiographics. 2005;25(6):1609–27.
27. Wong-You-Cheong JJ, Wagner BJ, Davis CJ Jr. Transitional cell carcinoma of the urinary tract: radiologic-pathologic correlation. Radiographics. 1998;18(1):123–42.
28. Kirkali Z, Tuzel E. Transitional cell carcinoma of the ureter and renal pelvis. Crit Rev Oncol Hematol. 2003;47(2):155–69.
29. Caoili EM, et al. MDCT urography of upper tract urothelial neoplasms. Am J Roentgenol. 2005;184(6):1873–81.

30. Maher MM, et al. Multidetector CT urography in imaging of the urinary tract in patients with hematuria. Korean J Radiol. 2004;5(1):1–10.
31. Roy S, Baijal SS. Pancreatic adenocarcinoma presenting with ureteric metastases case report and review of literature. Clin Imaging. 1993;17(2):99–103.
32. Wasnik AP, et al. Multimodality imaging in ureteric and periureteric pathologic abnormalities. Am J Roentgenol. 2011;197(6):W1083–92.
33. Winalski CS, Lipman JC, Tumeh SS. Ureteral neoplasms. Radiographics. 1990;10(2):271–83.
34. Jaeger CD, et al. Diffuse large B-cell lymphoma in an adolescent male presenting as ureteral stricture. Case Rep Radiol. 2014;2014:239345.
35. Ni B-W, et al. Malignant lymphoma of the ureter: a case report and literature review. Exp Ther Med. 2014;7(6):1521–4.
36. Ghersin E, et al. Multimodality imaging of direct ureteric involvement in non-Hodgkin's lymphoma using PET/CT, CT urography and antegrade CT pyelography. Br J Radiol. 2007;80(959):e283–6.
37. Kubota Y, et al. Bilateral primary malignant lymphoma of the ureter. Int J Clin Oncol. 2007;12(6):482–4.
38. Lebowitz JA, et al. Ureteral lymphoma: MRI demonstration. Abdom Imaging. 1995;20(2):173–5.
39. Ruth K, et al. Primary diffuse large B-cell lymphoma of the ureter in a patient with HIV: a case report and review of literature. Clinical Lymphoma Myeloma Leuk. 2013;13(3):324–6.

Chapter 8
Physiology and Pharmacology of the Ureter

Leslie Ojeaburu, Francisco Escobedo, Sapna Thaker, Parth Patel, and Kymora B. Scotland

Abstract The purpose of the ureter is to perform peristalsis, which facilitates the transport of urine from the kidney to the bladder. In this chapter, we explore the molecular, biological, and physical principles responsible for the ureter's primary action as well as the basis for the pharmacologic management of ureteral function.

Keywords Peristalsis · Ureteral contraction · Smooth muscle cells · Pacemaker cells · Calcium ion channels

Abbreviations

ASMCs	Atypical Smooth Muscle Cells
COX-2	Cyclooxygenase-2
PGE2	Prostaglandin E2
TSMCs	Typical Smooth Muscle Cells
UVJ	Ureterovesical junction

Learning Objectives

- To understand the basis for contraction in the ureter
- To detail how peristalsis is propagated
- To discuss the effects of medications, hormones, and chemicals on the function of the ureter
- To understand the mechanisms underlying ureteral dysfunction

Test your learning and check your understanding of this book's contents: use the "Springer Nature Flashcards" app to access questions. To use the app, please follow the instructions in Chapter 1.

L. Ojeaburu · F. Escobedo · S. Thaker · P. Patel · K. B. Scotland (✉)
Department of Urology, University of California Los Angeles, Los Angeles, CA, USA
e-mail: kscotland@mednet.ucla.edu

M. Abdel-Gawad et al. (eds.), *The Ureter*,
https://doi.org/10.1007/978-3-031-36212-5_8

8.1 Introduction

The urinary collecting system utilizes various motility patterns that promote the anterograde transport of materials. The ureter's role in this system is specifically to transport urine. Ureteric pacemaker cells allow the ureter to function independently by facilitating spontaneous muscle contractions that encourage the passage of urine from the renal pelvis to the ureter and into the bladder [1]. This spontaneous activity, occurring in a wave-like pattern, is known as peristalsis. Functioning through a combination of contraction, relaxation, and stretching of ureteral smooth muscle, ureteral peristalsis is integral to the transport of urine from the kidneys to the urinary bladder [2].

8.2 Mechanics of Peristalsis

8.2.1 Ureteral Motility

The primary function of the ureter is to transport urine from the kidneys to the urinary bladder, which is accomplished by means of peristalsis [2]. This process of peristalsis is thought to be myogenic, initiated at the pacemaker cells of the renal pelvis [3]. Urine is transported across the ureter to the bladder for storage until micturition. The mechanical aspects of peristaltic rate, rhythm, pressure, and amplitude are affected by the size and pattern of urine boluses [3].

8.2.2 Propagation of Urine Bolus

The proximal ureter maintains a collapsed state before the urine is expelled from the renal pelvis [4]. As the renal pelvis fills under normal conditions, a rise in pressure occurs and urine enters the ureter. Contraction waves at the proximal ureter move the bolus of urine distally. For propulsion to occur successfully, the contraction wave must sequentially collapse the ureteral walls [4] as seen in Fig. 8.1. Finally, the bolus enters the bladder due to the advancing contraction wave that dissipates at the ureterovesical junction (UVJ). However, when at extremely high flow the ureteral walls do not coapt and a continuous flow of urine is transported, unlike the series of boluses that form from a normal flow [4].

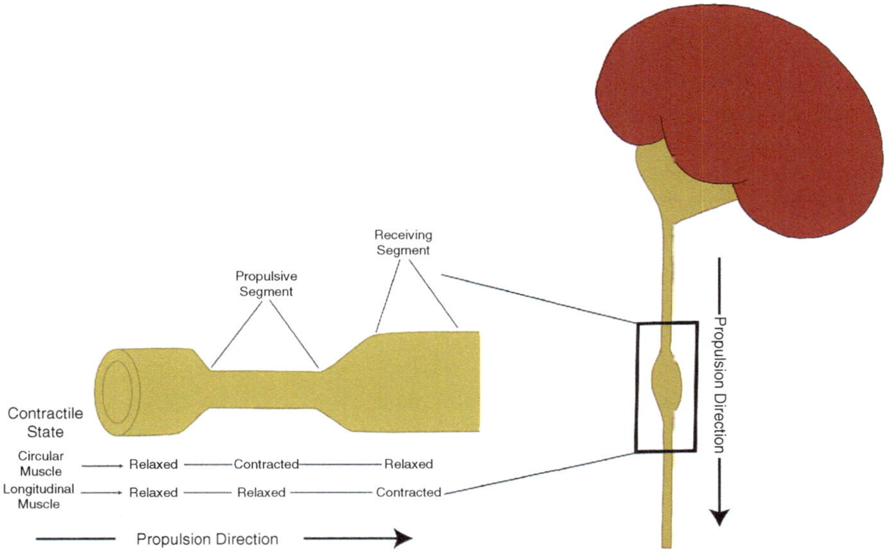

Fig. 8.1 Direction of propulsion of peristaltic waves

8.2.3 Effects of Diuresis/Heavy Flow Rates

When urine production increases, peristaltic frequency increases as well. Eventually, there is a plateau effect. Thus, when the maximum frequency is reached, further increases in the quantity of urine transported occur by increasing the volume of the urine bolus. If the urinary flow continues to rise, boluses coalesce and the ureter becomes filled with fluid and dilates, creating an open non-peristaltic channel [4].

8.2.4 Function at the Ureterovesical Junction

The UVJ facilitates one-way transport using a valve mechanism. Once the urine is transported across the UVJ, the trigone and detrusor muscle typically provide the necessary resistance to prevent the urine from refluxing [4]. However, bolus transfer from the UVJ to the bladder can be impeded during periods of high urinary flow or elevated intravesical pressure, preventing further propagation of the contraction wave and creating the possibility of retrograde flow [4]. Griffiths presented theoretical evidence of a similar situation (impediment of efficient bolus transfer) with a normal UVJ and a ureter that was too wide or experienced weak contractions. In essence, the wider the ureters or weaker the contractions, the lower the UVJ resistance must be in order not to impede bolus transport [5].

8.3 Automaticity of the Ureter

8.3.1 Shape and Nature of Ureteral Smooth Muscle Action Potential

Contraction takes place at the smooth muscle layer of the ureter (Fig. 8.2). Contractions result as a function of the coordinated activity of the circular and longitudinal smooth muscle fibers.

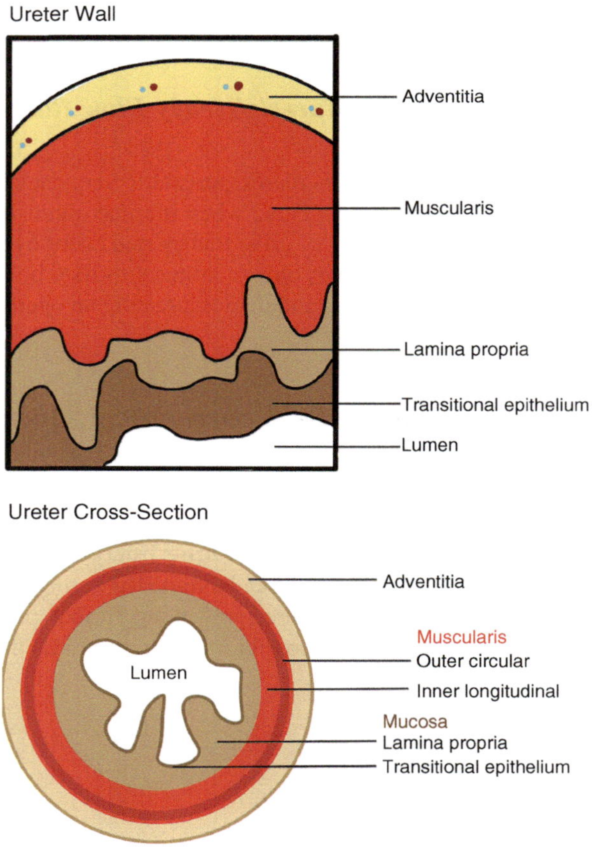

Fig. 8.2 Tissue layers of the ureter

Ureteral smooth muscle function relies on biochemical principles seen in other smooth muscle organs like the heart or intestines. These organs rely on a system of ion movement across cell membrane channels. Currently, the ionic basis for the electrical activity of the ureteral smooth muscle is not completely understood. However, work by several groups has provided key insights into the process. The selective permeability of membrane channels to different ions, their propensity to open at set voltages, as well as principles of voltage and concentration gradients all contribute to the flow of ions seen at different stages of this electrochemical cycle. The cycle can be divided into four important phases: resting potential, action potential (upstroke), plateau, and repolarization.

Resting potential is the voltage at which a cell is in a non-excitable phase and no electrical impulse is being generated across that cell. In terms of ion movement, it is the phase by which an electrical equilibrium is reached and there is no net flow of ions across the cell membrane. For ureteral smooth muscle cells, this resting potential has been measured to be −30 to −70 mV [6, 7], with variability across animal models (Fig. 8.3). Maintenance of this resting potential starts with the action of a Na^+/K^+ pump that couples passive inward K^+ flow to actively pump Na^+ out of the ureter [8]. This pump is necessary given the propensity of K^+ to flow passively across its concentration gradient outside the cell (K^+ is stored at larger concentrations within cells). This leads to a positive charge on the outside of the cell and a relatively negative charge on the inside [8].

Depolarization, also known as the upstroke, occurs when the cell receives a sufficiently large external impulse from its surrounding environment. This impulse may be electrical, mechanical (such as the stretch resulting from a urine bolus), or conduction from an adjacent cell. The impulse decreases the negative charge within the cell until it exceeds its threshold potential [8]. At that point, there is a temporary closure of inward K^+ channels and activation of L-Type voltage-gated Ca^{2+}

Fig. 8.3 Action potential in ureteral smooth muscle

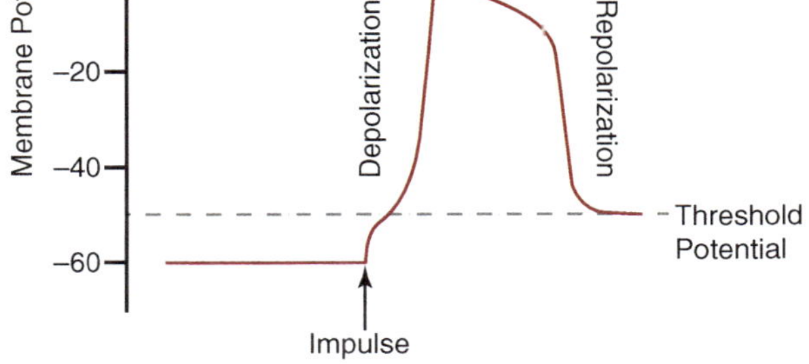

channels, thereby enabling Ca^{2+} passage into the cell [7, 9]. The result is a rapid decrease in the negative charge within the cell.

The plateau phase proceeds with continued inward Ca^{2+} along with an inward Na^{+} flow, which is balanced by Ca^{2+}-mediated activation of an outward K^{+} channel [7, 9, 10]. This balance maintains the cell membrane at a fixed voltage, enabling greater muscle contraction. The final stage of the ureteral smooth muscle cell action potential consists of a return to the electrochemical resting potential in a process termed repolarization (Fig. 8.3). This is achieved by reactivation of an inward K^{+} channel (Lang 1989). Ureteral action potential refractory periods are quite long compared to other tissues [6, 11–13]. This is likely to allow each peristaltic wave while preventing reflux and resulting kidney injury [4]. While the mechanism is not entirely understood, it appears to be mediated by calcium [14].

Although the principles remain the same, there are key differences in the electrochemical cycle of cell excitement between putative pacemaker cells and non-pacemaker cells. Peristalsis is thought to originate as a result of the electrical activity of so-called pacemaker cells. These cells are characterized by their ability to generate their own impulse and self-initiate an action potential. They have lower resting membrane potentials enabling depolarization with a smaller external impulse required [1]. The key differences driving pacemaker cell functionality lie in the loss of a plateau phase in pacemaker cells and "leaky calcium channels".

8.3.2 Site of Pacemaker Cells and Ureter Automaticity

The presence of pacemaker cells is a defining feature of smooth muscle systems. This feature enables rhythmic, coordinated peristalsis and is a major factor that differentiates smooth muscle from the skeletal muscle systems. While mechanisms of automaticity have been described, consensus on the location and identity of pacemaker cells within the urinary collecting system is still an evolving area of research. Ureteral pacemaker cells are thought to be primarily located in the proximal portion of the collecting system.

In comparative renal anatomy, two distinct models exist: the uni-calyceal and the multi-calyceal collecting system. Unicalyceal systems are typically found in smaller mammalian organisms like mice, rats, guinea pigs, and dogs [15]. These collecting systems are characterized by a single common calyx that drains into the ureter. The site of automaticity has been demonstrated to originate along the pelvicalyceal border extending to the ureteropelvic junction [15, 16]. Studies measuring the contraction frequency in circumferentially cut strips of unicalyceal systems demonstrate decreasing concentration of pacemaker cells along the ureter [1].

On the other hand, multi-calyceal systems have been identified in larger mammalian organisms like pigs and humans. They consist of minor calyces that coalesce into major calyces and eventually lead into the ureter. In these systems, automaticity is driven by special populations of pacemaker cells that are thought to reside in the region starting from the major calyces and extending to the pelvicalyceal area [15, 17] (Fig. 8.4). There may also be additional regions of automaticity throughout

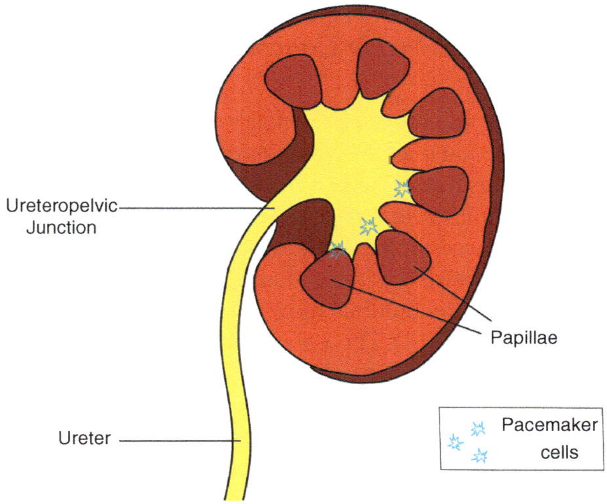

Fig. 8.4 Location of putative pacemaker cells

the urinary tract system that result from the activity of a population of latent pacemakers [18]. Thus, multiple pacemaker sites are thought to exist.

8.3.3 Characteristics of Pacemaker and Non-Pacemaker Cells

Two major cell types in the ureter interact closely to initiate electrical impulses and to generate the muscle contractions that characterize ureteral peristalsis. They consist of Atypical Smooth Muscle Cells (ASMCs) and Typical Smooth Muscle Cells (TSMCs). ASMCs and TSMCs are distinguished histologically and functionally [17, 1]. ASMCs are loosely arranged cells that appear to function as pacemaker cells, initiating action potentials and propagating impulses to the closely packed TSMCs to drive ureter contraction. The location of these cell populations within the broader pyelo-ureteral anatomy further highlights their function. ASMCs are found in the region from the major calyces to the pelvi-ureteric junction and decrease in concentration distal from the major calyces [17]. TSMCs make up the largest population of cells in the ureters with their concentration increasing in indirect proportion to ASMC concentration. Notably, some studies have demonstrated that TSMCs are the only cell population below the pelvi-ureteric region in human ureters [17].

Interstitial cells of cajal (ICC) -like cells are another cell population believed to play a key role in the transmission of the action potential to ureter muscle contraction [19]. These cells, first characterized in the GI system, have demonstrated pacemaker capabilities and reside throughout the entire ureter [20]. While their function is still being elucidated, current understanding places ICC-like cells as a signal relay system helping to transmit the action potentials from the ASMC to populations of TSMCs [15]. They are also believed to function as latent pacemakers.

8.3.4 Ureteral Peristaltic Movement - Propagation of Activity and Muscle Contraction

Peristalsis does not depend on nerve conduction; it is an electromechanical process. Cell excitation couples with contraction to form the peristaltic wave. Thus ureteral contractions directly result from action potentials. The goal of peristalsis is to propel fluid boluses in a coordinated fashion down the central lumen of the ureter. In order to successfully guide a bolus in this fashion, the ureter relies on varying degrees of resistance in the muscle walls. Greater resistance to transverse movement compared to longitudinal movement generates a force vector of motion perpendicular to peristalsis [4]. This coordinated motion relies on the successful propagation of signal to functional muscle units. These units must then act in unison to produce the necessary action.

First proposed by Engelmann in 1869 [21], the myogenic theory postulated that the ureteral action potential spread from cell to cell [22].Later studies identified intermediate gap junctions as permissive avenues for action potentials spread between cells. These junctions serve as channels connecting the cell membrane of adjacent cells, thereby enabling free flow of ions and small molecules (Fig. 8.5). This encourages rapid propagation of signals to groups of cells near the origin of the

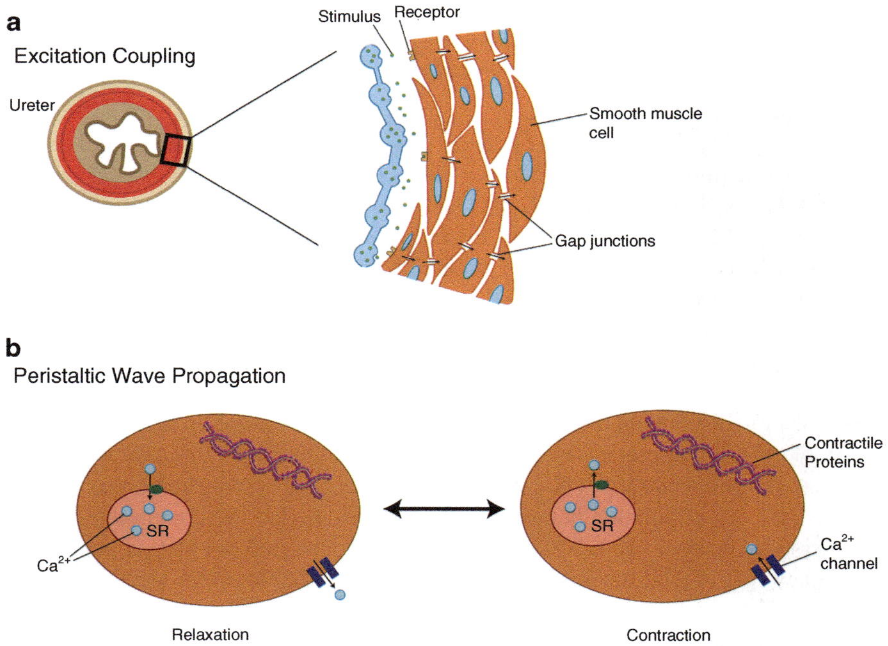

Fig. 8.5 Excitation-contraction coupling in ureteral peristalsis. (**a**) Process of excitation-contraction coupling (**b**) Propagation of a peristaltic wave

action potential signal. In that way, the ureter acts as a syncytium, with numerous cells receiving and acting on the same signal with only minimal delay.

Once the action potential reaches the TSMC, this signal is translated into a smooth muscle contraction through a calcium-mediated process. Depolarization leads to the release of calcium into the sarcoplasmic reticulum of smooth muscle cells. This activates calmodulin-dependent myosin light-chain kinases that phosphorylate other light-chain myosins and actins, eventually leading to the phosphorylation of a myosin-ATPase [1]. The smooth muscle then shortens in an ATP-dependent manner. Several groups have demonstrated that calcium administration increases the force of ureteral contraction [23–25].

8.3.5 Mechanical Properties Driving Peristalsis: Force-Length Relationship

Force developed by the muscle when stimulated (under isometric conditions) and the resting length of the muscle at the time of stimulation [4] both influence peristalsis. Isometric force-length measurements depend on the number of linkages between myosin and actin (active in contraction) [4]. When the ureter is stretched, the resting force increases. However, if the stretch is maintained at a constant level, the resting force decreases, leading to stress relaxation [4].

8.4 Biochemistry and Pharmacology of the Ureter

8.4.1 Sympathetic Activity

Both alpha and beta-adrenergic receptors have been identified in the ureter [8, 26]. Alpha 1A and 1D receptors are the dominant alpha receptors in the ureteral system, with clear implications for the pharmacologic management of ureteral obstruction [27]. Stimulation of alpha-adrenergic receptors plays an excitatory role in ureteral peristalsis by activating phospholipase C (PLC) and the downstream IP3/Dag pathway [28]. This leads to greater availability of Ca^{2+} and thereby greater contraction strength. Norepinephrine, a nonselective alpha agonist with B1 receptor activity, has consistently been shown to increase peristaltic contraction strength [8, 29]. Its effects are further enhanced by pharmacologic inhibition of its B1 activity.

Alpha 1 receptor inhibition has a dampening effect on ureteral peristalsis. Adrenergic antagonists such as phentolamine and phenoxybenzamine attenuate the contraction-strengthening effects produced by alpha agonists [26]. Similar results have been demonstrated with doxazosin and tamsulosin, both selective alpha-1 antagonists. Tamsulosin in particular has a higher affinity for alpha 1D and has been shown to decrease the force of ureteral contraction [25, 30]. Alpha 1 inhibitors are heavily used in combination with NSAIDs in managing renal colic caused by urolithiasis by promoting stone expulsion. However, the efficacy of alpha-blockers like tamsulosin in improving stone passage rates remains unclear [31, 32].

Beta-adrenergic receptors activate G proteins leading to increased cAMP and PKA, which promote smooth muscle relaxation. Although their role has been better studied in bladder detrusor muscle activity, they also modulate ureteral activity. There are three types of Beta receptors: Beta 1, Beta 2, and Beta 3. Beta 2 and 3 are the more prevalent beta receptors in pig and human ureters and play a more significant role in relaxation than B1 receptors [33, 34]. The agonist KUL-7211 with stimulating effects on both B2 and B3 has been shown to be a more potent inhibitor of peristaltic contractions in a dog ureteral system than selective alpha-1 antagonists, calcium channel blockers, and muscarinic antagonists [35]. Other agents like isoproterenol, a B1 and B2 agonist, have shown similar effects. However, Mirabegron, a beta 3 agonist, has not been shown to significantly affect ureteral stent symptoms or stone expulsion rates [36, 37].

8.4.2 Parasympathetic Activity

Although all five muscarinic receptor subtypes (M1-M5) have been identified in human ureters, M2, M3, and M5 are predominant [38]. Activation of these receptors increases ureter contraction strength and duration through the PLC and IP3/DAG pathway, in a similar mechanism as alpha 1 agonists. Select cholinergic stimulating agents like acetylcholine, methacholine, carbachol and bethanechol can induce this excitatory effect in various animal models. Methacholine and carbachol increase both the smooth muscle tone as well as the frequency of contractions, while bethanechol has been shown to only increase tone. Notably, Morita et al. demonstrated that acetylcholine can stimulate pelviureteric activity and accelerate the ureteral pace by initially increasing the rate of pacemaker discharge [29]. However, over time the pacemaker discharge frequency is shortened with acetylcholine. Acetylcholinesterase inhibitors like pyridostigmine further increase muscarinic activity by inhibiting the breakdown of acetylcholine.

Muscarinic antagonists like atropine have a relaxing effect on ureteral peristalsis, decreasing tonic and phasic contractile activity. However, several meta-analyses comparing the effects of antimuscarinic agents as monotherapy and in combination with alpha-blockers have shown variable benefits of antimuscarinics [39–42].

8.4.3 Prostaglandin Pathway

Prostaglandins are a group of lipid-based molecules that act on G-coupled protein receptors. They are metabolites of COX-2; an important inflammatory mediator. There are four groups of prostaglandins PGE2, PGI2, PGD2, and PGF2a.

PGE2 increases the strength of contraction in obstructed ureters while decreasing muscle tone in *unobstructed* ureters [43]. In unobstructed ureters, urothelial cells have been demonstrated to inhibit smooth muscle cell contractility, likely via a COX-2 metabolite such as PGE2 [44]. PGE2 is significantly increased in pigs' urine with ureteral stents compared to the unstented control population [45]. This aligns with other work postulating COX-2 is released in response to chronic stretch in the ureter walls. These studies provide data supporting the role of PGE2 as a target of pharmacologic modulation in partially or wholly obstructed ureters.

Understanding prostaglandin function in ureteral peristalsis has clear implications for clinical management. Non-steroidal anti-inflammatory drugs (NSAIDs) work by directly inhibiting COX-2 leading to a reduction in PGE2, likely resulting in a decrease in painful ureteral contractions around the site of stenting or obstruction [46]. NSAIDs like indomethacin and celecoxib, have long been utilized in the management of postoperative pain after ureteral procedures. Several randomized controlled trials have further indicated the effectiveness of NSAID agents in managing pain after various urologic procedures including lithotripsy, stent placement, and stent removal [47]. Additionally, guidelines on ureteral stone pain management recommend NSAIDs in the management of renal colic pain while waiting for stone expulsion [48].

8.4.4 Other Biochemical Mediators of Peristalsis

Other pathways besides adrenergic, muscarinic, and prostanoid have been shown to modulate peristalsis. Several of these pathways are believed to act directly on the ion channels involved in action potential generation and contraction. For example, l-Type calcium channel blockers like nifedipine and verapamil reduce the strength of ureteral contractions and the duration of the action potential [30, 49] . This is thought to be achieved through direct inhibition of Ca^{2+} flow into pacemaker cells. Caffeine has also been shown to reduce spontaneous ureteral contraction through action on Ca^{2+} flow. Potassium channel activation by channel openers such as cromakalim and nicorandil causes inhibition of ureteral activity. In contrast, the K-ATP channel blocker glibenclamide will prevent these relaxant effects on administration in the presence of channel openers, while having no effect on ureteral contraction on its own [50–52]. Potassium channels are also opened by amitriptyline, a tricyclic antidepressant, causing relaxation; this effect is inhibited by potassium channel blockers [53].

A recent study identified erythropoietin and Gli family proteins as mediators of ureteral contractility. Administration of erythropoietin causes a rapid decrease in ureteral contractile force, while inhibition of Gli family proteins leads to a similar decrease in contractility [25].

Though limited data exist, corticosteroids have been utilized in managing ureteral obstruction, particularly in combination with alpha-1 blockers. Their anti-inflammatory effects are believed to reduce the inflammation surrounding sites of

Table 8.1 Summary of Pharmacological Agents and Activity

Class	Agent Examples	Impact on Peristalsis	Clinical Uses
Alpha Agonists	Norepinephrine	Contraction Enhancement	No current clinical uses in the urinary tract
Alpha Antagonists	Tamsulosin	Relaxation	Medical expulsive therapy for ureteral stones; reduction in stent-related symptoms.
Beta Agonists	Mirabegron, Vibegron, KUL-7211, CL-316243	Relaxation	Increasing utility in overactive bladder; no clinically proven benefits in the ureter.
Beta Antagonists		Contraction Enhancement	No current clinical uses in the urinary tract
Muscarinic Antagonists	Solifenacin	Relaxation	Widely utilized for overactive bladder; some reduction in stent-related symptoms.
Calcium Channel Blockers	Nifedipine	Relaxation	Medical expulsive therapy for ureteral stones; reduction in renal colic.
NSAIDs	Tramadol, Diclofenac, Celecoxib, Indomethacin	Inhibit Ureteral Contractions	Widely utilized for the management of renal colic.

obstruction and enable improved peristalsis. Other hormones have demonstrated impact on ureteral contractility. Changes in progesterone levels during pregnancy have been shown to impact several aspects of kidney physiology, including ureter peristalsis. Progesterone is believed to decrease ureteral contraction and the frequency of peristalsis [54]. The table summarizes the effects of various pharmacological agents on the ureter (Table 8.1).

8.4.5 *Effect of Chemicals, Hormones, and Receptors on Ureteral Function*

Many chemicals have been proposed to influence ureteral function. However, much of this work was done in animal studies with unclear relevance to human ureteral functioning. In consequence, many chemicals have been shown to have both modulating and excitatory effects on the ureter. For instance, the hormone serotonin has been shown to have excitatory, inhibitory, and no impact on the ureter by various groups. Members of the kinin family of polypeptides have also variously been shown to increase the contractile frequency in one animal model while decreasing contractile force in another [3, 4].

Several groups have postulated that the effect of histamine on the ureter is excitatory, possibly acting via the H_1 receptor identified in the human ureter [50]. H_1 receptor antagonists such as mepyramine and pheniramine have been shown to inhibit the action of the ureter in some animals while the agonist 2-(2-pyridyl) ethylamine has the opposite effect [51, 52, 55]. Angiotensin receptors are also expressed in the ureter and are thought to mediate the stimulatory activity of angiotensin on ureteral function [56]. The AT2 receptor antagonist, losartan, was demonstrated to decrease both the amplitude and frequency of ureteral contractions [57].

8.4.6 Antibiotics

Some antibiotics have been reported to influence ureteral activity. Ampicillin administration results in ureteral relaxation, as do chloramphenicol, gentamicin, and isoxazoyl penicillins such as oxacillin. In contrast, tetracyclines have been shown to enhance contractility. The actions of these antibiotics were shown to be due to direct activity on the smooth muscle of the ureter [58].

8.5 Pathophysiology of Pain Response

Ureteral pain is a common cause of morbidity and urologic emergency room visits. Typically, this pain is caused by an obstruction that results in distension of the ureters and the kidney. The distension in the ureter leads to pain by both increased peristalsis around the site of the obstruction as well as an inflammatory process mediated by prostaglandins (as discussed in the prior section). For that reason, the management of ureteral pain relies heavily on anti-inflammatory agents like NSAIDs which inhibit the COX pathway and decrease prostaglandin presence [46]. Importantly, chronic NSAID use can cause worsening renal function in patients with underlying kidney disease. Pharmacologic relaxation of the ureter with agents like nifedipine or an alpha-1 antagonist is another important aspect of pain management [47].

Additionally, the ureters are innervated by afferent and efferent nerves that are sensitive to irritating stimuli and can modulate ureteral peristalsis in response. For example, different concentrations of capsaicin have been noted to have varying impact on ureteral activity. Low-dose capsaicin has an inhibitory effect on ureteral peristalsis, while higher doses have a stimulating effect. The inhibitory activity is believed to be impacted by calcitonin gene-related peptide (CGRP). This peptide's inhibitory action originates from its ability to increase cAMP. The stimulatory effect is believed to be mediated by several tachykinin molecules, including Substance P and neurokinin-2. These tachykinins induce contraction by increasing calcium ion sensitivity in both the membrane channel and the myofilament.

Finally, the effect of narcotics on ureteral function is unclear. While several groups have reported increases in the frequency or amplitude of contractions or the tone of the ureter with morphine and meperidine administration [23, 59], others have noted no effect [4]. Interestingly, there is little data to support a spasmolytic effect of narcotic medications, suggesting that their efficacy in treating renal colic is based mainly on their central nervous system activity.

8.6 Infection and Inflammation

There are some reports that upper urinary tract infection may delay or decrease the transport of urine by the ureter. For example, an inhibitory effect on ureteral peristalsis has been linked to pyelonephritis in an animal model. Similarly, some reports have associated bacterial endotoxins with decreased contractility [60]. However, others have shown no such association [61]. Uropathogenic *Escherichia coli* has been shown to decrease ureteral contractility via a mechanism thought to involve the activation of K^+ channels and subsequent blockage of calcium entry through the L-type calcium channels [62]. This uropathogen also inhibits contractility by its effect on urothelial cells. Urothelial cells that have been infected with bacteria release nitric oxide, which in turn acts to relax smooth muscle [63].

Urinary system infection as well as multiple periureteral inflammatory processes have been associated with ureteral dilation, decreased peristalsis, and even aperistalsis in humans [64, 65]. Additionally, there is evidence that procedures such as stent placement [66] or unilateral ureteral obstruction [67] lead to an inflammatory response in the porcine and murine ureters and an associated transient aperistalsis.

8.7 Pathophysiology of Ureteral Dilation and Hydroureter

8.7.1 Non-Obstructive Uropathy

Numerous non-obstructive uropathies can lead to complications in urine flow and infection. Vesicoureteral reflux (VUR) is the abnormal retrograde flow of urine from the bladder to the ureters and possibly the kidneys [68]. Most available studies focus primarily on the pediatric age group with few studies on adults. The lack thereof may have been associated with the implication that adults did not experience any serious symptoms or loss of renal function due to VUF. We focus here on the effect of VUR on the adult ureter and upper urinary tract.

The severity of VUR was characterized for the pediatric population and has been adopted for adult patients (Fig. 8.6).

VUR is ranked from Grades I–V:

1. Grade I: VUR does not reach the renal pelvis
2. Grade II: VUR extends up the renal pelvis with no dilation of the ureters
3. Grade III: Mild or moderate dilation of the renal pelvis and ureter. Little to no blunting of the fornices
4. Grade IV: Moderate dilation of the renal pelvis, ureter, and calyces. Complete obliteration of the sharp angle of the fornices but maintenance of the papillary impression in most calyces.
5. Grade V: Gross dilation and tortuosity of the ureter. Gross dilation of the renal pelvis and calyces. The papillary impressions are not visible in most calyces.

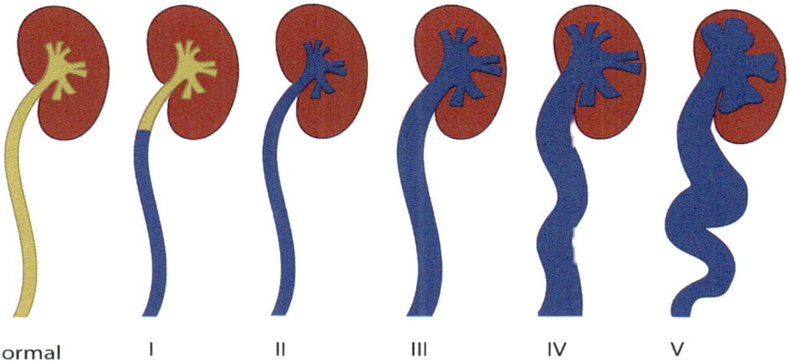

Grade

I	Urine refluxes into ureter. Ureter is not dilated.
II	Urine refluxes into ureter, pelvis, and calyces without dilation.
III	Ureter, pelvis, and calyces are mildly dilated. Fornicies have mild blunting.
IV	Moderate sinuosity of ureter. Ureter, pelvis and calyces are moderately dilated.
V	Ureter, pelvis, and calyces are severely dilated; papillary texture is lost; ureteral tortuosity.

Fig. 8.6 Vesicoureteral reflux grading

VUR is either acquired or congenital. The most common form seen in adult patients is primary congenital, which is a defect in the UVJ valve. One study followed the diagnosis after signs of urinary tract infections (infrequent or recurrent), arterial hypertension, back pain, or kidney stones [68]. The "gold standard" of diagnostic imaging is voiding cystourethrogram with an excretory urography (or intravenous pyelogram) being used in the past. Primary concerns of VUR and frequent indicators of treatment are the formation of renal scarring, pyelonephritis, and loss of renal function, which can develop regardless of the presence of urosepsis [68]. Medical treatment usually involves antibiotic therapy for the resolution of urinary tract infections secondary to VUR. VUR will be discussed in more detail in a separate chapter.

Megaureter is chronic dilation of the ureter's lumen for which no obstructive cause has been found [69]. In order for the diameter to be considered abnormal, the lumen must exceed a diameter greater than 8 mm. Megaureters can be classified as obstructive, refluxing, obstructive and refluxing, or neither [70]. Pathology can be either primary or secondary. Many studies have been performed to describe the histological appearance of the megaureter; the most common finding is consistent with an abundance of connective tissues in the abnormal ureter. There have been several findings that display a relationship between collagen and smooth muscle cells with the abnormal ureter. Lee et al. demonstrated a larger collagen-to-smooth muscle ratio in the megaureter when compared to a normal ureter. An increase in collagen production has also been seen in the abnormal ureter [71].

Most cases of megaureter are of non-obstructive, non-refluxing nature. The cases of secondary non-obstructive, non-refluxing megaureter are due to a cause unrelated to anatomy. It is in these cases that dilation is caused by high fetal urine output, increased compliance of the fetal ureter, or a partial or transient obstruction during development. Urinary tract infections may also cause megaureter [70].

8.7.2 *Obstructive Uropathy*

Obstructive uropathy is the blockage of urine flow anywhere along the urinary tract [72]. Obstruction in ureter function is evaluated on the degree and duration of the obstruction, rate of urine flow, and the presence of infection, or lack thereof. Once obstruction occurs, a backup of urine begins to appear, along with increased ureteral intraluminal pressure and ureteral size, both in diameter and length [4]. Hydroureter and hydronephrosis form proximal to the obstruction. Intraluminal pressure increases with the production of urine that cannot pass due to obstruction. Ureteral dimensions continue to grow with intraluminal pressure and retained urine. At first, peristaltic wave contractions increase (in frequency and amplitude) when accompanied by the initial changes in ureteral dimensions. Over time, these waves diminish and the ureter relies on the kidney's hydrostatic forces for urine transport [4]. As the obstruction continues, a considerable change in ureteral dimensions persists even when ureteral pressure remains low and constant.

The effect of ureteral calculi on ureter function is largely due to their relationship with ureteral obstruction. Spontaneous passage may occur based on the shape and size of the stone, ureteral peristalsis, hydrostatic pressure, and tissue abnormality caused at the site of the lodged stone. When passage does not occur, systemic inflammatory response syndrome (SIRS) is prevalent in patients entering the ED for renal colic. SIRS is one of several indicators of intervention for obstructing ureteral stones [73]. Calculi will be discussed in detail in a separate chapter.

8.7.3 *Renal Sequelae of Ureteral Obstruction*

Several complications can arise from an acutely or chronically obstructed ureter with short and long-term implications for renal function. In unilateral acute obstruction, there is an overall increase in ureteral pressure that is transmitted to the kidneys [74, 75]. This leads to decreased kidney function, evidenced by low GFRs. In response, prostaglandins cause vasodilation in an attempt to increase renal blood flow and improve the GFR. This increased flow further drives increased pressure leading to the renal colic seen clinically. Eventually, the renal blood flow decreases and the obstruction becomes more chronic in nature.

Chronic obstruction differs meaningfully from acute obstruction in that there is a reduction in blood flow. This decreases intrarenal pressure, thereby decreasing the pain experienced by patients [75]. Despite limited pain, chronic obstruction still has substantial negative effects on kidney function. For example, GFRs are decreased in unilateral chronic ureter obstruction. This may be due to several factors, but fibrotic changes in the obstructed kidney may play a contributory role. In chronically obstructed ureters the renin-angiotensin aldosterone system was found to be activated in the impacted kidney [76]. There was increased expression of angiotensin-converting enzyme 1 (ACE 1). This enzyme converts angiotensin I (Ang1) to angiotensin II (AngII). The increased angiotensin II then increases the expression of profibrotic factors like fibronectin and TGF-ß1 [76]. However, in the same obstructed kidney, an increase in angiotensin-converting enzyme 2 (ACE 2) leads to the increased expression of AngI which opposes the fibrotic effects of AngII. These findings suggest a delicate balance between pro and antifibrotic factors within a chronically obstructed kidney. There is likely a long-term consequence to the integrity and function of the ureter as a result. This will be explored in a separate chapter.

8.8 Conclusion

A basic understanding of ureteral physiology and pharmacology can have meaningful benefits in a clinical setting. Renal colic from ureteral obstruction is considered one of the worst pains a patient can experience. Even the stenting done to relieve obstruction can cause meaningful discomfort in select patients. Therefore, a thorough understanding of the agents that can induce relaxation in the ureters and limit pain can aid in reducing morbidity or ureteral obstructive pathologies.

Questions

1. How is ureteral peristalsis propagated?
   (a) Ureteral peristalsis is myogenic
   (b) Ureteral peristalsis is propagated via transcription factors
   (c) Ureteral peristalsis relies on the action of skeletal muscles

Answer: (a)
Peristalsis is a myogenic process that is initiated at the pacemaker cells

2. What ions are involved in contraction of the ureter?
   (a) Sodium
   (b) Potassium
   (c) Calcium
   (d) All of the above

Answer: (d)
The ion channels thought to be involved in peristalsis include the Na^+/K^+ pump and L-Type voltage gated Ca^{2+} channels. Peristalsis is also mediated via the activity of K^+ channels.

3. How does ureteral dysfunction contribute to renal colic?
   (a) It has no effect
   (b) Renal obstruction leads to colic
   (c) Decreased intrarenal pressure leads to renal colic

Answer: (b)
Renal colic is thought to involve increased spasmolytic activity in the ureter and elevated upper urinary system pressure associated with ureteral obstruction.

4. What is the proposed effect of alpha 1 receptor antagonist activity in ureteral obstruction?
   (a) Adrenergic antagonists increase the strength of ureteral contractions
   (b) Adrenergic antagonists decrease the strength of ureteral contractions
   (c) The effect of adrenergic antagonists on the ureter is unknown

Answer: (b)
Stimulation of alpha-adrenergic receptors results in excitation of ureteral peristalsis; antagonists of this receptor attenuate the strength of ureteral contractions.

5. What is the effect of urinary system infection on peristalsis?
   (a) Infection inhibits peristalsis
   (b) Infection has no effect on peristalsis
   (c) Infection increases peristalsis

Answer: (a)
Infection is thought to decrease the transport of urine by the ureter. The mechanism is still not fully understood.

References

1. Lang RJHH. Pacemaker mechanisms driving pyeloureteric peristalsis: modulatory role of interstitial cells. smooth muscle spontaneous activity. In: Advances in experimental medicine and biology. Singapore: Springer; 2019.
2. Weiss RM. Clinical implications of ureteral physiology. J Urol. 1979;121(4):401–13. https://doi.org/10.1016/s0022-5347(17)56799-3.
3. Boyarsky S, Labay P. Ureteral motility. Annu Rev Med. 1969;20:383–94. https://doi.org/10.1146/annurev.me.20.020169.002123.
4. Weiss RM, Martin DT. Physiology and pharmacology of the renal pelvis and ureter. In: Campbell-Walsh urology. Amsterdam: Elsevier; 2016.
5. Griffiths DJ. NC. The mechanics of urine transport in the upper urinary tract: 1. The dynamics of the isolated bolus. Neurourol Urodyn. 1983;2(2):155–66. https://doi.org/10.1002/nau.1930020209.
6. Kuriyama H, Osa T, Toida N. Membrane properties of the smooth muscle of guinea-pig ureter. J Physiol. 1967;191(2):225–38. https://doi.org/10.1113/jphysiol.1967.sp008247.

7. Lang RJ. Identification of the major membrane currents in freshly dispersed single smooth muscle cells of guinea-pig ureter. J Physiol. 1989;412:375–95. https://doi.org/10.1113/jphysiol.1989.sp017622.
8. Weiss RM, Bassett AL, Hoffman BF. Adrenergic innervation of the ureter. Investig Urol. 1978;16(2):123–7.
9. Kuriyama H, Tomita T. The action potential in the smooth muscle of the guinea pig taenia coli and ureter studied by the double sucrose-gap method. J Gen Physiol. 1970;55(2):147–62. https://doi.org/10.1085/jgp.55.2.147.
10. Burdyga TV, Wray S. The relationship between the action potential, intracellular calcium and force in intact phasic, guinea-pig uretic smooth muscle. J Physiol. 1999;520(Pt 3):867–83. https://doi.org/10.1111/j.1469-7793.1999.00867.x.
11. Cuthbert AW. The relation between response and the interval between stimuli of the isolated guinea-pig ureter. J Physiol. 1965;180(2):225–38. https://doi.org/10.1113/jphysiol.1965.sp007700.
12. Maggi CA, Giuliani S, Santicioli P. Effect of Bay K 8644 and ryanodine on the refractory period, action potential and mechanical response of the guinea-pig ureter to electrical stimulation. Naunyn Schmiedeberg's Arch Pharmacol. 1994;349(5):510–22. https://doi.org/10.1007/BF00169141.
13. Exintaris B, Lang RJ. Effects of nerve stimulation on spontaneously active preparations of the guinea pig ureter. Urol Res. 1999;27(5):328–35. https://doi.org/10.1007/s002400050159.
14. Burdyga T, Wray S. Action potential refractory period in ureter smooth muscle is set by Ca sparks and BK channels. Nature. 2005;436(7050):559–62. https://doi.org/10.1038/nature03834.
15. Lang RJ, Tonta MA, Zoltkowski BZ, Meeker WF, Wendt I, Parkington HC. Pyeloureteric peristalsis: role of atypical smooth muscle cells and interstitial cells of Cajal-like cells as pacemakers. J Physiol. 2006;576(Pt 3):695–705. https://doi.org/10.1113/jphysiol.2006.116855.
16. Hurtado R, Bub G, Herzlinger D. The pelvis-kidney junction contains HCN3, a hyperpolarization-activated cation channel that triggers ureter peristalsis. Kidney Int. 2010;77(6):500–8. https://doi.org/10.1038/ki.2009.483.
17. Dixon JS, Gosling JA. The musculature of the human renal calices, pelvis and upper ureter. J Anat. 1982;135(Pt 1):129–37.
18. Shiratori TKH. Electromyographic studies on urinary tract. Tohoku J Exper Med. 1961;73:159–69.
19. Hashitani H, Lang RJ. Functions of ICC-like cells in the urinary tract and male genital organs. J Cell Mol Med. 2010;14(6A):1199–211. https://doi.org/10.1111/j.1582-4934.2010.01043.x.
20. Lang RJ, Klemm MF. Interstitial cell of Cajal-like cells in the upper urinary tract. J Cell Mol Med. 2005;9(3):543–56. https://doi.org/10.1111/j.1582-4934.2005.tb00487.x.
21. Engelmann TW. Zur Physiologie des Ureters. Pflugers Arch. 1869;2:243–93.
22. Santicioli P, Maggi CA. Myogenic and neurogenic factors in the control of pyeloureteral motility and ureteral peristalsis. Pharmacol Rev. 1998;50(4):683–722.
23. Vereecken RL, Hendrickx H, Casteels R. The influence of calcium on the electrical and mechanical activity of the guinea pig ureter. Urol Res. 1975;3(4) 149–53. https://doi.org/10.1007/BF00261949.
24. Hong KW, Biancani P, Weiss RM. "On" and "off" responses of guinea pig ureter. Am J Phys. 1985;248(1 Pt 1):C165–9. https://doi.org/10.1152/ajpcell.1985.248.1.C165.
25. Scotland KB, Bidnur S, Wang L, Chew BH, Lange D. Mediators of human ureteral smooth muscle contraction-a role for erythropoietin, tamsulosin and Gli effectors Transl Androl Urol. 2021;10(7):2953–61. https://doi.org/10.21037/tau-20-1342.
26. McLeod DG, Reynolds DG, Swan KG. Adrenergic mechanisms in the canine ureter. Am J Phys. 1973;224(5):1054–8. https://doi.org/10.1152/ajplegacy.1973.224.5.1054.

27. Sasaki S, Tomiyama Y, Kobayashi S, Kojima Y, Kubota Y, Kohri K. Characterization of alpha1-adrenoceptor subtypes mediating contraction in human isolated ureters. Urology. 2011;77(3):762 e13–7. https://doi.org/10.1016/j.urology.2010.09.034.
28. Canda AE, Turna B, Cinar GM, Nazli O. Physiology and pharmacology of the human ureter: basis for current and future treatments. Urol Int. 2007;78(4):289–98. https://doi.org/10.1159/000100830.
29. Morita T, Ishizuka G, Suzuki T, Kondo S, Tsuchida S. Conduction velocity in various regions of the renal pelvis and ureter. Tohoku J Exp Med. 1983;141(2):245–6. https://doi.org/10.1620/tjem.141.245.
30. Troxel SA, Jones AW, Magliola L, Benson JS. Physiologic effect of nifedipine and tamsulosin on contractility of distal ureter. J Endourol. 2006;20(8):565–8. https://doi.org/10.1089/end.2006.20.565.
31. Davenport K, Timoney AG, Keeley FX Jr. Effect of smooth muscle relaxant drugs on proximal human ureteric activity in vivo: a pilot study. Urol Res. 2007;35(4):207–13. https://doi.org/10.1007/s00240-007-0100-x.
32. Meltzer AC, Burrows PK, Wolfson AB, Hollander JE, Kurz M, Kirkali Z, et al. Effect of tamsulosin on passage of symptomatic ureteral stones: a randomized clinical trial. JAMA Intern Med. 2018;178(8):1051–7. https://doi.org/10.1001/jamainternmed.2018.2259.
33. Michel MC. Beta-adrenergic receptor subtypes in the urinary tract. Handb Exp Pharmacol. 2011;202:307–18. https://doi.org/10.1007/978-3-642-16499-6_15.
34. Shen H, Chen Z, Mokhtar AD, Bi X, Wu G, Gong S, et al. Expression of beta-adrenergic receptor subtypes in human normal and dilated ureter. Int Urol Nephrol. 2017;49(10):1771–8. https://doi.org/10.1007/s11255-017-1667-y.
35. Wanajo I, Tomiyama Y, Tadachi M, Kobayashi M, Yamazaki Y, Kojima M, et al. The potency of KUL-7211, a selective ureteral relaxant, in isolated canine ureter: comparison with various spasmolytics. Urol Res. 2005;33(6):409–14. https://doi.org/10.1007/s00240-005-0475-5.
36. Tae BS, Cho S, Jeon BJ, Choi H, Park JY, Cho SY, et al. Does mirabegron relieve ureteric stent-related discomfort? A prospective, randomized, multicentre study. BJU Int. 2018;122(5):866–72. https://doi.org/10.1111/bju.14416.
37. Bayar G, Yavuz A, Cakmak S, Ofluoglu Y, Kilinc MF, Kucuk E, et al. Efficacy of silodosin or mirabegron in medical expulsive therapy for ureteral stones: a prospective, randomized-controlled study. Int Urol Nephrol. 2020;52(5):835–40. https://doi.org/10.1007/s11255-019-02368-y.
38. Sakamoto K, Suri D, Rajasekaran M. Characterization of muscarinic receptor subtypes in human ureter. J Endourol. 2006;20(11):939–42. https://doi.org/10.1089/end.2006.20.939.
39. Zhou L, Cai X, Li H, Wang KJ. Effects of alpha-blockers, antimuscarinics, or combination therapy in relieving ureteral stent-related symptoms: a meta-analysis. J Endourol. 2015;29(6):650–6. https://doi.org/10.1089/end.2014.0715.
40. Wang J, Zhang X, Zhang T, Mu J, Bai B, Lei Y. The role of solifenacin, as monotherapy or combination with tamsulosin in ureteral stent-related symptoms: a systematic review and meta-analysis. World J Urol. 2017;35(11):1669–80. https://doi.org/10.1007/s00345-017-2051-3.
41. Yan H, Wang Y, Sun R, Cui Y. The efficacy of antimuscarinics alone or in combination with alpha-blockers for the treatment of ureteral stent-related symptoms: a systematic review and meta-analysis. Urol Int. 2017;99(1):6–13. https://doi.org/10.1159/000449390.
42. Park J, Yoo C, Han DH, Shin DW. A critical assessment of the effects of tamsulosin and solifenacin as monotherapies and as a combination therapy for the treatment of ureteral stent-related symptoms: a 2 x 2 factorial randomized trial. World J Urol. 2015;33(11):1833–40. https://doi.org/10.1007/s00345-015-1544-1.
43. Lowry PS, Jerde TJ, Bjorling DE, Maskel JL, Nakada SY. Obstruction alters the effect of prostaglandin E2 on ureteral contractility. J Endourol. 2005;19(2):183–7. https://doi.org/10.1089/end.2005.19.183.
44. Mastrangelo D, Iselin CE. Urothelium dependent inhibition of rat ureter contractile activity. J Urol. 2007;178(2):702–9. https://doi.org/10.1016/j.juro.2007.03.099.

45. Huang ZA, Scotland KB, Li Y, Tan J, Kung SHY, Chew BH, et al. Determination of urinary prostaglandin E2 as a potential biomarker of ureteral stent associated inflammation. J Chromatogr B Analyt Technol Biomed Life Sci. 2020;1145:122107. https://doi.org/10.1016/j.jchromb.2020.122107.
46. Koprowski C, Kim C, Modi PK, Elsamra SE. Ureteral stent-associated pain: a review. J Endourol. 2016;30(7):744–53. https://doi.org/10.1089/end.2016.0129.
47. Hadibrata E, Farishal A, Ali Z, Danarto R. Tamsulosin and sodium diclofenac as an effective therapy to reduce pain after ureteral stent removal: a prospective, double blinded randomized placebo controlled trial. Urol J. 2020;18(1):111–6. https://doi.org/10.22037/uj.v0i0.5190.
48. Pearle MS, Goldfarb DS, Assimos DG, Curhan G, Denu-Ciocca CJ, Matlaga BR, et al. Medical management of kidney stones: AUA guideline. J Urol. 2014;192(2):316–24. https://doi.org/10.1016/j.juro.2014.05.006.
49. Forman A, Andersson KE, Henriksson L, Rud T, Ulmsten U. Effects of nifedipine on the smooth muscle of the human urinary tract in vitro and in vivo. Acta Pharmacol Toxicol (Copenh). 1978;43(2):111–8. https://doi.org/10.1111/j.1600-0773.1978.tb02244.x.
50. Floyd RV, Borisova L, Bakran A, Hart CA, Wray S, Burdyga TV. Morphology, calcium signaling and mechanical activity in human ureter. J Urol. 2008;180(1):398–405. https://doi.org/10.1016/j.juro.2008.02.045.
51. Smita K, Sushil Kumar V, Premendran J, Sharma ML. Goat ureter - an alternative model for measuring ureteral peristalsis. J Smooth Muscle Res. 2006;42(4):117–30. https://doi.org/10.1540/jsmr.42.117.
52. Dodel RC, Hafner D, Borchard U. Characterization of histamine receptors in the ureter of the dog. Eur J Pharmacol. 1996;318(2–3):395–402. https://doi.org/10.1016/s0014-2999(96)00765-0.
53. Achar E, Achar RA, Paiva TB, Campos AH, Schor N. Amitriptyline eliminates calculi through urinary tract smooth muscle relaxation. Kidney Int. 2003;64(4):1356–64. https://doi.org/10.1046/j.1523-1755.2003.00222.x.
54. Waltzer WC. The urinary tract in pregnancy. J Urol. 1981;125(3):271–6. https://doi.org/10.1016/s0022-5347(17)55008-9.
55. Benedito S, Prieto D, Rivera L, Costa G, Garcia-Sacristan A. Mechanisms implicated in the histamine response of the sheep ureterovesical junction. J Urol. 1991;146(1):184–7. https://doi.org/10.1016/s0022-5347(17)37749-2.
56. Santis WF, Peters CA, Yalla SV, Sullivan MP. Ureteral function is modulated by a local renin-angiotensin system. J Urol. 2003;170(1):259–63. https://doi.org/10.1097/01.ju.0000060848.61864.e1.
57. Fujinaka H, Miyazaki Y, Matsusaka T, Yoshida H, Fogo AB, Inagami T, et al. Salutary role for angiotensin in partial urinary tract obstruction. Kidney Int. 2000;58(5):2018–27. https://doi.org/10.1111/j.1523-1755.2000.00374.x.
58. Benzi G, Arrigoni E, Panceri P, Panzarasa R, Berte F, Crema A. Effect of antibiotics on the ureter motor activity. Jpn J Pharmacol. 1973;23(5):599–607. https://doi.org/10.1254/jjp.23.599.
59. Ockerblad NF, Hjalmar E, Carlson SJF. The effect of morphine on the human ureter. J Urol. 1935;3:356.
60. Roberts JA. Vesicoureteral reflux and pyelonephritis in the monkey: a review. J Urol. 1992;148(5 Pt 2):1721–5. https://doi.org/10.1016/s0022-5347(17)37013-1.
61. Struthers NW. The effect of E. coli and E. coli endotoxin on peristalsis in canine ureter. Urol Res. 1976;4(3):107–9. https://doi.org/10.1007/BF00257165.
62. Floyd RV, Winstanley C, Bakran A, Wray S, Burdyga TV. Modulation of ureteric Ca signaling and contractility in humans and rats by uropathogenic E. coli. Am J Physiol Renal Physiol. 2010;298(4):F900–8. https://doi.org/10.1152/ajprenal.00468.2009.
63. Poljakovic M, Persson K. Urinary tract infection in iNOS-deficient mice with focus on bacterial sensitivity to nitric oxide. Am J Physiol Renal Physiol. 2003;284(1):F22–31. https://doi.org/10.1152/ajprenal.00101.2002.
64. Ross JA, Edmond P. The effects of calculi on ureteral function. Br J Surg. 1972;59(1):45–9. https://doi.org/10.1002/bjs.1800590112.

65. Makker SP, Tucker AS, Izant RJ Jr, Heymann W. Nonobstructive hydronephrosis and hydropureter associated with peritonitis. N Engl J Med. 1972;287(11):535–7. https://doi.org/10.1056/NEJM197209142871104.
66. Janssen C, Buttyan R, Seow CY, Jager W, Solomon D, Fazli L, et al. A role for the hedgehog effector Gli1 in mediating stent-induced ureteral smooth muscle dysfunction and aperistalsis. Urology. 2017;104:242e1–8. https://doi.org/10.1016/j.urology.2017.01.029.
67. Park E, Cox M, Scotland K, Buttyan R, Lange D. Erythropoietin promotes functional recovery via anti-apoptotic mechanisms in mouse unilateral ureteral obstruction. Cell Stress Chaperones. 2020;25(2):245–51. https://doi.org/10.1007/s12192-020-01067-3.
68. Greenbaum LA, Mesrobian HG. Vesicoureteral reflux. Pediatr Clin N Am. 2006;53(3):413–27., vi. https://doi.org/10.1016/j.pcl.2006.02.010.
69. Williams DI. Mega-ureter. Postgrad Med J. 1958;34(389):159–62. https://doi.org/10.1136/pgmj.34.389.159.
70. Hodges SJ, Werle D, McLorie G, Atala A. Megaureter. ScientificWorldJournal. 2010;10:603–12. https://doi.org/10.1100/tsw.2010.54.
71. Lee BR, Silver RI, Partin AW, Epstein JI, Gearhart JP. A quantitative histologic analysis of collagen subtypes: the primary obstructed and refluxing megaureter of childhood. Urology. 1998;51(5):820–3. https://doi.org/10.1016/s0090-4295(98)00013-2.
72. Girardi M, Martin N. Obstructive uropathy. Hospital Med Clin. 2015;4(3):328–41. https://doi.org/10.1016/j.ehmc.2015.03.010.
73. Larkin S, Johnson J, Venkatesh T, Vetter J, Venkatesh R. Systemic inflammatory response syndrome in patients with acute obstructive upper tract urinary stone: a risk factor for urgent renal drainage and revisit to the emergency department. BMC Urol. 2020;20(1):77. https://doi.org/10.1186/s12894-020-00644-z.
74. Ucero AC, Benito-Martin A, Izquierdo MC, Sanchez-Nino MD, Sanz AB, Ramos AM, et al. Unilateral ureteral obstruction: beyond obstruction. Int Urol Nephrol. 2014;46(4):765–76. https://doi.org/10.1007/s11255-013-0520-1.
75. Capelouto CC, Saltzman B. The pathophysiology of ureteral obstruction. J Endourol. 1993;7(2):93–103. https://doi.org/10.1089/end.1993.7.93.
76. Washino S, Hosohata K, Miyagawa T. Roles played by biomarkers of kidney injury in patients with upper urinary tract obstruction. Int J Mol Sci. 2020;21(15) https://doi.org/10.3390/ijms21155490.

Chapter 9
Pathophysiologic Response of the Ureter to Obstruction

Alina Reicherz, Roman Herout, Ben H. Chew, and Dirk Lange

Abstract Ureteral obstruction results in a hydroureter and hydronephrosis. Depending on the degree and duration of the obstruction, ureteral obstruction causes morphological and functional changes. Acute ureteral obstruction impairs the urine outlet, and thus, a hydroureter develops. Initially, the peristaltic activity increases to overcome the obstruction; with prolonged obstruction, peristaltic waves decrease – ultimately leading to aperistalsis. Histologically, ureteral obstruction causes muscle hypertrophy and triggers an inflammatory response in the ureteral tissue. Chronically obstructed ureters show signs of fibrotic remodelling. Structural changes of the ureter likely impair ureteral functionality in the long term by affecting smooth muscle activity and electrical propagation. Evidence exists that the peristaltic activity of the contralateral ureter might also be affected.

Despite its high occurrence, pathophysiologic changes of the ureter in response to obstruction are poorly understood. Further studies are required to explore pathophysiologic changes in the ureter due to obstruction and the impact of ureteral dysfunction on kidney functionality.

Keywords Ureter · Peristalsis · Ureteral functionality · Histology · Pathophysiology · Smooth muscle functionality · Fibrosis

Learning Objectives
- Review morphological and functional changes of the ureter following ureteral obstruction
- Explore short- and long-term clinical implications of hydroureteric condition
- Discuss translation into clinical practice and open questions.

Test your learning and check your understanding of this book's contents: use the "Springer Nature Flashcards" app to access questions. To use the app, please follow the instructions in Chapter 1.

A. Reicherz · R. Herout · B. H. Chew · D. Lange (✉)
The Stone Centre at Vancouver General Hospital, Department of Urologic Science, University of British Columbia, Vancouver, BC, Canada
e-mail: Alina.reicherz@ruhr-uni-bochum.de; rherout@prostatecentre.com; ben.chew@ubc.ca; dirk.lange@ubc.ca

M. Abdel-Gawad et al. (eds.), *The Ureter*,
https://doi.org/10.1007/978-3-031-36212-5_9

9.1 Introduction

Ureteral obstruction is a common disorder impairing urine outlet. Obstruction can result from acute intraluminal blockage of the ureter, most commonly by a stone or acute extraluminal compression (e.g., retroperitoneal bleeding) or iatrogenic, by ligation. Furthermore, obstruction can develop chronically from partial intraluminal blockage by a stone or ureteral obstruction, e.g., inflammatory, posttraumatic, iatrogenic (e.g., strictures due to radiation or after ureteroscopies), ureteral malignancies or an extra ureteral compression. Pathophysiologic response of the ureter depends on the degree, partial or complete, and duration of obstruction as well as urine flow [1]. An impaired urine outlet and associated changes in pressure conditions cause a hydroureter and hydronephrosis. These conditions can cause acute and chronic kidney insufficiency and promote stone formation and urinary tract infection. As a complication of acute obstruction, a fornical rupture can occur and lead to extravasation of urine. Acute obstruction resulting from an immediate, high-grade obstruction causes severe pain, while gradually developing chronic obstruction can be without symptoms. Acute and chronic ureteral obstruction can severely affect the pathophysiology of the kidney. This chapter will focus on pathophysiologic changes of the ureter. Current knowledge originates mostly from animal trials — however, it is reasonable to assume that mechanisms can be largely applied to human pathophysiology.

9.2 Pathophysiologic Response of the Ureter to Acute Ureteral Obstruction

Rose and Gillenwater have contributed substantially to knowledge about hydrodynamics of the ureter and the effects of its complete obstruction [2, 3]. To better understand functional changes, one must differentiate between ureteral wall tension and intraluminal ureteral pressure at baseline (resting pressure between contractions) and during contraction.

Following acute ureteral occlusion, urine flow is impaired. As a result, baseline intraluminal ureteral pressure increases, and ureteral wall tension builds up slightly [4, 5]. Within minutes, the frequency of peristaltic waves rises [5, 6] as it attempts to overcome the obstruction. Both baseline and peak intraluminal ureteral pressure and wall tension increase; as the increase in peak pressure and peak tension are higher, the amplitude of the pressure waves increases [2, 6]. The mechanical stretch of the ureter is potentially responsible for COX-2 upregulation, which mediates prostaglandin (PGE) E_2 release and contributes to increased intrapelvic pressure [7] and is involved in pain perception. In the short term, baseline pressure increases gradually due to continued urine production and wall tension rises. These pressure changes lead to a decrease in ureteral pressure waves. After a peaking of intraluminal ureteral pressure within a few hours after obstruction, despite continued minimal urine flow, intraluminal ureteral pressure stabilizes. Reasons for that might be a decreased glomerular filtration rate, fluid reabsorption, and decreased wall tension [8].

9.3 Effect of Ureteral Obstruction on Morphological Changes

Anatomically, the ureters' dimensions (length and diameter) increase substantially as a result of obstruction. These changes are referred to as "creep"[9]. Computer tomography imaging in patients with acute flank pain has shown that the mean diameter of the ureter measures 7 mm ± 3.2 mm and 1.8 mm ± 0.9 mm for obstructed and asymptomatic sides, respectively [10]. The star-shaped lumen gradually flattens to a circular ring. Distension is associated with physical stretch and thereby causes ischemia and hence ischemic injury of ureteral tissue [11]. Ischemia is likely to trigger an inflammatory response. Submucosal mononuclear inflammatory cells following obstruction provide evidence [12]. A release of cytokines might contribute to the remodelling of ureteral tissue. To the best of our knowledge, inflammatory pathways that drive tissue alteration have not been studied comprehensively.

Various trials on partial and complete ureteral obstruction in animal models describe tissue remodelling within days to weeks following obstruction. Within days, hypertrophy of smooth muscle cells is present [2, 4, 13–16]. Within weeks, the number of elastic fibres increases, and fibrotic connective tissue is deposited in the muscle and adventitia layers.

Among others, these findings are based on results published in 1982 by Biancani and co-workers. They observed muscular changes in rabbit ureters after obstruction for two weeks: Hypertrophy of the muscle layer was present with an increase in the muscle layer by 248%, length by 24% and outer ureteral diameter by 100%. Segments from obstructed ureters developed higher contractile forces [4].

In more recent experiments by Tillig and co-workers in a model of chronic unilateral partial obstruction in guinea pigs, ureters were implanted into the psoas muscle and evaluated after 2–6 months [14]. Consistently, those chronically partially obstructed ureters showed an increased thickness of the muscular layer and an increase of connective tissue in the ureter proximal to the obstruction. Distal of the obstruction, thickness of the ureteral muscular layer was decreased while the connective tissue was increased, similar to the proximal ureter. After obstruction, rarefication and disorientation of the nerve fibres were present in the proximal ureter.

In a rat model of complete unilateral obstruction, apoptotic cells in the smooth muscle layer were observed 14 days after ligation of the ureter, and fibrotic changes were present after 21 days [15, 16]. These changes were associated with increased cytochrome c and caspases in the smooth muscle layer. Our work group demonstrated that erythropoietin treatment suppressed apoptosis in obstructed ureteral tissue and accelerated hydronephrosis resolution and ureteral peristalsis restoration [17].

9.4 Effect of Obstruction on Ureteral Peristalsis

Effective peristaltic waves are required to transport urine from the kidney to the bladder. Ureteral obstruction impairs efficient peristalsis. As described in *Effect of ureteral obstruction on morphological changes*, ureteric smooth muscle undergoes hypertrophic changes following obstruction and consecutively gains contractility. However, despite muscle hypertrophy and increased contractility: ureters have shown to be less able to coapt the ureteral wall due to a decreased ratio of ureteral wall thickness to ureteral diameter. Hence the ability to generate contractile pressure required for urine flow is decreased [2]. The LaPlace relationship has been employed to describe the underlying mechanism [1].

$$\text{Pressure} = \text{stress} \times \frac{\text{wall thickness}}{\text{radius}}$$

Peristaltic activity not only depends on ureteral motility but also electric impulses and transmission of impulses. The effect of obstruction on electric impulses and propagation alters between immediate, early and chronic stages.

In normal ureters, electric impulses are mainly generated in the kidney-pelvis-junction by typical and atypical smooth muscle cells and Cajal-like cells and propagated antegrade to the bladder [6]. Hammad and co-workers studied the propagation of electrical impulses in unilaterally obstructed ureters in rats [18]. They used 64 extracellular electrodes to record electrical activity proximal and distal of the obstruction for up to 2 weeks. Following the initial increase in the frequency of contractions in the proximal ureter, the frequency and velocity of contractions decreased gradually. In the distal ureter, antegrade propagation gradually faded.

One week after obstruction, one-third of the mice demonstrated retrograde electrical activity, whereas the velocity of impulses increased continuously with prolonged obstruction. These changes correlated with decreased peristaltic activity [18]. The findings indicate that in chronic stages when obstruction persists for days to weeks, propagation of excitation is likely inhibited by structural changes of the tissue as described in *Effect of ureteral obstruction on morphological changes*. Deposition of connective tissue might disrupt propagation and cause loss of coordination and impact frequency of contractions [6].

The model for partial chronic obstruction in guinea pigs supports the hypothesis of disrupted electric propagation by changes following dilatation of ureteral tissue. They showed increased spontaneous myogenic activity in the renal pelvis, ureteral-pelvic junction and distal ureter compared to the contralateral ureter, while spontaneous myogenic activity was decreased in the proximal ureter [14].

In vivo, experiments revealed that the number of interstitial Cajal-like cells in the submucosal layer of the ureteropelvic junction started to increase on day seven and peaked at day 14 after ureteral obstruction.

Interestingly, Hammad et al. found a transient increase in the frequency of peristalsis of the contralateral ureter immediately after obstruction [18]. Animal trials from our workgroup performing unilateral obstruction for 48 h observed reduced peristaltic frequency in the contralateral unobstructed ureter and hypothesized that the effect was driven by systemic acute inflammatory cytokine release [8, 19]. However, the systemic effect of obstruction and the inflammatory response to obstruction are poorly understood.

The COX-2-pathway is involved in altered contractility in obstructed ureters [20, 21]. As previously described, COX-2 is upregulated in obstructed ureters [7, 20]. The stretch-induced upregulation induces the synthesis of prostanoids, including PGE_2. In normal unobstructed ureters, PGE_2 has no effect or a relaxant effect. Ureteral obstruction seems to trigger changes that reverse the effect of PGE_2. In response to PGE_2, contractility increased in obstructed ureters, and contractility was accentuated with prolonged obstruction [21].

9.5 Long-term Effects of Ureteral Obstruction

Data on the long-term outcome concerning the impact of obstruction is limited. Typically, after resolving obstruction, patients present with transiently persistent hydronephrosis. Barbour et al. completed a retrospective review monitoring hydronephrosis in 324 patients who underwent ureterorenoscopy. [22] Four to 12 weeks after URS, 49 patients had evidence for hydronephrosis on computed tomography or ultrasound imaging, 24 patients had no evidence of obstruction, and underlying ureteral edema was suspected. To the best of our knowledge, no data on longer-term morbidity after ureteral obstruction is published. Moreover, it is unknown to what extent tissue damage and subsequent remodelling are irreversible. In 1992 Harada et al. published results on the loss of ureteral compliance following partial obstruction in dogs [13]. Ureters were partially obstructed by ligation for up to 26 weeks. Ureteral compliance increased until week eight of obstruction proportionally to muscle hypertrophy and decreased subsequently proportional to deposition of connective tissue. Furthermore, Lennon et al. demonstrated that the effect and recovery from complete and partial obstruction differs [23]. Partial obstruction of the ureter was induced in dogs by ligating a polyethylene stent into the lower end of the ureter for four weeks. Obstruction was relieved by dissecting the ureter above the ligature or stent, and ureters were reimplanted. Eight weeks after relief of obstruction, recovery was reevaluated. Ureters, both, after partial and complete obstruction, almost returned to pre-obstruction dimensions. While completely obstructed ureters returned to normal baseline ureteric pressure, peak pressure and peristaltic frequency, in those ureters that were partially obstructed, ureteric peak pressure was still increased compared to pre-obstruction, indicating persisting increased contractility.

In a rat model of 24 h complete unilateral obstruction, two weeks after the release of obstruction frequency and velocity of peristaltic waves returned to pre-obstruction levels after two weeks of recovery. After partial obstruction, restoration took a shorter time [6].

Interestingly, Chuang et al. analyzed myocyte regeneration in formerly obstructed ureters. PCNA, a marker for cell proliferation, was expressed 14 days after ligation of the ureter. Its increase correlated with an increase in epidermal growth factor, basic fibroblast growth factor and insulin growth factor-1. The authors hypothesized that these factors might contribute to ureteral regeneration [24].

9.6 Translation into Clinical Practice and Open Clinical Questions

Knowledge on the topic is mostly based on historical, scientific findings. Recently, little focus was put on ureteral pathophysiology, which is reflected in a minimal knowledge gain in the last decade.

In clinical practice, ureteral obstruction comprises a heterogeneous pathology. The degree of ureteral obstruction differs from patient to patient, and symptoms range from severe pain and symptomless. The question remains how the available research data can be translated into translated clinically. Experimental research is primarily based on animal models with complete ureteral obstruction by ligation or clamping of the ureter. Therefore, findings should be carefully translated. Applicability to the most common cause of ureteral obstruction, e.g. ureteral calculi, should be questioned, as obstruction by stones is considered to be predominantly partial. Existing data suggest that morphological and functional changes of ureteral stenting correspond to those of partial ureteral obstruction. Further research is required to understand the impact of stent insertion and optimize the duration of indwelling time.

The clinical question of the extent to which the ureter "can cope" with obstruction without losing pre-obstruction properties and how much loss of functionality can be tolerated remains unanswered. However, it can be concluded that the degree and duration of obstruction should be limited or prevented under ideal circumstances. This highlights the relevance of preventing the most common reason for obstruction – urinary stone disease.

Questions

1. Which of the following statements regarding smooth muscle cells is most accurate?
   (a) Complete obstruction of the ureter does not cause apoptosis of the smooth muscle cells in the ureter
   (b) Complete obstruction of the ureter does not have an impact on smooth muscle cells in the ureter
   (c) Ureteral smooth muscle cells have not been studied in obstructed ureters

(d) Complete obstruction leads to increased ureteral contractility
(e) Complete obstruction leads to tissue remodelling in the ureter, but this does not affect smooth muscle cells

2. Which of the following signaling pathways is involved in altered contractility in obstructed ureters?

(a) No pathway has been studied yet
(b) mTOR pathway
(c) Wnt pathway
(d) COX-2 pathway
(e) Sonic Hedgehoc (Shh) pathway

3. What is a dreaded complication of acute ureteral obstruction?

(a) Gross hematuria
(b) Forniceal rupture
(c) Intracapsular renal hematoma
(d) Urinary incontinence
(e) Hydrocele formation

4. Which of the following statements is false?

(a) Unilateral acute obstruction can lead to kidney failure
(b) Bilateral acute obstruction is a rare condition
(c) Obstruction of the ureter always causes severe pain in patients
(d) Retroperitoneal tumors can cause ureteral obstruction
(e) Urinary calculi are a common cause of acute ureteral obstruction

5. Which of the following hormones has been shown to have beneficial effects on hydronephrosis resolution and ureteral peristalsis restoration in an animal model?

(a) Testosterone
(b) Cortisol
(c) Erythropoetin
(d) Insulin
(e) Estrogen

References

1. Weiss RM. Effect of pathologic processes and pharmacologic interventions on ureteral function. Semin Urol. 1987;5:167–75.
2. Rose JG, Gillenwater JY, Rose JG, Gillenwater JY. Pathophysiology of ureteral obstruction. Am J Phys. 1973;225:830–7. https://doi.org/10.1152/ajplegacy.1973.225.4.830.
3. Rose JG, Gillenwater JY. Effects of obstruction on ureteral function. Urology. 1978;12:139–45. https://doi.org/10.1016/0090-4295(78)90323-0.
4. Biancani P, Hausman M, Weiss RM. Effect of obstruction on ureteral circumferential force-length relations. Am J Phys. 1982;243:F204–10. https://doi.org/10.1152/ajprenal 1982.243.2.F204.

5. Crowley AR, Byrne JC, Vaughan ED, et al. The effect of acute obstruction on ureteral function. J Urol. 1990;143:596–9. https://doi.org/10.1016/s0022-5347(17)40037-1.
6. Hammad FT. Electrical propagation in the renal pelvis, ureter and bladder. Acta Physiol (Oxf). 2015;213:371–83. https://doi.org/10.1111/apha.12392.
7. Nørregaard R, Jensen BL, Topcu SO, et al. Cyclooxygenase type 2 is increased in obstructed rat and human ureter and contributes to pelvic pressure increase after obstruction. Kidney Int. 2006;70:872–81. https://doi.org/10.1038/sj.ki.5001616.
8. Biancani P, Zabinski MP, Weiss RM. Time course of ureteral changes with obstruction. Am J Physiol. 1976;231(2):393–8.
9. Weiss RM. Effects of obstruction and age on the mechanical properties of the ureter. Nihon Heikatsukin Gakkai Zasshi. 1978;14(Suppl):47–9.
10. Natalie Zelenko, Deidre Coll, Arthur T. Rosenfeld et al. (2004) Normal Ureter Size on Unenhanced Helical CT // Normal ureter size on unenhanced helical CT. AJR Am J Roentgenol 182:1039–1041. https://doi.org/10.2214/ajr.182.4.1821039.
11. Dinlenc CZ, Liatsikos EN, Smith AD. Ureteral ischemia model: an explanation of ureteral dysfunction after chronic obstruction. J Endourol. 2002;16:47–50. https://doi.org/10.1089/089277902753483727.
12. Kuzgunbay B, Doran F, Bayazit Y, et al. The effects of ureteral obstruction on Cajal-like cells in rats. J Pediatr Urol. 2009;5:269–73. https://doi.org/10.1016/j.jpurol.2008.12.006.
13. Harada T, Issa MM, Kigure T, et al. Ureteral compliance and histology in partial obstruction in a canine model. J Urol. 1992;148:1274–8. https://doi.org/10.1016/s0022-5347(17)36891-x.
14. Tillig B, Mutschke O, Rolle U, et al. Effects of artificial obstruction on the function of the upper urinary tract of guinea pigs, rats and pigs. Eur J Pediatr Surg. 2004;14:303–15. https://doi.org/10.1055/s-2004-821019.
15. Chuang YH, Chuang WL, Liu KM, et al. Tissue damage and regeneration of ureteric smooth muscle in rats with obstructive uropathy. Br J Urol. 1998;82:261–6. https://doi.org/10.1046/j.1464-410x.1998.00725.x.
16. Chuang Y-H, Chuang W-L, Huang S-P, et al. Release of cytochrome c and activation of caspases related to myocyte apoptosis in obstructed ureters in a rat model of obstructive uropathy. BJU Int. 2003;92:113–8. https://doi.org/10.1046/j.1464-410x.2003.04288.x.
17. Janssen C, Jäger W, Moskalev I, et al. Erythropoietin accelerates the regeneration of ureteral function in a murine model of obstructive uropathy. J Urol. 2015;193:714–21. https://doi.org/10.1016/j.juro.2014.08.110.
18. Hammad FT, Lammers WJ, Stephen B, et al. Propagation characteristics of the electrical impulse in the normal and obstructed ureter as determined at high electrophysiological resolution. BJU Int. 2011;108:E36–42. https://doi.org/10.1111/j.1464-410X.2010.09793.x.
19. Park E, Cox M, Scotland K, et al. Erythropoietin promotes functional recovery via anti-apoptotic mechanisms in mouse unilateral ureteral obstruction. Cell Stress Chaperones. 2020; https://doi.org/10.1007/s12192-020-01067-3.
20. Nakada SY, Jerde TJ, Jacobson LM, et al. Cyclooxygenase-2 expression is up-regulated in obstructed human ureter. J Urol. 2002;168:1226–9. https://doi.org/10.1097/01.ju.0000023404.44796.2f.
21. Lowry PS, Jerde TJ, Bjorling DE, et al. Obstruction alters the effect of prostaglandin E2 on ureteral contractility. J Endourol. 2005;19:183–7. https://doi.org/10.1089/end.2005.19.183.
22. Barbour ML, Raman JD. Incidence and predictors for ipsilateral hydronephrosis following ureteroscopic lithotripsy. Urology. 2015;86:465–71. https://doi.org/10.1016/j.urology.2015.06.016.
23. Lennon GM, Ryan PC, Fitzpatrick JM. Recovery of ureteric motility following complete and partial ureteric obstruction // recovery of ureteric motility following complete and partial ureteric obstruction. Br J Urol. 1993;72:702–7. https://doi.org/10.1111/j.1464-410x.1993.tb16251.x.
24. Chuang Y-H, Chuang W-L, Huang S-P, et al. Expression of epidermal growth factor, basic fibroblast growth factor and insulin growth factor-1 and relation to myocyte regeneration of obstructed ureters in rats. Scand J Urol Nephrol. 2005;39:7–14. https://doi.org/10.1080/00365590510007649.

Chapter 10
The Ureteral Response to Ureteral Stents

Roman Herout, Alina Reicherz, Dirk Lange, and Ben H. Chew

Abstract Ureteral stents are an indispensable tool for urologists since these medical devices ensure urine flow from the kidney via the ureter into the bladder and are used for a myriad of indications. However, these ureteral stents can lead to changes in morphology and function and can cause significant morbidity in patients. First and foremost, ureteral stents interfere with the physiologic peristalsis and ultimately lead to aperistalsis. Due to the inhibition of physiologic, antegrade ureteral peristalsis, calculus expulsion is delayed in stented and previously stented ureters. Ureteral dilation is commonly observed, and the effect seems to be independent of size, shape and composition of the stent. The ureteral dilation seems to correlate with smooth muscle dysfunction and low contractility. Elevated intrapelvic and ureteral pressures after ureteral stent insertion are a consistent finding in the short term, but the upper urinary tract seems to adapt as persistent elevated pressures were rarely seen in animal studies. Clinicians should therefore be aware of the detrimental effects of ureteral stents on peristalsis, morphology, intrarenal pressure and contractility when the question is asked: "To stent or not to stent?"

Keywords Ureteral stents · Ureteral peristalsis · Ureteral dilation · Smooth muscle dysfunction · Intrarenal pressure

Learning Objectives
- Understand the basic principle of ureteral stents and their indications
- Describe the various phases of peristalsis after ureteral stent insertion
- Explain morphological changes of the ureter after stent insertion
- Understand the role of ureteral stents in changing intrarenal pressure

---

Test your learning and check your understanding of this book's contents: use the "Springer Nature Flashcards" app to access questions. To use the app, please follow the instructions in Chapter 1.

R. Herout · A. Reicherz · D. Lange · B. H. Chew (✉)
The Stone Centre at Vancouver General Hospital, Department of Urologic Sciences, University of British Columbia, Vancouver, BC, Canada
e-mail: rherout@prostatecentre.com; Alina.reicherz@ruhr-uni-bochum.de; dirk.lange@ubc.ca; ben.chew@ubc.ca

M. Abdel-Gawad et al. (eds.), *The Ureter*,
https://doi.org/10.1007/978-3-031-36212-5_10

- Mind the detrimental effects of stenting on ureteral contractility
- Identify histological changes in the ureteral wall caused by stenting
- Have an insight in molecular mechanisms pertaining to ureteral aperistalsis and smooth muscle dysfunction of the ureter as a result of stenting

10.1 Introduction

Ureteral stents have been extensively used in the field of urology for more than 50 years since their introduction in 1967 by Zimskind et al. [1] The modern "double pigtail" or "double J" ureteral stent was introduced 11 years later in 1978 by Finney and colleagues [2]. These hollow tubes ensure the flow of urine from the kidney via the ureter into the bladder. Indications for placing a ureteral stent can be either stone related or non-stone related. The former comprises patients who present with blocking ureteral calculi with signs of infection or pain and patients following an endoscopic procedure for urinary stones. The latter indication encompasses patients after endourological surgeries such as endoureterotomy, endopyelotomy, as well as reconstructive procedures such as uretero-ureterotomy or pyeloplasty. Moreover, patients with malignant obstruction rely on ureteral stents to ensure proper urinary drainage from the kidney to the bladder. Lastly, after ureteroneocystostomy as well as ileoureterostomy during cystectomy ureteral stents are inserted to provide proper drainage, protect the anastomosis, as well as to serve as a scaffold for healing. Ureteral stents are a very powerful tool in everyday practice for urologists worldwide. However, these ureteral stents are associated with a significant morbidity as they can lead to stent-related symptoms, hematuria, encrustation, infection and hence to an overall reduction in the quality of life of patients [3]. The scope of this chapter is to describe the various effects ureteral stents have on ureteral morphology, peristalsis, contractility, and on pressure in the upper urinary tract.

10.2 Effects of Stenting on Ureteral Peristalsis

Generally, data on the interaction between the ureter and ureteral stents is limited and our knowledge is mostly based on studies in animal models. The investigation of the pathophysiology of ureteral obstruction as well as the behavior of the ureter after the insertion of a ureteral stent in humans presents us with great challenges for anatomical and methodological reasons. Nonetheless, we do know that ureteral stents drastically affect the physiological and morphological properties of the upper urinary tract and, especially the ureter. The insertion of a stent itself induces a partial obstruction. After placement of a ureteral stent, a phase of hyperperistalsis is initiated that represents an attempt of the ureter to expel the foreign body. This hyperperistaltic phase is typically followed by complete aperistalsis.

Janssen et al. investigated molecular mechanisms involved in ureteral aperistalsis after double J stenting in a porcine model [4]. Therefore, 24 animals were stented unilaterally with 6F ureteral stents for 48 h, 1, 2, 4 and 7 weeks. Four animals served as controls, as well as the contralateral un-stented upper tract in each animal. Aperistalsis was evident in all stented ureters, irrespective of indwelling time (48 h versus 1 week). The animals were anesthetized, stents were removed transvesically, and ureters were observed but no spontaneous peristatic activity was regained after 30 min *in vivo*. However, upon mechanical stimuli, the ureters were excitable and contracted, but this resulted in irregular and uncoordinated peristalsis.

Venkatesh and colleagues studied ureteral peristalsis after insertion of double-pigtail ureteral stents in a porcine model in 2005 [5]. They deployed bipolar steel-wire electromyography electrodes as well as giant magneto resistive (GMR) sensors laparoscopically on the ureters of female pigs. Then, animals were randomly assigned to receive either 4.8F, 7F ureteral stents or serve as controls. A total of 12 pigs were stented unilaterally: 3 pigs received a 4.8F silicone, 3 pigs a 4.8F polyurethane, 3 pigs a 7F silicone and 3 pigs a 7F polyurethane stent. Ureteral peristalsis was initially monitored for 8 h under anesthesia with subsequent removal of the EMG electrodes and sensors. After 1 week, the animals were reevaluated in the same fashion under anesthesia and then sacrificed. The investigators observed a basic peristaltic rate of 2/min (range 1–6/min) with intervals between waves ranging between 3 and 45 s. An apparent activity occurred for 3–8 min and followed by a phase of inactivity for 2–6 min. In the first 2 h after stent insertion, an increase in ureteral peristalsis was observed. The contractions were visible to the naked eye but appeared weak. During the next 6 h, 4.8F-stented ureters showed a return of peristalsis to the basal rate. However, a dramatic decrease in ureteral peristalsis was seen in the 7F-stented ureters as early as 4–6 h post insertion. At the follow-up measurement after 1 week indwelling time of the ureteral stent, complete aperistalsis was seen in four ureters of the group with the smaller stents (4.8F), whereas two ureters of this group manifested occasional fasciculatory movements without organized peristalsis. All the 7F-stented ureters showed aperistalsis. In this study, smaller stents preserved some form of ureteral peristalsis while larger stents all resulted in aperistalsis.

Natalin and coworkers conducted a similar study in 2008 where they evaluated physiological and morphological changes of the ureter with a novel "ribbon stent" that the group developed against conventional 6F stents [6]. This "ribbon stent" consisted of a small diameter tube with two wings affixed in opposition to each other to minimize the contact area of the stent against the ureter. By applying the same method of measuring ureteral peristalsis in a porcine model as Venkatesh et al., they were able to measure ureteral peristalsis in 10 pigs. Hyperperistalsis was observed in all animals in the 6F group, whereas no change from baseline was seen after 2 h in the "ribbon stent" group. However, after three days peristalsis was significantly reduced or absent in both stented groups. These changes persisted at the 7 days post insertion timepoint.

The clinical impact of aperistalsis on stone transit time through the ureter was demonstrated by Ryan et al. in their work on the effect of ureteral stents on upper urinary tract motility and calculus transit in a canine model in 1994 [7]. They allocated 6 animals in their "acute" and 6 animals in their "chronic" study arms. Briefly, in the acute study model they inserted a 3.8F double-J stent in the right upper tract and 3 mm artificial calculi in both ureters (2 cm distal to the UPJ). Intrarenal pressure was measured via a 4F catheter that was inserted into the renal pelvis and ureter. To assess the transit of the calculi, daily X-ray imaging was performed. The authors found a significantly prolonged passage of the calculi in the stented ureters with 16.5 ± 2.2 days versus 3.4 ± 1.6 days for the unstented ureters ($p < 0.01$).

In the "chronic" study arm the authors inserted 3.8F DJ ureteral stents bilaterally. On day 28 the kidneys were exposed again, the left ureteral stent was removed, and 3 mm artificial calculi were inserted bilaterally, again 2 cm distal to the UPJ. Again, calculus transit time was measured via daily X-ray imaging. In 2 animals, serial renal pelvic motility measurements were carried out for 8 weeks; in 4 animals these measurements were done for 12 weeks. After these time points, animals were sacrificed and segments of ureters were studied *ex vivo* regarding motility and histologic examination. The authors found a baseline renal intrapelvic pressure of 2.8 ± 1.0 mmHg, a mean peristaltic rate of 10.8 ± 1.4 per minute and a mean peristaltic amplitude of 3.7 ± 0.5 mmHg. A reduced amplitude of renal pelvic motility was observed in some animals whereas it was completely absent in others. These findings persisted after 30 days. After unilateral stent removal, serial KUB X-rays showed a mean calculus transit time in the de-stented ureters of 7.2 ± 1.8 days compared to 24.1 ± 3.0 days in the stented upper tracts. Both pelvic and ureteric peristaltic activity were seen to recover but were not yet completely at baseline levels at the end of the study in two animals. The mean ureteric peristaltic rate was 7.5 ± 1.85 and a mean amplitude of 37.25 ± 3.68 mmHg. The presence of the stent presented not only a mechanical obstruction to stone passage, but also affected the peristaltic activity of the ureter.

Kinn and Lykkeskov-Andersen also investigated the impact of stents on ureteral peristalsis in pigs [8]. They stented five pigs unilaterally 6–8 weeks before the start of the study. The animals were anaesthetized, and kidneys were exposed. In animals that were stented 6–8 weeks before, the indwelling ureteral stent was removed. In all animals customized double-J ureteral stents with electrodes were introduced in the left upper tract. In pigs that have been stented for the previous 6–8 weeks, peristalsis was significantly lower when compared to pigs that were unstented. Besides a dramatic decrease in ureteral motility, they also showed a reduced amplitude of the contractions and altered directions of the peristaltic waves with long-term ureteral stenting. While these data show that a ureter stented for 6–8 weeks has impaired ureteric mobility immediately after stent removal, it is unknown how long ureteral recovery takes to occur after stent removal.

First evidence that ureteral peristalsis may recover with time while a ureteral stent is still in place was published by Soria et al. [9] They compared a new antireflux-biodegradable ureteral stent to a conventional 4.7F ureteral stent in a porcine model. After a study period of 5 months, peristalsis was evaluated via intravenous pyelography which showed full recovery of peristalsis in both stented groups. At an interim evaluation, 58% of animals with the biodegradable stent showed peristalsis at 3 weeks and 75% at 6 weeks whereas animals with the conventional stent showed aperistalsis. As the stent had partially degraded, it allowed ureteral function to partially recover and resume peristalsis.

10.3 Effects of Stenting on Ureteral Morphology

The ureter typically responds to foreign bodies such as an indwelling ureteral stent with dilation, as has been shown in several animal and human studies [4–8, 10–15]. Also, the dilation of the ureter seems to accrete with longer indwelling time [4].

The dilatation does not seem to be influenced by the size of the ureteral catheter as shown in the study by Venkatesh et al. where grossly dilated ureters with significant inflammation were observed in both stented pig groups (4.8F and 7F), whereas control ureters did not show any dilation [5].

Vogt et al. first investigated primarily the tolerance of a novel suture stent, but coincidentally found that all patients had dilated ureters. This finding was confirmed in a recent study by Majdalany et al. where all ureters that were stented with a conventional 4.8F ureteral stent and 83% of the ureters stented with a novel pigtail suture stent were dilated in a porcine model, irrespective of the indwelling time of 7 vs. 14 days [14]. Hence, ureteral dilation may be the physiologic response to any foreign body in the ureter, irrespective of size and configuration. With regards to timing, Lim et al. could demonstrate in humans that ureteral dilation increases within the first 5 days after DJ stent insertion and then seems to plateau [15]. However, the exact cause of the ureteral dilation remains unclear, although it was hypothesized that the dilation could be the result of initially increased intrapelvic pressures due to the acute partial obstruction. By dilating, the ureter seems to increase periprosthetic flow (flow around the outside of the lumen around the stent) that may eventually help lower intrapelvic pressures to baseline levels.

10.4 Effects of Stenting on Intrarenal Pressure

In a porcine model Cormio et al. compared renal pelvic pressure at the beginning of the study and after 6 weeks of DJ stenting in pigs. When they compared the baseline readings to pressures after 6 weeks of an indwelling DJ stent, they found that renal pelvic pressures remained at baseline levels in 17 of 19 studied animals [11].

However, Johnson et al. investigated the acute effects of stents on intrapelvic pressure and showed that pressures increased from 13.8 to 19.2 mmHg within 5 h after insertion of a stent in a porcine model [16].

Ryan et al. described a significantly elevated intrapelvic pressure 24 h after ureteral stent insertion in canines. In their work, baseline intrapelvic pressure was 2.8 mmHg and increased to 11 mmHg after DJ stent insertion. After 1 week, these elevated pressures returned to baseline again [7].

The most recent data were published by Majdalany et al. They observed an increase in intrapelvic pressure in both stented groups in a porcine model (pigtail suture stent vs. conventional 4.8F stent) [14]. After 7 days of stenting, intrapelvic pressure increased by 2.8 mmHg and ureteral pressure increased by 2.2 mmHg for the suture stent group and 1.5 mmHg and 0.8 mmHg in the DJ group, respectively. After 13–15 days, the increase in pelvic and ureteral pressure was significantly elevated when compared to baseline for the suture stent group (3.2 mmHg for pelvic pressure, $p = 0.02$; 3.8 mmHg for ureteral pressure; $p = 0.004$), whereas no significant increase was detected in the DJ stent group (3.6 mmHg for pelvic pressure, $p = 0.12$; 2.3 mmHg for ureteral pressure; $p = 0.14$). Generally, pressure increases in this study were mild compared to the increase in pressure in other animal studies.

In summary, insertion of stents seems to increase renal pelvic pressure for an initial period of time, but the upper urinary tract appears to adapt, as in most studies initially elevated pressures returned to baseline levels when measured at later timepoints.

10.5 Effects of Stenting on Ureteral Contractility

We tested ureteral smooth muscle contractility in stented and unstented ureters using a porcine model in our laboratory [4]. Briefly, 3 mm ureter strips were mounted in an organ bath containing Krebs-Henseleit solution at 37 °C. After equilibration, the maximum force was obtained after a 3-second supra-maximal electrical-field stimulation. The stress value was assessed by normalizing the isometric force from each ring to the smooth muscle cross-sectional area. The unstented animals as well as the contralateral unstented ureters in the unilaterally stented pigs served as controls. The exerted force by the 48 h stented ureters was minimal and significantly reduced when compared to the contralateral unstented ureters as well as the ureters of the control animals. The contractility was higher in the ureters that were stented for 7 days when compared to the 48 h stented ureters, but lower than contralateral and control animal ureteral forces. Furthermore, the response time to electrical stimuli was significantly delayed in stented ureters when compared to unstented ureters and peak force was obtained more slowly when compared to controls.

10.6 Histologic Findings in Stented Ureters

The study by Ramsay et al. where they stented pigs with ureteral stents for either 1 or 3 weeks, is one of the earliest reports of histologic changes after ureteral stenting. The investigators observed a thickening of the ureteral wall with degeneration of epithelium. Cells were shown to have multiple vacuoles and a patchy atrophy and hyperplasia of the epithelium was apparent [10].

Ryan et al. demonstrated persistent muscular hypertrophy and collagen deposition in the subepithelial layer upon histological assessment of canine ureters that were stented for 4 weeks and then recovered for 8 weeks following stent removal [7].

In another study, the number of smooth muscle cells in the ureter did not change when stented ureters were compared to control ureters [4]. However, stented ureters displayed signs of severe inflammation on histologic examination when compared to unstented ureters [4]. The peak of inflammation in the specimen was detected after 1 week post stent insertion and progressively returned to baseline with longer indwelling time of the stent.

Several groups have investigated new ureteral stents and compared severity of inflammation of surrounding tissues as a secondary objective [6, 9, 14, 17]. Soria et al. could demonstrate that their biodegradable stent was associated with less inflammation in the ureter when compared to a DJ stent, however the results were not statistically significant [9]. In the study by Majdalany et al. mild to moderate ureteral inflammation was observed in the mid ureter and in the uretero-pelvic junction in all animals irrespective of the stent used (suture stent vs. conventional 4.8F stent) [14].

10.7 Molecular Mechanisms of Aperistalsis in Stented Ureters

The Sonic Hedgehog (Shh) signaling pathway has been identified to regulate cell differentiation and morphogenesis in the development of the human ureters and kidneys [18, 19]. Sonic Hedgehog proteins bind to a specific receptor called Patched which results in inhibition of the repressor function of Gli2/Gli3 transcription factors. Because of this disinhibition, Gli1, a transcriptional activator, is expressed. Studies have shown that inhibition of the Shh pathway during development results in hydronephrosis, hydroureter, ureteral aperistalsis and a loss of smooth muscle cells within the ureter [19, 20].

Suspecting a role of the Shh pathway in ureteral aperistalsis, Janssen et al. investigated Shh and Gli1 protein expression in smooth muscle cells of stented ureters in a porcine model [4]. After 48 h, Gli1 expression was still present in smooth muscle cells of the ureter, but after one week a significant decline in Gli1 expression was observed in all smooth muscle cells of stented ureters. When the stents were removed after 7 weeks, Gli1 levels were shown to be similar to controls after a 3-week recovery period. Interestingly, Gli1 expression decreased while Shh levels were steadily increasing, presenting an inverse correlation that was not anticipated. The signaling might be more complex in the ureteral microenvironment with additional interacting proteins that may influence downstream molecules.

Vogt et al. investigated the role of Gli1 in human ureters in patients who underwent cystectomy for bladder cancer [21]. Nine ureteral segments of patients were investigated where a consistent finding was the decrease in Gli1 expression in ureters fitted with a double pigtail stent. However, Gli1 staining in the unstented controls, and the ureters fitted with the suture stent was heterogeneous and no clear conclusion could be drawn.

10.8 Summary and Translation into Clinical Practice

The interaction between the upper urinary tract and ureteral stents is extremely complex and not yet fully understood. Nevertheless, there are some conclusions that can be drawn from the available studies: First and foremost, ureteral stents interfere with the physiologic peristalsis and ultimately lead to aperistalsis. However, in the first few hours after DJ insertion a phase of hyperperistalsis can be observed which might represent an attempt of the ureter to expel the foreign body. Due to the inhibition of physiologic, antegrade ureteral peristalsis, calculus expulsion is delayed in stented and previously stented ureters. Ureteral dilation could be observed in all studies and the effect seems to be independent of size, shape and composition of the stent. The ureteral dilation seems to correlate with smooth muscle dysfunction and low contractility. Elevated intrapelvic and ureteral pressures after ureteral stent insertion are a consistent finding in the short term, but the upper urinary tract seems to adapt as persistent elevated pressures were rarely seen in animal studies.

Finally, clinicians should be aware of the detrimental effects of ureteral stents on peristalsis, morphology, intrarenal pressure and contractility when the question is asked: "To stent or not to stent?"

Key points

- Peristaltic activity initially increases within the first hours after ureteral stent insertion
- Ureteral stents disrupt ureteral peristalsis and ultimately lead to aperistalsis
- Full recovery of pelvi-ureteric contractility after stent removal appears to take time
- Smaller ureteral stents as well as stents with less contact area to the ureteral wall might have less adverse effects on ureteral peristalsis
- Ureteral stents cause ureteral dilation (irrespective of size and configuration)
- Ureteric stenting was associated with a significant delay in calculus passage down the ureter in an animal model
- Ureteral stents seem to cause inflammation of the ureter
- Renal pelvic pressures are initially elevated following ureteral stent insertion
- Most urine flow in the presence of a ureteral stent is periprostethic

Funding

Roman Herout and Alina Reicherz were funded by the Deutsche Forschungsgemeinschaft (DFG, German Research Foundation) - 447437311; 447617010.

Questions

1. Inserting a stent in the ureter typically leads to:
   (a) A Phase of aperistalsis followed by continuous hyperperistalsis
   (b) Immediate and complete aperistalsis
   (c) A Phase of hyperperistalsis followed by aperistalsis
   (d) No significant changes in peristaltic activity
   (e) A Phase of hypoperistalsis followed by complete aperistalsis
2. Inserting a stent in the ureter typically leads to:
   (a) No changes in ureteral morphology
   (b) Dilation of the proximal ureter and no changes in the distal and mid-ureter
   (c) Dilation of the renal pelvis, but no changes in the ureter
   (d) Dilatation of the ureter in all segments
   (e) Narrowing of the ureter in all segments
3. Which of the following statements regarding intrarenal pressure is true:
   (a) After stent insertion intrarenal pressure declines dramatically
   (b) After stent insertion intrarenal pressure does not change
   (c) Intrarenal pressure has not been studied with regards to intrarenal pressure
   (d) Elevated intrarenal pressures after stent insertion are a consistent finding in the short term, but the upper urinary tract seems to adapt as persistent elevated pressures were rarely seen in animal studies.
   (e) Elevated intrarenal pressures after stent insertion are a consistent finding in animal studies with no tendency towards normalization over time.
4. Which observations have been made in animal studies with regards to inflammation in stented ureters?
   (a) Severe inflammation was seen in all animal studies
   (b) Stenting did not cause any inflammation or histological changes
   (c) Ureteral stents smaller than 6F do not cause any inflammation
   (d) Only ureteral stents 6F or smaller caused inflammation
   (e) Stenting seems to cause inflammation in most animal studies
5. Which of the following signaling pathways has been studied in ureteral peristalsis?
   (a) mTOR pathway
   (b) Wnt pathway
   (c) JAK-STAT pathway
   (d) Sonic Hedgehoc (Shh) pathway
   (e) No pathway has been studied yet

References

1. Zimskind PD, Fetter TR, Wilkerson JL. Clinical use of long-term indwelling silicone rubber ureteral splints inserted cystoscopically. J Urol. 1967;97:840–4. https://doi.org/10.1016/s0022-5347(17)63130-6.
2. Finney RP. Experience with new double J ureteral catheter stent. J Urol. 1978;120:678–81. https://doi.org/10.1016/s0022-5347(17)57326-7.
3. Lange D, Bidnur S, Hoag N, Chew BH. Ureteral stent-associated complications-where we are and where we are going. Nat Rev Urol. 2015;12:17–25. https://doi.org/10.1038/nrurol.2014.340.
4. Janssen C, Buttyan R, Seow CY, Jager W, Solomon D, Fazli L, et al. A role for the hedgehog effector Gli1 in mediating stent-induced ureteral smooth muscle dysfunction and aperistalsis. Urology. 2017;104:242.e1–8. https://doi.org/10.1016/j.urology.2017.01.029.
5. Venkatesh R, Landman J, Minor SD, Lee DI, Rehman J, Vanlangendonck R, et al. Impact of a double-pigtail stent on ureteral peristalsis in the porcine model: initial studies using a novel implantable magnetic sensor. J Endourol. 2005;19:170–6. https://doi.org/10.1089/end.2005.19.170.
6. Natalin RA, Hruby GW, Okhunov Z, Singh H, Phillips CK, Humphrey PA, et al. Pilot study evaluating ureteric physiological changes with a novel 'ribbon stent' design using electromyographic and giant magnetoresistive sensors. BJU Int. 2009;103:1128–31. https://doi.org/10.1111/j.1464-410X.2008.08184.x.
7. Ryan PC, Lennon GM, McLean PA, Fitzpatrick JM. The effects of acute and chronic JJ stent placement on upper urinary tract motility and calculus transit. Br J Urol. 1994;74:434–9. https://doi.org/10.1111/j.1464-410X.1994.tb00418.x.
8. Kinn AC, Lykkeskov-Andersen H. Impact on ureteral peristalsis in a stented ureter. An experimental study in the pig. Urol Res. 2002;30:213–8. https://doi.org/10.1007/s00240-002-0258-1.
9. Soria F, Morcillo E, Serrano A, Budia A, Fernández I, Fernández-Aparicio T, et al. Evaluation of a new design of antireflux-biodegradable ureteral stent in animal model. Urology. 2018;115:59–64. https://doi.org/10.1016/j.urology.2018.02.004.
10. Ramsay JWA, Payne SR, Gosling PT, Whitfield HN, Wickham JEA, Levison DA. The effects of double j stenting on unobstructed ureters. An experimental and clinical study*. Br J Urol. 1985;57:630–4. https://doi.org/10.1111/j.1464-410X.1985.tb07021.x.
11. Cormio L, Koivusalo A, Mäkisalo H, Wolff H, Ruutu M. The effects of various indwelling JJ stents on renal pelvic pressure and renal parenchymal thickness in the pig. Br J Urol. 1994;74:440–3. https://doi.org/10.1111/j.1464-410x.1994.tb00419.x.
12. Lennon GM, Thornhill JA, Grainger R, McDermott TE, Butler MR. Double pigtail ureteric stent versus percutaneous nephrostomy: effects on stone transit and ureteric motility. Eur Urol. 1997;31:24–9. https://doi.org/10.1159/000474413.
13. Olweny EO, Portis AJ, Sundaram CP, Afane JS, Humphrey PA, Ewers R, et al. Evaluation of a chronic indwelling prototype mesh ureteral stent in a porcine model. Urology. 2000;56:857–62. https://doi.org/10.1016/S0090-4295(00)00734-2.
14. Majdalany SE, Aldoukhi AH, Jung H, Mehra R, Roberts WW, Ghani KR. In vivo evaluation of a novel pigtail suture stent. Urology. 2021;148:83–7. https://doi.org/10.1016/j.urology.2020.11.031.
15. Lim KS, Lim YW, Yong DZP, Hao Y, Ho HSS, Ng LG, et al. Two weeks too long: optimal duration for ureteral prestenting and its physiologic effects on the ureter in a Yorkshire-Landrace pig model. J Endourol. 2019;33:325–30. https://doi.org/10.1089/end.2018.0872.
16. Johnson LJ, Davenport D, Venkatesh R. Effects of alpha-blockade on ureteral peristalsis and intrapelvic pressure in an in vivo stented porcine model. J Endourol. 2016;30:417–21. https://doi.org/10.1089/end.2015.0251.
17. Vogt B, Chokri I. Histological inflammation in human ureter either healthy or fitted with double-pigtail stent or a thin 0.3 f suture thread: a preliminary study. Adv Urol. 2020;2020:1–5. https://doi.org/10.1155/2020/1204897.

18. Cain JE, Islam E, Haxho F, Chen L, Bridgewater D, Nieuwenhuis E, et al. GLI3 repressor controls nephron number via regulation of Wnt11 and ret in ureteric tip cells. PLoS One. 2009;4:e7313. https://doi.org/10.1371/journal.pone.0007313.
19. Yu J, Carroll TJ, McMahon AP. Sonic hedgehog regulates proliferation and differentiation of mesenchymal cells in the mouse metanephric kidney. Development. 2002;129:5301–12. https://doi.org/10.1242/dev.129.22.5301.
20. Cain JE, Islam E, Haxho F, Blake J, Rosenblum ND. GLI3 repressor controls functional development of the mouse ureter. J Clin Invest. 2011;121:1199–206. https://doi.org/10.1172/JCI45523.
21. Vogt B, Chokri I. Characterization of Sonic Hedgehog/Gli1 signal expression in human ureter either un-stented or fitted with double-pigtail stent or a thread. Res Rep Urol. 2021;13:529–33. https://doi.org/10.2147/RRU.S324192.

Chapter 11
Inflammatory Diseases of the Ureter

Zachary Dovey, Adriana M. Pedraza, Dhruti Patel, Swati Bhardwaj, Vinayak Wagaskar, Raghav Gupta, Akash Shah, and Ashutosh Tewari

Abstract There are multiple possible disease pathologies that can result in inflammation of the ureters. These include the presence of an infectious organism in the urine, hematogenous spread of infection from a distant site, and even direct infiltration from adjacent pelvic and/or abdominal viscera. Ureteral involvement, however, is most commonly caused by a secondary problem related to an existing pathology in the kidney (i.e. stone, pyelonephritis, malakoplakia, etc.), bladder, or uterus (endometriosis). It can also be caused by systemic auto-immune or inflammatory conditions such as amyloidosis or retroperitoneal soft tissue fibrosis. The ureter responds to inflammation by loss of contraction and hypotonia, mural thickening by edema and cell infiltration, ulceration, pseudo-diverticula formation, cystic degeneration, and desmoplastic reaction leading to narrowing and obstruction. Intravenous and retrograde pyelography, cystography, ultrasound, and computed tomography

Test your learning and check your understanding of this book's contents: use the "Springer Nature Flashcards" app to access questions. To use the app, please follow the instructions in chapter 1.

Z. Dovey · D. Patel
General Urology, Robotics, and Uro-oncology, Milton and Carroll Petrie Department of Urology, Icahn School of Medicine, The Mount Sinai Hospital, New York, NY, USA

A. M. Pedraza
Clinical Urologic Oncology, Milton and Carroll Petrie Department of Urology, Icahn School of Medicine, The Mount Sinai Hospital, New York, NY, USA

S. Bhardwaj
Anatomic and Clinical Pathology, Department of Pathology, Icahn School of Medicine, The Mount Sinai Hospital, New York, NY, USA

V. Wagaskar · R. Gupta · A. Tewari (✉)
Milton and Carroll Petrie Department of Urology, Icahn School of Medicine, The Mount Sinai Hospital, New York, NY, USA
e-mail: ash.tewari@mountsinai.org

A. Shah
Department of Uro-oncologic Surgery, Kokilaben Dhirubhai Ambani Hospital, Achutrao Patwardhan Marg, Four Bungalows, Mumbai, India

M. Abdel-Gawad et al. (eds.), *The Ureter*,
https://doi.org/10.1007/978-3-031-36212-5_11

(CT) scanning are the main contributory imaging methods used in the diagnosis of the underlying cause. Ureteroscopy is also a handy tool used for diagnostic and therapeutic purposes. Treatment of ureteral lesions should be done promptly so as to avoid deleterious effects on the renal parenchyma and ureteral wall. Here we present some of the common and uncommon inflammatory conditions of the ureter which require a clinician to maintain a high threshold of suspicion to enable rapid diagnosis and appropriate effective treatment.

Keywords Retroperitoneal fibrosis · Ureteritis cystica · Amyloidosis · Ureter · Endometriosis · Hydronephrosis · Ureteral inflammation

Learning Objectives
- To describe various inflammatory pathologies of the ureter and discuss their etiology, epidemiology, and clinical presentation
- To describe the imaging modalities that can be used to aid in the diagnosis of these various inflammatory pathologies of the ureter
- To provide a comprehensive review of the laboratory tests and/or laboratory work-up urologists and clinicians can perform to aid in the prompt diagnosis of these inflammatory conditions
- To summarize the current clinical treatment options that exist for the management of these inflammatory conditions of the ureter

11.1 Retroperitoneal Fibrosis

11.1.1 Background

Although Retroperitoneal Fibrosis (RPF) became known as Ormond's Disease after two cases were published by Dr. John Ormond in 1948, it had been described nearly five decades prior in 1905 in a case report by a French Urologist, Dr. Joaquin Albarran. All three of these landmark cases presented with bilateral ureteric obstruction, but it was Ormond who recognized this as a syndrome characterized by retroperitoneal inflammation [1, 2]. One of his cases subsequently died of end-stage renal failure, whilst the other was managed successfully by surgical ureterolysis after the presentation [1]. In keeping with Ormond's original insights, the pathophysiology is a retroperitoneal inflammatory process resulting in fibrosis around the abdominal aorta, proximal iliac vessels, and associated structures, including the ureters. The etiology for seconds or thirds of patients is not clear, but there are several secondary causes such as drugs and chemicals, inflammatory aortic aneurysms, malignancy, and radiation therapy. The disease parameters will all be discussed in more detail below.

11.1.2 Epidemiology

RPF remains rare with documented incidences of 0.1–1.3 per 100,000, with the higher incidence reported more recently, presumably as a result of raised awareness and more sensitive imaging studies. The Dutch incidence has been estimated at 1 in 200,000 [3], and based on a lack of familial clustering, genetics are not thought to have a major influence. Most cases occur in the fifth decade of life with a gender ratio of two to three men to one woman, although the disease may also present in children and much older patients [2, 4–6]. There is an association with HLA-BRB1*03, and RPF has recently been described as linked to IgG4-related disease affecting approximately 10% of patients and accounting for up to 60% of idiopathic RPF [7].

11.1.3 Etiology

A specific etiology for RPF is not found in up to 70% of cases, in whom the disease is termed idiopathic. Many secondary causes have been highlighted, not least of which is a malignancy that should definitely be excluded and may be found in up to 10% of patients [8]. Other secondary causes include drugs and chemicals, inflammatory diseases (for example, inflammatory bowel disease and sarcoidosis), local hemorrhage (from for example abdominal or pelvic surgery), periarteritis (including aneurysmal disease of the abdominal vasculature, inflammatory responses to atherosclerotic disease and systemic vasculitides), infection (for example tuberculosis), radiation as well as endometriosis or biliary disease [9]. The relationship between chronic peri-aortitis and idiopathic RPF is complex, and the latter may arise when there is no aortic aneurysmal dilation but rather as a localized inflammatory response to atherosclerotic antigens present in the plaque, such as ceroid and oxidized low-density lipoprotein (LDL) [2]. This is supported by the finding of elevated serum antibodies to these antigens in some idiopathic RPF patients, but does not explain the systemic symptoms, raised inflammatory markers, or elevated autoantibodies that some patients have, or the etiology of the disease in those who are not arteriopaths or when it arises in children [2]. The association to HLA-BRB*03 is mentioned above, and this HLA allele suggests a potential autoimmune etiology, itself being associated with, for example, myasthenia gravis and Hashimoto's thyroiditis [2]. More recently, another association of idiopathic RPF has been found with IgG4-related disease, a systemic fibro-inflammatory disease affecting a number of different organs and tissues. This is a rare condition characterized by single or multiple organ swelling, elevated serum IgG4 levels, and fibrosis with IgG4 plasma cell infiltration on histology [7], mainly limited to case reports in the literature.

11.1.4 Clinical Features

Because the symptoms are insidious in onset and relatively nonspecific in nature, patients may only present late in the disease course with clinical features secondary to either vascular or ureteric obstruction [8]. Patients will describe lower persistent dull backache, which may radiate into the upper legs and groin, initially improved with non-steroidal analgesics. Associated symptoms may include poor appetite, lethargy, low-grade fevers, and myalgia and arthralgia [9, 10]. As the inflammatory process continues and the fibrotic plaque develops mass effect, symptoms may develop from adjacent organ involvement with constipation, retroperitoneal lymphatic obstruction causing inguinoscrotal and peripheral limb edema, and vascular obstruction resulting in intestinal ischemia, claudication, and renal hypertension [2, 9, 10]. The commonly described ureteric obstruction with hydronephrosis and renal impairment with be seen in nearly half and all patients, and is bilateral in approximately 50% of the [9]. Bedside examination may reveal some abdominal tenderness, rarely a palpable abdominal mass, peripheral and scrotal edema, and potentially varicoceles [2].

11.1.5 Laboratory Investigations

Similarly, laboratory findings may at first seem nonspecific in nature. The disease process may affect the patient's hematology and biochemistry as well as cause elevation of inflammatory markers such as C reactive protein (CRP) and erythrocyte sedimentation rate (ESR). Both CRP and ESR may be elevated at presentation in greater than 50% of cases, but their use to monitor disease activity is unreliable when compared to changes in the disease pattern as assessed by imaging studies [11]. Patients may have anemia of chronic disease (normochromic and normocytic) and up to 50% will have elevated creatinine levels at presentation as a result of chronic renal obstruction [9]. Other abnormalities may include raised white count, eosinophilia, and elevated serum gamma globulins with concomitant hypoalbuminemia as well as urine analysis positive for blood and protein [6]. Autoantibodies will be positive in up to 40% of patients [12], with specific elevations in rheumatoid factor, anti-smooth muscle, anti-thyroid, and anti-cytoplasmic antibodies. When autoantibodies are present, the associated auto-immune disease would need to be ruled out [6].

11.1.6 Imaging

Ultrasound (US): RPF may be seen in the US as an iso or hypoechoic retroperitoneal lesion in front of the lower lumber vertebrae and sacrum, however, with low sensitivity due to overlying bowel obscuring views in early case s [13]. There may also be varying degrees of hydronephrosis due to ureteric involvement in the inflammatory mass as well as other intra-abdominal abnormalities that may be associated with RPF including sclerosing pancreatitis or cholangitis and primary biliary sclerosis causing biliary dilation and distorting biliary or pancreatic anatomy [14].

Intravenous Urography (IVU): IVU was traditionally one of the investigative modalities of choice, demonstrating a characteristic appearance with bilateral or unilateral hydroureteronephrosis tapering to the middle third of the ureters at the level of the lower lumbar vertebrae or sacrum, with a medial deviation of the dilated ureters [15]. This appearance may be mimicked by several conditions including retroperitoneal lymphadenopathy, inflammatory ureteric structures, or ureteric tumors, and this modality of imaging has been superseded.

CT imaging studies: CT imaging is now the modality of choice for RPF diagnosis. Although there is considerable variation, typically both primary and secondary RPF produce a periaortic mass of soft tissue attenuation from renal to iliac vessels, sparing the aorta but potentially enveloping IVC and ureters depending on disease stage [16]. Enhancement after iv contrast may be seen in the inflammatory stage of the disease, but this may be contraindicated because of renal impairment. Other findings which may be present include DVT, renal vessel involvement, and autoimmune pancreatitis, and CT may help to differentiate between causes of secondary RPF e.g. malignancy [13].

MRI: the main advantage of MRI over CT is superior contrast resolution, regardless of whether iv gadolinium is contraindicated because of associated renal impairment and subsequent risk of nephrogenic systemic fibrosis. Typically, the soft tissue mass described above has low signal intensity on T1-weighted images and, in the acute inflammatory phase, high signal intensity on T2-weighted images. This feature has been used to assess response to treatment for idiopathic disease [13].

Positron Emission Tomography (PET): F-FDG PET has also been used as an imaging modality providing functional insight into the state of inflammatory tissues. It allows localization of tissue with high metabolic activity within the retroperitoneum, and so can not only accurately image both idiopathic and secondary RPF, but also may have value in follow-up and the assessment of response to treatment by the assessment of residual inflammatory tissue [17]. Its disadvantage is an inability to distinguish between benign and malignant causes of RPF [17].

11.1.7 Treatment

Management of RPF includes both medical treatment for the inflammatory stage to limit disease extent and progression as well as surgical treatment to prevent or reverse disease complications and restore urinary patency and flow. Prior to this, it is important to rule out any secondary causes and if there are atypical features on clinical investigation either on laboratory tests or clinical imaging, a CT-guided biopsy may be done and a subsequent treatment plan on the basis of the biopsy result.

Once established as Idiopathic RPF, the mainstay of treatment is steroids and other forms of immunosuppression. The use of corticosteroids was first reported by Ross and Tinkler in 1958, and apart from a randomized trial in 2011 comparing prednisolone with tamoxifen for the maintenance of remission following induction prednisolone, there have been no other therapeutic randomized controlled trials examining either steroid efficacy or dosing regimes [18]. The evidence base is taken from different case series, and treatment is largely individualized and empiric. An algorithm has been used, outlining treatment for those with or without ureteric entrapment, which essentially recommends those who have ureteric involvement at presentation which does not respond to steroids, or develop new or recurrent ureteric involvement during follow-up, require surgical intervention by ureterolysis [2].

The starting dose for induction prednisolone is 30–60 mg for 1–2 months, then reduced over the same time period to a maintenance dose of 5–10 mg per day for up to 2 years or longer, depending on the disease state as assessed by following laboratory and imaging tests [19]. Most patients will report improvement in symptoms after the first few weeks on steroids, followed by an improvement in laboratory parameters a month and a half later (ESR, CRP, creatinine) and, for most, variable regression of the fibrotic plaque on CT or MRI imaging studies between 6 months and 12 months following the start of treatment. Although the remission rate for patients after induction steroids is reported at over 90–100%, the relapse rate is also significant at over 70% [2, 6]. Several agents have been used to reduce the dose of long-term steroids, and so limit their side effects. Notwithstanding its thrombo-embolic complications, tamoxifen was not found to be effective as prednisolone at reducing relapse rate following induction steroids in a randomized controlled trial of 36 patients between the ages of 18 and 85 (50% verse 17% relapse rates) over 18 months following up after initial remission [18]. Methotrexate has been used effectively to help reduce relapse rates and lower steroid maintenance doses either in combination or as a single agent [20, 21]. Both azathioprine and cyclophosphamide in combination with steroids have been used effectively for the same reason or as induction therapy, although azathioprine was found to have fewer adverse effects than the additional use of cyclophosphamide, especially for older patients [19]. Daily azathioprine alone has been used for maintenance treatment [22] or with monthly cyclophosphamide injections for more severe forms of the disease [11]. Mycophenolate mofetil has been used in combination with low-dose maintenance steroids to reduce the relapse rate in patients with RPF in remission after induction high dose steroids [23]. Monoclonal antibodies to various elements of the immune cascade have also been studied such as infliximab, rituximab, and tocilizumab (monoclonal antibodies to TNF-alpha, CD20 on B lymphocytes and interleukin-6 and its receptor respectively), with potential to have specific efficacy IgG4 related disease. For example, rituximab has been shown to be effective for idiopathic RPF including those IgG4 related disease [24].

For those in whom medication is ineffective at improving ureteric entrapment and renal insufficiency, the options are ongoing medical treatment with nephrostomy placement or ureteric stenting to assess for more prolonged improvement or surgical treatment by ureterolysis. The clear indications for surgical treatment are failure of medical treatment to resolve renal outflow obstruction with a dependence on nephrostomies for urine drainage, or a failure of ureteric stents to improve renal function. Other than that, some patients may not tolerate long-term stents, or once explained management options, opt for surgery electively [25]. Whichever approach is chosen, bilateral ureterolysis is recommended regardless of whether the disease is unilateral at the time of the procedure [25]. The surgical treatment of choice is ureterolysis, and by the time patients come to surgery most will have had stents or nephrostomies in for some time. Open, laparoscopic, and robotic approaches have been used successfully

[26, 27], and the fundamental technique includes dissecting out the ureter laterally, then closing it in an intraperitoneal position, with the peritoneum posteriorly, often with the ureter wrapped in a sleeve of omentum. Using the open approach in a team set up for high volume ureterolysis, [25] in a series of 50 patients, found 94% were stent free at 12 months with an overall improvement in GFR across all indication groups of +6 (−4 to +22 $p < 0.05$), with the conclusion that surgical treatment should be offered to all patients with medically refractory ureteric obstruction. The progress of minimally invasive options has led to the first ureterolysis performed laparoscopically in 1992 by Kavoussi [28]. Subsequently a retrospective analysis of open (36 patients) versus laparoscopic (34 patients) approaches was done by the same group, with 50% of patients having primary RPF and the rest having secondary RPF primarily mostly resulting from gynecological cancers. Both groups had comparable improvements in renal obstruction (97.1% vs 94.3% as assessed by post-operative imaging respectively) and although complication rates were similar (8.3% vs 8.8% respectively), the laparoscopic approach may have shown improvements in other surgical outcomes with lower transfusion requirements postoperatively (13.7% vs 3.7% respectively) and shorter hospital stay (10.8 days v 3.4 days respectively). A more recent retrospective laparoscopic series in 17 patients demonstrated similar outcomes with no patients requiring transfusion, mean LOS 4 (2–6), and mean change in GFR +7.5 (−8 to +23). Interestingly, for those patients who had stents or nephrostomies prior to ureterolysis, the median time was 13 months (range 3–44 months), [26] and the authors concluded that, rather than waiting, patients should be referred early to a specialized center to allow maximum preservation of renal function. Using the robotic approach for ureterolysis was first performed in 2006 by Mufarrij and Stifelman in 2006, with a retrospective series of 17 patients undergoing the procedure, three of whom were subsequently found to have lymphoma. One patient had a perioperative complication, and three patients required secondary procedures for recurrent renal outflow obstruction. At 20.5 months, all patients had improved symptoms or were symptom-free with no clinical evidence of persistent renal obstruction. Similarly, encouraging results were found in a more recent series of 18 patients demonstrating low perioperative complication rates and excellent longer-term outcomes with regard to improvements in renal outflow obstruction and function [29].

11.1.8 Conclusion

Primary idiopathic RPF is the commonest form and may have an autoimmune etiology. Nevertheless, secondary causes are common, requiring exclusion, which will likely need a biopsy of inflamed tissue and histological examination. Significant morbidity stems from renal outflow obstruction potentially causing irreversible renal damage, and if patients do not respond to medical immunosuppression, they should be referred early for consideration of surgical treatment by ureterolysis. Retrospective series suggest this is best done by high volume centers with specific expertise and may be performed by open or minimally invasive approaches. The results of ureterolysis suggest favorable long-term outcomes, allowing patients to live stent and nephrostomy free with stable renal function.

11.2 Ureteritis (Fig. 11.1)

11.2.1 Ureteritis Cystica (UC)

It is a benign condition related to chronic inflammation of the urothelium with the secondary cystic transformation of the epithelial nest of Brunn, most commonly affecting the proximal ureter [30]. Authors have found a strong association between recurrent urinary tract infections, lithiasis, and ureteritis cystica [31] predominantly affecting females, although it has also been reported in males and children. Diagnosis is usually incidental through endoscopic or radiographic studies, showing multiple millimetric hemispheric lesions or filling defects with a scalloped appearance [32]. No specific treatment is required in these cases except for the management of the associated infection of lithiasis. Regarding prognosis, urinary tract complications such as obstruction or renal failure are extremely unlikely.

11.2.2 Eosinophilic Ureteritis

It is a rare cause of ureteral obstruction although vesicoureteral reflux has also been described. The etiology is unclear. Nonetheless, eosinophilia, atopy, trauma, and autoimmune diseases seem to be related. In fact, decreased complement as well as

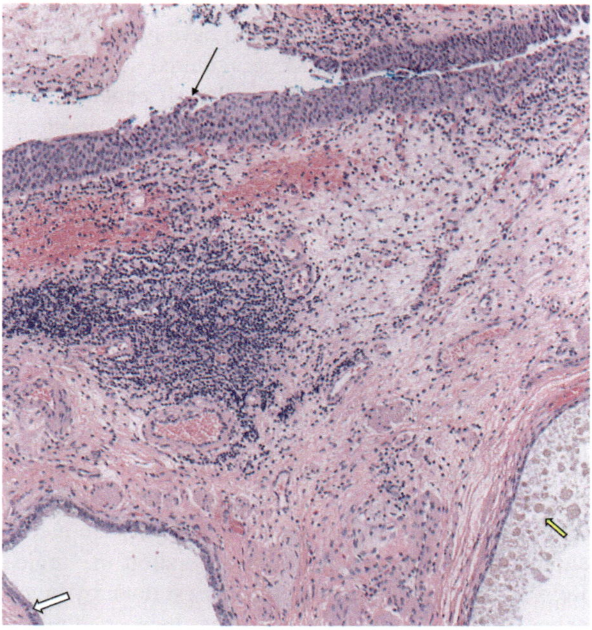

Fig. 11.1 Ureteral endometriosis: The surface shows transitional epithelium (black arrow) of the ureter, with the ureteral wall showing two endometriotic cysts. The one on the left shows columnar endometrial lining epithelium (Solid white arrow with a black outline). The one on the right shows the flattening of the epithelium by cyst contents that include hemosiderin-laden macrophages (solid yellow arrow with black outline)

decreased IgG, and elevated IgE have been reported in patients with eosinophilic ureteritis [33, 34]. The diagnosis is histological, and treatment implies surgical resection of the stenotic segment. However, prolonged use of oral corticosteroids has been reported as a possible alternative [35].

11.3 Malakoplakia

Malakoplakia is derived from the Greek words "malacos" and "placos" to describe a "soft plaque". It is a granulomatous condition, rare in incidence, and primarily affecting the genito-urinary tract but also less commonly, the gastrointestinal, musculoskeletal, and pulmonary systems as well as the skin, mesenteric lymph nodes, and thyroid gland [36]. Macroscopically, malakoplakia may be seen in the bladder, demonstrated by soft yellow plaques on mucosal tissue which on biopsy demonstrate pathognomonic histological lesions known as Michaelis-Guttman bodies, originally described in 1902 by Michaelis and Guttman. These consist of lysosomal basophilic inclusions seen on histiocytes, which are themselves known as Von Hansemann cells, described by Von Hansemann in 1903. These histopathological features are thought to result from defective macrophage function in association with E. Coli infection [37].

11.3.1 Etiology

The disease tends to predominantly affect those over the age of 50 years with a female-to-male ratio of 4:1, and as mentioned is commonly seen in association with E. Coli infection but also other organisms such as staphylococcus aureus, proteus, and klebsiella as well as mycobacteria and fungi [38–40]. The gender disparity seems specific to urinary malakoplakia but the etiology has not been clearly defined. Theory suggests it may arise from microbial urinary tract infection (UTI) in patients with an already weakened immune system from autoimmune disease, iatrogenic immunosuppression, or acquired syndromes of immunodeficiency, lymphoma, or another systemic disease such as diabetes [38–40]. Most patients will have a background of recurrent UTIs, and in a series of 93 patients with malakoplakia, nearly 90% of patients had urine cultures positive for E. Coli, and 40% had a history of systemic disease as above. On the basis of this, it was suggested there may be an abnormality in intracellular phagosomal bacterial breakdown resulting from bacterial fragments that act as a nidus for calcium phosphate deposition that is characterized by Michaelis-Guttman bodies [38]. More specifically macrophages are believed to have reduced intracellular cyclic guanine monophosphate which impairs lysosomal and microtubular functioning which underlies deficient bacterial breakdown [37].

11.3.2 Clinical Features

Ureteric malakoplakia is a rare manifestation of the disease which ultimately may result in bilateral hydronephrosis [41] with acute renal failure secondary to the disease process producing ureteric stricture and stenosis. More commonly patients present with urinary bladder involvement, causing irritative lower urinary tract symptoms, hematuria, and systemic upset with fever, often with a prior history of immunosuppression or chronic disease. The clinical presentation will lead to a cystoscopy, potentially with retrograde studies and ureteroscopic examination. This demonstrates characteristic yellow mucosal plaques which may progress to sessile lesions or masses showing up as filing defects on retrograde studies. Ureteric involvement in isolation is rare, and as well as bladder disease, malakoplakia may also cause renal parenchymal masses, complicated by renal vein and inferior cava thrombosis as well as prostatitis and epididymo-orchitis. Overall clinical diagnosis may be challenging without histology and given the association of multi-system disease, with for example lung involvement, the presentation may give the appearance of metastatic disease [37]. The differential diagnosis includes transitional cell carcinoma of the ureters or bladder, lymphoma, sarcoidosis, and microbial infections such as tuberculosis and fungal infections e.g. histoplasmosis or actinomycosis [42]. The presence of the multifocal renal parenchymal disease may also suggest multifocal renal cell carcinoma and von Hippel Lindau syndrome, and if there is renal obstruction with urinary tract calculi, depending on the clinical state of the patient, multiple focal renal abscesses.

11.3.3 Investigations

The diagnostic process focuses on imaging and histological analysis since there are no blood biomarkers for the disease. Since the disease is commonly multifocal ureteric involvement in isolation is rare, and usually in association with disease elsewhere in the urinary tract. In terms of basic laboratory investigations, depending on the prior history and associated medical comorbidities, there may be anemia of chronic disease, with hypoalbuminemia, biochemical evidence of renal impairment with raised blood urea nitrogen and creatinine as well as raised inflammatory mediators resulting from concomitant urosepsis. Urine analysis will likely demonstrate pyuria and microscopic hematuria and routine culture may be positive for bacterial organisms such as E. Coli or other gram-negative bacteria such as proteus or klebsiella and gram-positive organisms such as staph aureus [43]. Ureteric malakoplakia will likely cause obstruction, so urinary tract ultrasound with show hydronephrosis, but is relatively poor for distal ureteric imaging. Any associated renal parenchymal lesions may show parenchymal engorgement with distorted calyces and parenchymal hyperechogenicity. Similarly, CT imaging will also show appearances that depend on whether the disease is uni- or multi-focal. An isolated ureteric lesion may show some ureteral wall thickening, with enhancement, and secondary hydronephrosis, with enlarged kidneys and penal pelvic filing defects, if the disease is multi-focal with renal parenchymal lesions. Typically on arteriography multifocal malakoplakia lesions are hypovascular, but a focal lesion may show neovascularity [44]. Formal diagnosis requires histological examination by cystoscopy and ureteroscopy. If there are lesions within the bladder, they will be seen as yellow plaques on the mucosa, although larger lesions may become more sessile with ulceration and necrosis on their surface. Retrograde studies will show a filling defect at the site of any ureteric lesions, which may have a similar appearance under the direct vision [43]. Biopsy and histological examination of these lesions will demonstrate the characteristic appearances discussed above. There will be "von Hansemann cells", which are aggregated histiocytes with granular cytoplasm, containing "Michaelis-Gutmann bodies", which are pathognomonic. These are basophilic fragments of bacteria from incomplete degradation, which contain iron and calcium, the iron staining blue with Prussian blue stain, and the calcium staining black with von Kossa's reagent [37].

11.3.4 Treatment

Modalities of treatment may be both medical and surgical. Medical treatment is primarily antibiotics to treat the supposed causative bacteria, starting with any one of trimethoprim, rifampicin, tetracyclines, sulphonamides, or fluoroquinolones adjusting according to sensitivities if urine or blood cultures are positive [38]. All of these antimicrobials have a specific bactericidal action that is intracellular and, moreover, fluoroquinolones are often favored as first-line treatment because they are taken up by macrophages, which are involved in the pathogenesis [45]. With regards to etiology, other agents have been tried with the aim of improving macrophage function and intra-phagocytic bacterial degradation by increasing macrophage cytosolic GMP levels, including both ascorbic acid or anticholinergics such as bethanechol [46]. Ureteric Malakoplakia has a high chance of causing renal outflow obstruction, and in the context of associated urosepsis, with or without upper and lower urinary tract malakoplakia, may need surgical intervention by either insertion of double j stent or anterograde nephrostomy. If a retrograde approach is undertaken, it may be possible to laser fulgurate and resect ureteric malakoplakia lesions by ureteroscopy under direct vision at the same time. Nevertheless, there is also a subsequent risk of ureteric structuring which may then require reconstructive surgery. If the stricture is in isolation, without malakoplakia elsewhere in the upper tracts, depending on its position in the ureter, ureteric reimplantation, excision, and direct re-anastomosis, trans-uretero-ureterostomy, as well as psoas hitch and boari flap, may all be undertaken, either by open or minimally invasive approaches. Occasionally initial surgical intervention and renal disobstruction followed by a combined medical regime of antimicrobials, bethanechol, and ascorbic acid for up to 6 months by cause resolution of the disease, but in multifocal malakoplakia with more significant renal parenchymal involvement had significant mortality and surgical nephrectomy may be necessary [37].

11.3.5 Conclusion

Malakoplapkia is a rare condition, but nevertheless a potentially devastating one. Given its rarity, its association with other systemic diseases, and its multifocal presentation, a high index of suspicion is required to make a diagnosis. Histopathological examination is necessary and for ureteric malakoplakia, this will need ureteroscopy and biopsy under direct vision, which may be combined with a double J stent if renal unblocking is required. Treatment will likely need combined antimicrobials and surgery management. Although this may help to resolve the disease successfully, ultimately the long-term prognosis will be determined by multifocality at the time of presentation and the presence or absence of unilateral or bilateral renal involvement.

11.4 Amyloidosis of the Ureter

Virchow described in 1854 amyloid or "starch-like" deposits in tissue [47, 48].

11.4.1 Epidemiology

Primary localized amyloidosis of the ureter is a rare disease first described in 1937 [49]. About 200 cases of genitourinary amyloidosis have been described in the literature [50]. The prevalence is unknown. It is very difficult to radiographically distinguish from upper tract urothelial carcinoma [49]. Many patients undergo nephroureterectomy for this benign disease.

11.4.2 Etiology

Amyloidosis is a set of diseases caused by the extracellular deposit of insoluble protein, amyloid, in any area of the body causing organ dysfunction [51, 52]. It is classically known as the "great imitator" [49]. The etiology is unknown but postulated to be related to chronic inflammation. Disease symptoms are determined by the location of amyloid deposits, most commonly being seen in the kidney and heart [52]. Primary, secondary, familial, local, and systemic versions of this disease have been described [49, 51, 52]. Primary amyloidosis has elevated amyloid light chains while the secondary is an amyloid A protein variant. This is commonly seen in the skin, soft tissues, genitourinary tract, respiratory system, and gastrointestinal tract [49]. Primary amyloidosis is about 56% of cases, secondary amyloidosis is 8% of cases, localized amyloidosis is 9%, and familial (1%). Secondary amyloidosis is related to chronic infections or inflammatory disorders like rheumatoid arthritis, Crohn's disease, or tuberculosis [52]. Secondary amyloidosis could also be an indication of multiple myeloma [52].

Localized amyloidosis consists of two types: immunoglobulin light chain and senile amyloidosis [53]. This is overall very rare. There are rare reports of localized amyloidosis that is caused by the secondary type amyloid A protein variant.

Symptoms are related to the organ affected. Localized amyloidosis is about 10–20% of cases [51]. Amyloidosis of the genitourinary tract is rare and it is even rare to note this only affects the ureter [51]. Amyloidosis of the bladder, prostate, or seminal vesicles is commonly incidental [51, 53].

11.4.3 Clinical Features

Disease symptoms are determined by the location of amyloid deposits, most commonly being seen in the kidney and heart [51, 52]. Flank pain and gross hematuria are the most common symptoms. Additionally, hydroureteronephrosis elevated the serum creatinine [51]. Uncommon symptoms include renal failure, ureteral colic, or UTI with ureteral colic [54]. Absence of retroperitoneal lymphadenopathy in the imaging [52]. This is predominantly noted in females of all ages with the mean age being 58 years old [49]. Patients can have polypoid masses within the ureter, renal collecting system, or extrinsic compression by a large pelvic mass encompassing the ureters [50]. Intraureteric masses inside the renal pelvis are typically smooth and do not have characteristics of a transitional cell carcinoma [50]. It is imperative to distinguish these masses from malignancy which can be done only with biopsy and staining of tissue.

A rare presentation of this includes osseous metaplasia which has been described in 6 cases [49]. Ureteral masses can be seen with or without calcifications with an obstruction [50].

Typically, ureteral amyloidosis masses are unifocal, but bilateral and multifocal involvement has been described. If calcifications are present around the mass, tuberculosis, and schistosomiasis should be considered [54].

11.4.4 Laboratory Investigations

Congo red staining confirms the diagnosis of amyloid which is pink-red under light microscopy [52, 53]. Biopsy of the mass with hematoxylin and eosin staining shows pale eosinophilic deposits suggestive of amyloidosis [49]. Further staining with thioflavin shows apple-green birefringence which is also pathgnostic of amyloidosis.

Kappa and lambda light chains are elevated in the serum in these patients at similar levels [53]. Rarely ureteral amyloidosis is the second type with the secretion of serum amyloid A protein also known as AA-type amyloidosis [47].

Urine cytology can also help determine if these ureteral masses are benign or malignant [55].

11.4.5 Imaging

CT imaging studies: CT imaging of the abdomen and pelvis with contrast allows for evaluation of the ureter and rules out any lymphadenopathy. Other than hydronephrosis, the ureter may have linear calcifications from the amyloidosis [56].

Intraureteric retrograde pyelography, Ureteroscopy, Ureteral biopsy: Cystoscopy and retrograde pyelography with or without ureteroscopy allow identification of the location of the obstruction, amount of hydroureteronephrosis and possible ureteral mass secondary to amyloidosis [50, 57]. Ureteral involvement can be stricture, polypoid mass, or mucosal ulceration [56, 57] Hydronephrosis may be due to direct ureteral or periureteral amyloid infiltration or extrinsic compression from a large amyloid mass [56]. All ureteral masses should be assessed with a ureteroscopy and biopsy. That tissue should be evaluated using Congo Red staining.

MRI: For patients that present with a pelvic mass, MRI will allow delineation of the involved structures including the ureters, bladder, and prostate [51].

11.4.6 Treatment

Options for treatment are dependent on the size of the mass, location, surgical urgency, and comorbidities. Overall prognosis is excellent in the surgical management [58]. Patients with ureteral obstruction should undergo a ureteral biopsy to determine pathology prior to consideration of the surgical management [49, 55]. Segmental ureteral excision and anastomosis which is either ureteroneocystostomy or ureteroureterostomy.

11.5 Endometriosis of the Ureter

11.5.1 Epidemiology

The estimated prevalence of endometriosis is 5–10% [59]. The prevalence of ureteral endometriosis is 0.01–1.7% of women with endometriosis [60]. Overall, this is not an accurate assessment as this is commonly noted incidentally [60].

Endometriosis is an estrogen-dependent disease with its peak incidence between 24 years and 29 years old, while ureteral endometriosis peaks in the age 30–35 group [59, 60].

Ureteral endometriosis is the second most common organ involved in the urinary tract [59]. It is rarely seen with 1.2–6% of all endometriosis cases involving the urinary tract and 0.5–10% of those cases known to involve the ureter [61]. The estimate of ureteral endometriosis is about 0.08–1% of patients with deep infiltrating endometriosis [62].

11.5.2 Etiology

Endometriosis is the presence of functional endometrial tissue outside of the uterus. The tissue deposits are known as endometriomas. Overall endometriosis is a spectrum of diseases including superficial, deep, peritoneal, or extraperitoneal, ovarian endometriomas, and adhesions in the pelvic peritoneum and retroperitoneum. Deep infiltrating endometriosis is a peritoneal implant into the retroperitoneum at least 5 mm in depth. Pelvic pain and infertility are caused by this type of endometriosis.

The etiology of endometriosis is unclear but three main theories exist metastatic, metaplastic and induction [59]. The metastatic theory is the most accepted with viable endometrial tissue spreading retrograde out of the uterus during menstruation or via lymphatics, bloodstream, or iatrogenic spread. The metaplastic theory is that peritoneal cells can differentiate into endometrial tissue. The induction theory is a combination of metastatic and metaplastic theories with ectopic endometrium secretes tissue that causes differentiation.

11.5.3 Clinical Features

Ureteral endometriosis can be intrinsic or more commonly extrinsic. Intrinsic lesions involve the full thickness of the tunica muscularis of the ureter while extrinsic lesions only involve the ureteral adventitia (Fig. 11.2) [63].

The ureter is typically involved below the pelvic brim with and without associated hydroureteronephrosis [59]. Typically, hydroureteronephrosis is associated with a fibrotic pattern which histologically shows fibrosis [59]. The other noted type is endometriotic which includes endometrial glands within the ureteral wall and periuterine tissues [59].

Symptoms typically include lower back pain or renal colic, though up to 30% are asymptomatic [63, 64]. It can also be associated with nonspecific symptoms such as dysmenorrhea, dyspareunia, and non-menstrual pelvic pain [60]. Due to the slowly developing long-term ureteral obstruction that can be caused, patient symptoms do not correlate with the severity of the hydroureteronephrosis [63].

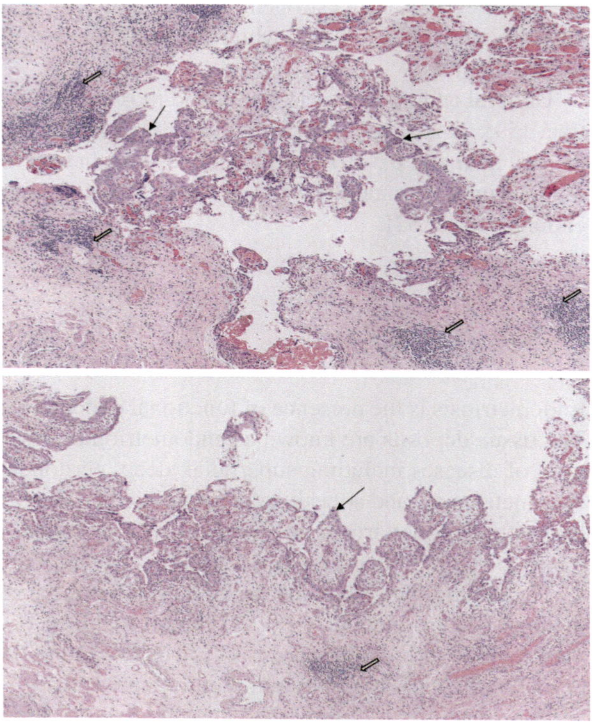

Fig. 11.2 This is a case of papillary ureteritis. Note the presence of papillary projections of the epithelium (black arrows) and lymphoid aggregate in the lamina propria (Solid white arrows with black outline)

Ureteral endometriosis is associated with other sites being affected 90% of the time [60]. These associated sites are ovarian endometriosis, uterosacral ligament involvement, gastrointestinal nodules, and retrocervical space nodules [64]. The left distal ureter 3–4 cm above the ureterovesical junction is the most commonly involved ureteral site [60, 63]. Rectovaginal endometriosis with lesions over 3 cm has a 12–18% prevalence of ureteral endometriosis [60]. It is also noted patients with ureteral endometriosis have had surgery in the past for endometriosis and typically have a lower BMI [60].

11.5.4 Laboratory Investigations

Renal function assessment and pre-operative blood counts are the only laboratory investigations needed in ureteral endometriosis. There are no urine markers.

11.5.5 Imaging

There is no consensus regarding the best diagnostic tool for ureteral endometriosis [60].

Transvaginal and transrectal ultrasound: Transvaginal ultrasound is the best first line imaging modality and can assess the rectovaginal and rectosigmoid septum for implants of 1.5 cm or more [59]. This is a cost-effective option [60].

Abdominal ultrasound: Given the non-invasive nature, this is an easy cost-effective way to assess for ureteral obstruction, assess renal parenchyma, and degree of hydronephrosis [60].

Ureteroscopy with Intravenous Urography and ureteral biopsy: Much of the literature is from the perspective of gynecology. As a result, ureteroscopy and biopsy are not recommended as part of the diagnostic workup due to invasiveness and risk of missing the extrinsic ureteral endometriosis [60, 62]. However, it is a modality that would allow the diagnosis of intrinsic ureteral endometriosis with a biopsy [60]. Those patients that undergo endoscopic excision have noted recurrence and high failure rates [60]. This may be best as a diagnostic not a management strategy.

MRI with IV contrast: MRI is the best imaging technique with can be used with or without vaginal gel and has a few distinct characteristics [59]. There is a T2 shading effect showing a high signal on the superior portion with a low signal on the dependent portion [59]. This is related to repeated hemorrhage cycles. Dark spots on T2 are also noted along the edges of endometriomas, which are also due to the hemorrhage [59].

Ureteral endometriosis is classified as a deep endometriosis with a hypointense pattern on T2W images [59]. MRI reporting of endometriosis includes lesion size, location: intrinsic/extrinsic, distance from the UVJ, and hydronephrosis.

While MRI has a grade A recommendation for diagnostic use, computed tomography is a close second when there is bowel involvement [60].

11.5.6 Treatment

Due to the rarity of this condition, there continues to be a debate regarding how best to manage ureteral endometriosis. The goals of treatment include the preservation of renal function and the management of symptoms. Medical treatment has been shown to have some short-term benefits but to be overall ineffective [62]. Hormonal contraceptives are the first-line therapy for endometriosis-related pain, however, due to obstruction, this is not the recommended first-line treatment for ureteral endometriosis [60]. No studies have evaluated the efficacy of medical treatment for ureteral endometriosis [60]. Given the growth of minimally invasive surgical options, laparoscopic or robotic ureterolysis, ureteroureterostomy, Boari flap with or without a Psoas hitch, or ureteroneocystostomy are the mainstay for ureteral endometriosis [63]. The initial surgical treatment is laparoscopic ureterolysis with or without ureteroneocystostomy [60, 62]. Surgical management has been shown to have long-term relief without many complications other than ureteral fistula which was due to lack of ureteral stent placement [62].

11.5.7 Conclusion

Ureteral endometriosis is a very rare disease that is best managed surgically, either with ureterolysis or excision of the endometriosis and ureteral reimplant or ureteroureterostomy.

Questions

1. What is the imaging modality of choice used to diagnose retroperitoneal fibrosis?
   (a) MR imaging
   (b) PET scan
   (c) US
   (d) CT imaging

Answer: (d)

CT imaging can be used to detect a periaortic mass of soft tissue attenuation

2. On biopsy what are the pathognomonic histological lesions seen in malakoplakia?
   (a) Psammoma bodies
   (b) Henderson-Paterson bodies
   (c) Michaelis-Guttman bodies
   (d) Keratin pearls

Answer: (c)

3. What is the best *first-line imaging modality* for the diagnosis of ureteral endometriosis?
   (a) CT imaging
   (b) MR imaging
   (c) PET scan
   (d) Transvaginal ultrasound

Answer: (d)

4. What form of staining is used to specifically aid in the diagnosis of amyloidosis?
   (a) Congo Red staining
   (b) Giemsa staining
   (c) Hematoxylin staining
   (d) Silver nitrate staining

Answer: (a)

5. Ureteritis cystica affects most commonly which part of the ureter?
   (a) Distal ureter
   (b) Mid-segment of the ureter
   (c) Proximal ureter
   (d) Vesiculo-ureteral junction

Answer: (c)

References

1. Ormond JK. Bilateral ureteral obstruction due to envelopment and compression by an inflammatory retroperitoneal process. J Urol. 1948;59(6):1072–9. https://doi.org/10.1016/s0022-5347(17)69482-5.
2. Runowska M, Majewski D, Puszczewicz M. Retroperitoneal fibrosis - the state-of-the-art. Reumatologia. 2016;54(5):256–63. https://doi.org/10.5114/reum.2016.63667.
3. Debruyne FM, Bogman MJ, Ypma AF. Retroperitoneal fibrosis in the scrotum. Eur Urol. 1982;8(1):45–8. https://doi.org/10.1159/000473477.
4. Brandt AS, Kamper L, Kukuk S, Haage P, Roth S. Associated findings and complications of retroperitoneal fibrosis in 204 patients: results of a urological registry. J Urol. 2011;185(2):526–31. https://doi.org/10.1016/j.juro.2010.09.105.
5. Uibu T, Oksa P, Auvinen A, Honkanen E, Metsarinne K, Saha H, et al. Asbestos exposure as a risk factor for retroperitoneal fibrosis. Lancet. 2004;363(9419):1422–6. https://doi.org/10.1016/S0140-6736(04)16100-X.
6. van Bommel EFH, Jansen I, Hendriksz TR, Aarnoudse A. Idiopathic retroperitoneal fibrosis: prospective evaluation of incidence and clinicoradiologic presentation. Medicine (Baltimore). 2009;88(4):193–201. https://doi.org/10.1097/MD.0b013e3181afc420.
7. Lian L, Wang C, J T. IgG4-related retroperitoneal fibrosis: a newly characterized disease. Int J Rheum Dis. 2016;19(11):1049–55.
8. Amis ES Jr. Retroperitoneal fibrosis. AJR Am J Roentgenol. 1991;157(2):321–9. https://doi.org/10.2214/ajr.157.2.1853816.
9. Vaglio A, Salvarani C, Buzio C. Retroperitoneal fibrosis. Lancet. 2006;367(9506):241–51. https://doi.org/10.1016/S0140-6736(06)68035-5.
10. Kermani TA, Crowson CS, Achenbach SJ, Luthra HS. Idiopathic retroperitoneal fibrosis: a retrospective review of clinical presentation, treatment, and outcomes. Mayo Clin Proc. 2011;86(4):297–303. https://doi.org/10.4065/mcp.2010.0663.
11. Warnatz K, Keskin AG, Uhl M, Scholz C, Katzenwadel A, Vaith P, et al. Immunosuppressive treatment of chronic periaortitis: a retrospective study of 20 patients with chronic periaortitis and a review of the literature. Ann Rheum Dis. 2005;64(6):828–33. https://doi.org/10.1136/ard.2004.029793.
12. Corradi D, Maestri R, Palmisano A, Bosio S, Greco P, Manenti L, et al. Idiopathic retroperitoneal fibrosis: clinicopathologic features and differential diagnosis. Kidney Int. 2007;72(6):742–53. https://doi.org/10.1038/sj.ki.5002427.
13. Caiafa RO, Vinuesa AS, Izquierdo RS, Brufau BP, Ayuso Colella JR, Molina CN. Retroperitoneal fibrosis: role of imaging in diagnosis and follow-up. Radiographics. 2013;33(2):535–52. https://doi.org/10.1148/rg.332125085.
14. Cronin CG, Lohan DG, Blake MA, Roche C, McCarthy P, Murphy JM. Retroperitoneal fibrosis: a review of clinical features and imaging findings. AJR Am J Roentgenol. 2008;191(2):423–31. https://doi.org/10.2214/AJR.07.3629.

15. Koep L, Zuidema GD. The clinical significance of retroperitoneal fibrosis. Surgery. 1977;81(3):250–7.
16. Vaglio A. Retroperitoneal fibrosis: new insights into clinical presentation and diagnosis. Medicine (Baltimore). 2009;88(4):208–10. https://doi.org/10.1097/MD.0b013e3181afc4d1.
17. Young PM, Peterson JJ, Calamia KT. Hypermetabolic activity in patients with active retroperitoneal fibrosis on F-18 FDG PET: report of three cases. Ann Nucl Med. 2008;22(1):87–92. https://doi.org/10.1007/s12149-007-0077-0.
18. Vaglio A, Palmisano A, Alberici F, Maggiore U, Ferretti S, Cobelli R, et al. Prednisone versus tamoxifen in patients with idiopathic retroperitoneal fibrosis: an open-label randomised controlled trial. Lancet. 2011;378(9788):338–46. https://doi.org/10.1016/S0140-6736(11)60934-3.
19. Li KP, Zhu J, Zhang JL, Huang F. Idiopathic retroperitoneal fibrosis (RPF): clinical features of 61 cases and literature review. Clin Rheumatol. 2011;30(5):601–5. https://doi.org/10.1007/s10067-010-1580-6.
20. Scavalli AS, Spadaro A, Riccieri V, Ricciuti GP, Taccari E, Marini M, et al. Long-term follow-up of low-dose methotrexate therapy in one case of idiopathic retroperitoneal fibrosis. Clin Rheumatol. 1995;14(4):481–4. https://doi.org/10.1007/BF02207688.
21. Alberici F, Palmisano A, Urban ML, Maritati F, Oliva E, Manenti L, et al. Methotrexate plus prednisone in patients with relapsing idiopathic retroperitoneal fibrosis. Ann Rheum Dis. 2013;72(9):1584–6. https://doi.org/10.1136/annrheumdis-2013-203267.
22. Marcolongo R, Tavolini IM, Laveder F, Busa M, Noventa F, Bassi P, et al. Immunosuppressive therapy for idiopathic retroperitoneal fibrosis: a retrospective analysis of 26 cases. Am J Med. 2004;116(3):194–7. https://doi.org/10.1016/j.amjmed.2003.08.033.
23. Adler S, Lodermeyer S, Gaa J, Heemann U. Successful mycophenolate mofetil therapy in nine patients with idiopathic retroperitoneal fibrosis. Rheumatology (Oxford). 2008;47(10):1535–8. https://doi.org/10.1093/rheumatology/ken291.
24. Khosroshahi A, Carruthers MN, Deshpande V, Unizony S, Bloch DB, Stone JH. Rituximab for the treatment of IgG4-related disease: lessons from 10 consecutive patients. Medicine (Baltimore). 2012;91(1):57–66. https://doi.org/10.1097/MD.0b013e3182431ef6.
25. O'Brien T, Fernando A. Contemporary role of ureterolysis in retroperitoneal fibrosis: treatment of last resort or first intent? An analysis of 50 cases. BJU Int. 2017;120(4):556–61. https://doi.org/10.1111/bju.13915.
26. Uddin M, Varley R, Napier-Hemy R. Our experience in laparoscopic ureterolysis and omental wrapping as a definitive surgical management of ureteric obstruction related to retroperitoneal fibrosis. J Clin Urol. 2021:205141582110222. https://doi.org/10.1177/20514158211022215.
27. Keehn AY, Mufarrij PW, Stifelman MD. Robotic ureterolysis for relief of ureteral obstruction from retroperitoneal fibrosis. Urology. 2011;77(6):1370–4. https://doi.org/10.1016/j.urology.2010.11.025.
28. Kavoussi LR, Clayman RV, Brunt LM, Soper NJ. Laparoscopic ureterolysis. J Urol. 1992;147(2):426–9. https://doi.org/10.1016/s0022-5347(17)37257-9.
29. Fernando A, Challacombe B, O'Brien T. Robotic ureterolysis for ureteric obstruction from retroperitoneal fibrosis (RPF). Eur Urol Suppl. 2017;16(3):e2144.
30. Menendez V, Sala X, Alvarez-Vijande R, Sole M, Rodriguez A, Carretero P. Cystic pyeloureteritis: review of 34 cases. Radiologic aspects and differential diagnosis. Urology. 1997;50(1):31–7. https://doi.org/10.1016/S0090-4295(97)00205-7.
31. He YR, Kam J, Chan HF. A rare case of extensive unilateral ureteritis cystica. Urology. 2020;138:e3–4. https://doi.org/10.1016/j.urology.2020.01.017.
32. Muraki PH, Donin NM. Ureteritis cystica mimicking upper tract urothelial cancer in a patient with bladder cancer. Urol Case Rep. 2021;39:101822. https://doi.org/10.1016/j.eucr.2021.101822.
33. Stormont G, Makari J, Bedrnicek JB, Berrondo C. Eosinophilic ureteritis in a child with ureteropelvic junction obstruction and vesicoureteral reflux. Cureus. 2020;12(7):e9214. https://doi.org/10.7759/cureus.9214.

34. Eguiluz Lumbreras P, Herrero Polo M, Palacios Hernandez A, Heir Zorzo O, Martin Parada A, Grinard De Leon E, et al. Eosinophilic ureteritis. Report of a case. Arch Esp Urol. 2012;65(7):706–8.
35. Sergeant G, Slabbaert K, Werbrouck P. Recurrent flank pain caused by eosinophilic ureteritis mimicking urinary stone disease: a case report. Int Urol Nephrol. 2004;36(1):23–5. https://doi.org/10.1023/b:urol.0000032678.84766.70.
36. Hina S, Hasan A, Iqbal N, Shabbir MU, Sheikh AAE. Malakoplakia of the urinary bladder and unilateral ureter. J Coll Physicians Surg Pak. 2019;29(6):582–4. https://doi.org/10.29271/jcpsp.2019.06.582.
37. Sanchez LM, Sanchez SI, Bailey JL. Malacoplakia presenting with obstructive nephropathy with bilateral ureter involvement. Nat Rev Nephrol. 2009;5(7):418–22. https://doi.org/10.1038/nrneph.2009.86.
38. Stanton MJ, Maxted W. Malacoplakia: a study of the literature and current concepts of pathogenesis, diagnosis and treatment. J Urol. 1981;125(2):139–46. https://doi.org/10.1016/s0022-5347(17)54940-x.
39. Dobyan DC, Truong LD, Eknoyan G. Renal malacoplakia reappraised. Am J Kidney Dis. 1993;22(2):243–52. https://doi.org/10.1016/s0272-6386(12)70313-x.
40. Long JP Jr, Althausen AF. Malacoplakia: a 25-year experience with a review of the literature. J Urol. 1989;141(6):1328–31. https://doi.org/10.1016/s0022-5347(17)41297-3.
41. Sexton CC, Lowman RM, Nyongo AO, Baskin AM. Malacoplakia presenting as complete unilateral ureteral obstruction. J Urol. 1982;128(1):139–41. https://doi.org/10.1016/s0022-5347(17)52789-5.
42. Stamatiou K, Chelioti E, Tsavari A, Koulia K, Papalexandrou A, Efthymiou E, et al. Renal failure caused by malakoplakia lesions of the urinary bladder. Nephrourol Mon. 2014;6(4):e18522. https://doi.org/10.5812/numonthly.18522.
43. Chen Y, Kuo H. Malakoplakia of ipsilateral kidney, ureter and bladder. Tzu Chi Med J. 2010;22:103–5.
44. Hartman D. Radiologic pathologic correlation of the infectious granulomatous diseases of the kidney: III and IV. Monogr Urol. 1985;6:26.
45. Vallorosi CJ, Putzi MJ, Wolf JS Jr. Renal malacoplakia. Tech Urol. 1999;5(1):43–4.
46. Stanton MJ, Lynch JH, Maxted WC, Chun BK. Malacoplakia of the bladder: a case report of resolution with bethanechol, trimethoprim-sulfamethoxazole and ascorbic acid. J Urol. 1983;130(6):1174–5. https://doi.org/10.1016/s0022-5347(17)51742-5.
47. Mantoo S, Hwang JS, Chiang GS, Tan PH. A rare case of localised AA-type amyloidosis of the ureter with spheroids of amyloid. Singap Med J. 2012;53(4):e77–9.
48. Sipe JD, Cohen AS. Review: history of the amyloid fibril. J Struct Biol. 2000;130(2–3):88–98. https://doi.org/10.1006/jsbi.2000.4221.
49. Shaker N, Tynski Z, Hudlak M, Brown RR, Qasem S, Parwani A. Primary localized amyloidosis of the ureter with osseous metaplasia presenting as a suspicious ureteral mass. Urol Case Rep. 2022;41:101967. https://doi.org/10.1016/j.eucr.2021.101967.
50. Hanna DN, Levy JA, Marshall JS. Amyloidosis and acute hemorrhage of the kidney, ureter, and bladder. Can J Urol. 2017;24(4):8934–6.
51. Al-Obaidy KI, Grignon DJ. Primary amyloidosis of the genitourinary tract. Arch Pathol Lab Med. 2021;145(6):699–703. https://doi.org/10.5858/arpa.2020-0102-RA.
52. Banerji JS, Gopalakrishnan G, Sriram K, Manipadam MT. Localised retroperitoneal amyloidosis mimicking retroperitoneal fibrosis: a rare cause of obstructive uropathy. Singap Med J. 2009;50(9):e332–5.
53. Zhou F, Lee P, Zhou M, Melamed J, Deng FM. Primary localized amyloidosis of the urinary tract frequently mimics neoplasia: a clinicopathologic analysis of 11 cases. Am J Clin Exp Urol. 2014;2(1):71–5.
54. Mark IR, Goodlad J, Lloyd-Davies RW. Localized amyloidosis of the genito-urinary tract. J R Soc Med. 1995;88(6):320–4.

55. Callaghan P, Asklin B. Ureteral obstruction due to primary localized amyloidosis. Scand J Urol Nephrol. 1993;27(4):535–6. https://doi.org/10.3109/00365599309182290.
56. Kawashima A, Alleman WG, Takahashi N, Kim B, King BF Jr, LeRoy AJ. Imaging evaluation of amyloidosis of the urinary tract and retroperitoneum. Radiographics. 2011;31(6):1569–82. https://doi.org/10.1148/rg.316115519.
57. Hadfield MJ, Lyall V, Ristau B, Patel V, Hundal J, Kennedy H, et al. Amyloid deposition of the bilateral ureters in a patient with chronic systemic al amyloidosis. Urology. 2020;146:e10–e1. https://doi.org/10.1016/j.urology.2020.08.024.
58. Kim SH, Park WS, Joung JY, Lee KH, Chung J, Seo HK. A surgically treated case of uretero-vesical amyloidosis of the bladder in a patient with idiopathic thrombocytopenia. Case Rep Urol. 2018;2018:1059349. https://doi.org/10.1155/2018/1059349.
59. Sud S, Buxi TBS, Sheth S, Ghuman SS. Endometriosis and its myriad presentations: magnetic resonance imaging-based pictorial review. Indian J Radiol Imaging. 2021;31(1):193–202. https://doi.org/10.1055/s-0041-1729670.
60. Barra F, Scala C, Biscaldi E, Vellone VG, Ceccaroni M, Terrone C, et al. Ureteral endometriosis: a systematic review of epidemiology, pathogenesis, diagnosis, treatment, risk of malignant transformation and fertility. Hum Reprod Update. 2018;24(6):710–30. https://doi.org/10.1093/humupd/dmy027.
61. Philip CA, Froc E, Chapron C, Hebert T, Douvier S, Filipuzzi L, et al. surgical management of urinary tract endometriosis: a 1-year longitudinal multicenter pilot study at 31 french hospitals (by the FRIENDS group). J Minim Invasive Gynecol. 2021;28(11):1889–97 e1. https://doi.org/10.1016/j.jmig.2021.04.020.
62. Camanni M, Bonino L, Delpiano EM, Berchialla P, Migliaretti G, Revelli A, et al. Laparoscopic conservative management of ureteral endometriosis: a survey of eighty patients submitted to ureterolysis. Reprod Biol Endocrinol. 2009;7:109. https://doi.org/10.1186/1477-7827-7-109.
63. Ceccaroni M, Ceccarello M, Caleffi G, Clarizia R, Scarperi S, Pastorello M, et al. total laparoscopic ureteroneocystostomy for ureteral endometriosis: a single-center experience of 160 consecutive patients. J Minim Invasive Gynecol. 2019;26(1):78–86. https://doi.org/10.1016/j.jmig.2018.03.031.
64. Froc E, Dubernard G, Bendifallah S, Hermouet E, Rubod-Dit-Guillet C, Canis M, et al. Clinical characteristics of urinary tract endometriosis: a one-year national series of 232 patients from 31 endometriosis expert centers (by the FRIENDS group). Eur J Obstet Gynecol Reprod Biol. 2021;264:155–61. https://doi.org/10.1016/j.ejogrb.2021.06.018.

Chapter 12
The Ureter and Schistosomiasis

Bedeir Ali-El-Dein and Ahmed M. Harraz

Abstract Schistosomiasis (Bilharzia) is one of the most common parasitic infestations. It is endemic in certain areas, including South America, Africa and the Middle East. The genus responsible for genitourinary pathology is Schistosoma haematobium which inhabits the venous channels around the urinary bladder. The infection starts with cercarial penetration of the skin and migration through the blood stream to mature to adult worms which lay eggs. The reaction to the eggs causes acute and chronic inflammatory and immune responses that result in ureteral fibrosis, stenosis, dilatation, secondary calcification, or stone formation. Patients commonly present with manifestations of ureteral obstruction. The diagnosis is made by finding the eggs in urine, in histopathological specimens, and/or via the detection of serum antibodies. The clues to diagnosis include bladder and/or ureteral wall thickening with or without calcification on abdomino-pelvic ultrasound and intravenous contrast imaging modalities such as intravenous urography (IVU), computerized urography (CTU), and magnetic resonance urography (MRU) to define the location, laterality, multiplicity, and extent of the ureteral pathology. Treatment is made by the anti-helminthic medication, pranziquantel, and surgical correction of the resulting complications, including ureteral stricture.

Keywords Ureter · Bilharzia · Schistosomiasis · Ureteral thickening · Hydronephrosis

Learning Objectives

- After reading this chapter, the readers will be able to describe the pathophysiology, the lifecycle, and mode of infestation of bilharziasis. In addition, the readers will be able to discuss how the ureter is affected by bilharziasis, its clinical pre-

Test your learning and check your understanding of this book's contents: use the "Springer Nature Flashcards" app to access questions. To use the app, please follow the instructions in chapter 1.

B. Ali-El-Dein (✉) · A. M. Harraz
Urology Department, Urology and Nephrology Center, Faculty of Medicine, Mansoura University, Mansoura, Egypt

M. Abdel-Gawad et al. (eds.), *The Ureter*,
https://doi.org/10.1007/978-3-031-36212-5_12

sentation, and the radiological and other signs of the bilharzial ureter. An additional objective is to describe a plan for the diagnosis and treatment of the disease.

12.1 Introduction

Schistosomiasis (Bilharzia) is one of the common tropical diseases in some parts of the world. It follows malaria as the second most prevalent parasitic infestation and it has been endemic in many areas in the world including Africa, the Middle East, South America, Asia, and more recently Southern Europe [1]. Based on the World Health Organization (WHO) website with the last update on the third of December 2021, Schistosomiasis affects almost 240 million people worldwide, and more than 700 million people live in endemic areas. Schistosomiasis prevails in less developed areas, where there is frequent exposure to fresh water and absence of effective primary health care facilities [2]. It is important to increase the index of suspicion for travelers to endemic areas who present with urinary symptoms [3, 4]. Figure 12.1 demonstrates the recent WHO organization status of schistosomiasis as of the 8th of January 2022.

Out of the six species that can cause diseases in humans [5], *Schistosoma haematobium*, residing in the peri-vesical venules, is the main culprit. It lays eggs in the bladder and ureteral walls causing chronic inflammation and fibrosis with characteristic calcifications. The sequelae included a variety of diseases, including benign (stenosis), malignant (squamous cell carcinoma), obstructive uropathy, and renal failure [6]. In this chapter, a focus on the discussion of the life cycle of schistosomiasis, pathophysiology, diagnosis, and treatment options of the bilharzial ureter is carried out.

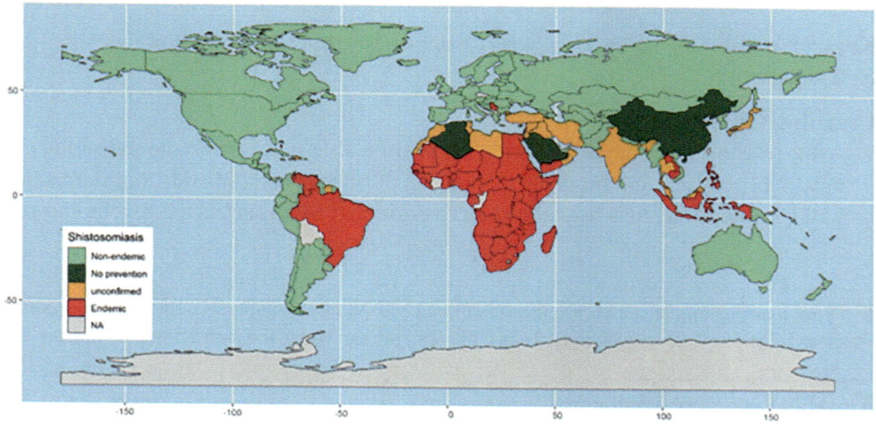

Fig. 12.1 The status of schistosomiasis in the world based on the latest WHO website. The figure was based on the data downloaded from the WHO site and was constructed using R programing language version 4.1.2. https://apps.who.int/neglected_diseases/ntddata/sch/sch.html

12.2 Schistosoma Life Cycle

The lifecycle starts with mating of male and female trematode bilharzia worms in the human blood vessels (the definitive host). On releasing eggs, some are shed through the urinary or fecal routes, and the others are retained and cause tissue damage and fibrosis. The released eggs in the freshwater hatch and release miracidia that target the suitable snail, where it undergoes asexual replication producing thousands of cercaria (the infective stage) through mother and daughter sporocysts. Whether shed or remain in tissues, the eggs die within 1–2 weeks. The process takes approximately 4–6 weeks in the snail and the cercariae remain active for 1–3 days. The cercariae penetrate the human skin and reach the target venous system where they mature into larvae (schistosomula) in 5–7 weeks [7]. Schistosoma haematobium larvae continue growing in the host's venous system [8]. When they become mature, the coupled worms travel to bladder and pelvic plexus veins, make their habitat, mate, and then eggs are laid by the female worm [8].

Because the venous circulation is so rich, the corresponding organs are significantly affected. Therefore, the urinary bladder, distal ureters, and seminal vesicles are the most frequently affected organs of the urinary and genital tracts; with 90%, 80%, and 19% egg distribution in the bladder, seminal vesicles, and prostate gland, respectively [9]. Similarly, the tissue burden of egg deposition was noted [10]. It is stated that when the tissue level of egg deposition is high, a severe reaction of the tissue is noted on histological sections [8].

The adult worm can live from 3 to 10 years, and for several decades in some reports [11]. The repeated infection with cercariae as well as the longevity of the adult worm is responsible for the chronicity of the disease. **The lifecycle is illustrated in** Fig. 12.2.

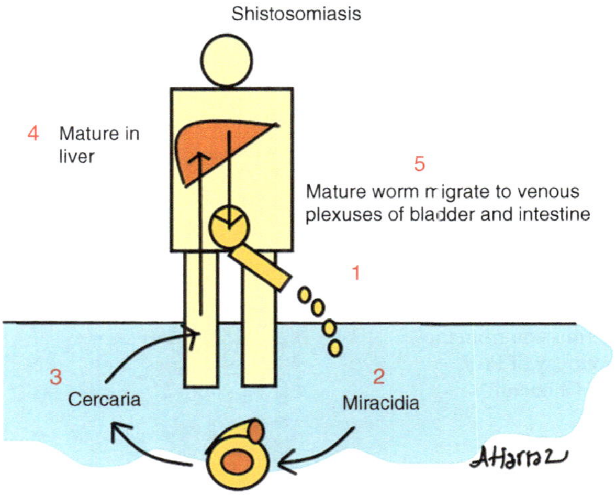

Fig. 12.2 Diagrammatic representation of the life cycle of schistosomiasis

12.3 Pathophysiology, Characteristic Lesions, and Sequelae

12.3.1 The Initial Response [8]

The hallmark pathology of the disease is the immune response against lodged eggs in the body with minimal effect from the adult worms [7]. The tissue-embedded eggs release soluble egg antigens (SEA) which chronically stimulate the immune system. In addition, the host defense of granuloma formation gradually causes fibrosis. This limits blood supply to the organs and causes strictures or a contracted bladder. The in-vitro studies mainly done through intestinal infestation with *S. Mansoni* showed that macrophage activation played an important role in granuloma formation [12]. Furthermore, the CD4+ T-helper cells-derived IL-4 and IL-13 are responsible for the initiation of granuloma formation [13, 14]. Such chronic stimulation and inflammation can lead to subtle morbidity such as anemia, growth disturbances, malnutrition, and cognitive impairment [11, 15].

The egg-induced granuloma develops in the lamina propria (Fig. 12.3). Multiple risk factors have been described to determine the severity of the lesions and the sequelae, namely the load of tissue egg deposition, the number of re-infections, the timing and efficacy of treatment, and the presence/absence of secondary infection [8].

12.3.2 Subsequent Lesions

Subsequent lesions occur as a result of the epithelium reacting to changes in the submucosal connective tissue [8]. The histolytic antigen, secreted by the bilharzial eggs, induces intense cell-mediated immune changes in the tissue with abundant eosinophils with a resultant hyperemia and/or polyp formation of the covering epithelium. Subsequent lesions may be ~~described as~~ atrophic, proliferative, or metaplastic.

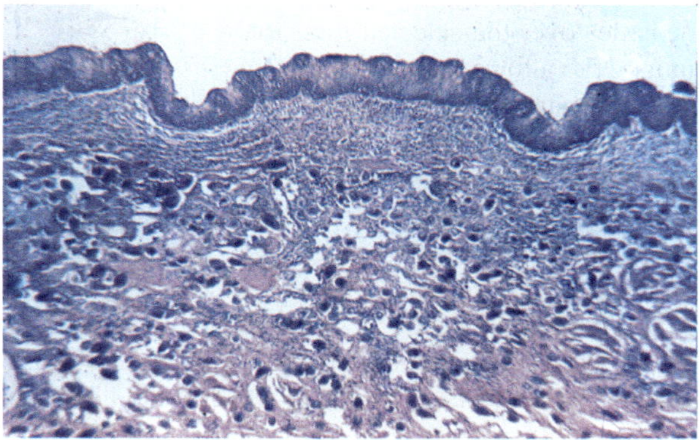

Fig. 12.3 Section of the bladder wall showing many calcified schistosomal ova at the lamina propria. There is associated inflammatory cell infiltrate, granulomas, and fibrosis. "With permission from the courtesy of Prof. M. Ghoneim"

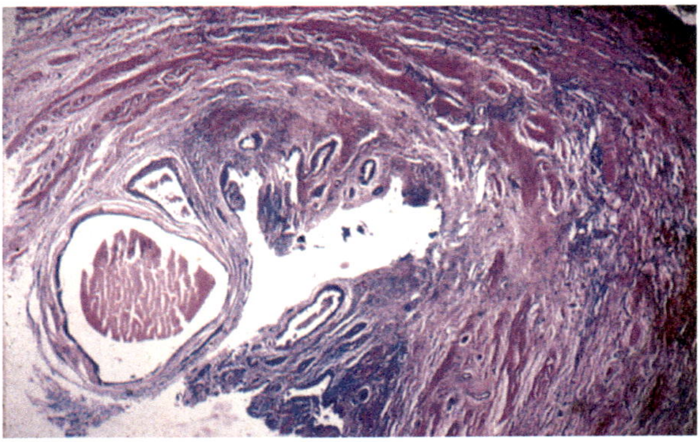

Fig. 12.4 Microscopical low power section of the ureteral wall, showing that the hyperplastic urothelial lining with proliferative lesion formation, ureteritis cystica. The wall demonstrates expanded fibrous tissue with reduction of the muscle layer. "With permission from the courtesy of Prof. M. Ghoneim"

Development of what is called bilharzial ulcer is the ultimate result of the atrophic changes, which develop because of ischemic changes of the covering epithelium secondary to heavy deposition of eggs with subsequent fibrosis, with or without secondary infection, in the submucosa. Proliferative changes occur in the form of epithelial hyperplasia, where the thickness of epithelial layers increases beyond six cells with polypoid lesions. Sometimes, proliferative changes are associated with dysplasia, where nuclear atypia limited to the basal epithelial layers, develops [8]. Metaplastic changes occur in the form of squamous or columnar metaplasia. As a result, glandular and/or cystic changes may develop secondary to epithelial columnar metaplasia [8] (Fig. 12.4).

12.3.3 *Secondary Bacterial Infection, Healing*

Superadded or secondary bacterial infection may occur on top of bilharzial lesions. They depend on ~~the~~ host age and severity and frequency of re-infections [8]. Escherichia coli accounts for 50% of these secondary bacterial infections [10]. Bacterial infections lead to worsening of the symptoms, ascending urinary tract infections, impairment of the kidney function, and increased rate of complications, such as stones, fistula formation, obstruction, and cancer.

Healing of the granulomatous lesions may be favorable or unfavorable. Favorable healing with mild mural fibrosis and/or calcification is achieved when infestation is occasional, and proper treatment is given on time. These factors are of special importance, particularly in children and young adults in whom the bilharzial granulomatous lesions are usually reversible [16].

12.3.4 *Ureteral Complications*

Unfavorable healing with subsequent complications occurs when re-infection is frequent, and/or treatment is delayed and improper, especially among farmers in endemic regions. The list of ureter-related complications includes ureteral strictures, ulceration, obstruction, and chronic kidney disease with eventual loss of kidney function.

The disease can spread through retrograde diffusion into the ureter causing bladder wall and distal ureteral wall thickening. The ureter can be involved in approximately 66% of cases which starts with ureteral dysfunction causing dilatation followed by inflammation and thickening with stenosis [17]. The initial site of pathology is the intravesical ureter followed by 1–2 inches above the ureterovesical junction in nearly 80% of patients [18]. However, the lumbar ureter may be affected as well [19]. Deposition of bilharzial ova usually occurs in all the layers of the ureter, especially in the submucosa and between the muscle layers; however, in one study ova were found mainly in the peri-ureteral layer [20].

The final picture can be a dilated thickened ureter like a pipestem, stenosed or dilated atonic ureter, or any combination [20, 21]. Latent in the disease, upper tract obstruction with renal failure can ensue notably if presented in school-age children with limited access to health facilities [6]. Therefore, early treatment of the disease might prevent long-term sequelae. Late presentation usually requires corrective surgery and close surveillance for squamous cell carcinoma of the urinary bladder [18, 22, 23].

12.4 Clinical Presentation

Earlier in the disease course, dermatitis induced by cercarial penetration of skin is the initial sign. Dermatitis is followed by bronchopulmonary and/or gastrointestinal manifestations usually associated with fever, headache, myalgia, weight loss, and eosinophilia commonly known as Katayama syndrome. The incubation period can range from two weeks up to approximately three months [24]. These manifestations are reactions to larval migration through the bloodstream. In chronic urinary schistosomiasis, patients usually present with hematuria, dysuria, suprapubic pain, and hematospermia [17, 18, 25].

Ureteral bilharziasis usually presents with loin pain, renal colic with or without symptoms of acute pyelonephritis. In addition, palpable kidney because of hydronephrosis, or even anuria may be the presenting manifestation [8].

12.5 Diagnosis

12.5.1 Role of Ultrasound

Ultrasound is an invaluable tool in suspected cases of schistosomiasis. The findings of bladder and/or ureteral walls thickening with or without calcifications are key radiological signs that are easily detected. In 118 young adult patients presenting with hematuria, a focused assessment with sonography for urinary schistosomiasis (FASUS) was performed in an endemic African territory [23]. The authors diagnosed 43% of ureteral pathologies based on the ultrasound findings. The WHO has developed the Niamey-Belo Horizonte Protocol, a standardized scoring system to assess the ultrasound-based morbidity of schistosomiasis in endemic areas [26]. Pathological changes in the ureter were detected in 34.4% of 157 school-aged children previously diagnosed with schistosomiasis in Angola using the WHO protocol [15]. In addition, an echogenic snow sign, defined as small scattered innumerable echogenic foci floating in bladder lumen, has increased the detection rate of the WHO protocol [27].

12.5.2 X-ray and Computed Tomography Scan (CT)

In the ureter, the diagnosis is suspected when mural calcification is found on X-ray, which is pathognomonic for calcified bilharzial eggs [25]. A computerized tomography (CT) scan is obtained in most patients. **Ureteral calcifications are important clues to the diagnosis**; they are initially sporadic, but coalesce with the progress of the disease giving a characteristic parallel linear pattern on plain-X ray (Fig. 12.5) or reformatted CT images, and a circular pattern on axial images.

12.5.3 Urography Studies

CT, MRI, or intravenous urography, retrograde or antegrade ureteropyelography can make the diagnosis of ureteral lesions, essentially stricture and obstruction (Fig. 12.6). In addition, ureteritis cystica and pyelitis cystica can cause air bubble-like filling defects in the ureteral lumen which are pathognomonic of ureteral schistosomiasis (Fig. 12.7) [17, 18].

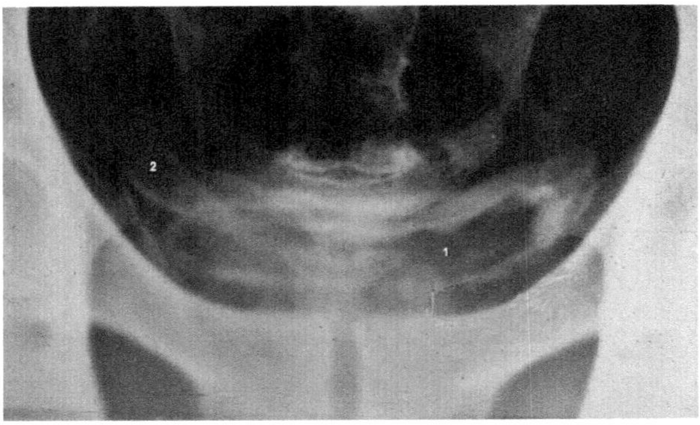

Fig. 12.5 Plain X-ray of the lower part of the pelvis. It shows the characteristic bilharzial curvilinear bladder (1) and linear ureteral (2) calcification

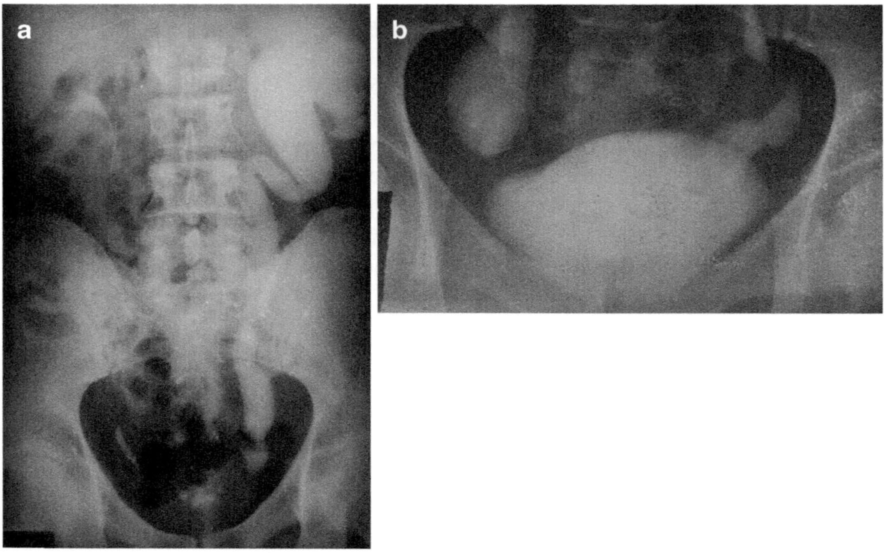

Fig. 12.6 IVU showing: (**a**) bilharzial stricture of the lower end of left ureter & (**b**) Bilateral lower end bilharzial ureteral strictures with spindle shaped lower ureter. "With permission from the courtesy of Prof. M. Ghoneim"

Furthermore, nuclear medicine (renogram) is very important to assess the kidney function, detect obstruction, and to evaluate the outcome of surgery on follow-up [28].

12.5.4 Confirming the Diagnosis

When the diagnosis is suspected based on imaging, urinary examination for the detection of eggs is diagnostic (Fig. 12.8) [29]. If not found, calcified dead eggs can be detected by bladder or ureteral biopsies [25, 30]. On certain occasions, the diagnosis can be only confirmed via the detection of bilharzial antibodies in the serum using enzyme-linked immunosorbent assay (ELIZA), Western blot, complement fixation, or indirect hemagglutination [29].

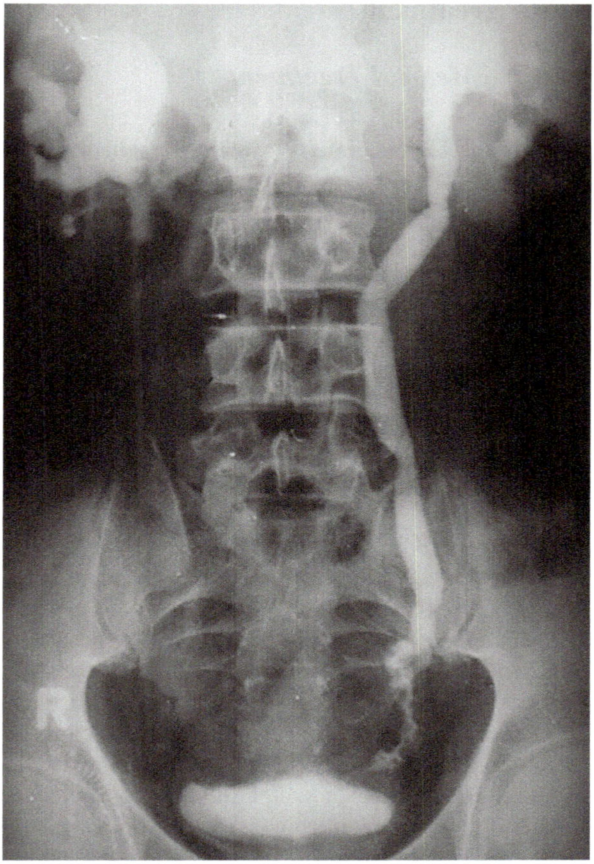

Fig. 12.7 Intravenous urography showing multiple air bubble-like filling defects in the lumen caused by bilharzial ureteritis cystica of the lower part of the left ureter

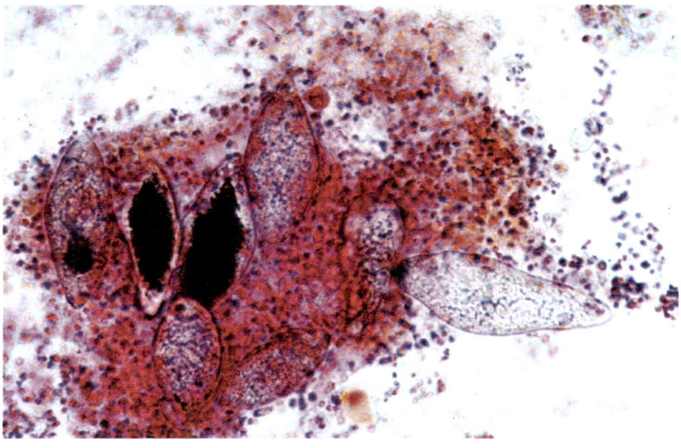

Fig. 12.8 Cytologic smear showing multiple viable Schistosoml ova associated with inflammatory cells and RBCs. "With permission from the courtesy of Prof. M. Ghoneim"

12.6 Treatment

12.6.1 Medical Treatment

Praziquantel is the main treatment for schistosomiasis infection, although there have been other old and recent treatments, such as Antimony compounds, Oxamniquine, Niridazole, and Mirazid. Praziquantel works by inducing paralysis and vacuolation of the parasite and ultimately detaching it from the mucosa. It is administered in a single dose of 40 mg/kg and is safe during pregnancy [25, 31]. It is recommended to have a second dose 2–4 weeks later to enhance its action [24]. Despite its effectiveness in the primary treatment of bilharziasis, it might be administered again if complications develop later [32].

In addition, corticosteroids have been recommended by some investigators to minimize the inflammatory response and to limit subsequent fibrosis [33].

12.6.2 Surgical Treatment

Endoscopic and endourological treatments, in the form of stone disintegration, dilation, endoureterotomy with stenting, may be tried for stones or short-segment ureteral strictures, which develop early in the disease, and they were attended with a fair success rate [34]. Laser incision has been tried to treat bilharzial stricture in some case reports [30]. However, failures and morbidity are to be considered when there is extensive periureteral fibrosis [20]. While stone disintegration in the bilharzial ureter is feasible, ureteral stenting has not been advocated postoperatively because the voiding loin pain and lower urinary tract symptoms might be exaggerated in the context of dilated ureter [35].

Reconstructive open surgery is usually required to manage well established ureteral strictures secondary to chronic bilharzial infestation. Table 12.1 summarizes the various treatment options for ureteral strictures. Ureteroureterostomy is indicated for mid- or proximal short-segment ureteral strictures. On the other hand,

Table 12.1 Treatment of short-, long-segment and multiple bilharzial ureteral strictures

Parameter	Treatment options
Short-segment stricture: –Proximal ureter –Mid-ureter –Distal ureter	•Trial of endourerotomy, dilation, stenting in some cases •Ureteroureterostomy or ureteropelvic anastomosis •Ureteroureterostomy •Ureteroneocystostomy, Psoas hitch, Boari flap (± antireflux technique)
Multiple or long-segment strictures	•Classic ileal ureter •Tailored ileal ureter •Ileal ureter with Yang-Monti principle •Transureteroureterostomy or autotransplantation (rarely feasible)

ureteroneocystostomy is the best option for distal ureteral strictures. A grossly dilated atonic ureter with associated bilharzial bladder lesion is not uncommon. This will make performing an anti-reflux mechanism very difficult. In these situations, a Boari flap is the best alternative when there is acceptable bladder capacity. However, some researchers have recommended anti-reflux anastomosis, such as the inverted nipple anti-reflux ureteroneocystostomy, with high success rate [36].

Replacement of the ureter, using an isoperistaltic ileal segment (ileal ureter) is the last resort for treatment of multiple and/or long segment ureteral strictures. Other alternatives of ileal ureter with less frequent complications have been successfully utilized with good outcome [37–39]. In cases of hydronephrosis with kidney function loss, nephrectomy is indicated.

Recently, minimally invasive techniques have been used as alternatives to open surgery with successful outcomes. In one study, laparoscopic ureterolithotomy/ ureterouretetostomy were successfully used to extract impacted stones and repair strictures of the ureter in 51 bilharzial patients [40].

Questions

1. The infective stage in schistosomiasis is:
   a. Adult male worm
   b. Ovum.
   c. Cercaria.
   d. Adult female worm.
   e. Larvae.

Answer: (c)

2. The hallmark pathology of scistosomiasis is:
   a. Neutrophil infiltration of the infected tissue.
   b. Direct trauma caused by cercarial penetration.
   c. secondary bacterial infection on top of infestation.
   d. Hematuria.
   e. The immune response against lodged eggs in the tissue.

Answer: (e)

3. Development of what is called bilharzial ulcer occurs on top of:
   a. Atrophic lesions.
   b. proliferative lesions.
   c. Metaplastic lesions.
   d. Both atrophic and proliferative lesions.
   e. Atrophic, proliferative, or metaplastic lesions.

Answer: (a)

4. The usual presentation of ureteral bilharziasis (schistosomiasis) is:

   a. Dermatitis.
   b. Asymptomatic bacteriuria.
   c. Hematuria.
   d. Loin pain or renal colic.
   e. Pallor.

Answer: (d)

5. Which of the following statements regarding the radiological diagnosis of ureteral bilharziasis is correct?

   a. Ureteral calcifications on KUB or Noncontrast CT are important clues to the diagnosis.
   b. Vesicoureteral reflux is always present.
   c. Ultrasound is sufficient for the diagnosis.
   d. Scattered calcifications at the kidney site are common.
   e. Filling defects on antegrade and retrograde studies.

Answer: (a)

6. Confirmation of the diagnosis of Scistosomiasis of the ureter is made by:

   a. Hydronephrosis on imaging.
   b. The triad of hematuria, loin pain, and hydronephrosis on imaging.
   c. CT or MR urography.
   d. A combination of CT/ MR urography and renogram.
   e. Urinary examination for the detection of eggs.

Answer: (e)

7. The main medical treatment for schistosomal infection is:

   a. Praziquantel
   b. Antimony compounds.
   c. Oxamniquine
   d. Niridazole
   e. Mirazid

Answer: (a)

References

1. Kincaid-Smith J, Tracey A, de Carvalho AR, et al. Morphological and genomic characterisation of the Schistosoma hybrid infecting humans in Europe reveals admixture between Schistosoma haematobium and Schistosoma bovis. PLoS Negl Trop Dis. 2021;15:e0010062.
2. Chitsulo L, Engels D, Montresor A, Savioli L. The global status of schistosomiasis and its control. Acta Tropica. 2000;77:41–51.

3. Vancauwenberghe T, Oyaert M, Termote JL, Mulkens T, Bellinck P. Ureteral obstruction caused by schistosomiasis. JBR-BTR. 2013;96:292–4.
4. Oyaert M, Lagrange W, Smet G, De Feyter K, Laffut W. Unexpected urinary Schistosoma infection in a Belgian travel group returning from Malawi. Acta Clin Belg. 2013;68:234–6.
5. Zheng L, Deng L, Zhong Y, Wang Y, Guo W, Fan X. Molluscicides against the snail-intermediate host of Schistosoma: a review. Parasitol Res. 2021;120:3355–93.
6. Antwi S, Aboah KE, Sarpong CK. The unacknowledged impact of urinary schistosomiasis in children: 5 cases from Kumasi, Ghana. Ghana Med J. 2014;48:228–33.
7. Colley DG, Bustinduy AL, Secor WE, King CH. Human schistosomiasis. Lancet. 2014;383:2253–64.
8. Ghoneim MA. Bilharziasis of the genitourinary tract. BJU Int. 2002;89(Suppl 1):22–30. https://doi.org/10.1046/j.1464-4096.2001.138.138.x.
9. Mohamed AS. Bilharziasis of the seminal vesicles. J R Egypt Med Assoc. 1952;35:613–26.
10. Smith JH, Kamel IA, Von Lichtenberg F. A quantitative post mortem analysis of urinary schistosomiasis in Egypt. Am J Trop Med Hyg. 1974;23:1054–71.
11. Colley DG, Secor WE. Immunology of human schistosomiasis. Parasite Immunol. 2014;36:347–57.
12. Barron L, Wynn TA. Macrophage activation governs schistosomiasis-induced inflammation and fibrosis. Eur J Immunol. 2011;41:2509–14.
13. Burke ML, Jones MK, Gobert GN, Li YS, Ellis MK, McManus DP. Immunopathogenesis of human schistosomiasis. Parasite Immunol. 2009;31:163–76.
14. Isnard A, Kouriba B, Doumbo O, Chevillard C. Association of rs7719175, located in the IL13 gene promoter, with Schistosoma haematobium infection levels and identification of a susceptibility haplotype. Genes Immun. 2011;12:31–9.
15. Bocanegra Garcia C, Pintar Z, Serres X, et al. Ultrasound findings and associated factors to morbidity in Schistosoma haematobium infection in a highly endemic setting. Tropical Med Int Health. 2018;23:221–8.
16. Farid Z, Miner WF, Higashi GI, Hassan A. Reversibility of lesions in schistosomiasis: a brief review. J Trop Med Hyg. 1976;79(7):164–6.
17. Cozzi D, Bertelli E, Savi E, et al. Ultrasound findings in urogenital schistosomiasis: a pictorial essay. J Ultrasound. 2020;23:195–205.
18. Shebel HM, Elsayes KM, Abou El Atta HM, Elguindy YM, El-Diasty TA. Genitourinary schistosomiasis: life cycle and radiologic-pathologic findings. Radiographics. 2012;32:1031–46.
19. Fergusson AR. Associated bilharziasis and primary malignant diseases of the urinary bladder, with observations on a series of 40 cases. J Pathol Bacteriol. 1911;16:76–94.
20. Zahran MM, Kamel M, Mooro H, Issa A. Bilharziasis of urinary and ureter. Comparative histopathologic study. J Urol. 1976;8:73–9.
21. Khalaf I, Shokeir A, Shalaby M. Urologic complications of genitourinary schistosomiasis. World J Urol. 2012;30:31–8.
22. Hatz CF, Vennervald BJ, Nkulila T, et al. Evolution of Schistosoma haematobium-related pathology over 24 months after treatment with praziquantel among school children in south-eastern Tanzania. Am J Trop Med Hyg. 1998;59:775–81.
23. Remppis J, Verheyden A, Bustinduy AL, et al. Focused Assessment with Sonography for Urinary Schistosomiasis (FASUS)-pilot evaluation of a simple point-of-care ultrasound protocol and short training program for detecting urinary tract morbidity in highly endemic settings. Trans R Soc Trop Med Hyg. 2020;114:38–48.
24. Nelwan ML. Schistosomiasis: life cycle, diagnosis, and control. Curr Ther Res Clin Exp. 2019;91:5–9. https://doi.org/10.1016/j.curtheres.2019.06.001.
25. Duan M, Popat S, Coburn M, Woc-Colburn LE. A 26-year-old woman with cysuria and hematuria. Urology. 2021;148:e25–e6.
26. Akpata R, Neumayr A, Holtfreter MC, et al. The WHO ultrasonography protocol for assessing morbidity due to Schistosoma haematobium. Acceptance and evolution over 14 years. Systematic review. Parasitol Res. 2015;114:1279–89.

27. Kim MJ, Ryu K, Jin Y, et al. Significance of echogenic snow sign as an ultrasonography finding for diagnosis of urogenital schistosomiasis. Am J Trop Med Hyg. 2016;95:842–8.
28. Husain I, Al Ali IH, Kinare AS. Evaluating bilharzial ureteropathy for surgery. Br J Urol. 1980;52(6):446–50. https://doi.org/10.1111/j.1464-410x.1980.tb03087.x.
29. Lee HJ, Sung WS. Calcification of the urinary bladder and ureter in schistosomiasis. Kidney Res Clin Pract. 2018;37:304–5.
30. Pal PO, Smith RD, Allen S, et al. Schistosomiasis-A disobedient ureter, a disobedient diagnosis. J Endourol Case Rep. 2017;3:114–8.
31. WHO Expert Committee on the Control of Schistosomiasis (2001: Geneva, Switzerland) & World Health Organization; 2002. Prevention and control of schistosomiasis and soil-transmitted helminthiasis: report of a WHO expert committee. World Health Organization. https://apps.who.int/iris/handle/10665/42588.
32. Badmos KB, Popoola AA, Buhari MO, Abdulkadir AY. Ureteric schistosomiasis with obstructive uropathy. J Coll Physicians Surg Pak. 2009;19:456–8.
33. Miller MJ, Reid EC. Steroid therapy in chronic urinary schistosomiasis (bilharziasis). Can Med Assoc J. 1967;97(11):594–9.
34. Ghoneim MA, Nabeeh A, El-Kappany A. Endourologic treatment of ureteral strictures. J Endourol. 1988;2:263–70.
35. Hussein A, Rifaat E, Zaki A, Abol-Nasr M. Stenting versus non-stenting after non-complicated ureteroscopic manipulation of stones in bilharzial ureters. Int J Urol. 2006;13:886–90.
36. Abou-Elela A, Torky M, Salah E, Morsy A, Elsherbiny M. Inverted ureteral nipple as antireflux technique in surgical management of bilharzial ureteral strictures. Urology. 2010;76:983–7.
37. Ali-El-Dein B, Ghoneim MA. Bridging long ureteral defects using the Yang-Monti principle. J Urol. 2003;169(3):1074–7. https://doi.org/10.1097/01.ju.0000050151.66653.cc.
38. Ali-El-Dein B, El-Hefnawy AS, D'Elia G, El-Mekresh MM, Shokeir AA, Gad H, Bazeed MA. Long-term Outcome of Yang-Monti Ileal Replacement of the Ureter: A Technique Suitable for Mild, Moderate Loss of Kidney Function and Solitary Kidney. Urology. 2021;152:153–9. https://doi.org/10.1016/j.urology.2020.09.061. Epub 2021 Jan 14
39. Bakari AA, Gadam IA, Aliyu S, Suleiman I, Ahidjo AA, Pindiga UH. Use of mitrofanoff and yang-monti techniques as ureteric substitution for severe schistosomal bilateral ureteric stricture: a case report and review of the literature. Niger J Surg. 2012;18:30–3.
40. Nour HH, Elgobashy SE, Elkholy A, et al. Laparoscopic management of distal ureteric stones in a bilharzial ureter: results of a single-centre prospective study. Arab J Urol. 2015;13:182–6.

Chapter 13
The Ureter and Tuberculosis (TB)

Ravindra Sabnis, Pavan Surwase Jain, Rohan Batra, and Niramya Pathak

Abstract Background: Tuberculosis is one of the most common infectious diseases in the world. Genitourinary TB is often diagnosed late due to nonspecific symptoms, chronic manifestations, and only subtle clinical signs. The incidence of GUTB varies from 15% to 20% in Africa, Asia, Eastern Europe, and the Russian Federation to 2–10% in western Europe and the USA. However, the true incidence of GUTB is difficult to ascertain as GUTB can remain subclinical.

Clinical presentation: The symptoms of ureteral TB are non-specific and can include hematuria, colicky abdominal pain, and pain associated with ureteric obstruction. The cornerstones of diagnosis are detailed history, clinical examination, laboratory and radiographic diagnosis, and in some cases, by a provocative test with therapy *ex juventabius*.

Treatment: Management of tuberculosis of the ureter is challenging as the outcome of ureteral involvement is also dependent on the extent of renal involvement. Confirmation of TB on investigations warrants initiation of multidrug antituberculosis treatment (ATT). Standard treatment duration is 2 months of intensive phase with Isoniazid (INH), Rifampicin (RIF), Ethambutol (ETH), and Pyrazinamide (PYR) daily, followed by 4 or 7 months of continuation phase with only two drugs (INH + RIF), in total 6–9 months. Ureteral stricture, as a sequel to GUTB, is associated with both concentric and longitudinal fibrosis, pipe-stem ureter, and poor vascularity. The management of ureteric stricture depends on the status of the patient and the degree of involvement of other organs, particularly the urinary bladder. Depending upon stricture characteristics such as length, location, and renal function, surgical options vary from endoscopic to open or laparoscopic surgery.

Test your learning and check your understanding of this book's contents: use the "Springer Nature Flashcards" app to access questions. To use the app, please follow the instructions in chapter 1.

R. Sabnis (✉) · R. Batra
Consultant Urologist, Muljibhai Patel Urological Hospital, Nadiad, Gujarat India

P. S. Jain · N. Pathak
Fellow in Endourology, Muljibhai Patel Urological Hospital, Nadiad, Gujarat India

M. Abdel-Gawad et al. (eds.), *The Ureter*,
https://doi.org/10.1007/978-3-031-36212-5_13

Keywords TB ureter · Ureteric stricture · Antituberculosis treatment · Genitourinary Tuberculosis

Abbreviations

GUTB	Genitourinary tuberculosis
MTB	Mycobacterium tuberculosis

Learning Objectives
After studying this chapter, the reader will be able to:

- Enumerate the incidence of tuberculosis of the ureter.
- Describe the pathophysiology of the urogenital spread of Tuberculosis of the ureter.
- Explain the presentation of patients with tuberculosis of the ureter.
- Enlist the investigations required to diagnose tuberculosis of the ureter.
- Chart the diagnostic algorithm of tuberculosis of the ureter.
- Discuss the differential diagnosis of tuberculosis of the ureter.
- Explain the treatment options available for tuberculosis of the ureter.

13.1 Introduction

Tuberculosis is one of the most common infectious diseases in the world [1]. In 2020, an estimated 9.8 million people suffered from Tuberculosis, according to the WHO Global Tuberculosis report 2021 [2]. Two-thirds of these cases were reported from South-East Asia and Africa. Only 6% of global incidences occur in the European Region and the WHO Region of the Americas. Overall, 214,000 people with HIV also had TB, of whom 72% were from Africa. TB occurs in all countries and age groups, with 90% of infections reported in adults. The most intriguing part of this infection is that it can affect any organ in the human body. It has been described as the 'great imitator' and can mimic other diseases [3]. However, the watershed moment in the history of tuberculosis was the successful isolation and identification of tubercle bacilli by Robert Koch [4]. Around 5% to 45% of patients have features of extrapulmonary tuberculosis [5] . The most common sites of extrapulmonary tuberculosis are lymph nodes, pleura, urinary tract, bones, and meninges. The Genitourinary TB (GUTB) includes infection of the whole urinary tract in males and females [6].

Genitourinary TB is often diagnosed late due to nonspecific symptoms, chronic manifestations, and only subtle clinical signs. Many times, it is a diagnosis of exclusion [7–9]. Due to this delayed diagnosis and untreated infection, patients may present with advanced and progressive conditions with ureteral strictures, small bladder, small shrunken kidneys or irreversible organ damage and end-stage renal disease (ESRD) [6].

Tuberculosis is caused by Mycobacterium tuberculosis complex (MTBC) bacilli [10]. These bacilli include Mycobacterium tuberculosis (MTB), M. Bovis, M. Africanum, M. Caprae, Mycobacterium Microti, and Bacillus Calmette-Guérin (BCG). MTB, M. Africanus, and M. Bovis are the most common causes of tuberculosis in humans [11]. The incidence of GUTB varies from 15–20% in Africa, Asia, Eastern Europe, and the Russian Federation to 2–10% in Western Europe and the USA. However, the true incidence of GUTB is difficult to ascertain as GUTB can remain subclinical. GUTB can occur concurrently with Pulmonary TB in 20% of individuals [12–14].

TB is more prevalent in people with malnutrition, HIV infection, diabetes, chronic renal and liver disease, alcohol and substance abuse, smoking, vitamin deficiency, immunosuppressive drugs, and renal transplantation [5].

TB bacilli can be transmitted to humans in several ways. The most common route is person-to-person transmission through inhalation of infected aerosols of people with active pulmonary TB and ingestion of M. Bovis-infected raw unpasteurized dairy products [10]. Other modes of TB infection are congenital transmission, sexual transmission, vaccination and therapeutic instillation [15, 16]. Vaccination with live BCG vaccine in HIV-infected and immunosuppressed individuals can result in local and disseminated BCG [17]. It can also spread through the intravesical instillation of BCG which is used as an adjuvant treatment for transitional cell carcinoma. TB of the bladder, epididymis, prostate and kidney have been reported following intravesical instillation with BCG for bladder cancer [15–17].

13.2 Pathology

The pathogenesis of the natural tuberculosis infection in humans is derived from animal models [18, 19]. Following primary infection through inhalation or ingestion, the bacilli multiply locally in the tissues and evoke a complex immune response, resulting in either elimination (eradication) or containment via primary granuloma formation (The primary Ghon's focus,) or progression. Primary TB lesions are found in the lungs or gut, but any organ can shelter the primary focus like primary genital TB of the cervix, vagina or vulva [20].

Primary granulomas consist of inflammatory and immune cells like neutrophils, lymphocytes, epithelioid cells, macrophages, Langhans giant cells, fibroblasts, and central caseous necrosis [18]. If it is not controlled at this stage, then the mycobacteria can spread through the lymphatics to regional lymph nodes (causing lymphangitis and lymphadenitis). At this stage, the lymph nodes can undergo caseous necrosis [19].

The primary disease progresses in 5–10% of people, leading to local spread or widespread dissemination of bacilli. Seeding of tissues of all body organs outside the lung can occur, known as Extra-pulmonary, which includes infection of the urological and reproductive tract also. Many patients with extra-pulmonary TB do not show any signs of the disease and continue to have a subclinical infection. GUTB can present in any age group, but due to the long latency period, it commonly affects people of age group 30–50 years. It is infrequently reported in children [21].

13.3 Urogenital Spread

Primary TB of the urogenital system is usually caused by hematogenous route affecting the kidneys first. After primary TB infection, it causes direct spread from primary lesions in the kidneys which leads to bacilli seeding into various parts of the urogenital tract. Bacilli from the kidney can enter and lodge in the urothelium, ureter, bladder, urethra, seminal vesicles, and testes [22]. Unilateral involvement is common, but bilateral disease of the genitourinary tract can occur.

13.4 Presentation

The most common part of the ureter to be involved with TB is the lower third followed by the ureteropelvic junction [23]. Ureteric involvement is almost always associated with renal involvement. 50% of patients with renal TB also have ureteric involvement. TB bacilli spread downstream with the urine to the ureters, the ureterovesical junction, and the bladder [24]. Ureteritis occurs due to mucosal involvement. This downstream spread leads to inflammation, granulomatous changes, small ulcerations, and fibrosis. These changes lead to ureteric strictures, segmental dilation, obstruction, and reflux [25]. These changes can lead to progressive hydroureteronephrosis. Ureteric calcifications may occur.

The symptoms of ureteral TB are non-specific and can include hematuria, colicky abdominal pain, and pain associated with ureteric obstruction.

13.5 Investigations

Primary and precise diagnosis of Urogenital Tuberculosis (UG-TB) is vital for its treatment to be successful. Unfortunately, this remains a challenge hence this condition is often underdiagnosed [26–29]. This is due to the inherent paucibacillary nature of UG-TB, insidious onset, poor health awareness among patients, non-specific clinical features, technical difficulties to isolate Mycobacterium tuberculosis (MTb), long culture times and lack of awareness of the physician [27–29]. This is highlighted by a study which showed that in an autopsy series, only 50% of the patients with renal and ureteral tuberculosis had symptoms and only 18% were diagnosed clinically [30]. There is no single specific diagnostic test for UG-TB and the gold standard for diagnosis is by identifying the presence of UG-TB from a clinical sample [27]. In the global literature, in 64.2% of cases of UG-TB, the diagnosis was thorough identification of MTB in the urine via a positive culture [14]. The cornerstones of diagnosis are detailed history, clinical examination, laboratory and radiographic diagnosis, and in some cases, by a provocative test with therapy *ex juventabius* [31, 32]. Generally, non-specific lower urinary tract symptoms, with abnormalities in urine analysis in the setting of a past medical history of pulmonary tuberculosis are crucial in the initial diagnostic workup. The imaging is useful only in the later stages of UG-TB [33]. The optimal microbiological or molecular diagnostic methods are dependent on available laboratory capacity, resources and clinical context. In developing countries, there is diversity in practice standards due to the medical facilities and services which are disproportionately available [34].

13.6 Microbiological and Molecular testing

13.6.1 Urine

Since the last few years, the urine confirmatory diagnostic tests have been undergoing step-wise upgradation from the microscopy of urine smear to urine culture using solid media (Lowenstein-Jensen medium) to culture using liquid media (rapid automated liquid culture systems such as Becton Dickinson BACTEC MGIT 960), to rapid molecular nucleic acid amplification systems like Line probe assay (LPA) and GeneXpert MTB/RIF Assay (Cepheid, Sunnyvale, CA, USA) which provide rapid diagnosis and identifies rifampicin resistance (within 24–48 h) [27].

13.6.1.1 Routine Urine Examination

Abnormal urinalysis is present in up to 90% of patients with GUTB with a range of findings from mild changes to severe pyuria. The common findings are acidic urine with low specific gravity and sterile pyuria, proteinuria, with or without microscopic hematuria in the setting of a negative urine culture for standard bacterial infection. These should raise the suspicion of a diagnosis of GUTB [12].

13.6.1.2 Smear Microscopy

Smear microscopy means a microscopic examination of body fluids and biopsy tissue for acid-fast bacilli (AFB) using Ziehl-Nelson (ZN) or auramine staining. Patients who are evaluated for UG-TB should collect three early morning urine samples on consecutive days for AFB microscopy and culture. This test gives rapid results in 24–48 h and is has been the first-line diagnostic method of pulmonary tuberculosis for many decades. It can be done using light microscopy or LED-based fluorescent microscopy with similar sensitivities and specificities but a faster reading time with LED microscopy [27]. Specificity is 97% and sensitivity is 20–40% [33].

13.6.1.3 Microscopy and Culture – Solid Media and Radiometric Media

Clinical specimen culture for MTB remains the gold standard for diagnosing active tuberculosis in general with a sensitivity of 65% and specificity of 100% [35]. Two types of culture media are used. The older used solid Lowenstein-Jensen culture medium which is cheap and readily available but takes 6–8 weeks to detect the growth of MTB and is being gradually phased out. The newer liquid automated Mycobacterial growth indicator tube (MGIT) culture system using BACTEC MGIT 960 system (Becton Dickinson) based on modified Middlebrook 7H9 broth which is expensive but gives results in 2 weeks with a better sensitivity, species identification and ability to do Drug sensitivity test (DST). The genotyping is recommended now by WHO as the gold-standard confirmatory test for TB diagnosis [27]. The overall disadvantage of culture methods is that it is time-consuming with even liquid cultures needing to wait for 6 weeks before giving a negative result.

13.6.1.4 Nucleic Acid Amplification Test (NAAT)

Nucleic acid amplification tests (NAAT) are classified by their working mechanisms into Polymerase Chain reaction tests (PCR), Ligase chain reaction tests (LCR), and variants of PCR such as Xpert MTB/RIF. These tests have the advantage of higher sensitivities and specificities, detection of resistance to Rifampin (a surrogate for MDR TB diagnosis and treatment), and faster reporting in 2–48 h. The disadvantages are cost, availability, and false positive results even after the eradication of live mycobacteria [36]. GeneXpert MTB/RIF assay is now the World Health Organization's recommended initial diagnostic test for patients with a clinical suspicion of TB [37]. A systematic review and meta-analysis reported sensitivity ranging from 83% to 95% and specificity from 79% to 99% [38]. For GUTB, the sensitivity of GeneXpert MTB/RIF for urine sample was 63% versus conventional microscopy 18.5% and culture 45.7% in a study [17].

13.6.1.5 Lateral Flow Assay – Detection of Mycobacterial Cell Wall Glycolipid Lipoarabinomannan (LAM) - LAM Assay

Lipoarabinomannan (LAM) is detected by Lateral flow urine LAM assay (Alere, Waltham, MA, USA) from the urine of patients having active TM using an immunochromatographic assay. The present recommendation by WHO is for diagnosis of HIV-associated TB in people with low CD4 lymphocyte count as immunosuppressed patients have more risk of disseminated TB and renal involvement releasing MTB in urine [39]. But its usefulness in the diagnosis of GUTB is under evaluation.

13.6.1.6 TB Drug Susceptibility Testing (DST)

Drug sensitivity testing is very important in MTB so that the appropriate treatment for MDR TB can be given. It is two types; Culture based phenotypic DST which has the advantages of cheap, and easy availability and the disadvantages of consumption of more time, and requiring strict quality control and another type which is Molecular Genotypic DST methods such as Next Generation sequencing using Line probe assays (LPA) which has the advantages of giving rapid results but disadvantages of the cost and availability [27]. WHO recommends molecular DST as the initial tests to detect drug resistance before initiation of therapy for all cases of TB. If there is Rifampicin resistance, further molecular tests for resistance of Isoniazid, Fluoroquinolones, and Amikacin should be performed promptly to detect drug resistance before starting treatment [40].

13.6.1.7 Whole Genome Sequencing (WGS)

Whole Genome Sequencing (WGS) is an emerging investigations for improvements in understanding MTB transmission patterns, rapid molecular diagnosis and identification of drug resistance [41, 42]. WGS is presently performed only on strains grown in culture since it requires a high viral load. Despite the potential advantages, the disadvantages are cost limitations, the need for specialized and well-trained staff, and the lack of infrastructure in low- and middle-income countries.

13.6.2 Histological Tests

13.6.2.1 FNAC or Biopsy Specimen

Histological examination of specimens sent from fine-needle aspirate and biopsies, or excised specimens can identify MTB bacilli and granulomas which is a hallmark of TB infection and is an adjunct to culture for diagnosis of TB infection. The specimens should also be sent for culture and processed simultaneously through GeneXpert MTB/RIF to increase the identification of MTB and confirm if antibiotic-resistant MTB strains are present [27]. The yield of biopsy for TB is around 45% and for FNA AFB may be detected in about 60% of cases [43]. Granulomas have central Langerhans cells surrounded by lymphocytes, fibrocytes, and epithelioid cells which advance to central caseous necrosis and a variable amount of fibrosis and calcification [43].

13.6.2.2 Blood tests

Blood tests are non-specific adjuncts to the management of GUTB. They are a marker of disease activity and severity and can gauge response to treatment and monitor the adverse effects of ATT.

1. Hematologic abnormalities
   Complete blood count may reveal anemia, leukocytosis, thrombocytosis, neutropenia, and thrombocytopenia in some cases. There may be elevated CRP and ESR levels [34].
2. Biochemical abnormalities
   Biochemical abnormalities may reveal hypoalbuminemia, impaired renal function, and electrolyte abnormalities such as hyponatremia, hypercalcemia, hypokalemia, and hyperkalemia [34]. Liver function tests are also required as a baseline before starting ATT.

13.6.3 Imaging Findings

The importance of imaging studies in GUTB is to localize the site of disease, check the extent of involvement, serially monitor the effect of treatment, detect relapse, detect complications, and take targeted biopsy/FNAC.

13.6.3.1 X-Ray

Plain Abdominal and chest X-rays are important first-line investigations in the diagnosis of GUTB and may be abnormal in 50% of cases [25]. GUTB patients can have concomitant active pulmonary TB with changes such as patchy or lobar consolidation, hilar lymph node enlargement, linear and nodular opacities, endobronchial thickening, cavities, tuberculoma formation, and military TB [25]. Abdominal X-ray may show changes such as renal calcification or nephrocalcinosis, granular opacification, dense punctate calcification in healed tuberculomas, lobar calcification, lymph node calcification, intraluminal ureteral wall calcification [25]. Renal parenchyma calcifications are amorphous, collecting system calcifications are granular or curvilinear, and ground glass or 'putty kidney' calcification is calcified caseous kidney tissue [43] (Fig. 13.1).

13.6.3.2 USG

Early GUTB generally has normal ultrasound findings. Hyperechoic areas suggestive of ureteral calcification may be seen in a later stage. Hydroureteronephrosis in cases of ureteral stricture or VUR due to VUJ involvement [44] (Figs. 13.2 and 13.3).

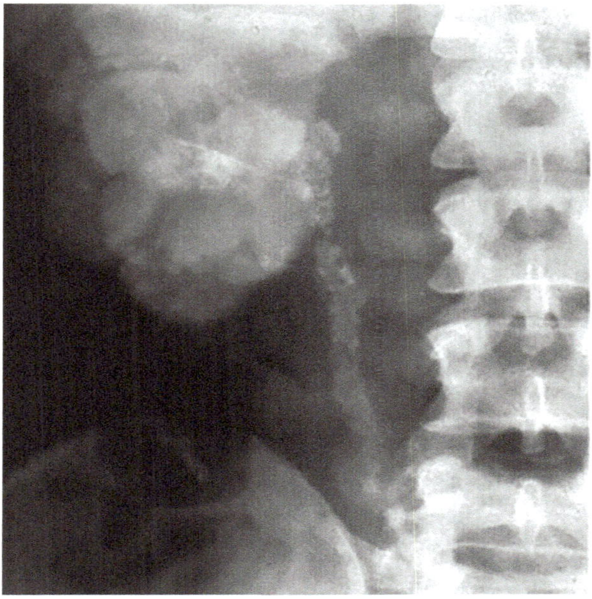

Fig. 13.1 A X-ray–showing renal lobar calcifications and ureteral calcification

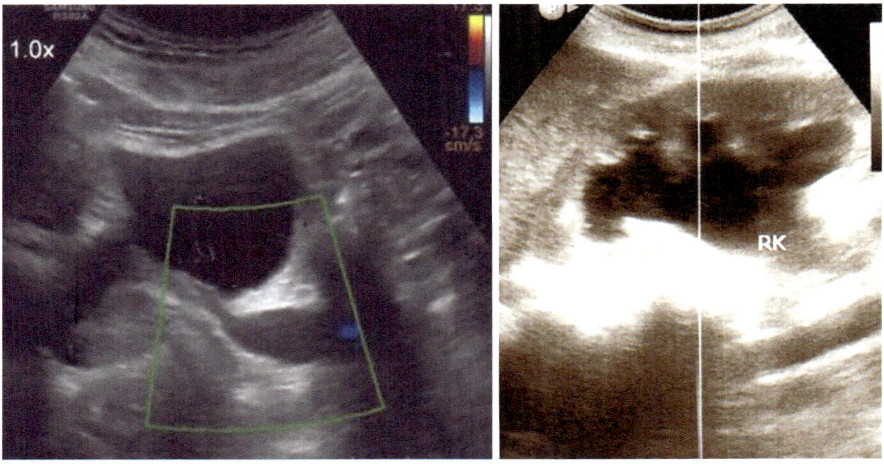

Fig. 13.2 Right lower ureteral narrowing with proximal hydroureter. Right hydroureteronephrosis

13.6.3.3 IVU

Intravenous Urography (IVU) is a non-specific but useful imaging that is infrequently used and provides anatomic details and drainage of the pelvicalyceal system and gives an estimate of the extent and severity of the disease. The early

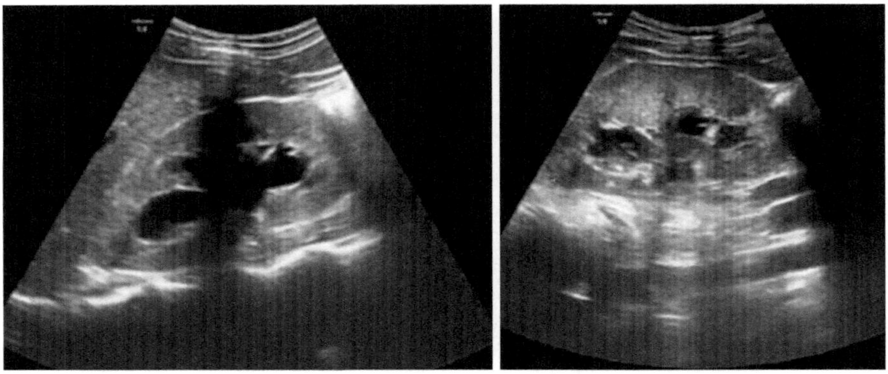

Fig. 13.3 Right hydro nephrosis with irregular caliectasis with ureteral wall thickening

involvement site in the ureter is in the distal ureter followed by the upper ureter and the mid ureter. Early changes are mucosal edema resulting in loss of sharpness, fuzzy calyx, calyceal erosion, moth-eaten calyx, calyceal dilation, initial cavitation, and papillary necrosis. Late changes are extensive cavitation, cortical scars, fibrotic strictures, mass lesions, calcifications, autonephrectomy, perinephric abscess, and fistula formation. Kinking of the renal pelvis due to traction from a strictured infundibulum and parenchymal fibrosis forms Kerr's kinks. Stricture of the inferior margin of the renal pelvis and its cephalic traction forms a 'hiked-up pelvis' [25]. Sawtooth ureter due to irregular mucosal ulcerations. Beaded or corkscrew ureter due to alternate areas of ureteral fibrosis and dilation of normal segments. Pipestem ureter due to fibrosis along the length of the ureter.

13.6.3.4 CT and CT IVP

CT scan is a better imaging modality than IVU for showing GUTB abnormalities. It is indicated in patients with suspicion of GUTB and normal other imaging findings with the most common findings being hydroureter, hydrocalyx and hydronephrosis which are secondary to ureteral stricture formation [27]. Common signs of ureteral involvement are ureteral thickening, ulcerations, strictures, calcifications, and granulomas presenting as filling defects. Plain CT – Figs. 13.4, 13.5, 13.6, and 13.7. CT IVU – Figs. 13.8 and 13.9.

13.6.3.5 MRI

MRI has a low sensitivity for detecting early lesions of GUTB but is good as an imaging modality in advanced disease and is primarily used for the evaluation of renal TB due to superior soft tissue resolution [27]. Indicated in pediatric or

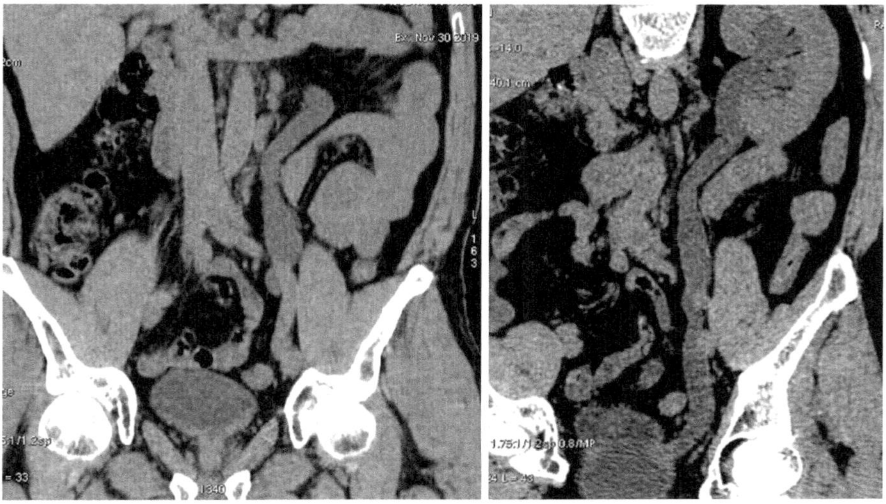

Fig. 13.4 Left mild hydronephrosis and hydroureter upto lower end

pregnant patients when radiation and contrast exposure is to be avoided, non-contrast MRI in patients with renal failure. It provides more information about the ureter and is preferably performed with a distended bladder [43] (Fig. 13.10).

13.6.3.6 Nuclear Medicine Imaging

18F FDG PET imaging provides functional information about places where the cells are metabolically active and using glucose and if combined with a CT scan provides anatomical and functional data in a single scan but it can not differentiate TB from cancer and other infections hence present-day use is limited to detecting extrapulmonary TB disease sites to obtain biopsies and monitor treatment response [27]. Radioisotope renal drainage study is also used to assess split function and the degree of obstruction in an advanced stage of GUTB [45].

13.6.3.7 Retrograde Pyelogram (RGP) and Antegrade Pyelogram (AGP)

Retrograde pyelogram is done in cases with compromised renal function and when distal ureteral obstruction level, extent and severity is to be estimated and obtain urine sample for culture after ureteral catheterization (Fig. 13.11). Antegrade pyelogram is required if retrograde access is not possible and kidney drainage is not adequate and to obtain a urine sample from the renal pelvis. It is also done in patients already having a percutaneous nephrostomy to accurately delineate ureteral pathology [45] (Fig. 13.12).

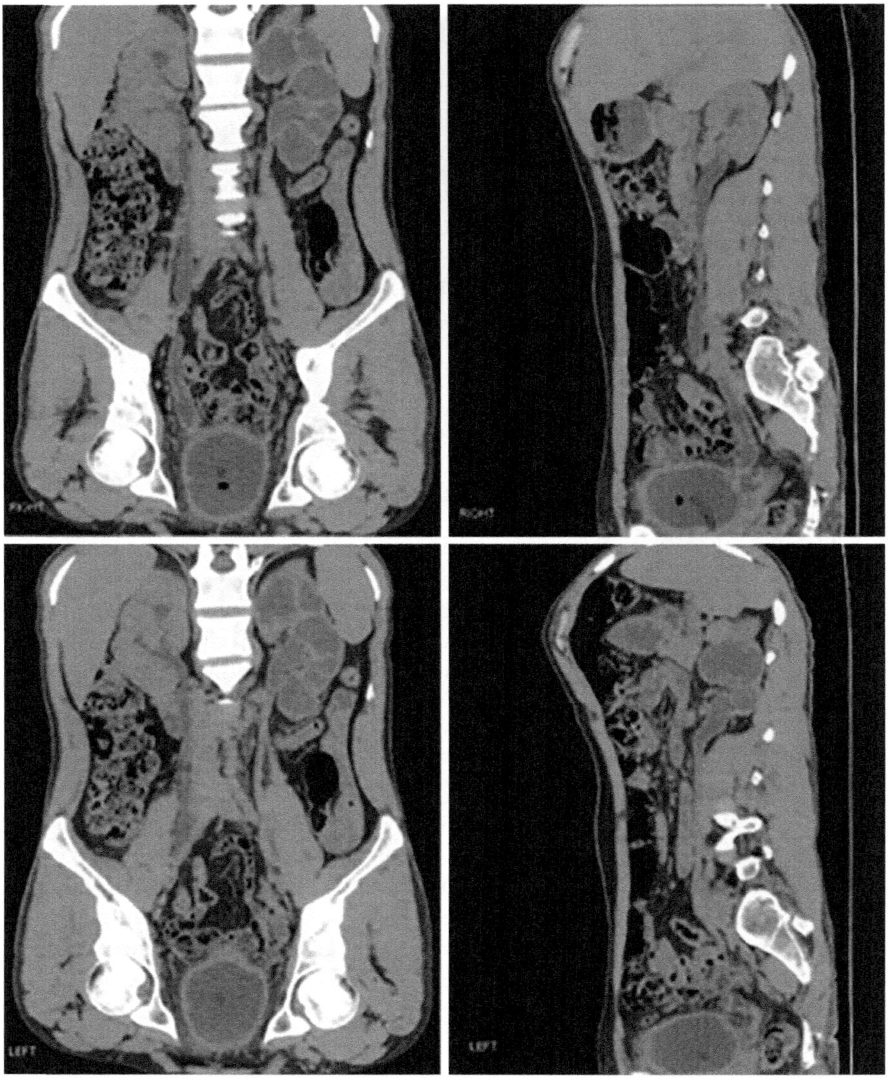

Fig. 13.5 Right hydroureteronephrosis with mucosal thickening of right ureter. Significant calyceal dilation and mild dilation of renal pelvis on left side with thinning of renal cortical parenchyma. Left ureteral mucosal wall thickening. Diffuse bladder wall thickening

13.6.3.8 Cystogram

Cystogram is used in cases of clinical suspicion GUTB to demonstrate small capacity urinary bladder. In later stages of fibrosis and trigonal involvement, the ureteral orifices are pulled medially resulting in golf hole ureter and vesicoureteral reflux (Fig. 13.13).

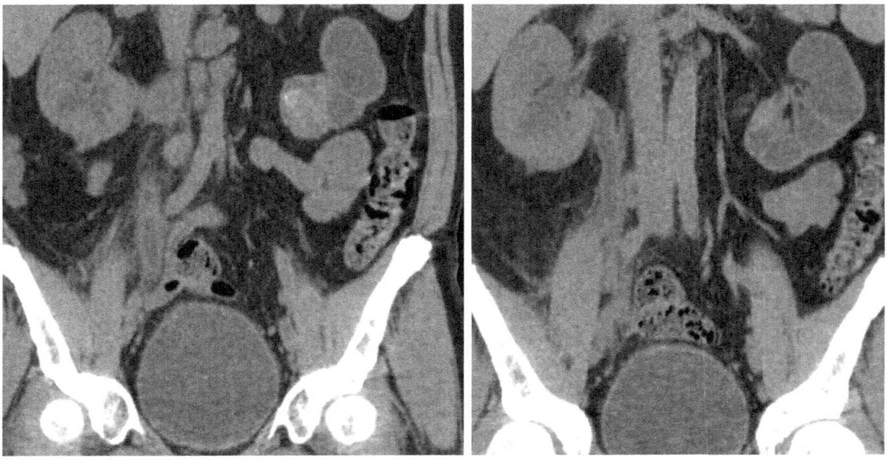

Fig. 13.6 Right kidney appears slighlty bulky in size as compared to left side with mild perinephric fat stranding. Circumferential wall thickening with periureteric fat stranding involving right ureter in its entire course associated with mild degree hydroureteronephrosis on right side. Moderate to gross hydronephrosis with thinning of cortical renal parenchyma & subtle perinephric fat stranding on left side. Area of calcification in lower pole of left kidney

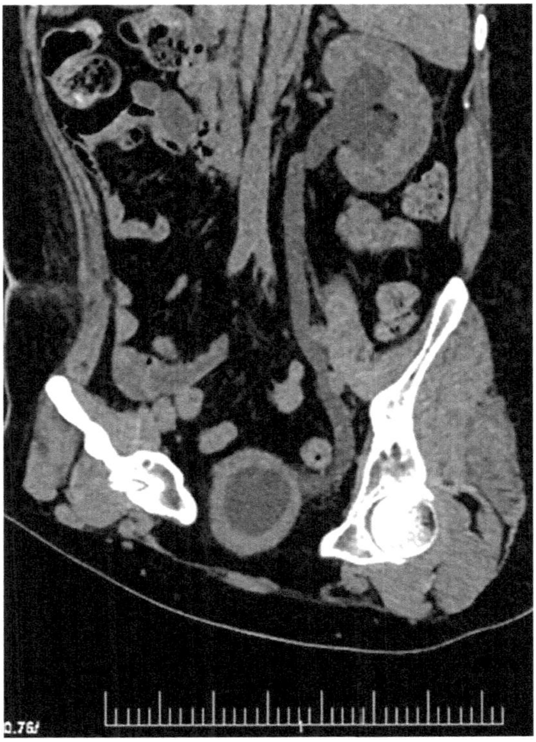

Fig. 13.7 Changes of cystitis causing left hydroureteronephrosis

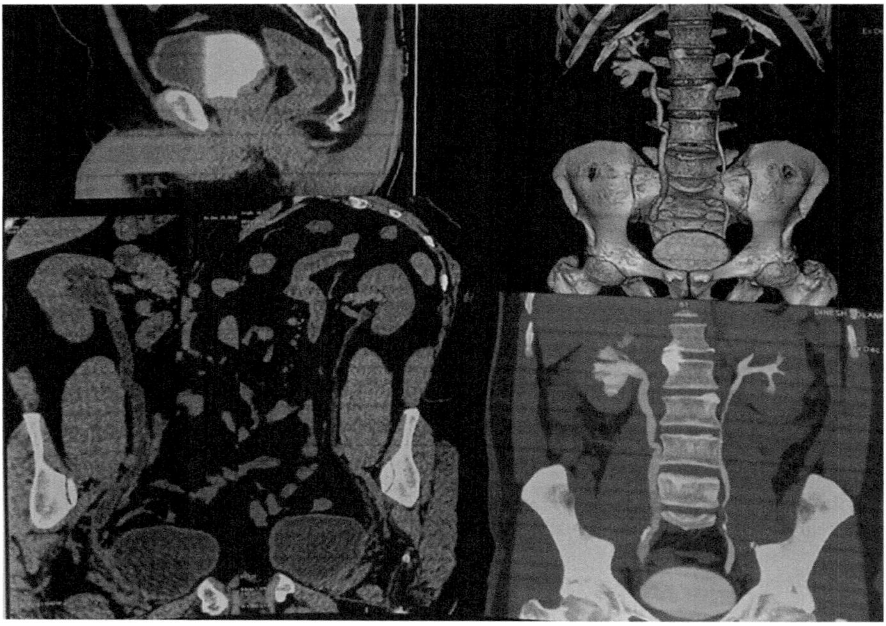

Fig. 13.8 Right kidney focal ill defined non enhancing areas representing extension of renal calyces with mild parenchymal thinning seen in upper pole. Right ureter and pelvis appear mildly dilated with mildly thickened and irregular enhancing wall. Thickened urinary bladder

13.6.4 Other Investigations

13.6.4.1 Endoscopy

Cystoscopy and ureteroscopy are very sparingly used with diagnostic aims. It is used if there is malignancy suspicion, for detecting anatomical abnormalities and lesion localization and biopsy tissue samples. Endoscopic signs are hyperemia, granulomas, ulcerations, reduced bladder capacity, and patulous or golf hole ureteral orifices [45] (Fig. 13.14).

13.6.4.2 Detection of Latent TB Infection

Immunosuppression increases the risk of reactivation of latent TB infection. Screening especially in the pretransplant and post-transplant setting is important. There are no gold-standard diagnostic tests available. Before initiation of treatment for such detected cases, active TB must be ruled out [27].

1. Tuberculin skin test (TST)

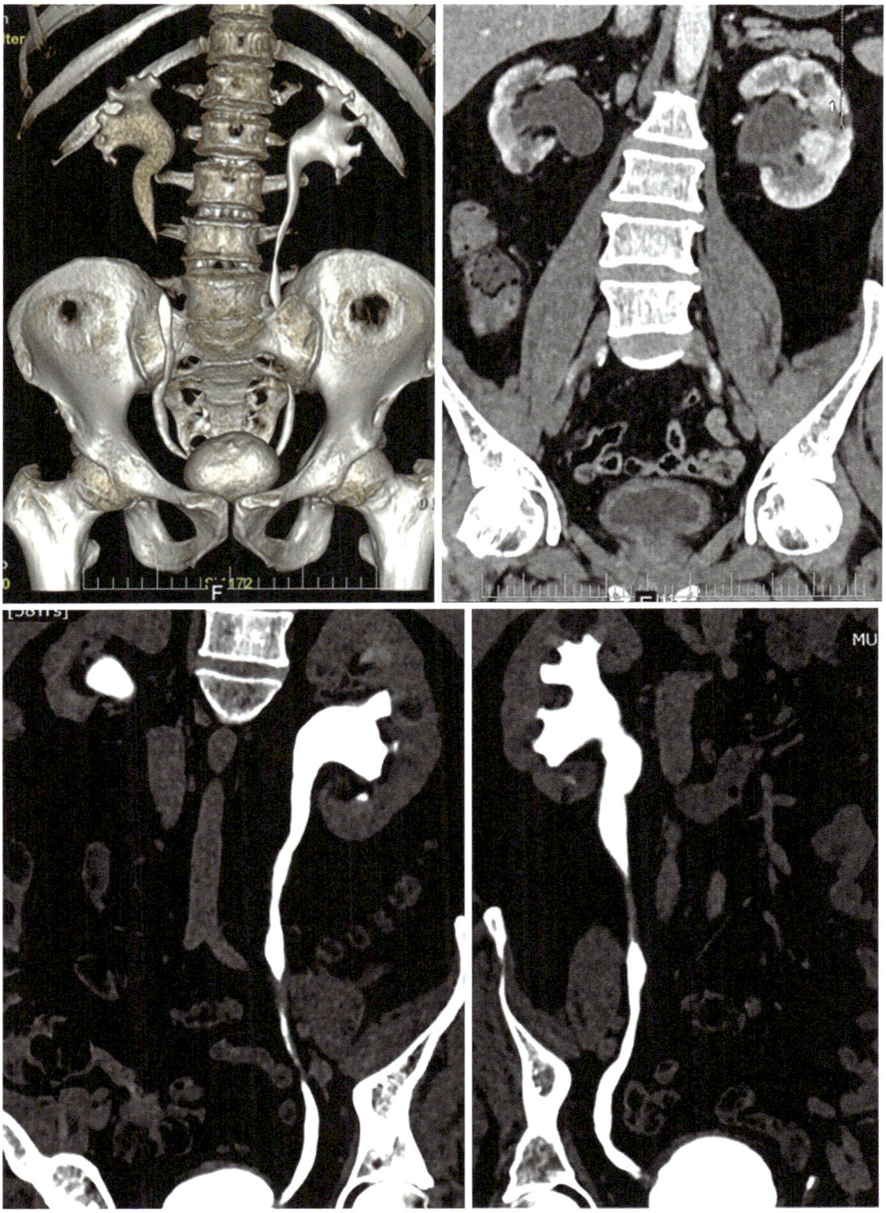

Fig. 13.9 Bilateral Mild hydronephrosis with long segment smooth narrowing of the both ureters, as described above with contracted Urinary bladder with marked generalised thickening of the urinary bladder. Few bilateral renal cysts

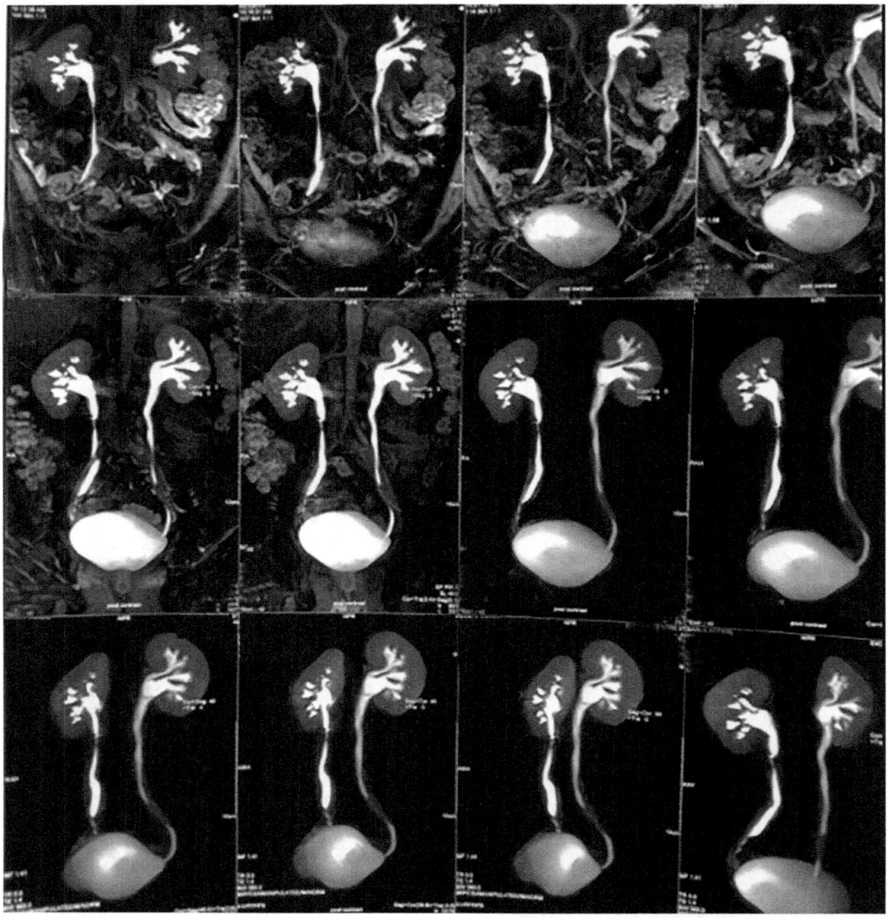

Fig. 13.10 Segment of mural thickening with enhancement at the junction of mid and distal third of left ureter with fullneess of proximal ureter

2. Interferon Gamma release assay (IGRA) – QuantiFERON-TB Gold In-Tube test (Q) and T-SPOT TB

DIAGNOSTIC CRITERIA GUTB [45, 46] – 1 Major/2 Minor criteria as given below:

1. Major criteria
   (a) Granulomatous lesion on histopathology
   (b) AFB positivity in urine or histopathology
   (c) Positive PCR

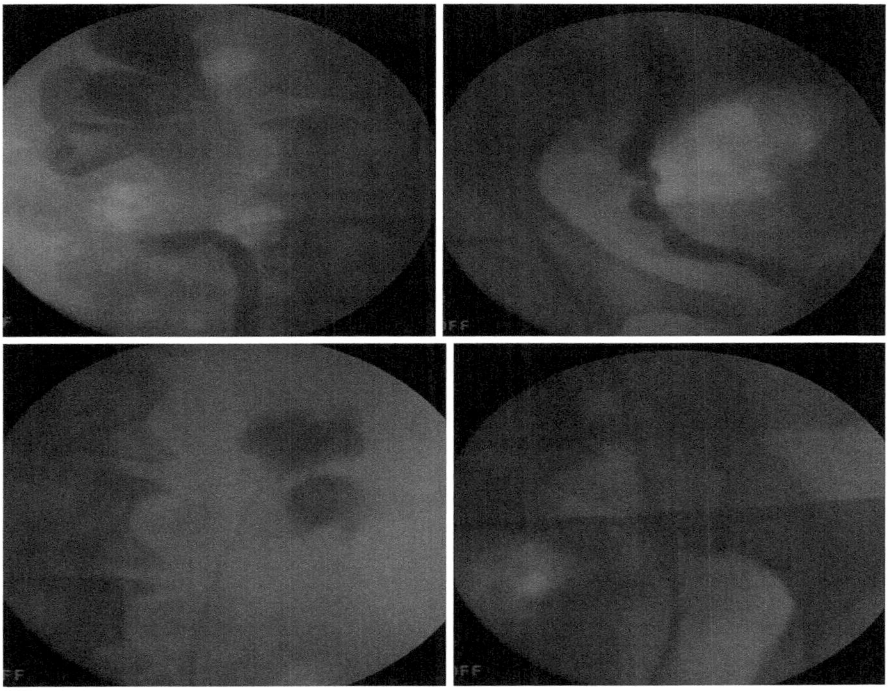

Fig. 13.11 Right RGP done s/o grossly dilated Right HUN till VUJ with Right upper ureteric kink. Left RGP done left side- Pipe stem beaded ureter with dilated calyces in kidney-pelvis not differentiated well

2. Minor criteria
   (a) Changes suggestive of tuberculosis on IVU/CT/MRI
   (b) Hematuria
   (c) Raised ESR
   (d) Pulmonary changes of old healed granulomas

DIAGNOSTIC ALGORITHM: Fig. 13.15 [45].

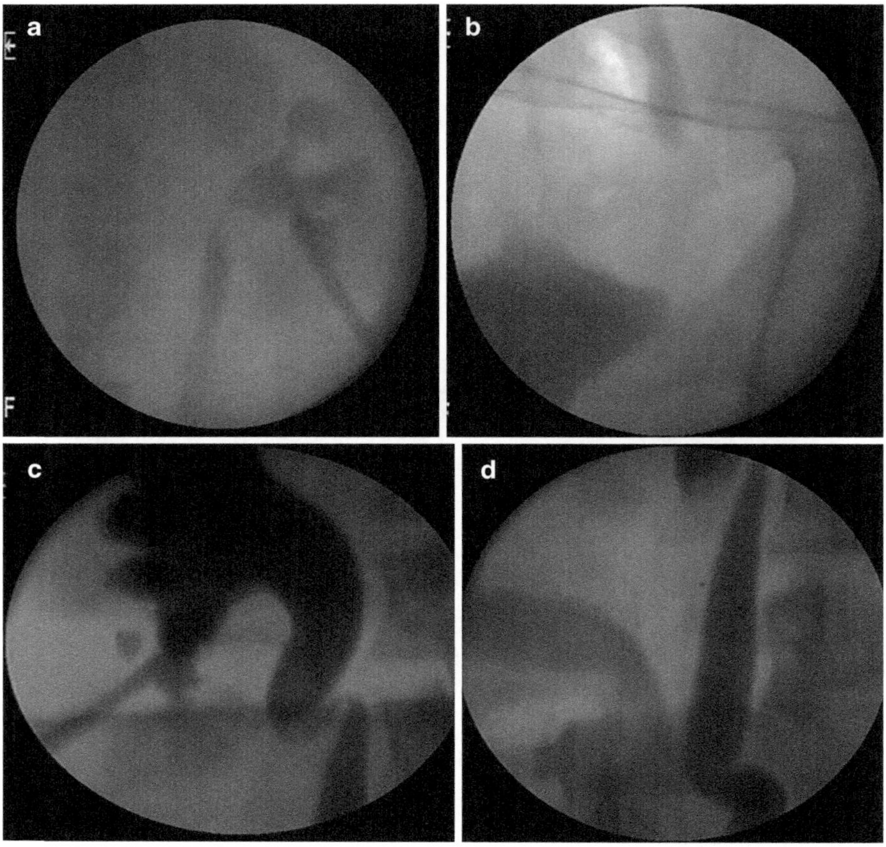

Fig. 13.12 (a) AGP GUTB with right lower ureteral stricture. (b) Right upper ureteric kink

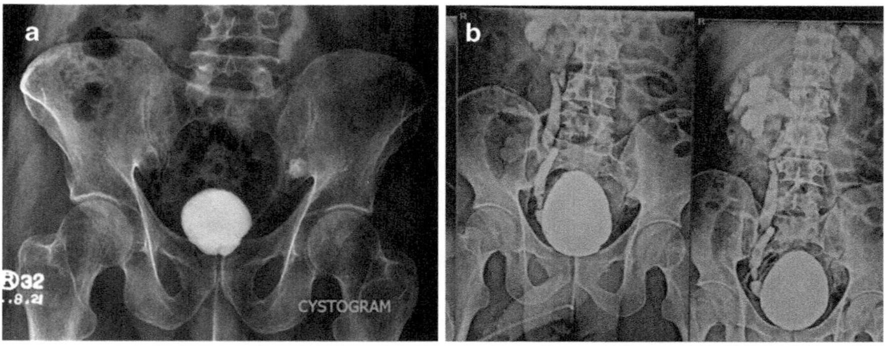

Fig. 13.13 (**a**) Small capacity urinary bladder. (**b**) Right grade 4 reflux diffuse irregular wall thickening of urinary bladder

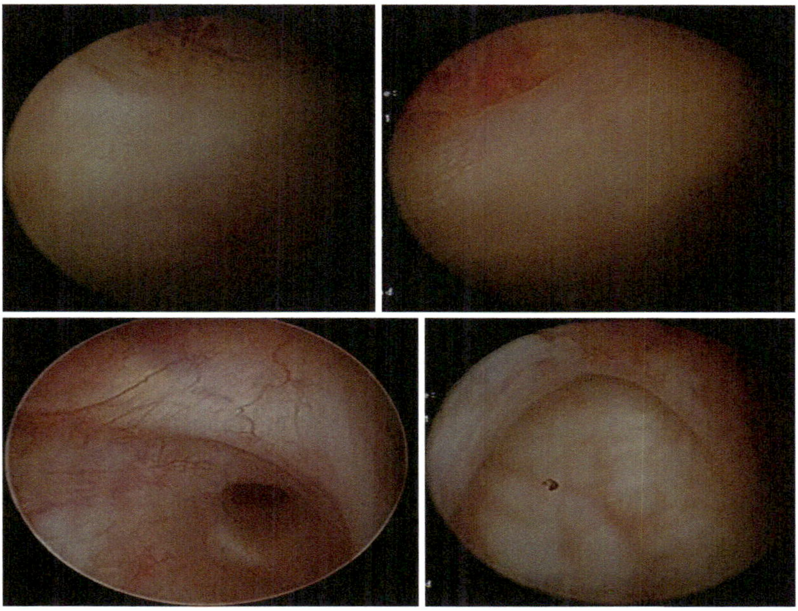

Fig. 13.14 Hyperemia, B/L Golf hole ureter identified

Fig. 13.15 Diag algo

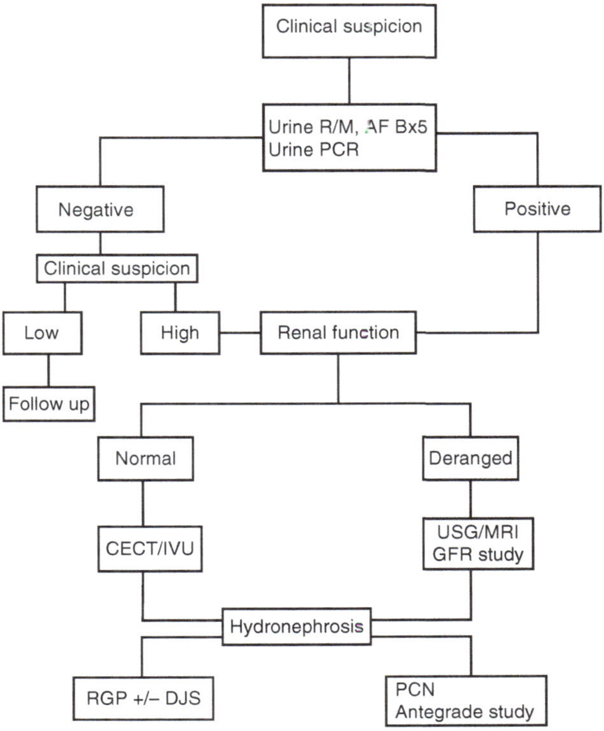

13.7 Differential Diagnosis [27]

1. Calcified ureter: Schistosomiasis has intramural calcification and lower ureteral calcification and discontinuous calcification. GUTB has intraluminal calcification, upper and mid ureteral calcification, and continuous calcification extending from the kidney and PCS
2. Stricture ureter: Post calculus stricture/Iatrogenic stricture – Post calculus ureteral stricture or post-URS stricture is generally at the site of stone impaction or site of ureteral injury during URS. Ureteral strictures may happen anywhere along the ureter. It typically involves the lower ureter followed by the upper ureter followed by the mid ureter, the occasionally whole length of the ureter may also be affected, and ureteral stricture is generally accompanied by renal changes of GUTB on imaging.
3. Mucosal granuloma: Renal papillary necrosis, benign ureteral lesions, urothelial tumors. These can be differentiated by imaging studies and cytology and biopsy

Types of ureteral lesions [27]

1. Radiological classification
   (a) Beaded or corkscrew ureter
   (b) Pipe stem ureter
   (c) Sawtooth ureter
2. Pathological classification
   (a) Inflamed ureter
   (b) Ulcerated ureter
   (c) Fibrosed or strictured ureter
   (d) Calcified ureter

13.7.1 Treatment of Tuberculosis Ureter

Management of tuberculosis ureter is challenging as the outcome of ureteral involvement is also dependent on the extent of renal involvement. Owing to the wide disparity prevailing in the involvement of the structures and severity of the disease, treatment should be tailor-made. Healing of ureteral tuberculosis leads to stricture formation observed in the distal ureter in 56% of cases, mid ureter in 13%, and multiple strictures in 17.19% of cases [47].

Confirmation of TB on investigations, warrants initiation of multidrug antituberculosis treatment (ATT). Medical therapy of UGTB is in general similar to treatment for pulmonary TB. Treatment according to WHO guidelines with four drugs is used: Isoniazid (INH), Rifampicin (RIF), Ethambutol (ETH) and Pyrazinamide (PYR). The standard treatment duration is 2 months of intensive phase with all four drugs daily, followed by 4 or 7 months of continuation phase with only two drugs

Table 13.1 Treatment regimen for UGTB

Initial 2 months	
Isoniazid (INH)	300 mg
Rifampicin[a] (RIF)	600 mg
Ethambutol (ETH)	1200 mg
Pyrazinamide (PYR)	2000 mg
Pyridoxine/B-combin F	20 mg per day or 50 mg every 2nd day
Continuation phase the following 4 months	
Isoniazid (INH)	300 mg
Rifampicin*(RIF)	600 mg
Pyridoxine/B-combin F	20 mg per day or 50 mg every 2nd day

[a]Rifampicin should be taken fasting preferably half an hour before the meal.

(INH + RIF), in total 6–9 months [48]. The dosage and schedule are depicted in Table 13.1 adopted from the article onedical treatment for urogenital Tuberculosis (UGTB)" authored by Wejse et al. [2] Since the advent of modern anti-tuberculosis chemotherapy, concepts regarding extirpative surgeries for unilateral renal tuberculosis have undergone considerable change. Patients refractory to or intolerant of chemotherapy and unable to stay on long-term chemotherapy for any reason may still require surgical interventions.

The use of corticosteroids is controversial. Horne et al. [49] advocated its use in the initial phaseofs an acute tuberculous disease to decrease inflammatory edema and stricture formation. The dictum to be followed in the treatment of genitourinary TB is to conserve the organs by reconstruction and excise diseased tissue only if mandatory.

13.7.2 Treatment in Early Disease

When the investigations show early ureteric disease, every attempt should be made to place a DJ stent. If DJ stent placement is not done, these patients should be followed closely monthly by limited IVU film or renal scan. If there is no improvement or deterioration then early intervention [DJ stenting or Percutaneous nephrostomy (PCN)] has to be done [50].

13.7.3 Treatment of Ureteric Stricture

Ureteral stricture as a sequel to GUTB is associated with both concentric and longitudinal fibrosis, pipe stem ureter, and poor vascularity. The management of ureteric stricture depends on the status of the patient and the degree of involvement of other organs, particularly the urinary bladder. Depending upon stricture characteristics such as length, location, and renal function, surgical options vary from endoscopic to open or laparoscopic surgery. Balloon dilatation and endoureterotomy have less success rate compared with surgical treatment and the patient may require surgery when overall renal function is poor (<25%), longer stricture length (>1 cm) and lumen stricture is tight (<1 mm) [51]. The patients of tuberculous ureteric stricture may be grouped into two broad categories:

1. Simple/uncomplicated: Short segment passable stricture with salvageable renal function and good bladder capacity.
2. Complex/complicated: Long segment, extensive/bilateral, or impassable stricture with or without salvageable kidney and bladder.

13.7.4 Management Options for Short Segment Stricture

Double-J stent placement: This gives the best outcome if the ureteric stricture is short and not dense with a functioning kidney and reasonable bladder capacity. The stent can be kept for 6–12 months and usually by that time the stricture stabilizes. The placement of the DJ stent is not always successful. If the DJ stent placement fails or if the obstruction is getting worse, other options have to be tried.

Retrograde balloon dilatation: The first case of effective balloon dilation of tuberculous ureteral stricture was performed by Waller et al. [52] in 1983. This technique is rarely definitive and usually requires repeated dilatations regularly. The dilatation is repeated every 2 weeks initially, later every 1–2 months, until the upper renal tract has stabilized. Contraindications include active infection and a length of stricture of more than 2 cm because dilatation alone will rarely be successful in this setting [53]. This treatment can be done only if it is possible to pass a guide wire across the stricture using transurethral techniques. After dilation, a DJ stent is placed. The drawbacks of this technique are high failure rates and repeated procedures requiring anesthesia. Lang et al. [54] in their work, stated that ureteral tuberculosis is prone to cause end-arteritis obliterans causing ischemia implying that the condition may have a poor response to balloon dilation. Therefore, it is unclear whether the ureteral strictures secondary to tuberculosis are good candidates for balloon dilation or not. In general, strictures of shorter length and shorter duration had better outcomes on dilation than those of longer length and longer duration [55].

Antegrade balloon dilation: If retrograde access fails, an antegrade approach may be attempted particularly if the patient already has nephrostomy in situ.

Endoureterotomy: Like balloon dilation, this procedure can be done either through the retrograde or the antegrade approach. Davies et al. [56] demonstrated both experimentally and clinically that upper ureteric strictures could be successfully treated by making a ureterotomy at the stricture site and leaving an indwelling ureteric splint. The usefulness of this technique for tuberculous ureteric strictures has been subsequently confirmed by Moore e al. [57]. The procedure can be performed either under direct vision using a ureteroscope or it can be guided fluoroscopically using hot-wire cutting balloon catheter.

Ureteroureterostomy: A short defect involving the upper or mid-ureter can be treated by ureteroureterostomy. The anastomosis should be tension-free, hence enough ureteral mobility is an essential prerequisite.

Ureteropyelostomy: Ureteropyelostomy is largely theoretical because if the stricture is at the pelviureteric junction it usually involves the kidney to the extent that this procedure becomes impossible.

Ureterocalicostomy is preferred as there is often associated with caliceal dilatation.

Psoas hitch: If the bladder capacity is normal, the psoas hitch can be performed for small-length strictures of the lower ureter.

13.7.5 Management Options for Long Segment Stricture

Endoureterotomy is recommended as a more successful endourologic procedure for long-segment strictures. The position for the endoureterotomy incision is chosen as per the level of the ureter involved. Lower ureteral strictures are incised in an anteromedial direction, taking care to stay away from the iliac vessels. Upper ureteral strictures are incised laterally or posterolaterally, again away from the great vessels [58]. The incision should involve the full thickness of the ureter including the periureteral fat. The balloon dilation is a useful adjunct either to gain access for endoureterotomy or to wide open the incision.

Boari flap: may be employed for long lower ureteric stricture.

Intubated ureterotomy: This procedure is popular for long upper and mid-ureteric strictures wherein the incised ureter is left to heal by regeneration over a stent.

Transureteroureterostomy: If the ureter can be mobilized sufficiently transureteroureterostomy is an option. However, if the other ureter is also diseased this should be attempted cautiously.

Ileal ureteral substitution: long ureteric strictures involving almost the whole length of the ureter or upper ureteric strictures require ileal replacement of the ureter.

Autotransplantation: For proximal or multiple ureteric strictures when other methods of repair fail or are not feasible, autotransplantation is the last and feasible option.

Questions

1. The most common part of ureter to be involved with TB is:

   (a) Lower third of ureter
   (b) Ureteropelvic junction
   (c) Ureterovesical junction
   (d) Upper third of ureter

Answer: (a)
The most common part of ureter to be involved with TB is the lower third of ureter followed by the ureteropelvic junction.

2. Delayed diagnosis of Genitourinary TB is often due to:

   (a) Nonspecific symptoms
   (b) Chronic manifestations
   (c) Subtle clinical signs
   (d) All of the above

Answer: (d)
Genitourinary TB is often diagnosed late due to nonspecific symptoms, chronic manifestations, and only subtle clinical signs. Many times, it is a diagnosis of exclusion.

3. Which of the following routes of infection is the most common in genitourinary tuberculosis?

   (a) Hematogenous seeding
   (b) Lymphatic spread
   (c) Direct inoculation
   (d) Sexual transmission

Answer: (a)
Primary TB of the urogenital system is usually by the hematogenous route affecting the kidneys first. After primary TB infection, it causes direct spread from primary lesions in the kidneys which leads to bacilli seeding into various parts of the urogenital tract. Bacilli from the kidney can enter and lodge in the urothelium, ureter, bladder, urethra, seminal vesicles, and testes.

4. Which of the following investigations is most sensitive to diagnose genitourinary tuberculosis?

   (a) b. CBNAAT Test for AFB
   (b) Mantoux test
   (c) Urine culture for AFB
   (d) Renal biopsy for AFB

Answer: (c)
Urine culture growing acid-fast bacilli is the most sensitive test for genitourinary TB.

5. Which of the urological interventions is not used in short segment stricture?

   (a) Ureteroureterostomy
   (b) Boari flap
   (c) Double-J stent placement
   (d) Psoas Hitch

Answer: (b)
Boari flap is employed for long lower ureteric stricture.

References

1. The top 10 causes of death [Internet]. [cited 2022 Apr 6]. Available from: https://www.who.int/news-room/fact-sheets/detail/the-top-10-causes-of-death
2. World Health Organization. Global tuberculosis report 2021. Geneva: World Health Organization; 2021.
3. Sievers ML. The second great imitator—tuberculosis. JAMA. 1961;176(9):809–10.
4. Sakula A. Robert Koch: the centenary of the discovery of the tubercle bacillus, 1882. Thorax. 1982;37(4):246–51.
5. Furin J, Cox H, Pai M. Tuberculosis. Lancet Lond Engl. 2019;393(10181):1642–56.
6. Kulchavenya E, Naber K, Johansen TEB. Urogenital tuberculosis: classification, diagnosis, and treatment. Eur Urol Suppl. 2016;15(4):112–21.
7. Abbara A, Davidson RN. Etiology and management of genitourinary tuberculosis. Nat Rev Urol. 2011;8(12):678–88.
8. Krishnamoorthy S, Palaniyandi V, Kumaresan N, Govindaraju S, Rajasekaran J, Murugappan I, et al. Aspects of evolving genito urinary tuberculosis-A profile of genito urinary tuberculosis (GUTB) in 110 patients. J Clin Diagn Res. 2017;11(9):PC01.
9. Gow J, Barbosa S. Genitourinary tuberculosis. A study of 1117 cases over a period of 34 years. Br J Urol. 1984;56(5):449–55.
10. Grange JM. The genus Mycobacterium and the Mycobacterium tuberculosis complex. Tuberc Compr Clin Ref (Phila PA Saunders). 2009:44–59. https://doi.org/10.1016/B978-1-4160-3988-4.00006-8.
11. Silva MR, Rocha ADS, Araújo FR, Fonseca-Júnior AA, de Alencar AP, Suffys PN, et al. Risk factors for human Mycobacterium bovis infections in an urban area of Brazil. Mem Inst Oswaldo Cruz. 2018;113:e170445.
12. Zachoval R, Nencka P, Vasakova M, Kopecka E, Borovička V, Wallenfels J, et al. The incidence of subclinical forms of urogenital tuberculosis in patients with pulmonary tuberculosis. J Infect Public Health. 2018;11(2):243–5.
13. Yadav S, Singh P, Hemal A, Kumar R. Genital tuberculosis: current status of diagnosis and management. Transl Androl Urol. 2017;6(2):222.
14. Figueiredo AA, Lucon AM, Junior RF, Srougi M. Epidemiology of urogenital tuberculosis worldwide. Int J Urol. 2008;15(9):827–32.
15. Klebanov N, Raghavan A. Tuberculous orchitis following intravesical Bacille Calmette-Guérin (BCG) therapy. Cureus. 2018;10(5):e2703.
16. Menzies NA, Wolf E, Connors D, Bellerose M, Sbarra AN, Cohen T, et al. Progression from latent infection to active disease in dynamic tuberculosis transmission models: a systematic review of the validity of modelling assumptions. Lancet Infect Dis. 2018;18(8):e228–38.
17. Angus BJ, Yates M, Conlon C, Byren I. Cutaneous tuberculosis of the penis and sexual transmission of tuberculosis confirmed by molecular typing. Clin Infect Dis. 2001;33(11):e132–4.
18. Hunter RL. Tuberculosis as a three-act play: a new paradigm for the pathogenesis of pulmonary tuberculosis. Tuberculosis. 2016;97:8–17.
19. Rao M, Ippolito G, Mfinanga S, Ntoumi F, Yeboah-Manu D, Vilaplana C, et al. Latent TB Infection (LTBI)–Mycobacterium tuberculosis pathogenesis and the dynamics of the granuloma battleground. Int J Infect Dis. 2019;80:S58–61.
20. Lamba H, Byrne M, Goldin R, Jenkins C. Tuberculosis of the cervix: case presentation and a review of the literature. Sex Transm Infect. 2002;78(1):62–3.
21. Arora N, Saha A, Kaur M. Tuberculous pyelonephritis in children: three case reports. Paediatr Int Child Health. 2017;37(4):292–7.

22. Schubert G, Haltaufderheide T, Golz R. Frequency of urogenital tuberculosis in an unselected autopsy series from 1928 to 1949 and 1976 to 1989. Eur Urol. 1992;21:216–23.
23. Puigvert A. The ureter in renal tuberculosis. Br J Urol. 1955;27(3):258–66.
24. Corbishley C, Crange J. Tuberculosis and the kidney. J Am Soc Nephrol. 2001;12(6):1307–14.
25. Merchant S, Bharati A, Merchant N. Tuberculosis of the genitourinary system-Urinary tract tuberculosis: Renal tuberculosis-Part I. Indian J Radiol Imaging. 2013;23(01):46–63.
26. Kulchavenya E. Best practice in the diagnosis and management of urogenital tuberculosis. Ther Adv Urol. 2013 Jun 1;5(3):143–51.
27. Muneer A, Macrae B, Krishnamoorthy S, Zumla A. Urogenital tuberculosis—epidemiology, pathogenesis and clinical features. Nat Rev Urol. 2019;16(10):573–98.
28. Figueiredo AA, Lucon AM. Urogenital tuberculosis: update and review of 8961 cases from the world literature. Rev Urol. 2008;10(3):207.
29. Ghaleb K, Afifi M, El-Gohary M. Assessment of diagnostic techniques of urinary tuberculosis. Mediterr J Hematol Infect Dis. 2013;5(1):e2013034.
30. Medlar EM, Spain D, Holliday R. Post-mortem compared with clinical diagnosis of genitourinary tuberculosis in adult males. J Urol. 1949;61(6):1078–88.
31. Kulchavenya E. Best practice in the diagnosis and management of urogenital tuberculosis. Ther Adv Urol. 2013;5(3):143–51.
32. Lewinsohn DM, Leonard MK, LoBue PA, Cohn DL, Daley CL, Desmond E, et al. Official American Thoracic Society/Infectious Diseases Society of America/Centers for Disease Control and Prevention clinical practice guidelines: diagnosis of tuberculosis in adults and children. Clin Infect Dis. 2017;64(2):e1–33.
33. Mantica G, Ambrosini F, Riccardi N, Vecchio E, Rigatti L, De Rose AF, et al. Genitourinary tuberculosis: a comprehensive review of a neglected manifestation in low-endemic countries. Antibiotics. 2021;10(11):1399.
34. So PNH, Villanueva ART. Serologic and urinary characteristics of laboratory-confirmed genitourinary tuberculosis at a tertiary hospital in the Philippines. BMC Urol. 2021;21(1):1–34.
35. Reid MJ, Arinaminpathy N, Bloom A, Bloom BR, Boehme C, Chaisson R, et al. Building a tuberculosis-free world: the Lancet Commission on tuberculosis. Lancet. 2019;393(10178):1331–84.
36. Walzl G, McNerney R, du Plessis N, Bates M, McHugh TD, Chegou NN, et al. Tuberculosis: advances and challenges in development of new diagnostics and biomarkers. Lancet Infect Dis. 2018;18(7):e199–210.
37. Global Tuberculosis Report s [Internet]. [cited 2022 Apr 3]. Available from: https://www.who.int/teams/control-of-neglected-tropical-diseases/lymphatic-filariasis/morbidity-management-and-disability-prevention/global-tuberculosis-programme
38. Altez-Fernandez C, Ortiz V, Mirzazadeh M, Zegarra L, Seas C, Ugarte-Gil C. Diagnostic accuracy of nucleic acid amplification tests (NAATs) in urine for genitourinary tuberculosis: a systematic review and meta-analysis. BMC Infect Dis. 2017;17(1):1–9.
39. Lawn SD, Gupta-Wright A. Detection of lipoarabinomannan (LAM) in urine is indicative of disseminated TB with renal involvement in patients living with HIV and advanced immunodeficiency: evidence and implications. Trans R Soc Trop Med Hyg. 2016;110(3):180–5.
40. WHO-CDS-TB-2018.19-eng.pdf [Internet]. [cited 2022 Apr 3]. Available from: https://apps.who.int/iris/bitstream/handle/10665/274443/WHO-CDS-TB-2018.19-eng.pdf
41. Colijn C, Cohen T. Whole-genome sequencing of Mycobacterium tuberculosis for rapid diagnostics and beyond. Lancet Respir Med. 2016;4(1):6–8.
42. Doyle RM, Burgess C, Williams R, Gorton R, Booth H, Brown J, et al. Direct whole-genome sequencing of sputum accurately identifies drug-resistant Mycobacterium tuberculosis faster than MGIT culture sequencing. J Clin Microbiol. 2018;56(8):e00666–18.
43. Amaya-Tapia G, Aguirre-Avalos G. Urinary tract tuberculosis. Tuberculosis. 2018;
44. Vijayaraghavan SB, Kandasamy SV, Arul M, Prabhakar M, Dhinakaran CL, Palanisamy R. Spectrum of high-resolution sonographic features of urinary tuberculosis. J Ultrasound Med. 2004;23(5):585–94.

45. Kapoor R, Ansari M, Mandhani A, Gulia A. Clinical presentation and diagnostic approach in cases of genitourinary tuberculosis. Indian J Urol. 2008;24(3):401.
46. Venugopal P. South Indian Consensus on the Diagnosis and Management of Genito-Urinary Tuberculosis. 9.
47. Satish K, Mittal A, Kumar S, Vikash K, Kim J, Usha P. Int J Sci Res.
48. Wejse C. Medical treatment for urogenital tuberculosis (UGTB). GMS Infect Dis. 2018;6:Doc04.
49. Horne NW, Tulloch WS. Conservative management of renal tuberculosis. Br J Urol. 1975;47(5):481–7.
50. Goel A, Dalela D. Options in the management of tuberculous ureteric stricture. Indian J Urol. 2008;24(3):376.
51. Stuart Wolf J, Elashry OM, Clayman RV. Long-term results of endoureterotomy for benign ureteral and ureteroenteric strictures. J Urol. 1997;158(3):759–64.
52. Waller RM, Finnerty DP, Casarella WJ. Transluminal balloon dilation of a tuberculous ureteral stricture. J Urol. 1983;129(6):1225–6.
53. Wein AJ, Kavoussi LR, Novick AC, Partin AW, Peters CA. Campbell-Walsh urology: expert consult premium edition: enhanced online features and print, 4-volume set. Amsterdam: Elsevier Health Sciences; 2011.
54. Lang EK. Glorioso 3rd L. Antegrade transluminal dilatation of benign ureteral strictures: long-term results. Am J Roentgenol. 1988;150(1):131–4.
55. Beckmann CF, Roth RA, Bihrle W 3rd. Dilation of benign ureteral strictures. Radiology. 1989;172(2):437–41.
56. Davis DM, Strong GH, Drake WM. Intubated ureterotomy: experimental work and clinical results. J Urol. 1948;59(5):851–9.
57. Moore CA, Diaz-ball FL. Management of ureteral stricture secondary to tuberculosis. J Urol. 1969;102(2):176–9.
58. Meretyk S, Albala DM, Clayman RV, Denstedt JD, Kavoussi LR. Endoureterotomy for treatment of ureteral strictures. J Urol. 1992;147(6):1502–6.

Chapter 14
Trauma of the Ureter

Ravindra Sabnis, Abhijit Patil, and Pavan Surwase Jain

Abstract The ureter originates from the renal pelvis as the most posterior structure in the renal hilum. Later it traverses caudally through the retroperitoneum along the anterior surface of the psoas muscle, posterior to the colonic mesentery, and lateral to the gonadal vein. Ureteric injuries from external trauma are rare owing to its mobility, narrow diameter, retroperitoneal location (between the spine and major muscle groups), and the overlying peritoneal contents making it an unlikely target for injury.

The most common cause is iatrogenic trauma during open surgery, laparoscopic, or endoscopic procedures. Penetrating trauma accounts for most non-iatrogenic ureteral injuries. Ureteral injuries can be missed, or the diagnosis can be delayed hence necessitating a high index of suspicion. Patients with ureteral injuries are usually asymptomatic, and the diagnosis can be challenging. Haematuria is a non-specific sign but frequently the only clue pointing towards ureteric injury.

Imaging studies are confirmatory in ureteral injury. A retrograde pyelogram (RPG) is the most accurate imaging test to evaluate the location and extent of the ureteral injury. CT urogram can precisely identify the ureteral injury. When possible, in a stable patient, primary repair of the injured ureter is preferred. Based on the location of the injury, surgical repair is done.

An unrecognized or mismanaged ureteral injury can lead to life-threatening complications, including urinoma, abscess, ureteral stricture, and potential loss of ipsilateral kidney or even death; hence accurate diagnosis and treatment of ureteric injury are crucial.

Test your learning and check your understanding of this book's contents: use the "Springer Nature Flashcards" app to access questions. To use the app, please follow the instructions in chapter 1.

R. Sabnis (✉) · P. S. Jain
Department of Urology, Muljibhai Patel Urological Hospital, Nadiad, India

A. Patil
Muljibhai Patel Urological Hospital, Nadiad, India

M. Abdel-Gawad et al. (eds.), *The Ureter*,
https://doi.org/10.1007/978-3-031-36212-5_14

Keywords Ureteric injury · Urine leak · CT urogram · Percutaneous nephrostomy · Ureterouretrostomy

Learning Objectives
- Understand the incidence of ureteral trauma.
- Understand the etiology and pathophysiology of ureteral trauma.
- Understand the diagnostic modalities for ureteral trauma.
- Understand the management of ureteral trauma.
- Understand the prognosis of ureteral trauma.

14.1 Introduction

Ureter is a thin tube that traverses the abdomen and pelvis. The ureter has a very delicate blood supply. The ureter can get easily injured due to many reasons. Ureteral trauma can be broadly divided as:

1. External trauma
   (a) Blunt injury
   (b) Penetrating injury
2. Internal Trauma
   (a) Intrinsic (Endoscopic)
   (b) Extrinsic (Iatrogenic due to surrounding organ surgery)

14.1.1 Incidence

Ureteral injuries occur in 0.2–1% of all pelvic surgeries, 0.3% of all gynecological surgeries [1], and 30% of radical hysterectomies [2, 3]. The incidence of ureteral injuries during colorectal surgeries is around 0.18% [4], whereas it is 0.6% for open surgeries and 1.0% for laparoscopic surgeries [5].

Ureteric injuries from external trauma are rare. The incidence is <106 per year, even in the busiest trauma centers, representing less than 1% of urologic injuries [6]. Penetrating trauma accounts for most non-iatrogenic ureteral injuries. Ureteral injuries are often subtle and easily missed. An unrecognized or mismanaged ureteral injury can lead to life-threatening complications, including urinoma, abscess, ureteral stricture, and potential loss of ipsilateral kidney or even death [7].

14.1.2 Ureteral Anatomy Pertinent to Trauma

The ureter is narrowest at the vesicoureteral junction and the pelvic-ureteric junction. These areas of the ureter are most prone to endoscopic trauma. The other areas prone to trauma are the ureteral kink at the crossing of the ureter over the iliac vessels or the exit of the ureter from the bladder muscle layer.

The pelvic ureter is susceptible to injury during gynecological, pelvic, gastrointestinal, or urological surgeries. The ureter here may get de-vascularised or transected. In cadaver studies, the blood supply of the distal ureter is via branches from the uterine artery in 10% of females. These branches are compromised when the uterine artery is ligated during a routine hysterectomy [8].

14.2 Etiology

Ureteroscopic injuries: the ureter could be injured during rigid ureteroscopy due to laser disintegration of calculus or forceful basketing of stone. The risk factors for ureteral injuries are surgeon inexperience, a larger impacted stone associated with mucosal edema, longer operative times, and previous irradiation around the ureter. In the era of flexible ureteroscopy, ureteral access sheaths also lead to ureteral trauma.

Minimal access surgery: The ureter may get injured during pelvic surgeries like gastrointestinal, urological, or gynecological surgeries. The ureter may get injured during pelvic lymph node dissection for urological malignancies. Laparoscopic or robotic colonic surgery may also injure the ureter. Interestingly, a recent series comparing laparoscopic and open colectomy found a lower rate of ureteral injury with minimally invasive techniques [9]. One-third of ureteral injuries are identified intraoperatively during open surgery, while most ureteral injuries are missed in minimal access surgery and usually are presented as delayed injuries [10].

Open surgeries: The possible causes of iatrogenic ureteric injuries include gynecologic procedures like abdominal or vaginal hysterectomy. Minimally invasive hysterectomy and anterior colporrhaphy are also involved [11]. The other risk factors include prior radiation therapy, pelvic adhesion due to previous surgeries, advanced abdominopelvic cancers, endometriosis, large uterus during hysterectomy, cervical or broad ligament fibroids, limited experience of the surgeon, bleeding, excessive use of diathermy [12–15]. Suture ligation of the ureter, sharp incision and transection, avulsion, devascularization, and heat energies can cause ureteral damage. Most iatrogenic ureteral injuries involve the pelvic ureter.

External trauma: Ureter is unlikely to get injured from external trauma due to its mobility, narrow diameter, retroperitoneal location, and protection from overlying peritoneal contents. Most external Ureteric injuries occur from Gunshot wounds. Penetrating abdominal injuries involving the ureters are usually associated with other injuries in 90% of cases and include injuries to the small bowel (75%), colon (40%), and inferior vena cava (IVC) (20%) [8]. Patients with blunt trauma with a ureteral injury are subject to extreme force applied over the entire body or a larger surface area [9]. Ureteric injuries due to blunt trauma usually occur in children during rapid deceleration causing excessing hyperextension and disruption at PUJ.

14.3 Presentation and Diagnosis

14.3.1 Intraoperative

The ureteroscopic injury would be identified intraoperatively as a mucosal injury or minor ureteral perforation. Sometimes, the ureter may get significantly injured or completely get avulsed during stone retrieval (Fig. 14.1).

The ureter transection may be identified intraoperatively by active urine leak (Fig. 14.2). Sometimes, the ureter devascularization or transection may be self-evident. The intraoperative detection of ureteral injury requires a high degree of suspicion.

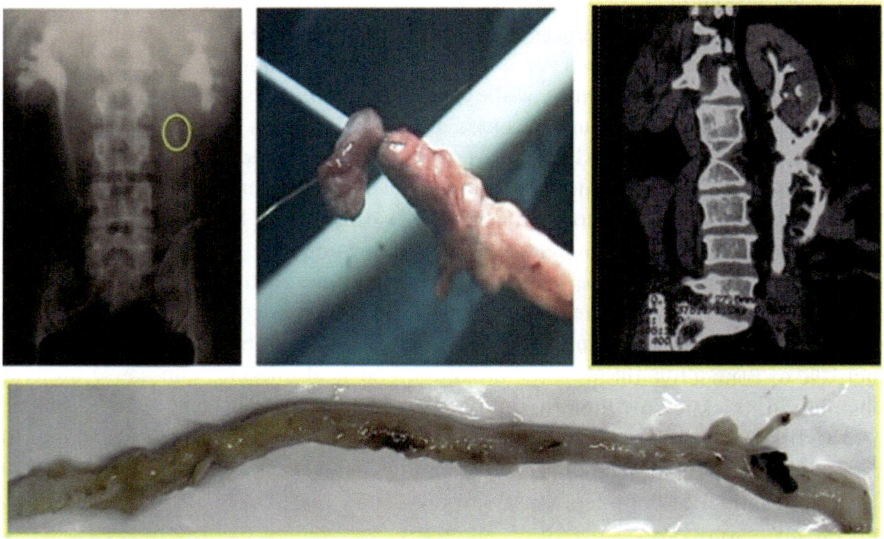

Fig. 14.1 Complete avulsion of the ureter in a 48-year-old female who underwent ureterorenoscopy for upper ureteric stone. Blind basketing led to complete degloving of the ureter

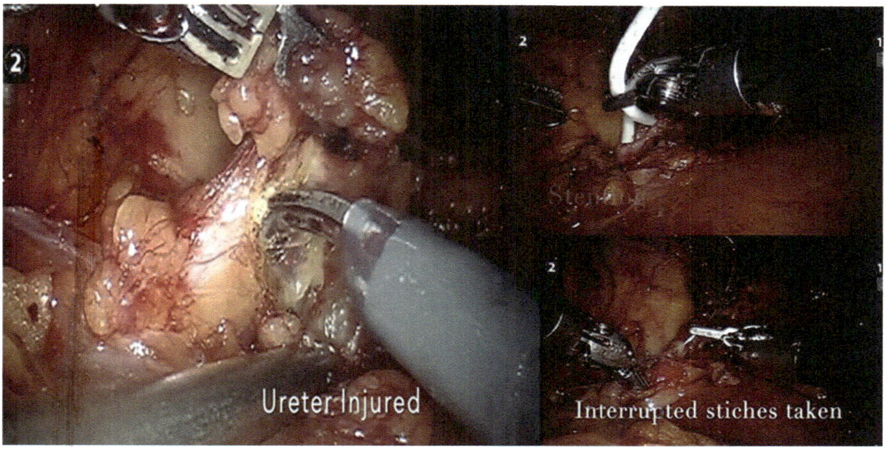

Fig. 14.2 Partial Ureteric injury during pelvic lymph node dissection in robotic-assisted radical prostatectomy. Ureter was repaired with absorbable sutures over a ureteric stent

14.3.2 Postoperative

Patients with postoperative or delayed presentation of ureteral injury present with increased drain output, abdominal pain, fever, or abdominal distention. Laboratory values may show increased blood leucocyte counts, sometimes increased serum creatinine (due to peritoneal absorption of urine), and drain fluid creatinine analysis will show an increased ratio of fluid: serum creatinine. The fluid creatinine would be around the value of urine creatinine.

14.3.3 Traumatic Ureteric Injury

Patients with ureteral injuries are usually asymptomatic, and the diagnosis can be challenging. Hematuria is a non-specific sign but frequently the only clue pointing towards ureteric injury. Any degree of hematuria warrants further investigation. The absence of hematuria doesn't exclude ureteric injury. Therefore, diagnosis relies on a high index of suspicion based on the mechanism and site of injury. Ureteral injuries can be missed, or the diagnosis can be delayed, usually due to prioritization of severe injuries, hemodynamic instability preventing radiographic imaging, or less clinical concern due to the misconception that the retroperitoneal location of ureters is completely protective [16].

A high index of suspicion and low threshold for imaging is warranted for early diagnosis. The commonest site for ureteral injuries is at the vesicoureteral junction and the upper part of the ureter [17]. In the case of delayed diagnosis of ureteral injuries, 59.5% of all the missed ureteral injuries involved the proximal ureter [18]. Surgical exploration and visual inspection are reliable and accurate methods of diagnosing penetrating injuries [19].

14.3.4 Differential Diagnosis

- Unknown bladder injury will result in urine leaking into the retroperitoneum, which can simulate ureteral injury symptoms. Bladder injury is treated by placement of a Foley catheter for 7 to 10 days. Cystogram should be obtained to ensure bladder healing.
- Lymphocele can present with flank pain.
- Hematoma can present with flank pain.
- In females, ureteral fistulae can present as a ureterovaginal fistula with continuous urinary incontinence.

14.3.5 Imaging

CT urography: This modality is best to diagnose delayed ureteral injuries. Delayed images must be obtained (10 min after contrast injection) to allow contrast material to extravasate from the injured collecting system, renal pelvis, or ureter (Figs. 14.3 and 14.4). The other findings could be ipsilateral periureteral urinoma leading to hydronephrosis or lack of contrast in the distal ureter. The traumatic ureteric injuries can be graded as shown in Table 14.1.

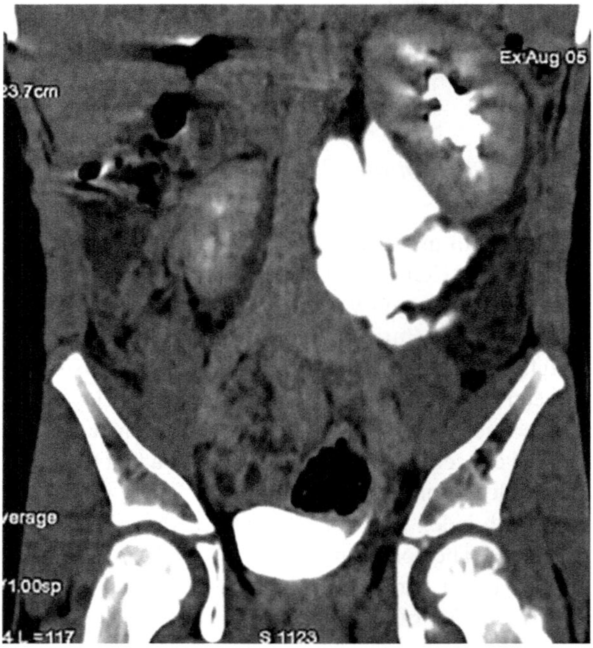

Fig. 14.3 CT Urography showing extravasation of contrast due to left ureteric injury with renal injury in an 8-year-old male child after road traffic

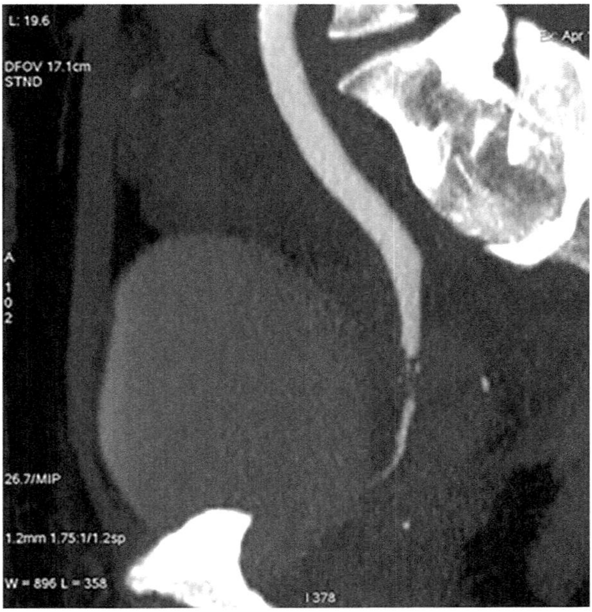

Fig. 14.4 CT Urography showing left ureteric stricture developed after a ureteric injury during laparoscopic hysterectomy

Table 14.1 American Association for the Surgery of Trauma Grading of ureter injury

Grade	Description of injury
I	Hematoma only
II	Lacerations less than 50%
III	Lacerations more than 50%
IV	Complete tear <2 cm of devascularization
V	Complete tear >2 cm of devascularization

A retrograde ureterogram is the most sensitive radiographic test for ureteral injury (Fig. 14.5). It is the best investigation to diagnose ureteral injury in stable patients. It allows the detection of the presence, location, and amount of ureteral injury. It also allows the simultaneous placement of a ureteral stent if possible. This test is also a useful tool when the serum creatinine is raised. Non-contrast CT would tell about collection and hydronephrosis, while retrograde ureterogram is useful for diagnosis.

Antegrade Ureterography and antegrade placement of stent could be performed if retrograde stent placement is not possible, usually secondary to a large gap in the two ends of the transected ureter. A percutaneous nephrostomy can be placed at the time of antegrade stent placement.

An intravenous pyelography can be performed in case of the non-availability of a CT scan. It has the same picture as CT urography but is a less sensitive diagnostic test. Ultrasound abdomen may reveal collection around the ureter and associated hydronephrosis.

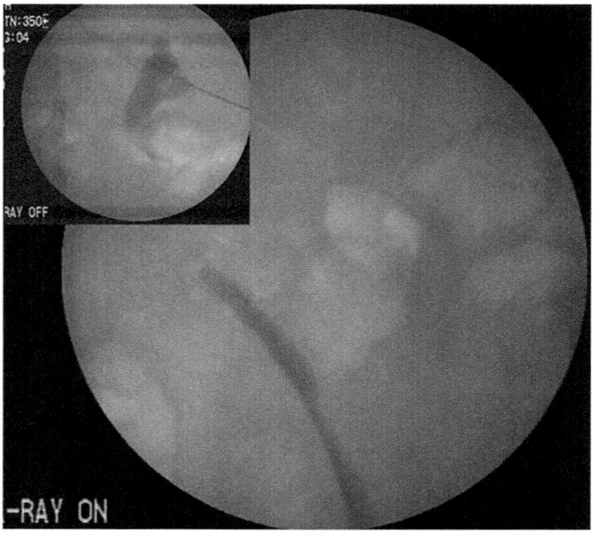

Fig. 14.5 Antegrade and retrograde dye study showing complete transection of pelviureteric junction after open partial nephrectomy done for right lower pole mass

14.4 Management

In a stable patient, primary repair of the injured ureter is preferred during initial laparotomy, and this may not be feasible in unstable, complex polytrauma patients. The principles of management of the injured ureter are as follows:

- The blood supply of the ureter is tenacious. Try to avoid devascularization of the ureter while dissection by avoiding adventitial stripping.
- In case of transection or thermal injury to the ureter, debride the ureter minimally until the edges bleed.
- The ureteral repair should be spatulated and tension-free.
- A stented watertight anastomosis, using fine absorbable sutures, is necessary.
- Retroperitonealize the ureteral repair by closing the peritoneum over it if possible and maintain a retroperitoneal drain.
- Perform a widely spatulated non-tunneled anastomosis, thus avoiding ureteral stenosis.
- If the patient is hemodynamically unstable, the better option is to ligate the ureter with a long silk suture and place a nephrostomy tube and plan for definitive repair later.
- With severely injured ureters, blast effect, concomitant vascular surgery, and other complex cases, consider omental interposition to isolate the repair when possible.
- Mid and upper ureteral defects can be bridged by appendicular interposition in an isoperistaltic manner or by ileum (Monti procedure).
- Complete avulsion of the ureter can be replaced by ileal interposition with proximal ileal anastomosis with the renal pelvis and distal anastomosis with the bladder.

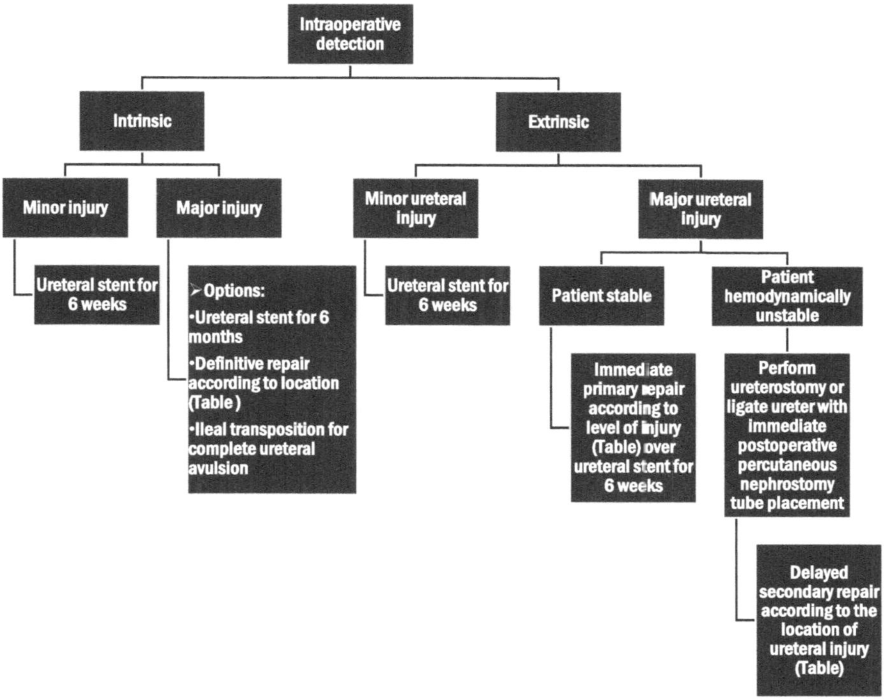

Fig. 14.6 Management algorithm for intraoperative detection of ureteric injuries

14.4.1 Traumatic Ureteric Injuries can be Managed as Follows

Penetrating injuries: Early treatment is preferred. Contusion and proximity of Gunshot wounds (GSW) can be successfully treated by ureteric stenting. Extensive contusions should be treated by segmental excision and ureteroureterostomy.

Blunt injuries: Blunt injuries are typically at the pelvi-ureteric junction and proximal ureter. Primary pelvi-ureteric injury can be treated by a primary repair or ureteric stenting with or without proximal urinary diversion. Complete transection can be successfully repaired by ureteroureterostomy or Ureteropyelostomy [19].

Iatrogenic ureteric injuries could be detected intraoperatively or postoperatively. The management algorithm for the intra and postoperative detection of ureteric injuries is depicted in Figs. 14.6 and 14.7. The management algorithm for traumatic ureteric injuries is described in Fig. 14.8.

The management options for ureteral injuries depending upon the location of injuries are described in Table 14.2.

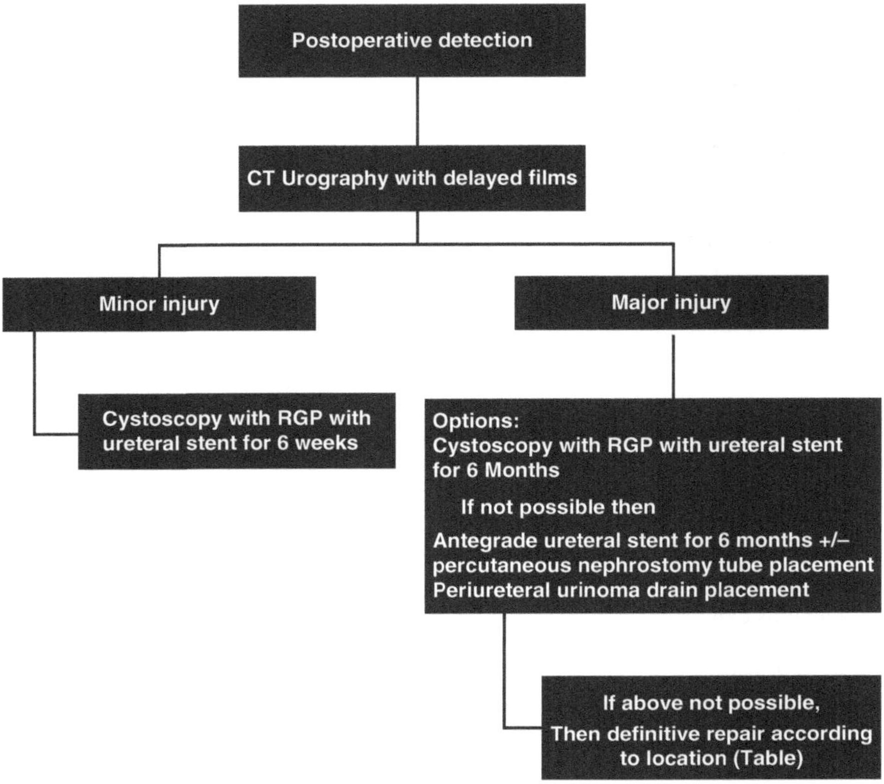

Fig. 14.7 Management algorithm for postoperative detection of ureteric injuries

14.4.2 Surgical Procedures for Ureteric Injuries

14.4.2.1 Ureteroureterostomy (UU)

When the ureter is identified, it can be looped to help in further atraumatic dissection. Minimal handling of the ureter is key to surgery, and care should be taken not to damage the adventitia. As mentioned above, we have abided by the general principles of ureteral repair.

Absorbable sutures are used for anastomosis, and care should be taken to make the knot lie outside. The opposite corner and apex are sutured and approximated. A Double J stent should be placed before the completion of the anastomotic closure. Retroperitoneal fat or omentum may be used to cover the site of anastomosis.

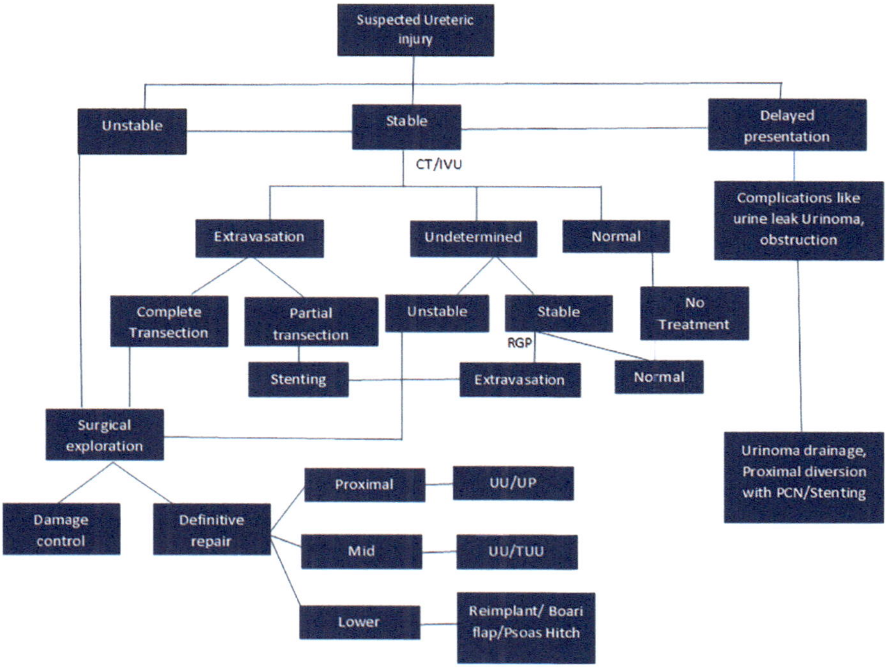

Fig. 14.8 Management algorithm for traumatic ureteric injuries

14.4.2.2 Transureteroureterostomy (TUU)

Lower vertical midline incision. Incise the white line of Toldt and reflect the sigmoid colon medially and trace the ureter. Mobilize the ureter by separating it with periadventitial tissue from the surroundings up to the superior vesical artery. Cut the ureter and ligate the lower end of the ureter. Create a tunnel in the retroperitoneum posterior to the sigmoid colon and mesentery and inferior to the inferior mesenteric artery. Cannulate the ureter. Spatulate the end of the cut ureter and do water-tight, tension-free anastomosis on the medial side of the opposite ureter with Vicryl 5–0 continuously.

Table 14.2 Management options depending upon location of ureteric injury

Location of injury	Procedure
Upper	Direct ureteroureterostomy
	Transureteroureterostomy
Middle	Direct ureteroureterostomy
	Transureteroureterostomy
Lower	Ureteric reimplantation
	Psoas hitch
	Boari flap

14.4.2.3 Ureteroneocystostomy (UNC)

The bladder is dissected. An area over the anterior surface of the bladder near the dome is selected for ureteric reimplantation. The detrusor is incised, and the bladder mucosa is dissected. The bladder mucosa is then incised. The ureter is then spatulated, and tension-free anastomosis is done between the ureteral mucosa and bladder mucosa over the ureteral stent. The anastomosis is covered by detrusurorrhy.

14.4.2.4 Psoas Hitch Procedure

A transverse-oblique cystotomy is made on the posterior bladder dome ipsilateral to the ureteral pathology. The bladder dome is displaced cephalad to the ipsilateral psoas muscle. The posterior wall of the bladder dome is sutured to the psoas minor tendon. A tunnelled ureteral anastomosis can be created by submucosal dissection toward the neo-orifice. The ureter is delivered through the submucosal tunnel into the bladder. The ureter is spatulated anteriorly and anastomosed to the neo-orifice in an interrupted fashion. The ureter may be loosely anchored to the extravesical surface of the bladder at its point of entry. A ureteral stent is placed, and a two-layer closure is commenced by first performing a mucosal closure. The detrusor muscle is closed.

14.4.2.5 Boari Flap

The colon is mobilized medially by freeing it along the line of Toldt, and the injured ureter is isolated. The ureter is then sharply transected 1 cm proximal to the injury and mobilized for 4 to 5 cm, A 3 to 4-mm-thick sheath of periureteral tissue preserved to protect the vascular supply. The bladder is visualized by filling it with 200 to 300 mL of saline. The anterior peritoneum overlying the bladder is incised using monopolar electrocautery, and the bladder is fully mobilized. The ureteral stump and intact bladder dome are approximated with graspers to measure the distance needed to bridge the two structures. Tissue contraction is to be anticipated. The flap length needs to be adequate to reach the ureter, and the distal flap edge to be wide enough to equal the ureteral diameter after tubularization. The flap is fashioned to be 1.5 times longer than the bridge defect. The distal flap edge measured 4 to 5 cm to provide an adequate diameter for tubularization.

The ureter is spatulated anteriorly for 1 to 1.5 cm. Interrupted full-thickness 4–0 Vicryl sutures are used to construct the posterior wall of the anastomosis. A 6F double-J ureteral stent is placed into the ureter. Full-thickness sutures are placed to complete the anastomosis circumferentially. Psoas hitch sutures are generally added to confer protection against tension on the anastomosis.

14.4.2.6 Cat Tail ureter

This procedure is performed for bilateral long-length ureteric injuries, using single segment ileal interposition in cat tail configuration. After urinary diversion, the best possible renal function can be achieved by waiting 2–3 weeks, after which definitive surgery can be planned. A lower Midline vertical incision taken. Mobilize the Sigmoid and descending colon to identify the left lower ureter, which is isolated until cm of the healthy ureter can be identified. Similarly, on the right side-side, the ascending colon is mobilized medially, and the ureter is isolated and dissected freely up to the level of the common iliac artery. Then 15 cm ileal segment is isolated, approximately 15 cm proximal to the ileocecal junction. This 15–20 cm segment is used for cat tail configuration for simultaneous bilateral ureteric replacement. Both ureters are spatulated, and unhealthy segments are removed. Proximal end of the isolated ileum passed through the sigmoid mesentery to the left side so that ileal segment could reach up to the left renal pelvis. Then left healthy ureter was spatulated and anastomosed to the isolated ileum end with an absorbable suture in an end-to-end manner. The cat tail ileal segment then routed towards the right ureter. Approximately 8–10 cm from left uretero-ileal anastomosis, right ureteral end anastomosed to the side of the ileum with absorbable suture. The uretero-ileal anastomosis is completed over a 6 Fr/30 cm double J stent. The distal ileal end is anastomosed to the bladder dome with absorbable sutures. Ileum fixed to the posterior wall. Sigmoid colon fixed to left posterolateral wall.

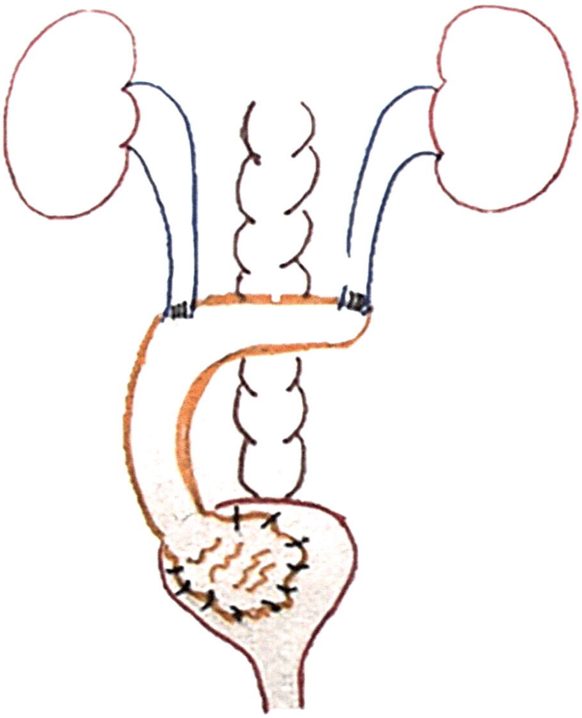

14.5 Prognosis

If the injury is identified immediately, the patients will have an exceptional outcome, as a urologic surgeon can immediately repair the ureter. Early diagnosis is considered the single most important prognostic factor. Patients with a delayed diagnosis of ureteral injury have a much higher rate of complications.

Questions

1. Most common cause of ureteral injury is:

   (a) Blunt trauma
   (b) Iatrogenic
   (c) Gunshot
   (d) Penetrating abdominal injuries

Answer: (b)
The most common cause is iatrogenic trauma during open surgery, laparoscopic, or endoscopic procedures. Penetrating trauma accounts for most non-iatrogenic ureteral injuries.

2. The commonest site for ureteral injuries is the:

   (a) Vesicoureteral junction
   (b) Middle third of the ureter
   (c) Pelviureteric junction
   (d) Lower third of the ureter

Answer: (a)
The commonest site for ureteral injuries is at the vesicoureteral junction and the upper part of the ureter.

3. Which is the most sensitive radiographic test for ureteral injury?

   (a) X-Ray Intravenous Pyelogram
   (b) Retrograde ureterogram
   (c) CT urography
   (d) Renal angiogram

A retrograde ureterogram is the most sensitive radiographic test for ureteral injury. It is the best investigation to diagnose ureteral injury in stable patients. It allows the detection of the presence, location, and amount of ureteral injury. It also allows the simultaneous placement of a ureteral stent if possible.

4. What are the surgical options available for ureteric injuries?

    (a) Cat tail ureter
    (b) Transureteroureterostomy
    (c) Psoas hitch
    (d) All of the above

Answer: (d)
Surgical options available for ureteric injuries are Ureteroureterostomy, Transureteroureterostomy, Psoas hitch, Boari Flap, and Cat tail ureter.

5. What is grade IV according to the American Association Grading of ureter injury?

    (a) Laceration <50%
    (b) Complete tear<2 cm of devascularisation
    (c) Laceration>50%
    (d) Complete tear>2 cm of devascularisation

American Association for the Surgery of Trauma Grading of ureter injury.

Grade	Description of injury
I	Hematoma only
II	Laceration less than 50%
III	Laceration more than 50%
IV	Complete tear <2 cm of devascularization
V	Complete tear >2 cm of devascularization

References

1. Wong JMK, Bortoletto P, Tolentino J, Jung MJ, Milad MP. Urinary tract injury in gynecologic laparoscopy for benign indication: a systematic review. Obstet Gynecol. 2018;131(1):100–8. https://doi.org/10.1097/AOG.0000000000002414.
2. Jha S, Coomarasamy A, Chan KK. Ureteric injury in obstetric and gynecological surgery. Obstet Gynaecol. 2004;6(4):203–8.
3. Kumari Rani A. Urological injury in obstetric and gynecological surgery: a retrospective analysis of five years. Indian. J Obstet Gynecol. 2020;8(2):18–22. https://doi.org/10.21088/ijog.2321.1636.8220.2.
4. Eswara JR, Raup VT, Potretzke AM, Hunt SR, Brandes SB. Outcomes of iatrogenic genitourinary injuries during colorectal surgery. Urology. 2015;86(6):1228–34.
5. Marcelissen TA, Den Hollander PP, Tuytten TR, Sosef MN. Incidence of iatrogenic ureteral injury during open and laparoscopic colorectal surgery: a single center experience and review of the literature. Surg Laparosc Endosc Percutan Tech. 2016;26(6):513–5.

6. Chou M, Wang C, Lien RC. Prophylactic ureteral catheterization in gynecologic surgery: a 12-year randomized trial in a community hospital. Int Urogynecol J. 2009;20:689–93.
7. Ledderose S, Beck V, Chaloupka M, Kretschmer A, Strittmatter F, Tritschler S. [Management of ureteral injuries]. Urologe A. 2019;58(2):197–206.
8. Fraga GP, Gustavo MB, Mantovani M, et al. Penetrating ureteral trauma. Int Braz J Urol. 2007;33(2):142–50.
9. Engelsgjerd JS, LaGrange CA. Ureteral injury. Tampa, FL: StatPearls [Internet]; 2021 Jul 10.
10. Parpala-Spårman T, Paananen I, Santala M, Ohtonen P, Hellström P. Increasing numbers of ureteric injuries after the introduction of laparoscopic surgery. Scand J Urol Nephrol. 2008;42(5):422–7.
11. Mamik MM, et al. Risk factors for lower urinary tract injury at the time of hysterectomy for benign reasons. Int Urogynecol J. 2014;25(8):1031–6.
12. Silver R, et al. National Institute of child health and human development Maternal-Fetal medicine units network. Maternal morbidity associated with multiple repeat cesarean deliveries. Obstet Gynecol. 2006;107(6):1226–32.
13. Smith IA, Cooper M. Management of ureteric endometriosis associated with hydronephrosis: an Australian case series of 13 patients. BMC Res Notes. 2010;3(1):1–5.
14. E. Working group of ESGE and WES, et al. Recommendations for the surgical treatment of endometriosis. Part 2: deep endometriosis. Hum Reprod Open. 2020;2020(1):hoaa002.
15. Tohamy AZ, Samy HA, Salah T, Hussien MT, Hussein M. Ureteric injuries during cancer surgery presentation and management over a 20-year. Int Surg J. 2021;8(2):593–9.
16. Best CD, Petrone P, Buscarini M, Demiray S, Kuncir E, Kimbrell B, et al. Traumatic ureteral injuries: a single institution experience validating the American Association for the Surgery of Trauma-Organ Injury scale grading scale. J Urol. 2005;173:1202.
17. Burks FN, Santucci RA. Management of iatrogenic ureteral injury. Ther Adv Urol. 2014;6(3):115–24.
18. Kunkle DA, Kansas BT, Pathak A, et al. Delayed diagnosis of traumatic ureteral injuries. J Urol. 2006;176:2503–7.
19. Brandes S, Coburn M, Armenakas N, McAninch J. Diagnosis and management of ureteric injury: an evidence-based analysis. BJU Int. 2004 Aug;94(3):277–89.

Chapter 15
Ureteral Strictures: Etiology, Diagnosis and Treatment

Bedeir Ali-El-Dein

Abstract Ureteral stricture is defined as narrowing of the ureteral lumen due to a variety of diseases, such as stones, trauma, tumors, specific infection or inflammation, retroperitoneal fibrosis (RPF), and radiotherapy. Diagnosis and treatment of ureteral stricture is performed as urgent as possible in order to avoid the resulting loss of kidney function.

The diagnosis of ureteral stricture is suspected clinically by pain, fever, recurrent urinary tract infection (UTI), with or without hematuria, oliguria/anuria, or worsening of the renal function. Then, the diagnosis is confirmed by one or more of the following investigations: ultrasound, CT or MRI, radioisotope renography, antegrade, retrograde, and ureteroscopy (URS).

The treatment of ureteral strictures depends on the location, extent, multiplicity, and bilaterality of the lesion. The treatment includes endoscopic, open, and laparoscopic approaches. The common treatment strategies are intravesical/extravesical ureteroneocystostomy, psoas hitch, or Boari flap for the distal ureteral strictures, ureteroureterostomy for localized strictures of the middle and upper ureter, pyeloplasty for UPJO, and ileal ureter for multiple or long segment strictures.

Keywords Ureter · Ureteral stricture · Short segment stricture
Ureteroneocystostomy · Ureteroureterostomy · Boari flap · Long segment stricture
Transureteroureterostomy · Ureteral replacement · Ileal ureter · Monti principle

Test your learning and check your understanding of this book's contents: use the "Springer Nature Flashcards" app to access questions. To use the app, please follow the instructions in chapter 1.

Supplementary Information The online version contains supplementary material available at https://doi.org/10.1007/978-3-031-36212-5_15.

B. Ali-El-Dein (✉)
Urology Department, Urology and Nephrology Center, Faculty of Medicine, Mansoura University, Mansoura, Egypt

M. Abdel-Gawad et al. (eds.), *The Ureter*,
https://doi.org/10.1007/978-3-031-36212-5_15

Learning Objectives

- The learning objectives for this chapter are (1) to enlist the various causes of strictures of the ureter with a focus on the most common causes, (2) to compose a plan for diagnosis of the location, extent and multiplicity of ureteral strictures, and (3) to describe the various techniques used for treatment of short, long, and multiple strictures of the ureter.

15.1 Introduction

Ureteral (or ureteric) stricture means narrowing of the lumen of the ureter with subsequent obstruction and renal function deterioration if not treated. The various causes of ureteral ostruction can be classified into luminal, mural, and extramural or intrinsic and extrinsic or benign and malignant causes. The common causes include, but not limited to calcular disease, iatrogenic injuries and trauma, either induced by urologists or gynecologists and obstetricians, or blunt/penetrating external trauma, and specific inflammatory diseases, such tuberculosis and bilharziasis. This list also includes Post-radiotherapy strictures, retroperitoneal fibrosis, aortic aneurysm, endometriosis and malignant strictures. Post-ureteroscopy (URS) strictures are common because of the frequent use of it; however, with recent techniques, the incidence of post-URS stricture is getting less and less (1%) [1].

The diagnosis and treatment of ureteral stricture should be conducted as early as we can, in order to avoid the subsequent complications, such as sepsis, and loss of the kidney function.

In this chapter, the etiology, the various diagnostic tools and the treatment methods and approaches of ureteral strictures are discussed.

15.2 Etiology of Ureteral Stricture

Table 15.1 shows the various causes of ureteral strictures.

15.2.1 Congenital Causes

The commonest sites for congenital ureteral strictures are at both ends of the ureter, where the ureter joins the bladder, such as ureteroceles or megaureter, or at the junction between the ureter and renal pelvis which is called ureteropelvic junction obstruction (UPJO) (**see the chapters of congenital anomalies of the ureter and UPJO**). The presentation of these anomalies may be at childhood, adolescence, adulthood (Fig. 15.1).

Table 15.1 Etiology of ureteral strictures

Classification	Benign	Malignant
Mural (Intrinsic)	• Iatrogenic (following urologic, gynecologic, general surgical maneuvers). • Ureteral stones. • Post-traumatic strictures (blunt or penetrating). • Chronic inflammation/infections: Bilharziasis, tuberculosis. • Post-radiation ureteral strictures. • Post-chemotherapy strictures. • Ureteral strictures after renal transplantation. • Uretero-enteric strictures after urinary diversion. • Idiopathic. • Congenital.	• Urothelial carcinoma of the ureter (UTUC). • Urothelial carcinoma of the bladder infiltrating the ureter. • Other non-urothelial malignancies.
Extramural (Extrinsic)	• Retroperitoneal fibrosis (RPF) • Pelvic endometriosis	• Prostatic cancer • Cervical or endometrial cancer. • Colon cancer. • Lymphoma or metastasis in lymph nodes.

15.2.2 *Calcular Disease of the Ureter*

Stones in the ureter can lead to ureteral strictures, either by themselves or secondary to the treatment methods used for their removal.

15.2.3 *Iatrogenic Ureteral Strictures*

Ureteral strictures resulting from iatrogenic injuries to the ureter consist a major sector of the etiology of urteral stricture. Together with post-radiation stricture, they account for around 75% of the strictures [2]. Iatrogenic gynecological injuries, for example post-hysterectomy, or post-panhysterectomy, account for the majority of cases, followed by injuries inflicted during urological surgeries and during general surgical interventions. The location of iatrogenic stricture is most commonly at the lower third of the ureter, while the upper and middle thirds are rarely affected [3, 4]. The ureter is vulnerable to iatrogenic injury with subsequent stricture due to its unique anatomy with delicate periureteral vascular network and its close relationship to other organs, such as uterus, ovaries, cervix, sigmoid colon, and rectum [5].

Of the urologic interventions, endoscopic and endourologic techniques are responsible for most ureteral injuries [2]. Some studies have investigated the risk factors for ureteral stricture after endourologic maneuvers [1–10]. These include impacted ureteral stones, ureteral perforation, edematous ureter, mucosal damage, the limited working space with or without edema, stone fragments embedded in the

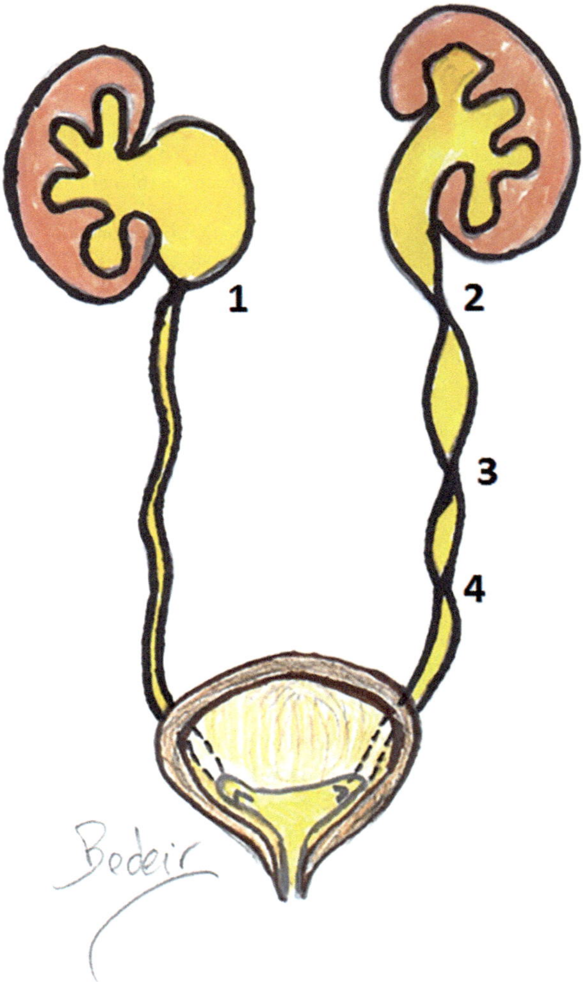

Fig. 15.1 Diagram showing sites of strictures in the ureter. The numbers (1–4) refer to UPJO, lumbar, mid-, and pelvic ureter stricture, respectively

mucosa with associated inflammation, and stone-induced fibrosis secondary to prolonged irritation, pressure ischemia, and/or immunological reaction to stone materials [1–10]. In addition, prolonged operative time, decreased surgeon experience and associated renal stones are among the risk factors of having more frequent post-URS complications [11].The rate of ureteral stricture after URS for ureteral stones ranges from 0.3% to 24% as shown in Table 15.2 [6, 12–19]. In the few studies conducted, the risk of ureteral stricture was higher after URS for proximal stones than for lower stones; however, in a global study including 9681 patients, ureteral stricture developed in 0.9%, 1.1%, and 0.7% for proximal, mid-ureteral and distal locations, respectively [20, 21].

Detailed information about iatrogenic ureteral injuries is provided in other chapters of this book.

Table 15.2 The rate of ureteral stricture after urteroscopy for treatment of ureteral stones

Authors	Patients no.	Type of URS	Incidence (rate) %
Roberts et al. [6]	21	Rigid	23.8
Fam et al. [9]	64	Rigid	7.8
Weizer et al. [12]	241	Rigid/flexible	1.2
Adiyat et al. [13]	214	Rigid/flexible	1.4
Binbay et al. [14]	80	Rigid	1.3
Li et al. [15]	982	Rigid	2.95
de la Rosette et al. [16]	10,511	Rigid/flexible	0.3
Darwish et al. [18]	251	Rigid	1.5
Shen et al. [19	447	Flexible	6.4–8
Ulvik et al. [17]	995	Rigid/flexible	3

15.2.4 *Post-radiation Stricture*

Although rare, ureteral stricture after radiotherapy for abdominal or pelvic tumors is a well-known complication [22, 23]. The list of the abdominal and pelvic tumors, which are treated with radiotherapy includes prostate cancer, bladder cancer, cervical cancer, lymphoma, pancreatic carcinoma, colorectal cancer, etc. Severe ureteral strictures with grade 4 or 5 hydronephrosis have been noted in 1.0, 1.2, 2.2, and 2.5% after 5, 10, 15, and 20 years from radiotherapy, respectively; so there is a continuous increase of the actuarial risk of around 0.15% per year, with 1.7% at 3 years and 2.1%, at 5 years [22, 23]. The risk factors for development of post-radiation ureteral strictures include advanced pelvic tumors with hydronephrosis at the initial diagnosis, and multiple radiation treatments [23]. Radiation-induced ureteral strictures usually present late and they may be asymptomatic or associated with renal function loss or severe sepsis [22, 23]. Radiation-induced injury may be attributed to radiotherapy alone or to radiotherapy and associated treatments, such as surgery and chemotherapy.

15.2.5 *Retroperitoneal Fibrosis (RPF)*

Retroperitoneal fibrosis (RPF) is a rare disease with characteristic development of chronic inflammatory process with marked fibrosis affecting the retroperitoneum in the peri-aortic and peri-ileal areas at the level of the lower four lumbar vertebrae [24, 25].

The incidence RPF is 1.4 per 100,000 individuals and it affects males more commonly than females [26]. RPF is an immune-mediated disease and may be primary or idiopathic and may be secondary RPF; the latter develops secondary to retroperitoneal malignancy, inflammation and infection, irradiation, abdominal surgeries, some drugs, and asbestos exposure [27]. Entrapment of the ureter with subsequent affection of the renal function or even acute renal failure is one of the most common complications of RPF [28]. It is a disease of ongoing debates, since a lot of questions regarding its pathogenesis, diagnosis, and treatment remains unanswered [28].

The treatment options will be discussed later in this chapter. They include steroid therapy, immunosuppressive drugs, ureteral stents or percutaneous nephrostomy tube (PCN), and ureterolysis/omental wrapping [24–28].

15.2.6 Malignant Obstruction

Malignant tumors may develop in the wall of ureter, or invade the ureter from extramural primary source. Both will lead to ureteral obstruction, which may not be an actual stricture (**see also chapter of ureteral tumors in this book**).

15.2.7 Chronic Inflammation

Chronic inflammatory diseases and infections, such as tuberculosis (TB) and bilharziasis, my cause stricture of the ureter. For example, tuberculous ureteral strictures are not uncommon in big hospitals treating a big number of patients with urinary TB [29] (see also Chap. 13 in this book).

Idiopathic: Sometimes the cause of ureteral stricture is unknown.

15.3 Sites of Ureteral Strictures

15.3.1 Strictures at the Distal Ureter

These strictures occur at the pelvic ureter, either close to the bladder or at the ureteral orifice. The latter is most commonly a congenital stricture; sometimes it is iatrogenic and occurs secondary to endoscopic manipulations of stones or bladder tumor. Overall, pelvic ureteral strictures are usually iatrogenic and develop due to pelvic surgeries, endoscopic stone retrieval, or radiotherapy for treatment of pelvic malignancies.

15.3.2 UPJO

UPJO is essentially a congenital stricture. However, it may develop secondary to treatment of stones impacted at the UPJ.

15.3.3 Strictures at the Upper Third of the Ureter

The commonest causes of upper third ureteral strictures are renal stones, either as an association or due to their treatment, and recurrence after pyeloplasty for UPJ.

15.3.4 Strictures Affecting the Whole Ureter or Multiple Sites

Multiple ureteral strictures or strictures affecting the whole ureter are rare and may develop due to RPF, specific infection, such as TB, or after treatment of multiple urinary tract stones.

15.4 Diagnosis of Ureteral Strictures

15.4.1 Clinical Presentation

Ureteral strictures may present with symptoms of urinary tract obstruction including flank pain, fever with associated constitutional manifestations such as nausea and vomiting, frequent or difficult urination, urinary tract infection, bloody urine or change in the urine color, or high blood pressure. Sometimes, ureteral strictures are asymptomatic, especially if they cause gradual obstruction and this may lead to serious consequences, such as deterioration in kidney function or sepsis.

15.4.2 Laboratory Tests of Blood and Urine

15.4.2.1 Urine Analysis for White and Red Blood Cells

Examination of the urine for white and red blood cells is often normal in cases of ureteral obstruction due to stricture, unless there is infection on top of obstruction.

15.4.2.2 Assessment of Creatinine, Blood Urea Nitrogen in Blood

Examination of the blood for creatinine, blood urea nitrogen or both usually shows normal levels, unless the strictures are bilateral, complete, and the resulting obstruction lasts for few hours.

15.4.3 Diagnostic Imaging of Ureteral Strictures

15.4.3.1 Ultrasound

Gray scale ultrasound is the initial imaging used in suspected ureteral obstruction due to stricture. It can assess the size, echogenicity of the kidney, detect hydronephrosis as back pressure effects, and can define ureteral dilation proximal to the stricture site. The sensitivity of ultrasound in diagnosing hydronephrosis is high, yet it has some limitations [30]. In addition, color Doppler duplex ultrasound can measure the resistive index in the intrarenal arteries, which becomes higher than the upper normal limit (0.7) in cases of obstruction due to stricture. Furethermore, ultrasound has a very crucial role in cases of ureteral strictures associated with chronic kidney disease (CKD). Also, ultrasound can be repeated many times without side effects.

Limitations

Among the limitations of ultrasound is that it gives false negative results in the early phase of ureteral obstruction, in the case of marked dehydration or severe CKD, or if the obstruction is progressing slowly and gradually as in the case of RPF [30]. In addition, the technique is operator dependent and can't diagnose the cause of ureteral stricture.

15.4.3.2 CT scan

CT scan gives better characterization of the ureteral strictures regarding the etiology, location, laterality, and stricture extent. Therefore, a proper decision on the mode of treatment can be achieved. CT associated with intravenous injection of a contrast material or what called CT urography (CTU) is the gold standard diagnostic tool for strictures of the ureter [31, 32]. Along with the above mentioned role, wall thickening, whether focal or diffuse, proximal hydronephrosis, luminal irregularities with nodularity or enhancement, and contrast excretion by the kidney can be shown by CTU [31, 32]. In addition, an approximate differentiation between benign and malignant strictures can be made by CTU. Furthermore, non contrast CT can show urine extravasation and perinephric fat stranding in cases of obstruction and/or infection.

Limitations

In cases of hypersensitivity to contrast or in chronic or acute renal impairment, the use of intravenous contrast is contraindicated.

15.5 Magnetic Resonance Imaging (MRI) and MR Urography (MRU)

MRI in the form of dynamic or gadolinium-enhanced MR urography can give the urologists important information about the anatomy and function of urinary tract secondary to obstruction by ureteral stricture [33–36]. This is of particular concern in children and it has the advantage of avoiding exposure to radiation. The changes in renal perfusion and diffusion can be non-invasively assessed by diffusion-weighted MRI in cases of unilateral obstruction of the ureter due to stricture [36].

Renal functional magnetic resonance imaging (fMRI), is a non invasive rapidly progressing technique, which has been proved to be accurate in evaluation of the glomerular filtration rate (GFR); it utilizes markers related to renal function, including water molecular diffusion, perfusion, and oxygenation [37]. Renal transit time for gadolinium on MRI can be used to detect ureteral and urinary tract obstruction [36]. In addition, the non dilated ureter with ureteral peristalsis can be assessed using special technique of T2-weighted MRU, where early obstruction can be diagnosed even before hydronephrosis is evident [38].

MRU is particularly helpful in cases of hypersensitivity to contrast material (with CTU or IVU), during pregnancy, dilated ureter with poorly functioning kidney, and when the cause of ureteral stricture and obstruction is not defined.

15.5.1 Intravenous Urography (IVU)

IVU was a common diagnostic technique of ureteral strictures in the past. Nowadays, CTU and MRU are usesd instead of IVU; however, in regions where these recent imaging tools are not available IVU still has a role.

15.6 Retrograde Pyelography and Antegrade Nephrostogram

Retrograde pyelography is a more invasive technique than the above mentioned tools. Retrograde pyelography (**or retrograde pyeloureterography**) is performed by injection of a radiocontrast material, similar to that used in IVU, into a ureteral catheter through cystoscopy in order to visualize the ureter and pelvicalyceal sytem. It has been the main imaging method of the ureter and collecting system before IVU was introduced in 1930.

15.6.1 Indications and Advantages

Invasive retrograde and/or antegrade studies are highly sensitive in diagnosing the location, extent, cause and in guiding the treatment of ureteral stricture. They are usually used in situations where the proper diagnosis of the extent, location, and cause of ureteral obstruction is not definite.

Antegrade pyelography is the technique conducted to visualize the renal pelvis, calyces and ureter, which is indicated when other imaging modalities have failed to make a diagnosis of the ureteral stricture. It is also indicated when injection of contrast material is contraindicated, when a percutaneous nephrostomy tube (PCN) is present, or when better visualization of the kidney and ureter is required.

Avoiding intravenous contrast is a major advantage of these techniques. This makes these techniques suitable for assessing ureteral pathology when the patient has a history of allergy to intravenous contrast or in cases of renal impairment. Retrograde and antegrade studies are often conducted intraoperatively.

15.7 Nuclear Medicine

Diuretic radioisotope renography or nuclear medicine diuretic imaging is used to assess the kidney function and whether the system is obstructed or not. It measures the glomerular filtration rate and split renal function; however, it has a little role in anatomical diagnosis of ureteral strictures. It has been noted that a baseline split renal function of 20% or more of the affected kidney is needed in order to have a good outcome after repair of the ureteral stricture [39, 40].

15.7.1 Other Imaging Modalities

Endoscopic intraluminal ultrasound and virtual endoscopy have been investigated in the diagnosis of ureteral strictures; however, they are not yet well studied [41, 42]. Voiding cystourethrography (VCUG) may be performed to exclude vesicoureteral reflux as the cause of hydronephrosis, especially in children.

Table 15.3 demonstrates the various diagnostic tests of ureteral strictures.

Table 15.3 A summary of various diagnostic tests used in cases of ureteral strictures

Test	Value	Limitations
Urine analysis	Can show white and red blood cells in cases of infection or tumors	Often normal in cases of obstruction
Serum creatinine & blood urea nitogen	One of the kidney function tests	May be normal, unless the ureteral stricture is bilateral, complete, and lasts more than few hours
Ultrasound (gray-scale & Doppler)	It can assess the kidney size, echogenicity, hydronephrosis, and hydroureter proximal to the stricture. Color Doppler duplex ultrasound can measure the resistive index. It has a very crucial role in CKD associated with ureteral strictures.	False negative results in the early phase of ureteral obstruction, in marked dehydration or severe CKD, or if the obstruction is gradual as in RPF. It is operator dependent and can't diagnose the cause of ureteral stricture.
CT scan	Better characterization of the ureteral strictures: etiology, location, laterality, and stricture extent. Ct with contrast or CTU can differentiate between benign and malignant strictures. Non contrast CT can show urine extravasation and perinephric fat stranding in cases of obstruction and/ or infection.	CT with contrast is contraindicated in cases of hypersensitivity to contrast or in chronic or acute renal impairment.
MRI/MRU	Can assess the anatomy and function of urinary tract secondary to obstruction by ureteral stricture, especially in children. It avoids exposure to radiation. Of special importance during pregnancy, dilated ureter with no definite diagnosis, and hypersensitivity to contrast materials.	Some people can't tolerate it. If used with contrast, may be dangerous in CKD.
Intravenous urography (IVU)	In regions where CT or MRI is not available IVU still has a role.	It is contraindicated in cases of hypersensitivity to contrast or in chronic or acute renal impairment.
Retrograde pyelography and antegrade nephrostogram	Retrograde and/or antegrade studies are highly sensitive in diagnosing the location, extent, cause and in guiding the treatment of ureteral stricture. They are of special value when the diagnosis is not definite.	They are invasive.
Nuclear medicine	It evaluates the kidney function and whether the system is obstructed or not. It measures the glomerular filtration rate and split renal function.	Fallacies in cases of dehydration and in severely dilated system.
Other imaging modalities	Endoscopic intraluminal ultrasound and virtual endoscopy have been tried, but not well studied. VCUG may be performed to exclude vesicoureteral reflux.	

15.8 Treatment

Treatment of ureteral strictures depends on the etiology, location, extent, multiplicity, bilaterality of the stricture, and the function of the affected kidney. **Malignant, tuberculous, bilharzial ureteral strictures have been discussed in separate chapters.** So, the following discussion is devoted to ureteral strictures other than those mentioned above.

The aim of any treatment method is to get rid of the obstruction and to maintain or improve the function of the kidney.

Treatment of ureteral strictures can be classified in three ways; either as endoscopic, open, minimally invasive or as treatment of short segment and long segment strictures or as treatment of lower, mid-, proximal ureteral stricture. In this chapter, a combination of these classification methods is used.

Open reconstructive techniques are still the gold standard for treatment of ureteral strictures, because of the high success rate and the lower possibility of a redo procedure. On the other hand, in special situations with proper selection criteria endoscopic maneuvers may provide a good choice [43, 44].

15.8.1 Endoscopic Treatment

Endoscopic or endourologic treatment of ureteral strictures is usually carried out as initial treatment by most urologists, because of being less invasive, less painful, with faster recovery, and shorter operative time compared to open surgery [43, 44].

The list of endoscopic treatment includes ureteral stents, percutaneous nephrostomy (PCN), retrograde or antegrade balloon dilation of the stricture, endoscopic meatotomy, acucise treatment, endoureterotomy, and combined antegrade and retrograde methods (rendezvous procedure) [45, 46].

15.8.1.1 Indications and Choice of Candidates

Endoscopic treatment of ureteral strictures is attended with high success rate in the following conditions: (1) short segment strictures less than 2 cm, (2) benign strictures, (3) non-ischemic stricture, (4) stricture affecting the upper or lower ureter, and (5) if there is no history of radiation [46, 47].

15.8.1.2 Ureteral Stents

Types

There are two major types of ureteral stents, namely the polymer or polytetrafluoroethylene (PTFE) stents and metallic stents [48, 49]. Nitinol alloy has recently been used in the synthesis of metallic stents. The Resonance, Memokath, Allium and the Uventa stents are examples of metallic stents. The polymer stents are fixed for a period of 3 to 6 months, while the metallic stents can stay longer (12 months).

Indications and Efficacy

Ureteral stents are usually used as an initial temporary procedure before definitive treatment is carried out. They can be inserted either by a retrograde or antegrade method with a very high success rate. Ureteral stents are especially indicated in cases of severe and/ or acute obstruction located at the ureter or renal pelvis, bilateral obstruction with oliguria/anuria and/ or elevated serum creatinine level. In addition, ureteral stents can be used when definitive surgical intervention can not be done because of poor performance status or contraindications. Luminal and mural (intrinsic) ureteral strictures are more favorable for ureteral stents than strictures caused by extramural lesions [50, 51]. However, metallic stents can be used in cases of extrinsic obstruction of the ureter, as in the case of post-radiation, and malignant stricture, with more favorable outcome compared to the polymer stents [48, 49].

Complications

In most patients, pain and irritative voiding symptoms occur due to bladder irritation by the lower coil of the stent. In addition, urinary tract infection, stent migration, malposition, encrustation, and stent breakdown may occur [52, 53]. Furthermore, failure of insertion, failure to relieve obstruction and fistula formation are among possible complications [52].

15.8.1.3 Percutaneous Nephrostomy (PCN)

Indications and its Choice Versus Retrograde Ureteral Stents:

Again, PCN is usually used as a temporary step until a more definitive treatment is conducted. PCN fixation has the same indications of ureteral stents, and there has been ongoing debate about the choice and safety of either technique versus the other. PCN is preferred to drain obstructed system secondary to ureteral stricture in cases of impending sepsis, failed negotiation of the ureteral orifice and in cases of extrinsic ureteral obstruction. On the other hand, with recent advances in the manufacture of ureteral stents, they may be the preferred option in patients with coagulopathy and in non-complicated cases [54]. PCN is fixed with a high success rate, with the patient is in the prone position, under guidance of either ultrasound and/ or fluoroscopy [55].

Limitations and Complications

Additional limiting factors of the use of PCN include its complications, diminished quality of life because of the presence of external collecting bag, and that it needs a qualified interventional radiologist or a certified urologist. The complications include pain at the insertion site, obstruction, and dislodgement [56].

15.8.1.4 Balloon Dilation

Balloon dilation of the strictured part of the ureter can be performed as antegrade or retrograde maneuver. The procedure is conducted by inflating a balloon at the stricture site, and leaving a stent thereafter.

Indications

Patients with short (less than 2 cm) and non-ischemic, non-radiated and benign strictures are suitable candidates for initial treatment with balloon dilation [57–60]. In addition, ureteral strictures developing early after renal transplantation can be treated with balloon dilation and ureteral stenting as initial step with moderate success rates of 40% to 70% [57–60]. Furthermore, balloon dilation has been carried out to treat iatrogenic ureteral strictures following pelvic surgery or ureteroscopy and to treat children and young adults with primary obstructive megaureter with wide variation in the reported success rates [61, 62]. The lowest success rates were obtained in cases of malignant strictures [63]. Proximal and distal ureteral strictures treated with balloon dilation have higher success rates than strictures of the mid-ureter [64].

Complications

The complications include failure of balloon dilation, recurrence of the stricture and perforation of the ureter [60].

15.8.1.5 Acucise Balloon Incision

The Acucise cutting balloon is one of the options of endoscopic treatment of ureteral strictures.

Indications and Contraindications

It can be used with fair rates of success for strictures at the lower and proximal ureter, including UPJO. It is indicated and is attended with relatively high success rates in short segment strictures (<2 cm), split renal function more than 20% and in the presence of mild to moderate hydronephrosis. It is relatively contraindicated in cases of massive hydronephrosis, crossing renal vessels causing UPJO, and/ or ureteral stricture associated with proximal renal calculi [65, 66].

Efficacy

When acucise balloon dilation is properly indicated a success rate of around 70% was achieved [65]. It has been used in treatment of post-renal transplant ureteric stricture with high success rate [67]; however, it gives poor results in cases of ureteroenteric or malignant strictures.

15.8.1.6 Endoureterotomy

It is one of the minimally invasive techniques. The basis of endoureterotomy is that the ureter after incision of the stricture can regenerate its epithelium. The first report of endoureterotomy was that of Davis and associates in 1948 [68].

15.8.1.7 Site and Technique of Endoureterotomy

The technique can be performed as a retrograde or antegrade maneuver, using cold knife, electrosurgical probe, or laser. The site of incision in the proximal ureter is posterolateral and is anteromedial in the distal ureter. This is to avoid injury of the vessels in the nearby area [69]. An incision including the whole wall thickness with proximal and distal 2–3 mm extension of into the healthy tissue is necessary.

15.8.1.8 Indications and Contraindications

The site, length, etiology, and function of the affected kidney are the major determinants of the success of endoureterotomy [40, 47]. As with other endoscopic techniques for treatment of ureteral strictures, the best results are achieved in short (less than 2 cm), upper, lower, and non-ischemic non-radiated ureteral strictures and when the split function of the affected kidney is 25% or more [40, 70]. Therefore, mid-ureteral, post-radiation, and strictures associated with poor function of the affected kidney may be considered as relative contraindications because of the resulting poor outcome [40, 70].

15.8.1.9 Success Rate

The reported success rate of appropriately indicated endoureterotomy for benign strictures is within the range of 50% to 80% [40, 71]. Endoureterotomy using laser (usually Holmium laser) becomes a preferred option because of the combined cutting and coagulation. However, other lasers such as Thulium laser can be used with good results [72].

Overall, endoscopic and endourological procedures can work as primary or secondary treatment alternatives to open surgery. They are indicated in cases of short segment, benign strictures especially those located proximally or distally and when there is good ureteral vascularity. However, the success rate is not that high and they are of limited role in malignant, post-radiation and uretero-enteric strictures.

Table 15.4 demonstrates the indications and different types of endoscopic treatment of ureteral strictures.

15.8.1.10 Open Surgical Interventions

Again, there are a variety of open procedures used to treat ureteral strictures and they depend on the etiology, site, extent, multiplicity and bilaterality of the stricture. They can be classified into two main categories: procedures used for short segment and those used for long segment strictures.

15.8.2 Open Procedures to Treat Short Segment Stricture

These can be further classified into refluxing and non-refluxing techniques.

15.8.2.1 Ureteroneocystostomy, Boari Flap and Psoas Hitch

The term, ureteroneocystostomy or ureterovesical anastomosis or ureterovesicoplasty, is used when the ureter is re-implanted into the bladder because of various reasons. It is the surgical technique of choice to treat strictures involving the lower ureter and within 3–5 cm from the bladder (Fig. 15.2).

Table 15.4 A summary of the indications and different methods of endoscopic treatment of ureteral strictures

Parameter	Indication/type	Notes
Indications	(1) short segment strictures less than 2 cm, (2) benign strictures, (3) non-ischemic stricture, (4) stricture affecting the upper or lower ureter, and (5) if there is no history of radiation.	Endoscopic treatment of ureteral strictures is attended with high success rate if these indications are adhered with.
Ureteral Stents	• Indicated in cases of severe and/ or acute obstruction, bilateral obstruction with oliguria/anuria and/ or elevated serum creatinine level, and if surgery is contraindicated, for example because of poor performance status.	• Special complications: Pain and irritative voiding symptoms, urinary tract infection, stent migration, malposition, encrustation, and stent breakdown.
Percutaneous nephrostomy (PCN)	• A temporary step until a more definitive treatment is conducted. PCN fixation has the same indications of ureteral stents. PCN is preferred in cases of impending sepsis, failed negotiation of the ureteral orifice and in extrinsic ureteral obstruction.	• Side effects: It needs special expertise for insertion. The complications include pain at the insertion site, obstruction, dislodgement, and decreased quality of life (bag).
Balloon dilation	It can be performed as antegrade or retrograde maneuver, by inflating a balloon at the stricture site, and leaving a stent thereafter.	Complications: Failure of balloon dilation, recurrence of the stricture and perforation of the ureter.
Acucise balloon incision	Can be used with fair success for strictures at the lower and proximal ureter, including UPJO.	It is relatively contraindicated in cases of massive hydronephrosis, crossing renal vessels causing UPJO, and/ or ureteral stricture associated with proximal renal calculi.
Endoureterotomy	Can be performed as a retrograde or antegrade maneuver, using cold knife, electrosurgical probe, or laser. The site of incision in the proximal ureter is posterolateral and is anteromedial in the distal ureter.	Mid-ureteral, post-radiation, and strictures associated with poor kidney function may be considered as relative contraindications because of the resulting poor outcome.

A variety of techniques have been described including refluxing and non-refluxing procedures; however, the commonest of which are Lich-Gregoir and its modifications and Boari flap. The list includes Lich-Gregoir, Politano-Leadbetter, Cohen cross-trigonal, Psoas hitch, Boari flap and other techniques.

15.8.2.2 Refluxing Versus Non-refluxing Ureteroneocystostomy

Whether to use a non-refluxing ureterovesical reimplantation is a matter of surgeon preference and ongoing controversy. Although some surgeons prefer the anti-reflux anastomosis, there was no difference between refluxing and non-refluxing

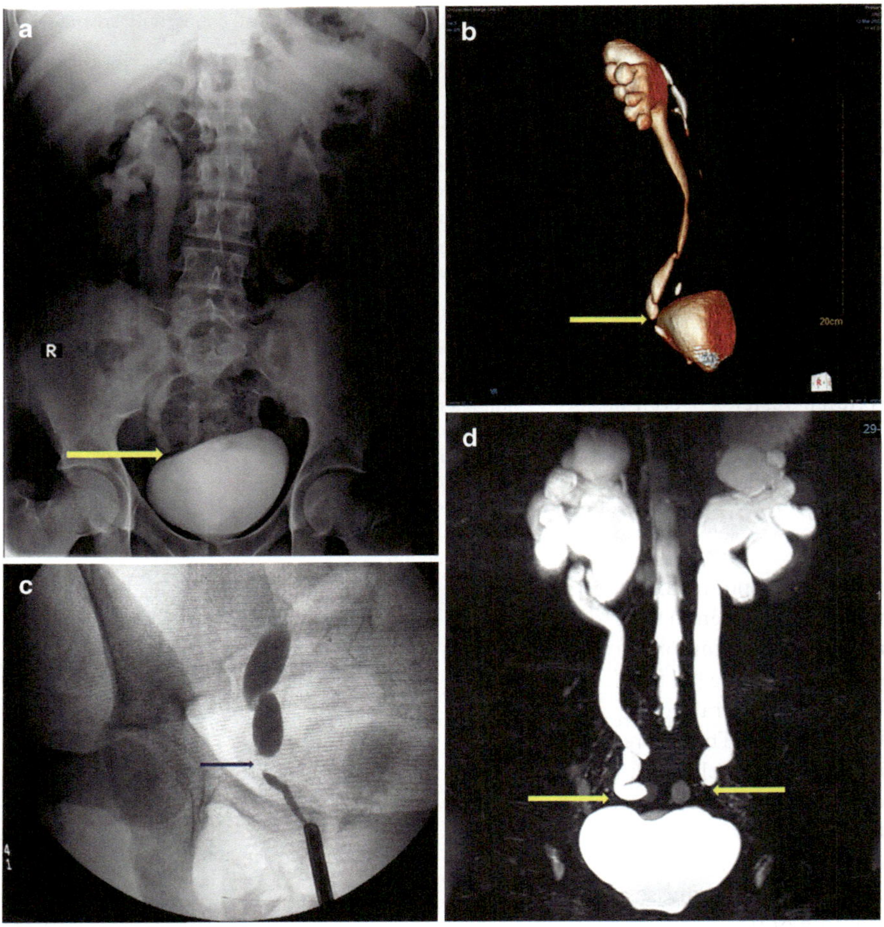

Fig. 15.2 Various imaging and radiological tests to diagnose stricture of the pelvic ureter. (**a**) is an IVU showing stricture of the pelvic part of the right ureter (arrow). (**b**) is a 3D CT scan showing stricture of the pelvic part of the right ureter (arrow) of the same patient. (**c**) is a retrograde ureterogram showing stricture of the pelvic part of the right ureter (arrow) of the same patient. (**d**) is an MRU showing stricture of the pelvic parts of both ureters (arrows) in another patient

techniques regarding kidney function or recurrence of the ureteral stricture, even in renal transplantation [77–79]. **However, in our opinion anti-reflux procedures are preferred for treatment of ureteral strictures in children, especially congenital strictures such as obstructed megaureter, in implanting the graft ureter in renal transplantation, and whenever the length of the healthy ureter is enough for a tension free anstomosis.**

15.8.3 General Hints on These Techniques

They are non-refluxing techniques, where the ureter is reimplanted into a submucosal tunnel created from outside as in extravesical Lich-Gregoir, or from inside as in transvesical Politano-Leadbetter or performed on both ureters as in the Cohen technique. The stricture segment is identified, the ureter transected, its distal end ligated and the proximal end is trimmed until a viable area is reached. The bladder is filled with an antibiotic solution with or without minimal mobilization, the submucosal tunnel for 2–3 cm is created and the ureter is implanted. Preservation of the periurетral adventitia with its vascular network is very important.

15.8.3.1 Extravesical Ureteroneocystostomy

Lich et al. described the original technique, Lich-Gregoir (Fig. 15.3) and thereafter multiple modifications were made to the technique, including the toe stitch used to fix the spatulated ureter toe to the bladder wall, one-stitch, two-stitch and parallel incision modifications [73–75] (See also Chap. 22: ureter and renal transplantation).

15.8.3.2 Transvesical Ureteroneocystostomy

The technique is known as Politano-Leadbetter. After anterior cystostomy, the submucosal tunnel for reimplantation of the ureter is created from inside the bladder, through one or two incisions in the mucosa [76] (see also Chap. 23: Ureter and Renal Transplantation).

Success Rate of Ureteroneocystostomy

The success rate of extravesical (Lich-Gregoir) and transvesical procedure (Politano-Leadbetter, Cohen) is very high (95–99%) [80].

Complications

The complications of non-refluxing ureteroneocystostomy include hematuria, bleeding, hematoma with subsequent ureteral compression, urinary tract infection, urinary leakage, inadvertent injury to adjacent organs such as intestine or blood vessels, renal impairment, bladder spasms especially with the transvesical procedure, ureteral obstruction, recurrence of the stricture, and complications of anesthesia.

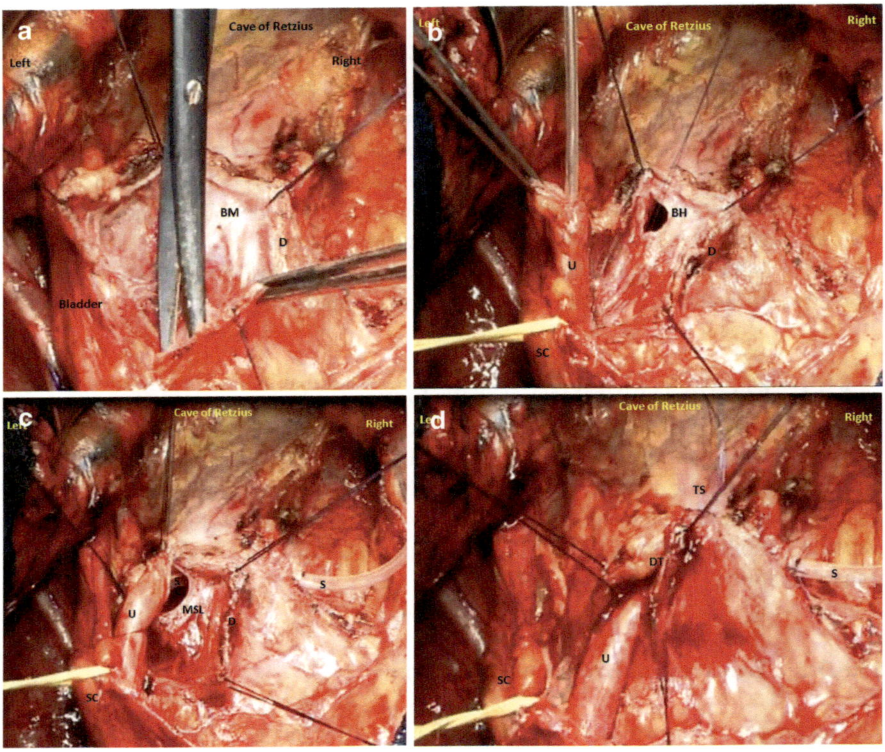

Fig. 15.3 Intraoperative photos of a Lich-Gregoir extravesical ureteroneocystostomy for treatment of a stricture in the left pelvic ureter. After ligation division of the ureter and limited dissection of the bladder on the right side and in the cave of Retzius, the bladder mucosa (BM) is dissecte off the detusor muscle (D) by sharp dissection (**a**). The ureter (U) is passed under the spermatic cord (SC) and spatulated posteriorly, a button hole (BH) is made in the distal part of the dissected BM, and multiple holding sutures are used as stays to retract the detrusor muscle (**b**). A mucosa to mucosa anastomosis is made, the lateral raw of sutures is completed first, a siliconized stent (S) is inserted, and the medial suture line (MSL) is performed later using 5/0 vicryl sutures (**c**). The ureter is now seen laid in the detrusor tunnel (DT), the tunnel is closed over the ureter using interrupted 3/0 vicryl sutures, and a toe stitch (TS) is used at the distal tunnel end to anchor the ureter (**d**)

15.8.3.3 Psoas (Vesico-psoas) Hitch

Indication

Psoas hitch is indicated when the ureteral stricture or ureteral defect is too long (around 5–10 cm) to perform ureteroneocystostomy. Other indications include fixed immobile ureter in a fibrous field, irradiated field such as in cervical cancer to get out of the latter, and in conjunction with Boari flap. The purpose of this technique is to avoid carrying out the uretero-vesical anastomosis under tension [81–83].

A hint on the Technique

Psoas hitch, which was introduced in the middle of the twentieth century, is considered as a universal technique for reimplantation of the ureter into the bladder. The procedure starts with mobilization of the bladder in the cave of Retzius and dissection on its contralateral side. Thereafter, three non-absobable sutures are used to hitch the bladder to the ipsilateral psoas muscle. The stitches should include the outer serosa and detusor muscle and should be taken with caution in order not to injure the genitofemoral nerve [81–83] (Fig. 15.4). The ureter is then implanted into the bladder with (sumucosal tunnel) or without an antireflux technique. Sometimes, psoas hitch is performed in conjunction of Boari flap if the defect in the ureter is too long to be bridged by a submucosal ureteral reimplantation.

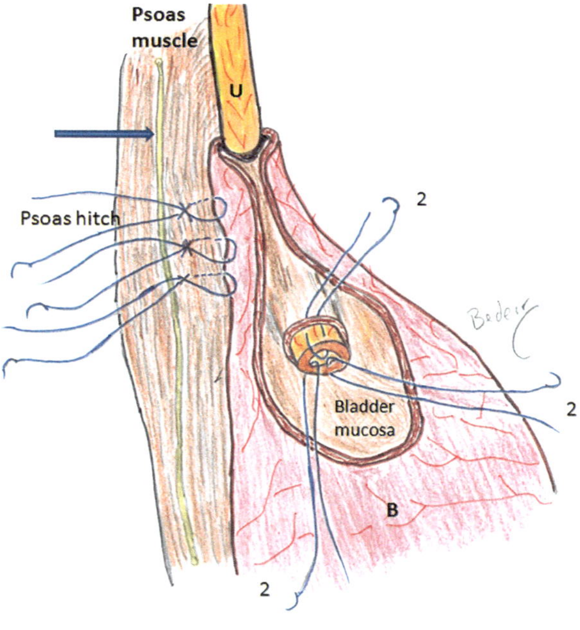

Fig. 15.4 Diagrammatic demonstration of psoas-hitch technique. Three non-absobable sutures are used to hitch the bladder to the ipsilateral right psoas muscle. The stitches include the outer serosa and detusor muscle and should be taken with caution to avoid injury of the genitofemoral nerve (arrow). The ureter (U) is then implanted into the bladder (B) with (sumucosal tunnel). A mucosal opening (button hole) is made in the distal end of the tunnel and a tension-free ureteral mucosa to bladder mucosa anastomosis is then carried out using 4/0 or 5/0 absrbable sutures (represented by the number 2)

Psoas hitch has the advantages of tension-free ureteroneocystostomy through bladder mobilization and hitching above the iliac vessels, possibility of performing a proper antireflux procedure through creation of sufficient submucosal tunnel, and prevention of ureteral kinking through implanting the ureter in fixed part of the bladder [82].

15.8.3.4 Contraindications

Psoas hitch is contraindicated in cases of neurpathic or non-compliant bladder and in cases of bladder outlet obstruction.

15.8.3.5 Boari Flap

Historically, Boari flap was introduced in the nineteenth century by the Italian surgeon, Achille Boari, and the technique was named after him [84].

Advantages and Indications

A Boari or Boari bladder flap is indicated when ureteroneocystostomy is not possible for bridging a ureteral defect arising from excision of the ureteral strictured segment. This can be seen in cases of lower or mid-ureteral strictures, which are more than five cm away from the bladder. **A properly designed and performed Boari flap can bridge a ureteral defect of up to 10–15 cm of the lower or mid-ureter** [83–85]. In addition, in exceptional cases, a spiral Boari flap can bridge a defect up to the renal pelvis, and an additional nephropexy can add 3–5 cm more [69, 86].

The advantages of the Boari flap include the repair of the ureteral defect from within the urinary tract using urothelial tissue, and its use is not contraindicated when the kidney function is impaired or in the case of bowel disease.

The indications of both psoas hitch and Boari flap include ureteral strictures/ureteral defects (5–12 cm) secondary to trauma, inflammation, fistula, or tumor, and in cases of high grade reflux, obstructive or reflexive megaureter, and duplex system provided that extravesical ureteroneocystostomy is not possible or when the ureteral mobility is too limited.

15.8.3.6 Hints on the Technique

An ascending cystogram is necessary preoperatively to assess the capacity and contour of the bladder. The procedure starts with identification and dissection of the ureter with preservation of the periureteral vascular network till a healthy segment is reached. Then, the bladder is mobilized with judicial dissection on its

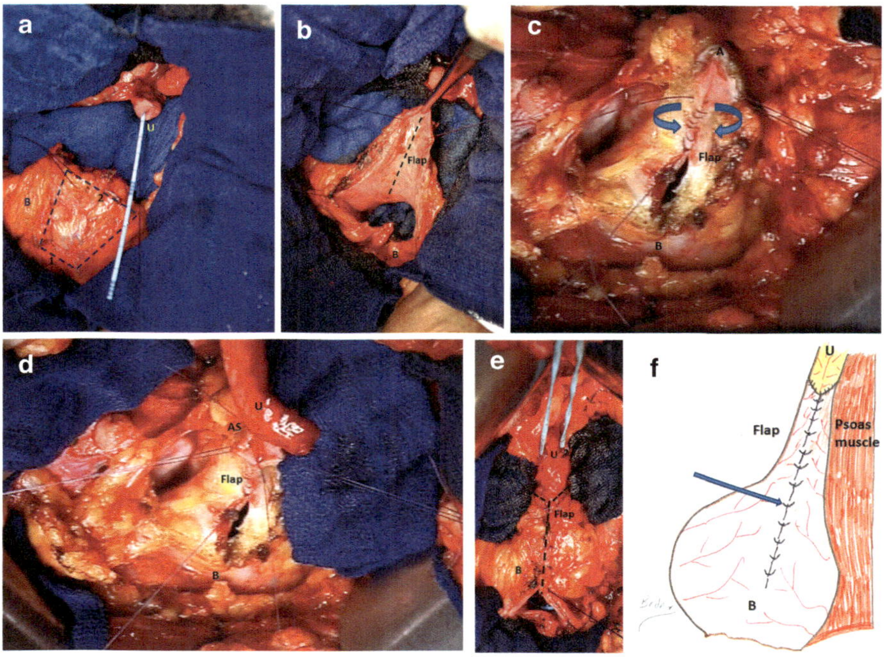

Fig. 15.5 After dissection of the bladder (B) in the cave of Retzius and on the contralateral side, a full thickness flap is then raised with the ratio of length to width (base) of the flap of 2 to 1 (**a** and **b**). Tubularization of the flap is then performed; the apex of the flap (A) and the anterior cystotomy in the bladder (B) are shown; the arrows refer to the direction of tubularization (**c**). The ureter (U) is anastomosed directly to the tubularized bladder flap, through a tension-free full thickness anastomosis including the mucosa, using 4/0 or 5/0 interrupted absrbable sutures, and starting with the apex stitch (AS) (**d**). The cystotomy is closed in two water-tight layers using running sutures (arrow), leaving a JJ stent and urethral catheter (**e** and **f**)

contralateral side. It is preferred not to dissect the bladder on the same side of the future Boari flap, in order to avoid flap ischemia. Mapping and marking the site of the Boari flap in the bladder wall is them made after defining the length of the defect in the ureter.

Figures 15.5, 15.6, and 15.7 show the technical steps of creation of a Boari flap. A full thickness flap is then raised with the ratio of length to width (base) of the flap of 2 to 1. The ureter is implanted either directly or with incorporation of antireflux procedure by implanting it in a submucosal tunnel in the raised bladder flap. The ureter is anastomosed, in a tension-free manner, to the full thickness of the flap in case of direct anastomosis or to the mucosa in case of submucosal tunnel, using interrupted absorbable sutures (4–0 or 5–0). An additional psoas hitch may be used to ensure a tension-free anastomosis. The flap is tabularized and the cystotomy s closed in two water-tight layers using running sutures. A urethral catheter and a stent are then left for one to two weeks, unless the stent is internal, where it can be removed later.

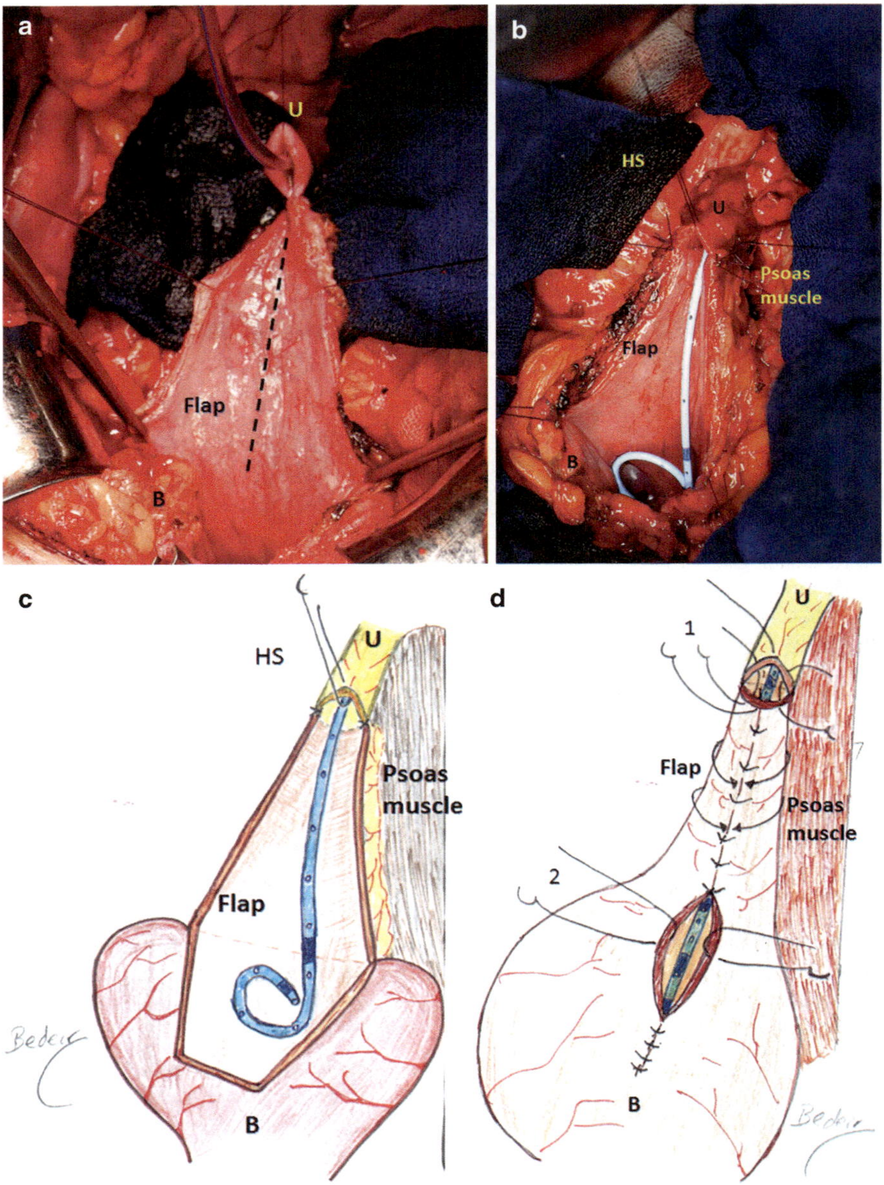

Fig. 15.6 A Modification of the Boari technique is shown. The ureter (U) is anastomosed to the raised bladder flap before the latter is tabularized (**a**). After completion of the posterior raw stitches, a JJ stent is inserted, and a holding suture (HS) is seen holding the apex of the anterior ureteral wall (**b** and **c**). The anterior raw stitches (1) are then performed using interrupted absorbable sutures (4–0 or 5–0), the flap is tabularized (arrows), and the anterior custotomy (2) is then closed (**d**)

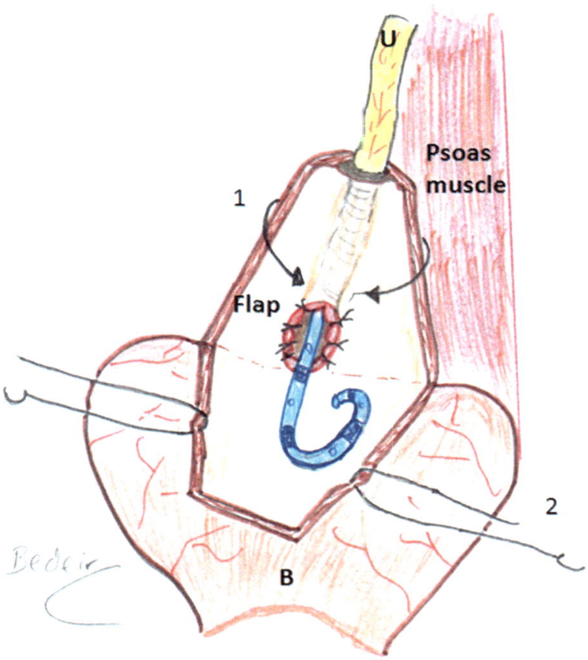

Fig. 15.7 Diagram showing Boari flap with antireflux ureteral reimplantation. The ureter (U) is implanted in a submucosal tunnel in the raised bladder flap. The ureteral opening is anastomosed, in a tension-free manner, to the bladder mucosa using interrupted absorbable sutures (4–0 or 5–0).

15.8.3.7 Contraindications

As in the case of psoas hitch, Boari flap is contraindicated in cases of neurpathic or non-compliant bladder and in cases of bladder outlet obstruction.

15.8.3.8 Outcome of Psoas Hitch and Boari Flap

In cases of pre-existing good kidney function the outcome is expected to be excellent with high success rates (80–95%), regarding resolution of hydronephrosis, alleviation of symptoms, and improvement of differential renal function [82, 87, 88]. However, in cases of chronic kidney disease or underlying chronic ureteral disorder such as in irradiated ureter, the post-operative renal function may not be improved [87, 88]. **The complications of psoas hitch/Boari flap are usually minimal and include urinary leakage requiring prolonged catheterization, stent-related complications such as dysuria and frequency, and recurrence of the disease** [87, 88].

15.8.3.9 Mininally Invasive Approaches Using Laparoscopy and Robot

Laparoscopic and robot-assisted approaches of ureteroneocystostomy, psoas hitch, Boari flap, and ureteroureterostomy have been studied extensively during the last years. It has been stated by some researches that laparoscopic Psoas hitch and Boari flap ican be performed safely and successfully with the advantages of shorter hospital stay, less blood loss, and less analgesic needs compared to the open approach [89–91]. However, such techniques are to be conducted in specialized hospitals and by highly expert laparoscopists [87]. Similarly, robot-assisted techniques are feasible for surgical treatment of ureteral strictures at all levels [91–95]. A long Boari flap up to the level of L3–L4 can be carried out by robot [92].

Overall, open surgical approaches are still the gold standard in surgical treatment of ureteral strictures, while minimally invasive laparoscopic or robot-assisted techniques are good alternatives, provided that they are carried out by high volume surgeons in high volume centers.

15.8.3.10 Ureteroureterostomy

Definition

Ureteroureterostomy (or ureteroureteral anastomosis or resection and reanastomosis of the ureter) refers to resection of a limited short segment stricture of the ureter, followed by an end-to-end reanastomosis of the two healthy segments. It is also called van Hook operation, after the name of the surgeon Weller van Hook.

Ureteroureterostomy (UU) can also be carried out in children with obstructed functioning upper moiety of a duplex system, where the healthy part of the upper moiety ureter is transected and anastomosed in an end-to-side way to the ureter of the lower moiety.

Indications

The indications of UU include short segment mid- or proximal ureteral stricture (less than 3 cm), injuries to the ureter above the pelvic brim causing a defect of less than 3 cm, and retrocaval ureter [69, 77].

Contraindications:

Long segment ureteral strictures or injury-induced defects and poor kidney function with split function of less than 15% of the total GFR are the main contraindications [77].

Technical Aspects

The technique is well known to all certified urologists (Figs. 15.8, 15.9, 15.10, and 15.11). A lumbar or flank incision is used for the proximal and a Gibson or pararectal or paramedian incision is used for the mid-ureteral stricture.

Dissection of the ureter is performed carefully in order not to devascularize the healthy segments, and then the unhealthy segment is identified. Resection of the unhealthy segment is then conducted, followed by simulation, so that the two healthy ends are reconnected without tension. Both proximal and distal ends are spatulated for about 1–1.5 cm, at 180 degrees apart (anterior and posterior or medial and lateral). This step is followed by placement of what is called the corner sutures (figure…). The corner and other sutures used for the anastomosis are absorbable 4/0 or 5/0 sutures. A tension free, water tight, mucosa-to-mucosa, and stented anastomosis is performed. Thereafter, the wound is closed in layers with tube drainage. The stent is usually endoscopically removed after four weeks.

Complications

When UU is properly conducted, the rate of complications is minimal. The complications include urinary leakage, recurrence of the stricture, and the general surgical complications such as hemorrhage, wound related complications, and adjacent organ injury.

Mininally Invasive Approaches Using Laparoscopy and Robot

Robot assisted UU has been reported and the success rate was comparable to the open approach [91].

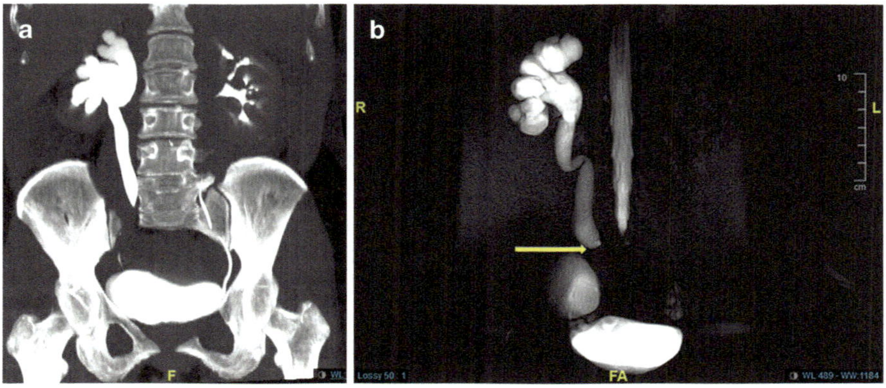

Fig. 15.8 The figure demonstrates a CTU with a stricture at the right iliac ureter (**a**), and MRU with a stricture at the same location (**b**). It was treated by UU

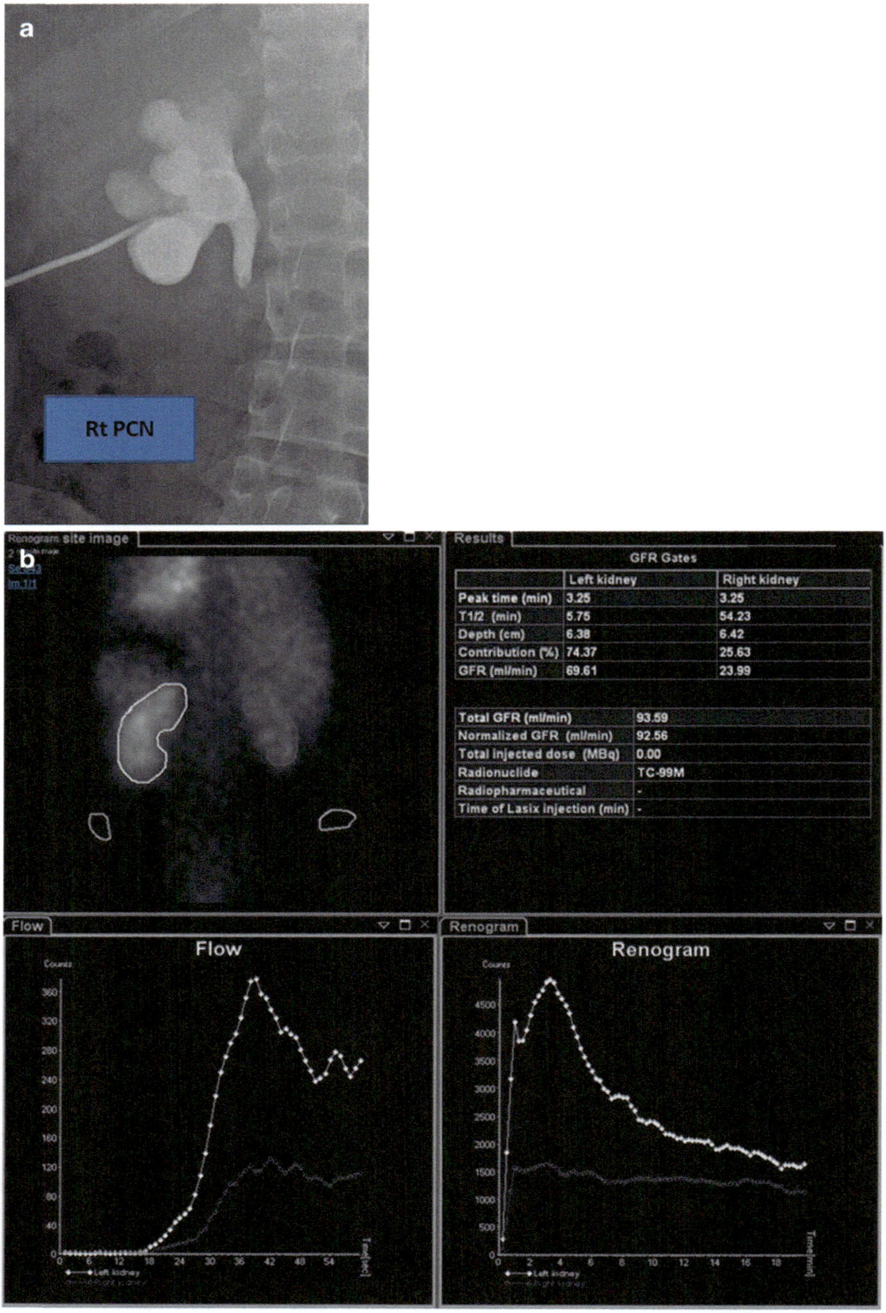

Fig. 15.9 An antegrade nephrostogram showing arrest of the dye at the level of the lumbar ureter, because of post-URS stricture (**a**). Renogram of the same case showed evidence of a decline in the right GFR with a differential function of 26% and obstructed excretory curve (**b**). The case was treated by UU

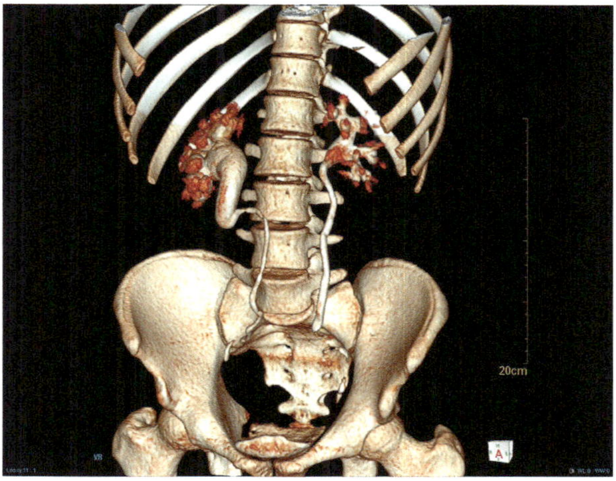

Fig. 15.10 CTU (3D CT) showing retrocaval ureter. It was treated by UU

15.8.4 Treatment of Long Segment or Multiple Ureteral Strictures

The most common techniques used to bridge long ureteral defects are the ileal ureter and its modifications. However, the list of treatment options includes transuretroureterostomy, renal autotransplantation, and ureteral substitution using a wide variety of procedures.

15.8.4.1 Transureteroureterostomy

Transureteroureterostomy (TUU) is one of the options to bridge long ureteral defect by discarding the unhealthy segment of the ureter, bringing the proximal healthy segment across the midline, and anastomosing it to the healthy contralateral ureter by an end-to-side technique (Fig. 15.12). TUU was first carried out in humans by Higgins [96].

Indications

TUU may be preferred in cases when there is extensive adhesions in the pelvis secondary to **previous complex pelvic surgery or pelvic irradiation, which makes psoas hitch or boari flap impossible** [97, 98]. It can be used in children as an alternative to complex cases of urinary reconstruction. However, the most important issue is good selection of cases [101]. In addition, when the distal ureter is affected with primary or secondary malignancy, TUU may be a suitable option of urinary diversion [99]. **The keys of success and the keys to avoid major complications are tension-free anastomosis, avoidance of ureteral kinking or angulation, and healthy non-devascularized ureter** [98].

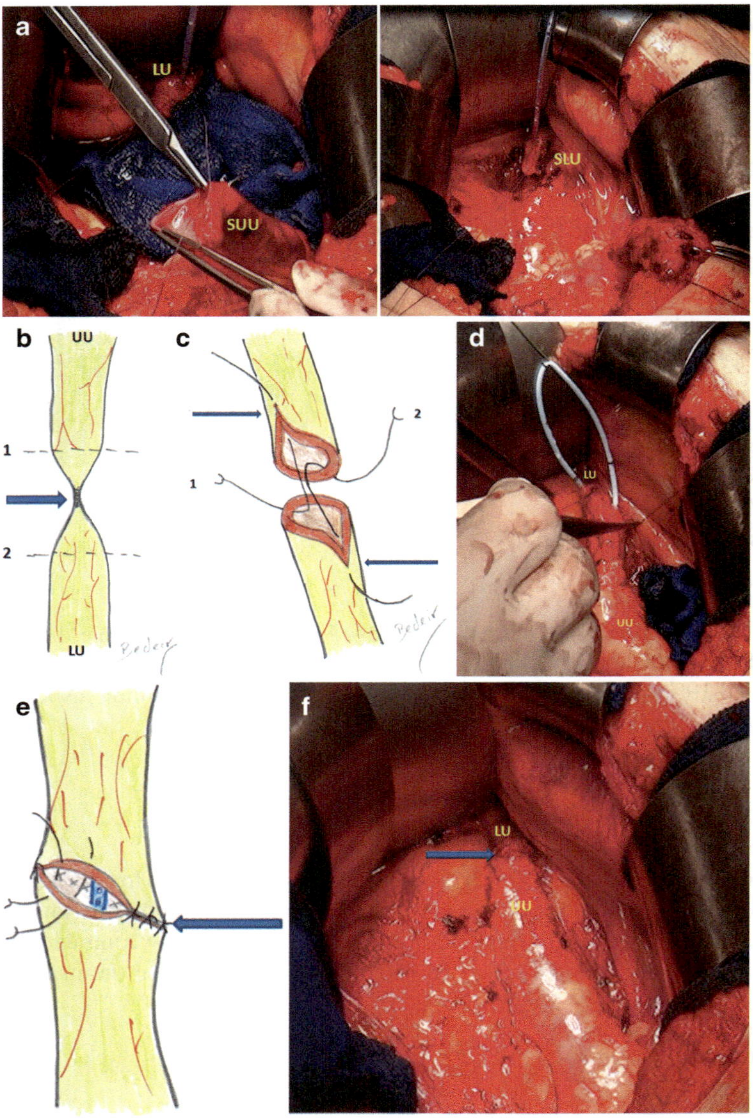

Fig. 15.11 (**a**) is an intraoperative photo demonstrationg that unhealthy segment of the left ureter was resected, followed by spatulation of the healthy upper ureter (SUU) and lower ureter (SLU) for 1–1.5 cm. (**b**) is a diagram showing the line of resection of the unhealthy segment in the upper ureter UU (1) and in the lower ureter LU (2). (**c**) is a diagram showing the direction of spatulation of the UU and LU at 180° apart (opposite direstions), with 2 holding stay sutures (5/0 absorbable) at both angles of the future anastomosis. (**d**) is an intraoperative photo showing that the posterior row suture line of the UU was completed and the JJ stent was inserted. (**e**) is a diagram demonstrating (**d**), and it shows that the anterior row sutures were started. (**f**) shows the final intraoperative scene of ureteroureterostomy, where the suture line (arrow) is seen completed between the upper ureter (UU) and lower ureter (LU)

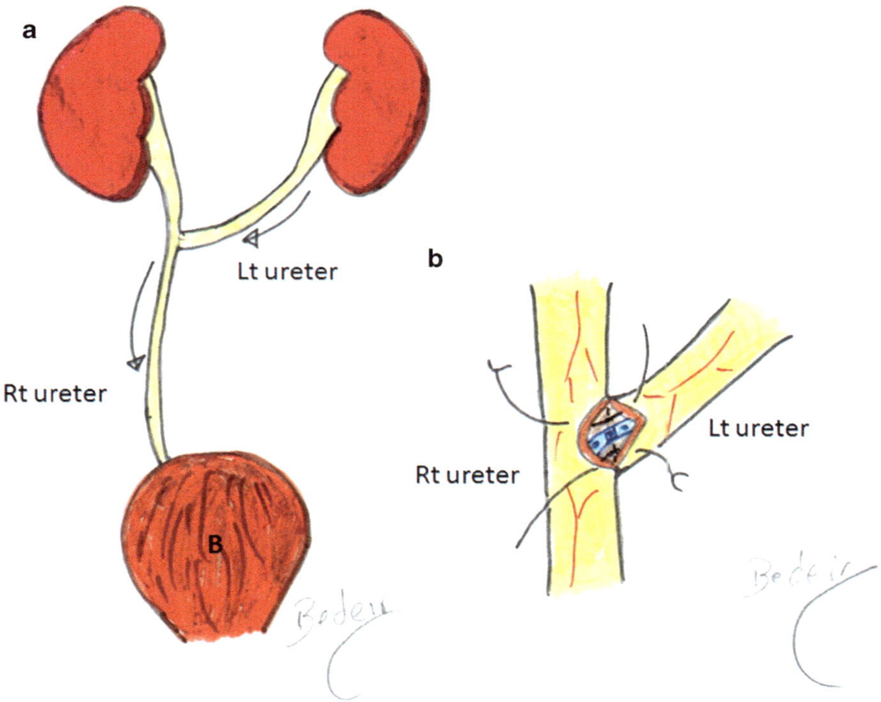

Fig. 15.12 Two diagrams demonstrating the technique of transureteroureterostomy (TUU). The unhealthy segment of the left ureter is dicarded, bringing the proximal healthy segment across the midline, and anastomosing it to the healthy right ureter by an end-to-side technique (**a**). The end-to-side anastomosis is made in 2 layers using interrupted absorbable sutures (4/0 or 5/0), beginning with the posterior row suture line, and followed by stent insertion as shown in (**b**). Then, the anterior suture line is completed

Complications

Nowadays, TUU is rarely performed since it poses both renal units at risk, especially the risk of obstruction on the contralateral healthy renal unit [102–104]. This may occur because of problems, mainly urinary leakage and stricture at the anastomotic site.

The list of complications include urinary leakage, strictures at the site of TUU or distal to it, and stone formation [100].

Contraindications

When the length of the transposed ureter is too short to reach the target site without tension, the technique is contraindicated. In addition, other contraindications include a diseased recipient ureter such as in cases of primary or secondary malignancy, RPF, stone disease, and chronic kidney disease [105, 106].

15.8.4.2 Renal Autotransplantation

Hardy in 1963 was the first one to describe the technique of renal autotransplantation or renal autotransplant; it was carried out for the treatment of high ureteral injury [107].

Technique

Renal autotransplantation for ureteral loss or ureteral stricture includes two subsequent steps, namely nephrectomy and transplantation of the kidney into the epsilateral iliac fossa using the iliac vessels for revascularization (Fig. 15.13). After revascularization, the proximal healthy ureteral segment or the renal pelvis is reimplanted into the bladder [108].

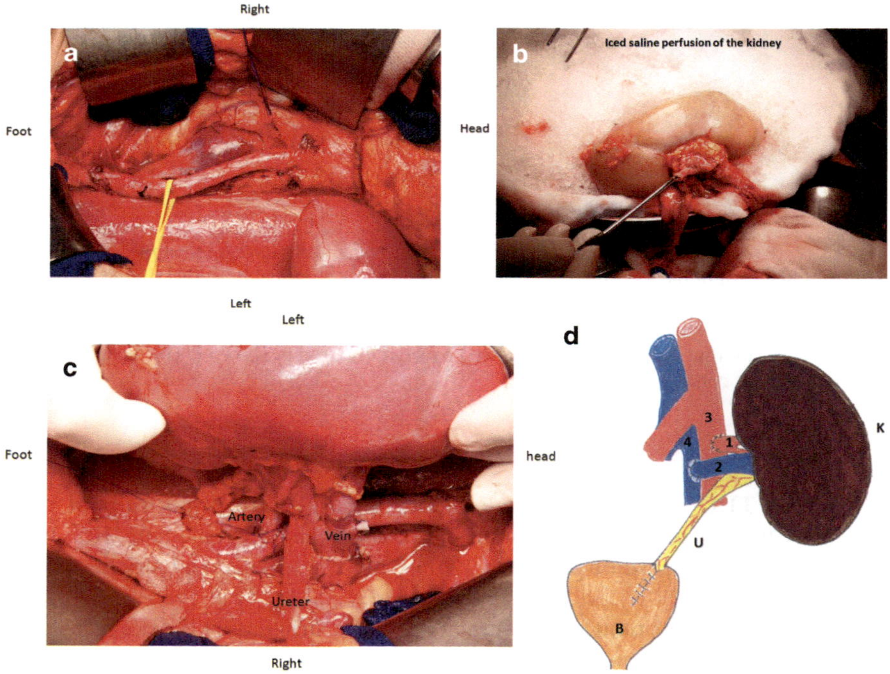

Fig. 15.13 Renal autotransplantation. (**a**) Shows that the left side iliac vessels were dissected in preparation for left kidney autotransplantation. (**b**) Shows perfusion of the kidney after nephrectomy. The perfusion is carried out using iced heparinized saline. (**c**) Demonstrates the technique of autotransplantation, where the renal vein was anastomosed end-to-side to the external iliac vein, the renal artery end-to-side to the external iliac artery, and the ureter to the bladder. (**d**) Is a diagram demonstrating the whole technique, where the kidney (K) is transplanted to the left iliac fossa, the renal artery (1) is anastomosed to the external iliac artery (3), the vein (2) to the external iliac vein (4), and the ureter (U) to the bladder (B)

The nephrectomy step can be performed laparoscopically in cases of long ureteral stricture or loss with good outcome, provided that a good cooperation between the laparoscopic and the transplant teams is conducted in for proper preparation of the harvested kidney and optimal urinary recontinuity [109].

Indications

Currently, the most frequent indications for renal autotransplantation are hematuria/loin pain syndrome or nutcracker syndrome, ureteral stricture and vascular anomalies, such renal artery aneurysm [110, 111]. In addition, the techniques may be rarely used to conduct a nephron sparing surgery (NSS) in complex renal tumors, in which NSS is not otherwise possible [112].

The technique carries the advantages of proper exposure of the bloodless surgical field, and preservation of the kidney by the induced hypothermia. **Nevertheless, renal autotransplantation is rarely performed because of the reported short term complications**, such as kidney function loss and because **many urologists are not familiar with the technique of vascular anastomosis.**

Contraindications

It is worth noting that this technique should be reserved to very highly selected cases [113, 114]. The contraindications to renal autotransplantation include previous radiotherapy or surgery on the kidney with subsequent extensive adhesions and fibrosis around the kidney. In addition, marked obstructive uropathy, chronic pyelonephritis, and marked atherosclerosis are among the contraindications, since they may lead to risky renal ischemia or risky arterial anastomosis.

15.8.4.3 Ureteral Replacement Using Techniques Other than the Ileal Ureter

Ureteroplasty Using Free Grafts

A long ureteral defect can be bridged using grafts, especially grafts from within the urinary tracts and buccal mucosa grafts. These grafts were tried in order to avoid the serious complications of either using the bowel for replacement or renal autotransplantation [115].

The donor tissue from which the graft is harvested should be hairless, easily accessible, immune to infection, and should remains viable in a wet environment [116]. There have multiple reports with somewhat promising results on the use of buccal mucosa, skin of the prepuce, mucosa of the bladder, and other grafts, such as synthetic grafts, in the treatment of long segment ureteral defects. Among these, buccal mucosa graft (BMG) is the most extensively studied [115–118].

The first experience on buccal mucosa ureteroplasty in animals was reported by Somerville and Naude, and the first human experience by Naude [119, 120].

Buccal mucosa is a very suitable graft to bridge a gap within the urinary tract because it is hairless, it resists infection, suitable to a wet invironment, and it has a thick lamina propria similar to that of the urinary tract, which augments nutrition of the graft mucosa by imbibitions [121].

BMG can be used as onlay or tabularized graft. Some authors stated that leaving the adventitia of the ureter to act as scaffold for the tabularized BMG and wrapping the graft with omentum or perinphric fat will augment the vascularization of the graft and enhance the success rate [122, 123]. However, regardless of the case series reported on successful outcome of BMG, a lot of authors are still skeptical about the use of tubularized BMG ureteroplasty because of the very poor outcome of the tabularized grafts in urethroplasty [124].

Indications

Free grafts to bridge ureteral defects are indicated in cases of strictures more than 2 cm in the mid- or upper ureter, which are not suitable for ureteroureterostomy and in cases of previously failed repair of ureteral stricture or ureteral defects [125].

Free grafts, particularly BMG, have the same indications as renal autotransplantation, TUU, and ileal ureter. However, some investigators reported that BMG may be a better choice than the others, because of the lower morbidity and less challenge associated with BMG [117, 118, 122].

Types of Free Grafts other than BMG

There have been a lot of free grafts other than BMG, which were used to reconstruct the urinary tract, including the ureter. The list includes free peritoneal graft [126], autogenous vein grafts [127], common iliac artery graft [128], a subcutaneous skin tube [129], free fascial grafts [130], and split-thickness or full thickness skin grafts [131, 132]. Overall, most of these free graft techniques were experimental, unsuccessful, and failed to gain any popular acceptance.

Grafts of Urinary Origin

Free grafts from the bladder mucosa and from autologous and homologous ureteral segment have been tested, both experimentally and clinically [133, 134]. However, the outcome was usually complicated with hydronephrosis, obstruction, and renal atrophy; therefore, their use was discontinued.

Limitations

BMG ureteroplasty and free grafts in general are of limited value and limited success when the ureteral stricture length is long, and ischemic as in the case of radiation-related stricture. Apart from BMC, all other free grafts for ureteroplasty have become historical with limited use nowadays.

Minimally Invasive Approaches for Free Grafts Used in Ureteroplasty

There are some recent reports on the use of robots in BMG for ureteroplasty, and the use of special techniques to refine the suturing technique and to precisely define the margins of the stricture [115, 117, 118]. However, most of these techniques are merely case reports or case series.

Synthetic Ureteral Substitutes

Some inert synthetic materials have been tried as ureteral prosthesis, including glass, Tantalum or Vitallium [135], Polyethylene [136], Teflon [137], silicon [138], and modified silicon prosthesis [139]. **All of these synthetic grafts are historical and are mentioned to be condemned**, because of the associated serious complications, such as encrustations, migration, obstruction, strictures, and urinary tract infections [139, 140].

Small Intestinal Submucosa

Small Intestinal Submucosa (SIS) is a xenogenic graft derived from the swine small intestine, in the form of a membrane. This biocompatible material was used for the purpose of augmentation of the bladder or for repairing a ureteral defect ureteral as an onlay and a tube [141, 142]. **It failed to gain general acceptance because of poor vascularization of the graft** [143].

Tissue Engineering and Use of Biologically Inert Materials

Tissue engineering has been recently used, where some biodegradable synthetic materials, either as polymers or collagen based, were utilized to augment regeneration of the urothelium in the urinary tract. These materials were introduced in experimental and clinical setting [144–146]. **The matrix materials act as scaffolds to enhance tissue regeneration after being seeded with cells, and these cell-based technologies of tissue engineering have been tried in the urology field and in ureteroplasty** [146].

Several experimental studies have been reported to date with positive results. The first trial to bridge a ureteral defect using collagen sponge tube graft in dogs was conducted by Tachibana et al. in 1985 [147]. However, in all dogs, proximal hydronephrosis and possibly progressive obstruction were observed. Nevertheless, because of the limited clinical studies and data on the use of these technologies in treating long segment ureteral strictures, tissue engineering in the field of ureteroplasty is still of limited value and further studies are needed to define its role.

15.8.5 Ureteral Replacement Using Pedicled Flaps

Several pedicled flaps have been reported to replace the strictured ureter, including the appendix [148, 149], fallopian tube [150], renal capsule [151], anterior abdominal wall, bladder flaps, and most commonly the pedicled bowel flaps. **Out of the pedicled bowel flaps, the ileal ureter is the most commonly performed technique**, although other intestinal segments, including the stomach, ileo-colonic segment, and the colon, have been used before [152–154].

15.8.5.1 Ileal Ureter

History

The ileal ureter describes the isolation of a pedicled ileal segment to replace the damaged or the structured ureter. The isolated ileal sements for ureteral replacement in three dogs were first described by Italian surgeons in 1900 [155]. The first ileal replacement of the ureter in humans was carried out by Shoemaker in 1906, in a woman with genitourinary tuberculosis [156]. However, the result was not satisfactory. Then, Bricker conduit as a method of urinary diversion was introduced and was successful. This led to revival of the interposition of the ileal segments into the urinary tract, until the technique of the ileal ureter has been popularized by Goodwin et al., who first used the name "ileal ureter"and stated that isolation of 15–25 cm ileal segment is necessary to achieve proper peristalsis and good drainage [157].

A Hint on Indications of the Ileal Ureter

In ureteral strictures, whatever their etiology may be, the ileal ureter is indicated when more conservative measures, such as ureteroneocystostomy, Boari flap, or psoas hitch have failed or deemed impossible to bridge a long ureteral defect [104, 158–160]. In addition, recurrent stone disease is one of the important historical indications of the ileal ureter [161, 162]. The assumption of these authors was that the reflux of urine through the refluxing ileal ureter will induce a urinary douche to washout the recurrent stones. Other indications include total ureterectomy for ureteral tumor in cases of solitary kidney [162], and in some selected cases of failed repair of ureteral stricture, or in cases of total ureteral necrosis after renal transplantation [163, 164].

Technical Aspects of the Ileal Ureter

The Classic Ileal Ureter

The technique of the classic ileal ureter is well known and entails the isolation of an isoperistaltic segment of the ileum, 20–25 cm long, to replace the strictured or damaged ureter on the right or left side [165–168]. After opening the peritoneum through a midline approach, mobilization of the cecum and ascending colon on the right, or of the sigmoid and descending colon on the left side is conducted. Sometimes, a window is made in the descending colon mesentery to facilitate proximal anastomosis of the ileum to the ureter and distal anastomosis to the badder. A full thickness button hole, sufficient to adapt the diameter of the isolated ileal ureter, is made in the posterior bladder wall. Then, the ileo-vesical anastomosis is carried out into one or two layers using (3/0 or 4/0) absorbable sutures.

The proximal uretero-ileal anastomosis is performed as a tension-free anastomosis, usually end-to-end and sometimed end-to-side. A stent, either external or internal, is left for 2 weeks (for external) and 2–6 weeks in internal stents (Fig. 15.14).

Various Arrangements of the Classic Ileal Ureter

According to Goodwin and co-workers, various arrangements of the proximal and distal anastomosis of the ileal ureter were reported [157]. Regarding the proximal anastomosis, the ileum is usually anastomosed to the proximal healthy ureter. Alternatively, it may be anastomosed to the renal pelvis or to the lower calyx. The ileal ureter may be used as a single or two loops for unilateral or bilateral ureteral defects. An augmentation ileocystoplasty may be done in a combination with ileal ureter. In addition, tailoring of the ileal ureter, or an antirefluxive ileovesical anastomosis may be carried out as alternatives to the classic ileal ureter.

Segmental Replacement of the Ureter by Ileum

When the stricture segment is located in the middle of the ureter and is too long to be repaired by ureteroureterostomy interposition of an ileal segment between the proximal and distal healthy parts of the ureter is possible (Fig. 15.15) [165, 169, 170]. Care should be taken proper spatulation of the proximal and distal ureteral segment and to tailor the distal ileal segment to make it comparable to the diameter of the distal spatulated ureter. This variation of the ileal ureter carries the advantages of isolation of a smaller ileal segment, with subsequent decline in the ileal absorption-related complications, and of preventing reflux through the natural antireflux mechanism of the distal ureter, with a further decline in reflux-related

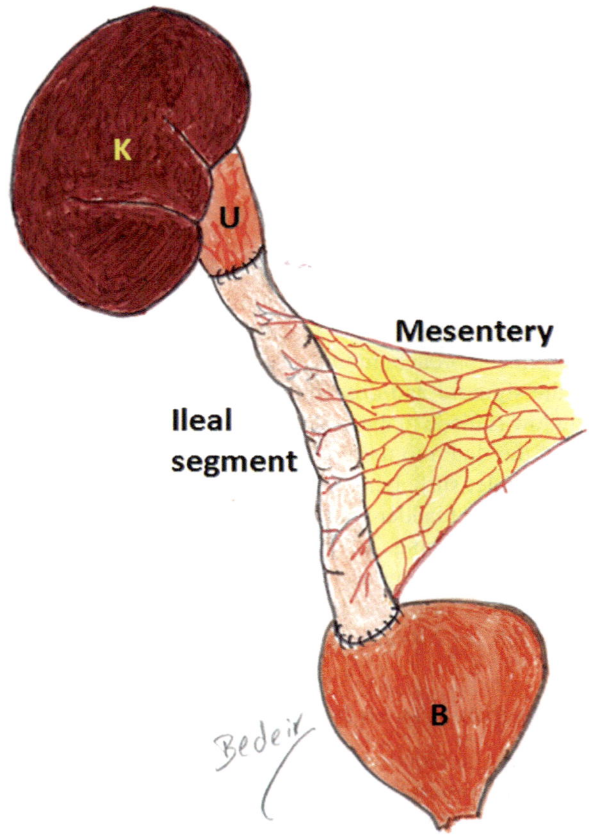

Fig. 15.14 A diagram demonstrating the classic ileal ureter. The unhealthy segment of the right ureter is dicarded, an isoperistaltic 20–25 cm segment of the terminal ileum is isolated, anastomosed proximally to the healthy segment of the ureter (U), and distally to the bladder (B)

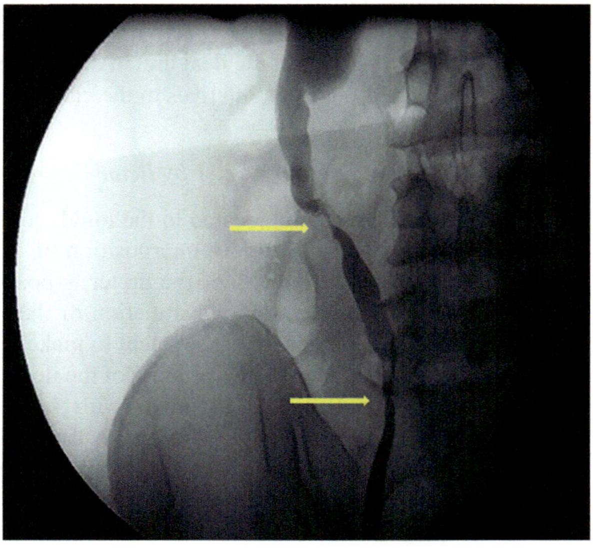

Fig. 15.15 Retrograde ureteropyelogram showing two ureteral strictures, at the iliac and low lumbar parts of the right ureter (arrows). The case was treated by ileal interposition between the two healthy parts of the ureter, after resection of the part between the two arrows

complications. An ileal patch graft has been used instead of the whole ileal loop interposition to repair ureteral stricture with good outcome and without metabolic complications [170].

Complications of the Ileal Ureter

Exposure of the ileal mucosa, which is characterized by its high absorptive potential, to the urine and reflux of urine account for the majority of important complications of the ileal ureter [162]. **The list of serious complications includes electrolyte imbalance and metabolic acidosis, especially with chronic kidney disease, stricture at the ileo-vesical anastomosis, and/or bladder outlet obstruction** [77, 162]. In addition, the condition is aggravated by the bicarbonate secretion of the ileal segment. It is worth noting that electrolyte imbalance on top of the classic ileal ureter is rare with normal kidney function, and if it ever occurs it can be easily corrected with liberal fluid intake and sodium bicarbonate [171]. In addition, deterioration of the renal function was reported in a significant sector of patients with the classic ileal ureter [172]. Furthermore, other surgery-related complications were reported, such as urinary leakage, vesico-enteric fistula, recurrent pyelonephritis, stones, and sepsis [172].

Excessive mucus secretion by the ileal segment may cause obstructive problems and may predispose to urinary tract infections. Late uro-ileal cancer may develop after ileal replacement of the ureter, usually after after a decade [173]. Therefore, it is recommended that annual surveillance of the urinary tract using cytology is to be considered in cases of ileal incorporation into the closed the urinary tract [173].

15.8.5.2 Modifications of the Classic Ileal Ureter

Because of the serious complications that may develop after the classic ileal ureter, certain technical modifications have been conducted. These modifications included incorporation of a reflux preventing procedure and decreasing the surface area exposed to the urine by tailoring of the ileal ureter or by stripping the ileal mucosa [174–177]. In addition, stripping the ileal ureter mucosa and the use of small intestinal submucosa were tried to obviate the use of ileal mucosa and prevent the uncontrolled absorption through the ileum.

Reflux Preventing Modifications

Whether an anireflux mechanism is needed in the adult population undergoing ileal ureter has been a matter of continuous debate with some investigators advocating it and others criticizing. Several modifications of the classic ileal ureter have been reported to prevent vesico-ileal reflux. The opinion of the advocates is that reflux leads to renal function deterioration on the long-term evaluation [177,

178]. Therefore, old studies stated that an antireflux procedure should be done in young patients with longer life expectancy and that reflux prevention is mandatory to prevent scarring of the kidney in animals [179–182]. In addition, an antirefluxive ureteroileal anastomosis in a Bricker conduit urinary diversion may be necessary for prevention of bacteriuria and renal scarring [181].

Several reflux prevention techniques have been reported in association with the ileal ureter and they include:

Intussuscepted Nipple Valve at the Vesico-Ileal Junction

An intussuscepted nipple valve fashioned in the terminal part of the ileum at the junction between the bladder and the ileal ureter was used to prevent vesico-ileal reflux [177]. This was performed together with tailoring of the ileal segment in a modification of the ileal ureter.

The nipple valve was originally fashioned using 3 to 4 raws of metal staples to maintain the fashioned intussusception, which were complicated in the long term with stone formation at the staples and valve desussception. To avoid the use of metallic staples, a stapleless antireflux nipple valve was reported with acceptable outcome, where the created intussusception was maintained with multiple raws of silk sutures [183].

Ileo-psoas Tunnel or Subserous Tunnel at the Proximal End

A group of investigators described the use of what they called ileo-psoas tunnel at the proximal end of the ileal ureter to prevent reflux [184]. The ureter was placed between the isolated ileal segment and the psoas muscle and the result was satisfactory.

Submucosal Bladder Tunnel (Mucosal Sulcus)

It is performed by implantation of the distal part of the isolated ileum into the bladder through a mucosal sulcus [185]. Later on, the bladder mucosa will grow over the ileal serosa to create a tunnel for reflux prevention. This technique showed satisfactory results both at experimental and clinical setting; however, the anastomotic stricture rate was high because of ischemia with subsequent failure of the antireflux procedure.

Proximal Submucosal Ileal Tunnel

In this technique the terminal ureter is implanted in a sulcus made in the mucosa of the ileal segmen over a length of more than 3 cm, where the implanted ureter is covered later on by the mucosa, thus fashioning a submucosal ileal tunnel at the proximal uretero-ileal anastomosis [186].

Yang Needle Tunneling Technique

This technique can be used to anastomose the terminal ureter, in a submucosal tunnel created by the Yang needle, into the ileal segment without making a sulcus in the ileal mucosa [187].

Tailoring of the Ileal Ureter

To decrease the diameter of the ileal ureter with subsequent decrease of the absorptive capacity, tailoring of the isolated segment was advocated by several authors [162, 177, 180, 188, 189]. The risk of electrolyte and acid-base disturbance is thus minimized. Another advantage of tailoring is that it improves the propulsive property of the ileal ureter and prevents stasis of the urine in the dilated ileum [180, 189]. Also, it allows minimal mucus production, which is of particular importance in children [162]. Similarly, a new variation of tailoring called amphora-like ileal ureter was described to replace the tuberculous ureter with good result [190]. However, tailoring of the ileal ureter may be attended with some limitations, because it is complex, time-consuming, and it may jeopardize the vascular supply of the ileum [185]. In addition, when the indication of the ileal ureter is recurrent stone formation, no reflux-preventing valve or tailoring is indicated. This is to facilitate easy passage of the stones through the wide-lumen refluxing ileal ureter. Furthermore, the refluxing urine will induce a washout effect on the renal and calyceal stones [162].

Critics of Antireflux Techniques

Recent investigators reported that an antireflux technique is not needed and that reflux seems to induce no harmful impact on the kidney function in adults undergoing ileal replacement of the ureter [191–195]. Furthermore, all reflux-preventing anastomotic techniques are attended with higher incidence of complications, especially strictures, compared to direct anastomotic procedures [191].

In one of the studies and over a long term follow-up, although reflux was present in 87% of the cases, the outcome of refluxing ileal ureter was good in 81% of the patients, and the majority of these patients showed static or improved serum creatinine and pelvicalyceal system dilation [192]. Similarly, another group of investigators stated that the use of ileal ureter without a reflux preventing procedure is safe, where all their patients maintained their kidney function without deterioration in a long-term assessment [193]. Also, radiographic studies showed stable or improved dilation of the ureter and pelvicalyceal system on long-term follow-up. In addition, the ileovesical anastomosis was performed as a direct refluxing and using an antireflux technique and both procedures were compared in dogs [194]. These authors concluded that an antireflux technique is not necessary to maintain the kidney function and morphology of the collecting system. Furthermore, the same conclusion was drawn by more recent researchers, where the kidney function was maintained or improved after the use of refluxing ileal ureter [195].

15.8.5.3 The Yang-Monti Principle-based Ileal Ureter

In principle, ileal replacement of the ureter using the Yang-Monti principle was introduced to overcome the problems and limitations of the classic ileal ureter and to minimize the complications associated with the latter. The Yang-Monti principle entails the construction of a long narrow tube from a short bowel segment, usually the ileum, through longitudinal incision of the bowel segment close to its mesenteric border, thus converting the circular muscle layer into a longitudinal one, followed by reconfiguration [187, 196]. **It was first described by Yang et al.** [187] **and then the experimental and clinical application of the technique was verified by Monti et al.** [196]. The reconfigured tube, in their studies, was used as a continent conduit connected to the skin. Because of the good results of this technique, it was widely recognized and accepted.

Few investigators used the same principle in reconfiguration of the colon, in order to bridge a ureteral defect and the constructed tube was connected either to the skin, ileal conduit, or to the pouch [197–199]. In all these trials, no ileovesical anastomosis was performed. However, colon handling is not that easy because its blood supply is precious, epiploic appendixes may be abundant in obese people, and the colon may be affected by various diseases, like ulcerative colitis or diverticulosis. All these reasons have limited the use of the colon and subsequently made the ileum a more suitable choice for replacement of the ureter, unless the ileum is affected by previous irradiation.

The first application of the Yang-Monti principle, in a closed urinary tract to replace the ureter by reconfigured ileal tube between the renal pelvis and the bladder, was conducted on dogs in the Urology and Nephrology Center, Mansoura University, by a group of investigators from Mainz, Germany and Mansoura, Egypt [200]. In the experimental setting, the technique was attended with excellent and encouraging results. **The first clinical application of the use of Yang-Monti ileal ureter in a closed urinary tract was reported by Ali-El-Dein and Ghoneim** [201]. The good functional results and the low rate of complications of this new technique have encouraged several authors to use it with satisfactory functional outcome [202–207].

The Technique

Initial Evaluation

Patients undergoing Yang-Monti ileal ureter were initially assessed by urine analysis, urine culture, serum creatinine, electrolytes, blood gases, and other routine laboratory investigations. In addition to serum creatinine, the renal function was evaluated by a renogram, in the form of DTPA or MAG-3, and/or eGFR [201, 208, 209]. A magnetic resonance urography (MRU), antegrade/ retrograde ureteropyelography were conducted to define the site, laterality, and extent of the ureteral pathology.

Technical Details

At first the length of the defect or gap in the ureter is detrmined. Based on this gap, isolation of 5 or 7.5 cm long terminal ileal segment is decided [201, 208, 209]. Restoration of the gut continuity is then performed. Then, subdivision of the isolated segment of the ileum into two or three units was done and their respective blood supply was preserved (Figs. 15.16, 15.17, 15.18, and 15.19). Longitudinal paramesenteric incision of the subdivided units is then made. If three units are to be used, the middle unit is incised at the antimesenteric border.

After incising the units (subdivided segment), unfolding of the intestinal wall into two or three sheets is carried out. This is followed by suturing of the two or three sheets together through their adjacent edges using 4/0 absorbable sutures. This will result in a uniform intestinal sheet 12 to 18 cm long and 2.5 cm in width. The isolation of 5 cm ileal segment i.e. two units will result in 12 cm sheet or plate, while isolation of 7.5 cm segment i.e. three units will result in 18 cm long sheet. Around 16-Charriere Nelaton tube, the common sheet is then tabularized. Proximally, the ileal tube is anastomosed to the terminal ureter or to the renal pelvis using 4/0 absorbable sutures. Distally, the ileal tube was implanted into the bladder by either a direct refluxing anastomosis, or by a Lich-Gregoir like extravesical antireflux ileovesical anastomosis. A siliconised stent is then fixed and removed after three weeks. The latter is removed after the suture line integrity has been tested using a contrast material injected either through the stent or through the PCN in cases with preoperative fixation of PCN.

Advantages of the Technique

After its creation, the Yang-Monti ileal tube will be devoid of mesentery at its proximal end, which facilitates appropriate anastomosis between the ureter and the ileum, and at its distal end, which gives the possibility of a Lich-gregoir technique, whenever needed. In addition, this technique has several advantages when compared with the classic or the modified ileal ureter [201, 208, 209]. **A shorter ileal segment is needed, from which a long narrow ileal tube is fashioned. This will lead to much less mucous production, and less transmucosal absorption with subsequent decline of the incidence metabolic acidosis and renal impairment** [201, 208, 209]. **Furthermore, this technique provides a unidirectional antegrade passage of the urine,** like the normal ureter, contrariwise to the to-and-fro irregular peristalsis of the older versions of the ileal ureter [210] (see Supplementary Video 15.1; video clip).

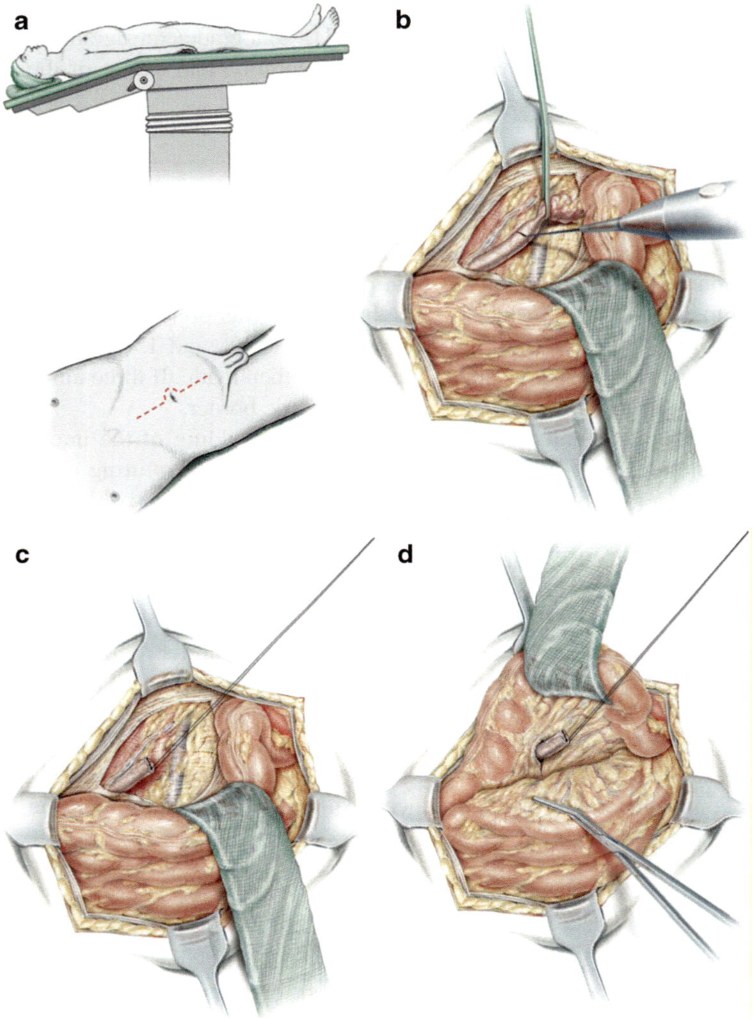

Fig. 15.16 Diagrammatic representation of the Yang-Monti ileal replacement of the ureter. Reproduced with permission from *"Ghoneim MA, Ali-El-Dein B. Replacing the ureter by an ileal tube, using the Yang-Monti procedure. BJU Int. 2005 Feb;95(3):455–70. doi: 10.1111/j.1464-410X.2005.05369.x. PMID: 15679821."* (**a**) The left ureter became obstructed after a complicated ureteroscopy. The patient is placed supine position and a median laparotomy performed. (**b**) The paracolic gutter is incised and the descending colon reflected medially to expose the retroperitoneum. The left ureter is exposed proximal to and away from the strictured segment to avoid difficult dissection of the dense adhesions with the possibility of injury to adjacent structures. A loop is passed beneath the ureter and held up for traction, to facilitate its dissection. (**c**) The ureter is transected at a healthy well vascularized segment and freed cranially, taking care to preserve its blood supply. A stay suture is applied which helps later in proper orientation to avoid the possibility of any axial rotation. (**d**) A sufficiently wide, properly placed buttonhole is created in the left mesocolon near its base; this site is carefully selected to avoid injury of the mesocolic vessels. With the help of the previously inserted stay suture, the ureter is pulled through this window and laid intraperitoneally

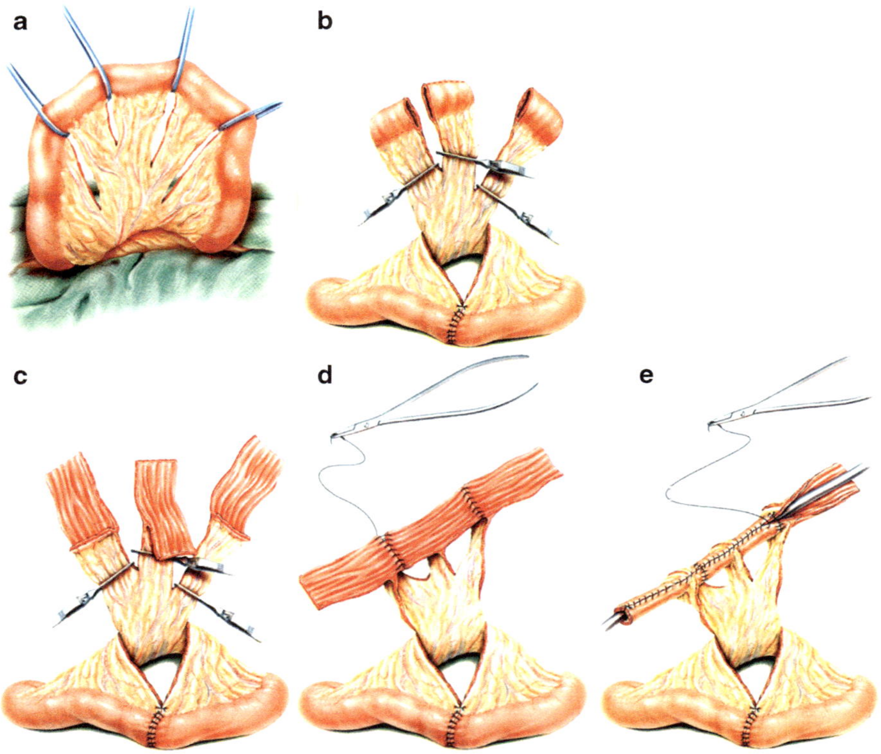

Fig. 15.17 Diagrammatic representation of the Yang-Monti ileal replacement of the ureter (continued). Reproduced with permission from *"Ghoneim MA, Ali-El-Dein B. Replacing the ureter by an ileal tube, using the Yang-Monti procedure. BJU Int. 2005 Feb;95(3):455–70. doi: 10.1111/j.1464-410X.2005.05369.x. PMID: 15679821."* (**a**) The intestinal substitute is derived from the terminal ileum; a segment 6–7 cm long is usually sufficient. The main operating room lights are switched off. With back transillumination, the arborization of the blood vessels within the mesentry is clearly visible. The selected segment is further subdivided into three equal parts, with preservation of the individual blood supply. (**b**) The isolated segments are then separated and the continuity of bowel re-established. The pedicles of the isolated ileal rings are temporarily controlled by a soft bulldog clamp. (**c**) Each ring is then incised along its longitudinal axis; the incisions of the most proximal and distal segments are not at the antimesenteric border but close to the mesenteric attachments. The incised segments are unfolded and their adjacent ends sutured together using 4/0 absorbable material. (**d**) The result is the creation of an intestinal plate of 2.5 cm wide and 16–18 cm long. (**e**) This plate is then tubularized around a 16 F Nelaton catheter using a continuous 4/0 absorbable material. The result is the formation of an ileal tube with a suitable cross-sectional diameter and of sufficient length. The ends of this tube are devoid of any mesenteric attachments, because of the asymmetric incisions of the proximal and distal rings. This facilitates anastomosis of the tube to the ureter proximally and its potential antirefluxive implantation in the bladder distally

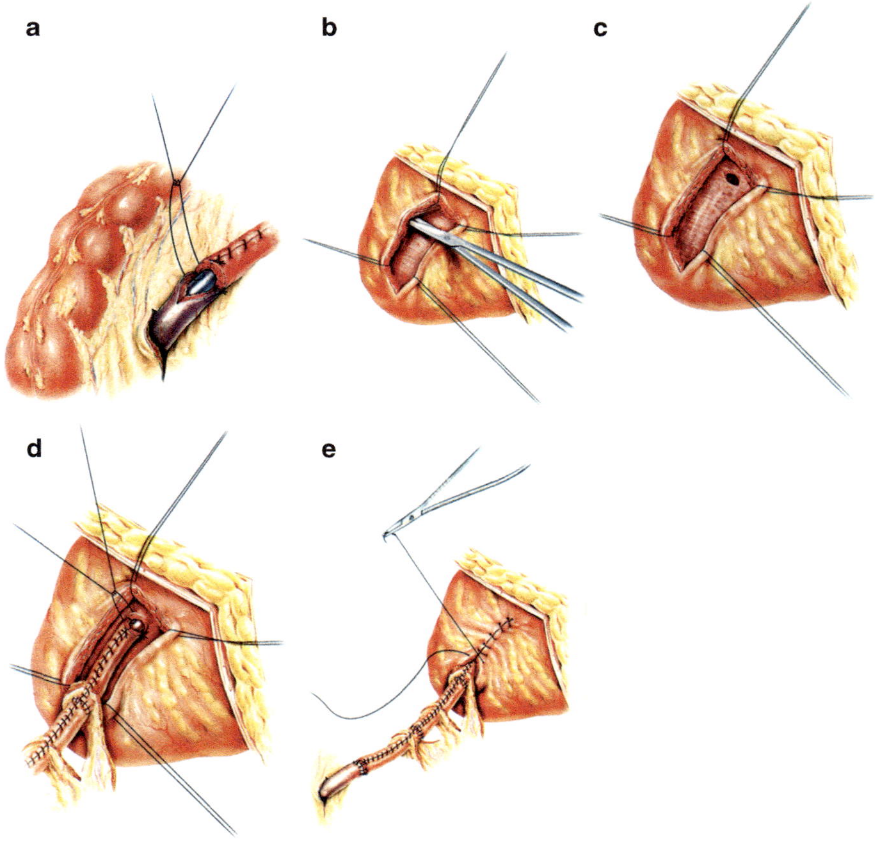

Fig. 15.18 Diagrammatic representation of the Yang-Monti ileal replacement of the ureter: proximal and distal anastomoses (continued). Reproduced with permission from *"Ghoneim MA, Ali-El-Dein B. Replacing the ureter by an ileal tube, using the Yang-Monti procedure. BJU Int. 2005 Feb;95(3):455–70. doi: 10.1111/j.1464-410X.2005.05369.x. PMID: 15679821."* (**a**) An end-to-end-anastomosis is now made between the cephalic end of the ileal tube and the spatulated proximal ureter. The previously inserted stay suture helps in orientation and prevents any tendency for axial rotation. The anastomosis is made using interrupted 4/0 absorbable sutures and stented using a silicone tube of suitable size (10–12 F). (**b**) The distal end of the ileal tube is then implanted into the bladder by a nonrefluxing ileo-vesicostomy, using the Lich-Gregoir principle. The bladder is moderately filled with saline solution. Exposing a 4–5 cm aspect of the bladder wall, the incision is carried out through the perivesical fascia, the detrusor muscle and down to the submucosa. The fascial muscular flaps are raised on either side by further dissection using a fine pair of scissors with a blunt tip. Care is taken to avoid injury of the underlying mucous membrane. (**c**) The bladder is then emptied of its fluid contents. A buttonhole is excised from the mucosa at the distal end of this trough. (**d**) A stented mucosa-to-mucosa anastomosis is then made between the vesical mucosal membrane and the distal end of the ileal tube, using interrupted 5/0 absorbable material. (**e**) The previously dissected flaps are joined together in front of the ileal tube using interrupted 3/0 absorbable sutures

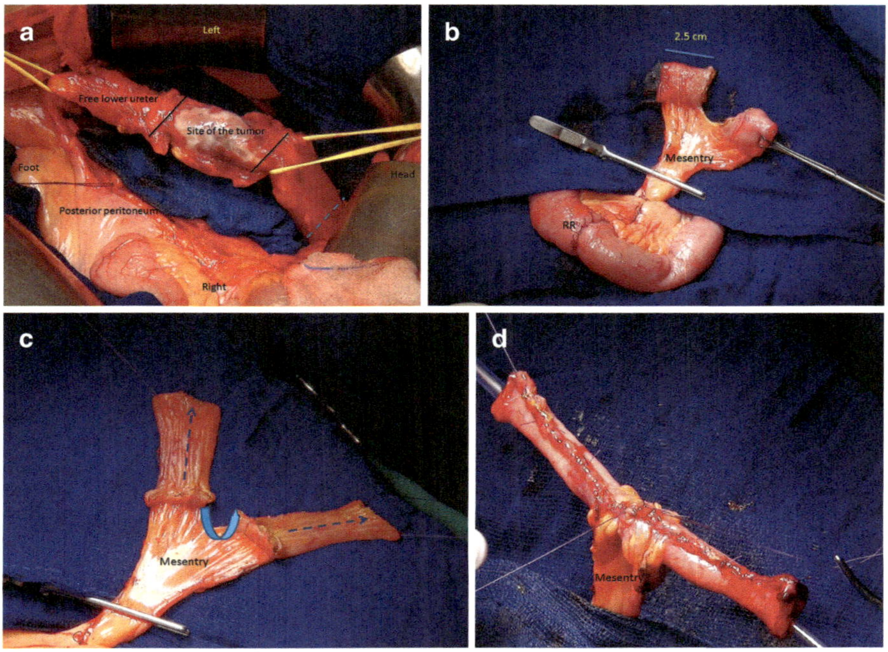

Fig. 15.19 Intraoperative photos of Yang-Monti ileal ureter. Reproduced with permission from *"Ali-El-Dein B, et al. Long-term Outcome of Yang-Monti Ileal Replacement of the Ureter: A Technique Suitable for Mild, Moderate Loss of Kidney Function and Solitary Kidney. Urology. 2021 Jun;152:153-159. doi: 10.1016/j.urology.2020.09.061. Epub 2021 Jan 14. PMID: 33359492."* (**a**) Intra-operative photo showing dissection of the whole left ureter in a 70-year old man with solitary left kidney. A tumor is seen involving 4 cm of the mid ureter. The dotted line on the upper ureter defines the line of transection in the healthy ureter (3 cm above the upper margin of the tumor). (**b**) The figure shows isolation of 5 cm. of the terminal ileum. This segment is further divided into 2 equal segments; each is 2.5 cm. long. Recontinuity of the ileum is made (RR). Sometimes, three segments (2.5 cm.) are isolated to bridge a longer defect. (**c**) Each segment is longitudinally incised close to its mesentery and then unfolded. The adjacent edges of the unfolded segments are subsequently sutured to each other using fine absorbable stitches to form a uniform (2.5 × 12 cm.) intestinal sheet. (**d**) Thereafter, the intestinal sheet (plate) is then tubularized around a 16 Fr Nelaton tube using fine absorbable sutures. The proximal end of the tube is then anastomosed to the proximal ureter, while the distal end is implanted into the bladder, with or without an antireflux Lich-Gregoir technique

Postoperative Evaluation and Follow-up

The patients are followed up by the same measures conducted at initial evaluation [201, 208, 209]. The laboratory investigations, including serum creatinine are performed every 3 months. Imaging studies, renogram, and eGFR are carried out 3 months after the operation and they are repeated after 1 year.

Outcome of the Technique

Excellent outcomes have been achieved, as reported by several authors [201, 207, 208, 210]. **It is a safe procedure and can be successfully utilized in patients with mild loss of the renal function, in whom the classic ileal ureter is contraindicated** [208] (Figs. 15.20 and 15.21). Long-term evaluation after Yang-Monti ileal ureter showed that the function of the kidney was preserved or improved in most cases [208].

Few complications may arise after this technique, most importantly urinary leakage, urinary tract infection, and localized peritonitis [207, 208, 210, 211]. Therefore, it is recommended that temporary urinary diversion using either external stent or PCN is indicated, along with perioperative broad spectrum antibiotic prophylaxis [168, 207, 208, 210, 211].

In summary, in long or multiple ureteral defects and when the psoas hitch and/or Boari flap are impossible, this technique can provide an effective solution much better than renal autotransplantation, transurteroureterostomy, or nephrectomy [208, 210, 211]. **Meticulous and close follow-up is mandatory after Yang-Monti ileal ureter to assess the kidney function. It is worth noting that the technique is contraindicated when eGFR is less than 40 ml/min/1.73 m^2** [208].

15.8.5.4 Minimally Invasive Approaches for Ileal ureter and Yang-Monti Technique

A few trials on the robot-assisted ileal ureter have been reported [91, 166, 212–216]. The first robot-assisted ileal replacement of the ureter was reported by Wagner *and co-workers in 2008 in a patient with a single kidney, cystinuria, and recurrent stricture of the ureter* [212]. They reported that the technique was performed partially intra- and partially extracorporeal. However, complete intracorporeal robotic ileal replacement of the ureter was performed by few investigators later on [213, 214]. In addition, the techniques of laparoscopic or robotic ileal ureter and Yang-Monti technique were carried out in children with satisfactory results [215, 216]. However, so far, the open approach is still the gold standard in performing such complex procedures.

Fig. 15.20 Outcome in one of the patients treated with Yang-Monti ileal ureter. Reproduced with permission from "*Ali-El-Dein B, Ghoneim MA. Bridging long ureteral defects using the Yang-Monti principle. J Urol. 2003 Mar;169(3):1074-7. doi: 10.1097/01.ju.0000050151.66653.cc. PMID: 12576849.*" (**a**) Preoperative antegrade study shows long stricture of low and mid ureter beginning from lower border of third lumbar vertebra. (**b**) Antegrade study in the same patient 3 weeks after operation demonstrates unidirectional nonobstructed antegrade passage of dye. (**c**) Postoperative magnetic resonance urography reveals improved configuration of left renoureteral unit without evidence of obstruction. (**d**) At 6 months gravity cystography showed no reflux

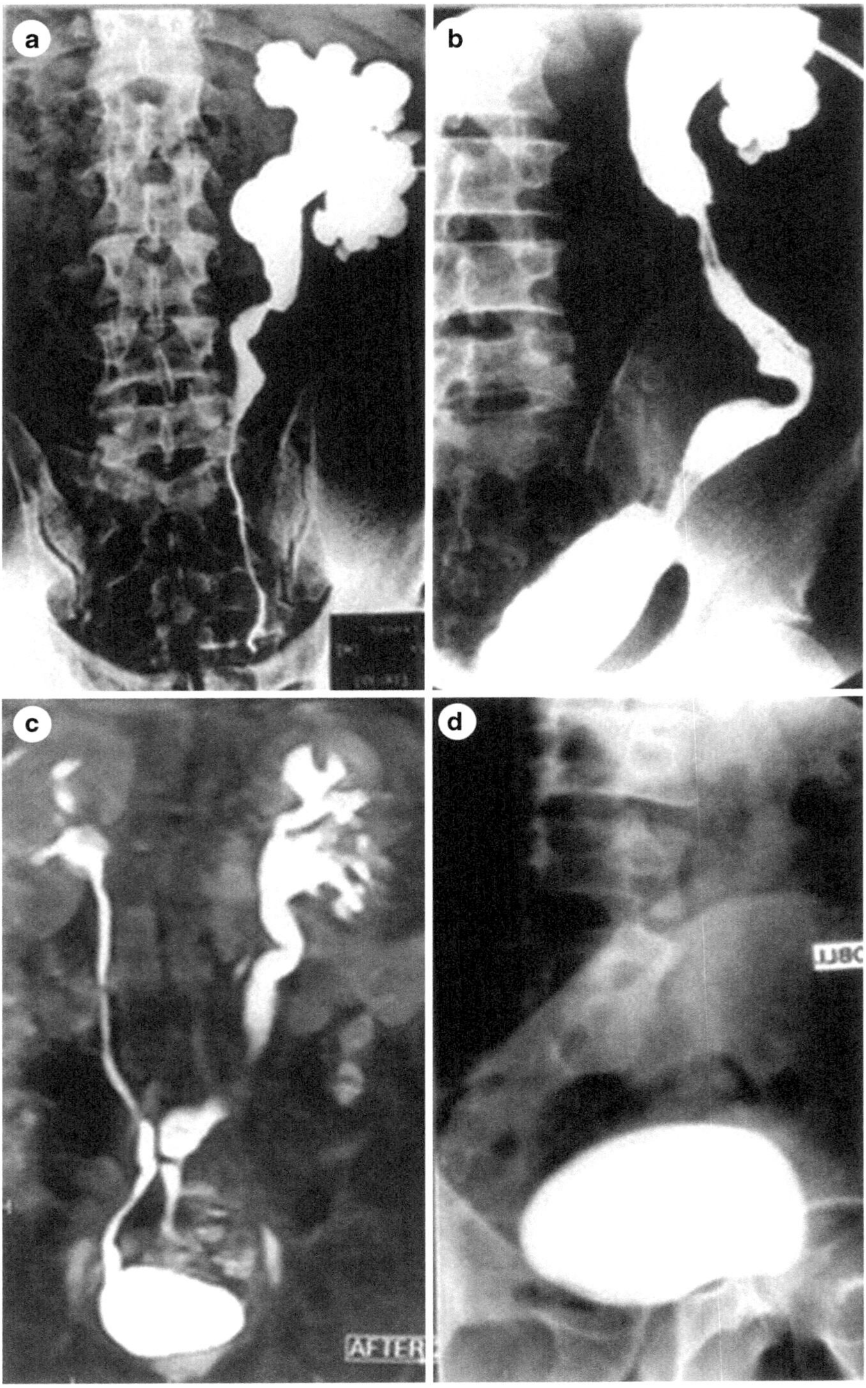
a
b
c
d
AFTER

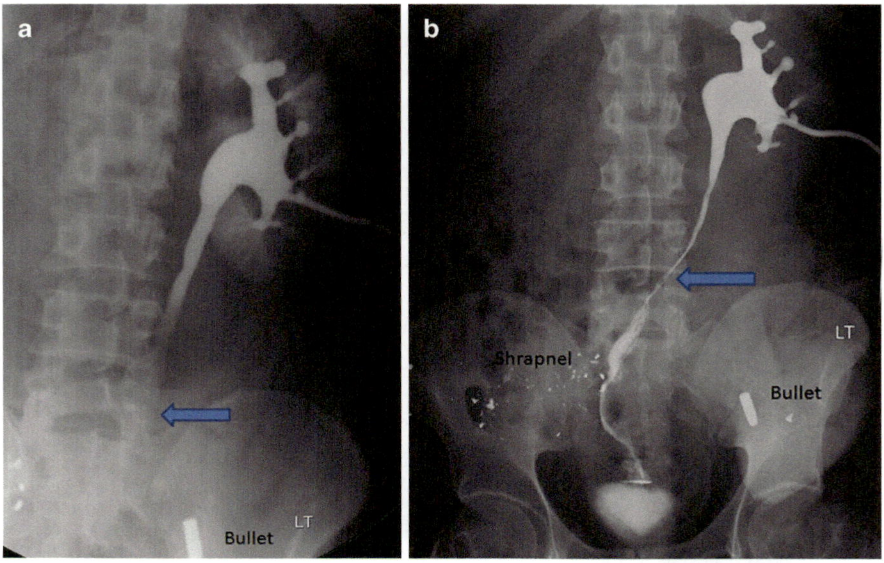

Fig. 15.21 Outcome in another patient treated with Yang-Monti ileal ureter. Reproduced with permission from *"Ali-El-Dein B, et al. Long-term Outcome of Yang-Monti Ileal Replacement of the Ureter: A Technique Suitable for Mild, Moderate Loss of Kidney Function and Solitary Kidney. Urology. 2021 Jun;152:153-159. doi: 10.1016/j.urology.2020.09.061. Epub 2021 Jan 14. PMID: 33359492."* 29-year old Yemeni man with multiple injuries because of gunshot presented with colostomy and left nephrostomy tube with history of abdominal exploration twice and failed left ureterovesical reimplantation. Pre-operative left antegrade nephrostogram (**a**) shows arrest of the contrast at the low lumbar ureter, with evidence of the bullet and shrapnel. Two months after ileal replacement of the damaged ureter using the Yang-Monti ileal ureter, post-operative antegrade nephrostogram (**b**) shows free passage of the contrast through the reconfigured ileal ureter to the bladder

15.8.5.5 Contraindications to the Ileal Ureter

Among the most important contraindications to the ileal ureter is chronic kidney disease or renal impairment. However, the Yang-Monti ileal ureter can be conducted safely in cases of mild to moderate loss of the kidney function, when it is the only available treatment option [208]. The cutoff value of serum creatinine or creatinine clearance, beyond which ileal replacement of the ureter is contraindicated, is still debatable. Most urologists stated that a serum creatinine of 2 mg/dL or more is a contraindication to the ileal ureter [217]. In another study, a threshold of 1.7 mg/dL was stated [218]. Furthermore, in the study of Ali-El-Dein et al. in 2021, a threshold of 2.4 mg/dL was stated if the Yang-Monti technique was used. Nevertheless, the use of serum creatinine as a kidney function cutoff is not accurate, and we recommend that the kidney function is to be assessed by preoperative renography and/or eGFR [208]. In this setting, if the eGFR is less than 40 ml/min/1.73 m^2, any sort of ileal replacement of the ureter is contraindicated [208].

The contraindications to ileal ureter also include neuropathic bladder, bladder outflow obstruction, and urethral stricture or obstruction, because in these situations a high pressure reflux is induced with subsequent deterioration of the kidney function [162]. In addition, short bowel syndrome or inflammatory bowel disease are definite contraindications to the ileal ureter [159]. Also, in cases of liver disease with hepatic functional disorders, the ileal ureter is contraindicated because hepatic encephalopathy may result from undue absorption of nitrogenous waste into the blood, particulary in cases of portocaval shunt [165].

15.8.5.6 Summary on the Ileal Ureter

Overall, ileal ureter is a complex procedure that should be performed as a last resort when replacement of the ureter can't be conducted using urothelium-lined tissue and techniques such as psoas hitch and/or Boari flap. It is a viable alternative to the ablative solution of nephrectomy and to the more demanding techniques of renal autotransplantation or transureteroureterostomy. The classic ileal ureter is attended with a lot of major complications on the long run. So, the Yang-Monti ileal ureter is considered as the best choice of the use of ileum in replacement of the damaged ureter.

15.8.6 A hint on the Treatment of RPF

Both ureters may be involved in RPF, leading to deviation of their middle parts to a medial position. The disease is sometimes called "Ormond's disease". What is called "**narrow-waisted maiden**" is thus produced when the ureters are opacified on IVU, CTU, or MRU [219]. Usually, blood levels of inflammatory markers are elevated in RPF, including erythrocyte sedimentation rate (ESR) and C-reactive protein [220, 221]. Most cases of RPF are idiopathic, and if it is diagnosed early and timely treated, the prognosis is good.

The most effective and classical treatment of RPF is urgical intervention [25, 201, 208]. However, when the RPF-related obstructive uropathy is initially relieved, medical treatment in the form of steroids, tamoxifen, and other immunosuppressive drugs may be used with somewhat satisfactory results if started early [219].

Surgical treatment ranges from cystoscopic guided fixation of JJ stents up to ileal replacement of the ureter [25, 201]. However, ureterolysis and omental or peritoneal wrapping is the most appropriate and specific treatment of idiopathic RPF after a period of steroid treatment (Figs. 15.22 and 15.23). Laparoscopic and open approaches have been descried for this mode of treatment [25, 222, 223].

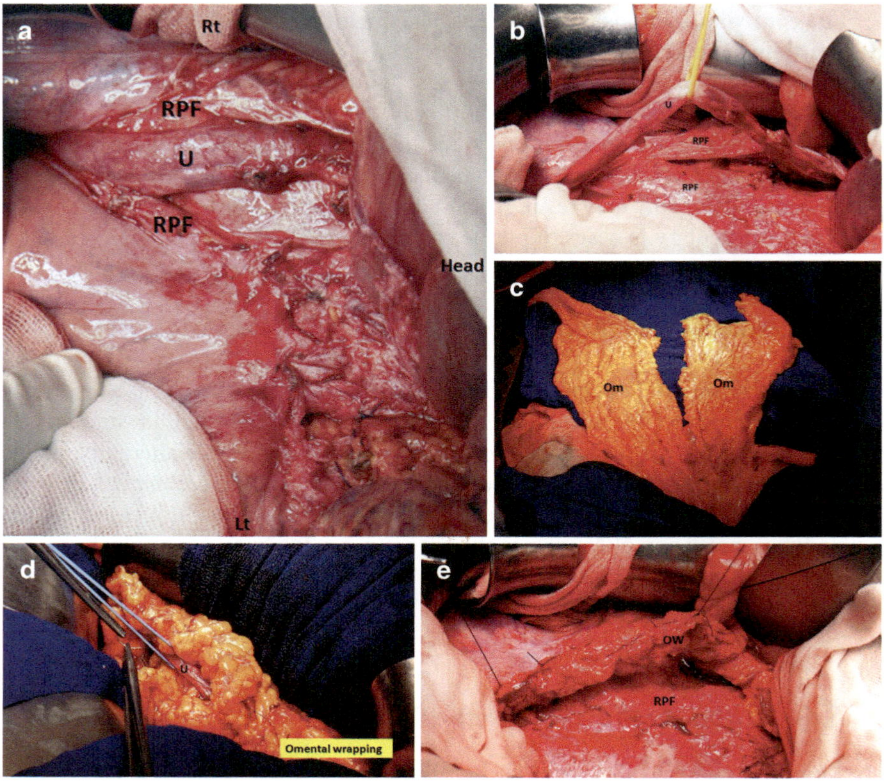

Fig. 15.22 Intra-operative photos demonstrating ureterolysis and omental wrapping in a man with RPF. (**a**) The right ureter (U) is seen surrounded by the dense fibrous mass of RPF. (**b**) The right ureter (U) was dissected out of the mass of RPF (ureterolysis). (**c**) Raising a pedicled omental flap (Om) and dividing it into 2 halves, one for each ureter. (**d**) After complete ureterolysis, the right ureter (U) is wrapped with omentum. (**e**) The final scene is shown. The right ureter (U) is completely wrapped with omentum (OW) and the same is repeated on the left side

Steroid therapy with or without other immunosuppressive drugs may be used in treatment of RPF [24, 25], although they have limited overall cure rate [28]. In addition, urterolysis and omental wrapping is recommended by some researchers as a first-line therapy [28]. Ureteral stents and/or renal decompression by percutaneous nephrostomy tube (PCN) is a well known procedure before starting medical treatment.

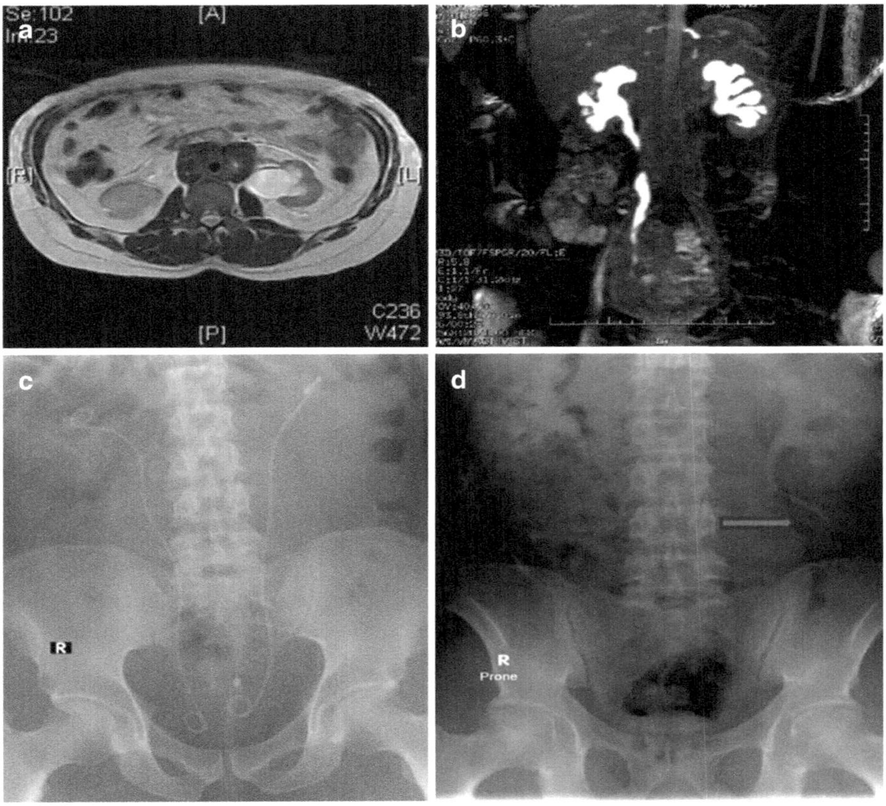

Fig. 15.23 Reproduced with permission from *"Zahran MH, et al. Idiopathic retroperitoneal fibrosis: clinical features and long-term renal function outcome. Int Urol Nephrol. 2017 Aug;49(8):1327-1334. doi: 10.1007/s11255-017-1608-9. Epub 2017 May 13. PMID: 28501912."* A 44-year-old male with bilateral obstructed kidneys caused by retroperitoneal fibrosis. (**a**) MRI (axial cut) showing the plaque encasing the major vessels and obstructing both ureter. (**b**) MRI (coronal image) showing the plaque. (**c**) Plain X-ray after drainage by bilateral JJ stents. (**d**) IVP showed lateralized ureters with no hydronephrosis after ureterolysis and omental wrapping

15.9 Summary

Ureteral stricture disease may be benign or malignant, intrinsic affecting the wall or extrinsic, and/or short segment or long segment stricture. The causes of ureteral stricture include iatrogenic, stones, trauma, tumors, specific infection or inflammation, retroperitoneal fibrosis (RPF), and radiotherapy. Urgent diagnosis and treatment is of paramount importance in order to preserve the renal function in cases of ureteral stricture. The diagnosis is made by a battery of investigations, including ultrasound, CT or MRI, radioisotope renography, antegrade, retrograde, and ureteroscopy (URS).

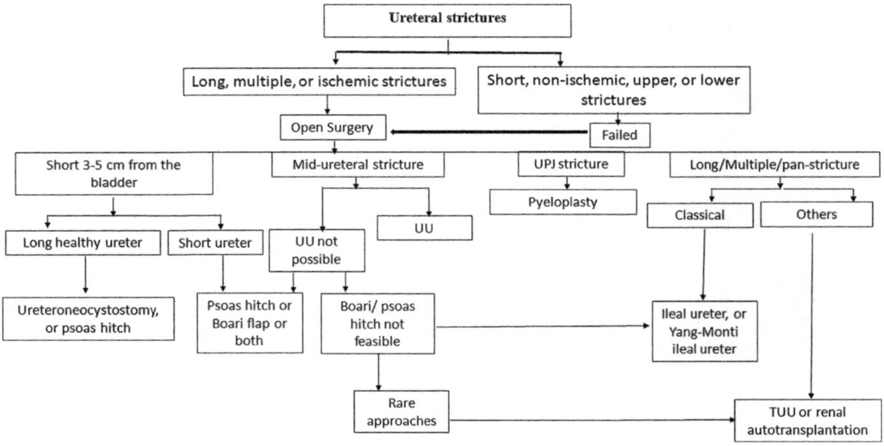

Fig. 15.24 A summary of the algorithm of the main treatment options in cases of ureteral stricture

The treatment of ureteral strictures depends on the site, extent, and whether the stricture is multiple or bilateral. Endoscopic treatment may be tried at first, although the gold standard treatment is performed by open reconstructive techniques. Robot assisted and laparoscopic approaches have been used with success to repair ureteral strictures.

A summary of the algorithm of the main treatment options in cases of ureteral stricture is shown in Fig. 15.24.

Questions

1. Post-ureteroscopy (URS) strictures are common because of the frequent use of it; however, with recent techniques, the incidence of post-URS stricture is within the range of:

   (a) 5%–10%
   (b) 10%–15%
   (c) 1%–3%
   (d) 5%–8%
   (e) 10%–12%

Answer: (c)

2. Regarding ureteral strictures resulting from iatrogenic injuries, choose the best statement of the following:

   (a) Injuries inflicted during urological surgeries account for the majority of cases.
   (b) Iatrogenic gynecological injuries account for the majority of cases.

(c) Injuries inflicted during general surgical interventions account for the majority of cases.
(d) Both iatrogenic gynecological injuries and iatrogenic urological injuries have the same rate of ureteral stricture.
(e) Both iatrogenic gynecological injuries and iatrogenic general surgical injuries have the same rate of ureteral stricture.

Answer: (b)

3. Which of the following statements is correct concerning radiation-induced ureteral strictures:

(a) The strictures are usually asymptomatic and may be associated with renal function loss.
(b) The strictures are usually symptomatic and present early after radiation exposure.
(c) The kidney function is usually preserved till a late stage.
(d) The symptoms of obstruction of the ureter are usually severe.
(e) The resulting strictures are ischemic and therefore, are not associated with sepsis.

Answer: (a)

4. The commonest causes of upper third ureteral strictures are:

(a) Renal stones and/or their management.
(b) Inflammatory diseases.
(c) Malignant disease.
(d) Retroperitoneal fibrosis.
(e) Congenital disease.

Answer: (a)

5. In the case of ureteral stricture associated with chronic kidney disease, the following statement may be true or false:

CT associated with intravenous injection of a contrast material and gadolinium enhanced MRI are the imaging modalities of choice.

True. False

Answer: False

6. Regarding radioisotope renography and split renal function, one of the following statements is the most appropriate:

(a) A baseline split renal function of 10% of the affected kidney is needed in order to have a good outcome after repair of the ureteral stricture.
(b) A baseline split renal function of 30% of the affected kidney is needed in order to have a good outcome after repair of the ureteral stricture.
(c) A baseline split renal function of 20% or more of the affected kidney is needed in order to have a good outcome after repair of the ureteral stricture.

(d) A baseline split renal function of 20% or more of the affected kidney is needed in order to have a good outcome after repair of the ureteral stricture.
(e) A baseline split renal function of 15% of the affected kidney is needed in order to have a good outcome after repair of the ureteral stricture.

Answer: (d)

7. In the treatment of ureteral strictures:

(a) Mid-ureteral strictures are best treated by endoscopic measures.
(b) A stricture 3 cm above the bladder is best treated by ureteroureterostomy.
(c) Open reconstructive techniques are the gold standard.
(d) Robot assisted and laparoscopic techniques are the gold standard, if properly indicated.
(e) Endoscopic techniques are the gold standard for short strictures.

Answer: (c)

8. Regarding the use of ureteral stents in treatment of post-radiation and malignant ureteral strictures:

(a) Polymer stents and metallic stents are contraindicated.
(b) Both metallic stents and polymer stents give poor outcome.
(c) Both metallic stents and polymer stents give favorable outcome.
(d) Polymer stents are preferred with more favorable outcome compared to the Metallic stents.
(e) Metallic stents are preferred with more favorable outcome compared to the polymer stents.

Answer: (e)

9. Regarding psoas hitch technique:

(a) Psoas hitch was introduced in the first decade of the twentieth century and is considered as a universal technique for reimplantation of the ureter into the bladder.
(b) Psoas hitch was introduced in the middle of the twentieth century and is considered as a universal technique for reimplantation of the ureter into the bladder.
(c) Psoas hitch was introduced in the end of the twentieth century and is considered as a universal technique for reimplantation of the ureter into the bladder.
(d) One of the complications of psoas hitch is ureteral kinking after the operation.
(e) Psoas hitch was introduced in nineteenth century and is usually performed as an augment to Boari flap.

Answer: (b)

10. Of the techniques described for ileal replacement of the ureter, one of the following is the best option when there is mild to moderate loss of the kidney function:
    (a) Classic ileal ureter.
    (b) The modified ileal ureter with tapering.
    (c) The modified ileal ureter with antireflux ileovesicostomy.
    (d) The modified ileal ureter with antireflux ureteroileostomy.
    (e) The Yang-Monti ileal ureter.

Answer: (e)

References

1. Johnson DB, Pearle MS. Complications of ureteroscopy. Urol Clin North Am. 2004;31(1):157–71. https://doi.org/10.1016/S0094-0143(03)00089-2.
2. Abboudi H, Ahmed K, Royle J, Khan MS, Dasgupta P, N'Dow J. Ureteric injury: a challenging condition to diagnose and manage. Nat Rev Urol. 2013;10(2):108–15. https://doi.org/10.1038/nrurol.2012.254. Epub 2013 Jan 15
3. Selzman AA, Spirnak JP. Iatrogenic ureteral injuries: a 20-year experience in treating 165 injuries. J Urol. 1996;155(3):878–81. https://doi.org/10.1016/s0022-5347(01)66332-8.
4. Brandes S, Coburn M, Armenakas N, McAninch J. Diagnosis and management of ureteric injury: an evidence-based analysis. BJU Int. 2004;94(3):277–89. https://doi.org/10.1111/j.1464-410X.2004.04978.x.
5. Gild P, Kluth LA, Vetterlein MW, Engel O, Chun FKH, Fisch M. Adult iatrogenic ureteral injury and stricture-incidence and treatment strategies. Asian J Urol. 2018;5(2):101–6. https://doi.org/10.1016/j.ajur.2018.02.003. Epub 2018 Feb 17
6. Roberts WW, Cadeddu JA, Micali S, Kavoussi LR, Moore RG. Ureteral stricture formation after removal of impacted calculi. J Urol. 1998;159(3):723–6.
7. Dretler SP, Young RH. Stone granuloma: a cause of ureteral stricture. J Urol. 1993;150(6):1800–2. https://doi.org/10.1016/s0022-5347(17)35899-8.
8. Mugiya S, Ito T, Maruyama S, Hadano S, Nagae H. Endoscopic features of impacted ureteral stones. J Urol. 2004;171(1):89–91. https://doi.org/10.1097/01.ju.0000100960.08768.81.
9. Fam XI, Singam P, Ho CC, et al. Ureteral stricture formation after ureteroscope treatment of impacted calculi: a prospective study. Korean J Urol. 2015;56(1):63–7. https://doi.org/10.4111/kju.2015.56.1.63.
10. Yamaguchi K, Minei S, Yamazaki T, Kaya H, Okada K. Characterization of ureteral lesions associated with impacted stones. Int J Urol. 1999;6(6):281–5. https://doi.org/10.1046/j.1442-2042.1999.00067.x.
11. Schuster TG, Hollenbeck BK, Faerber GJ, Wolf JS Jr. Complications of ureteroscopy: analysis of predictive factors. J Urol. 2001;166(2):538–40. https://doi.org/10.1016/s0022-5347(05)65978-2.
12. Weizer AZ, Auge BK, Silverstein AD, Delvecchio FC, Brizuela RM, Dahm P, Pietrow PK, Lewis BR, Albala DM, Preminger GM. Routine postoperative imaging is important after ureteroscopic stone manipulation. J Urol. 2002;168(1):46–50.
13. Adiyat KT, Meuleners R, Monga M. Selective postoperative imaging after ureteroscopy. Urology. 2009;73(3):490–3. https://doi.org/10.1016/j.urology.2008.09.064. Epub 2008 Dec 18. discussion 493

14. Binbay M, Tepeler A, Singh A, et al. Evaluation of pneumatic versus holmium:YAG laser lithotripsy for impacted ureteral stones. Int Urol Nephrol. 2011;43:989–95.
15. Li L, Pan Y, Weng Z, Bao W, Yu Z, Wang F. A prospective randomized trial comparing pneumatic lithotripsy and holmium laser for management of middle and distal ureteral calculi. J Endourol. 2015;29(8):883–7. https://doi.org/10.1089/end.2014.0856. Epub 2015 Feb 18
16. de la Rosette J, Denstedt J, Geavlete P, Keeley F, Matsuda T, Pearle M, Preminger G. Traxer O; CROES URS Study Group. The clinical research office of the endourological society ureteroscopy global study: indications, complications, and outcomes in 11,885 patients. J Endourol. 2014;28(2):131–9. https://doi.org/10.1089/end.2013.0436. Epub 2013 Dec 17
17. Ulvik Ø, Harneshaug JR, Gjengstø P. Ureteral strictures following ureteroscopic stone treatment. J Endourol. 2021;35(7):985–90. https://doi.org/10.1089/end.2020.0421. Epub 2020 Oct 21
18. Darwish AE, Gadelmoula MM, Abdelkawi IF, Abdellatif AM, Abdel-Moneim AM, Hammouda HM. Ureteral stricture after ureteroscopy for stones: a prospective study for the incidence and risk factors. Urol Ann. 2019;11(3):276–81. https://doi.org/10.4103/UA.UA_110_18.
19. Shen Y, Xiang A, Shao S. Preoperative hydronephrosis is a predictive factor of ureteral stenosis after flexible ureteroscopy: a propensity scores matching analysis. BMC Urol. 2021;21(1):153. https://doi.org/10.1186/s12894-021-00917-1.
20. Brito AH, Mitre AI, Srougi M. Ureteroscopic pneumatic lithotripsy of impacted ureteral calculi. Int Braz J Urol. 2006;32(3):295–9. https://doi.org/10.1590/s1677-55382006000300006.
21. Perez Castro E, Osther PJ, Jinga V, Razvi H, Stravodimos KG, Parikh K, Kural AR, de la Rosette JJ, CROES Ureteroscopy Global Study Group. Differences in ureteroscopic stone treatment and outcomes for distal, mid-, proximal, or multiple ureteral locations: the Clinical Research Office of the Endourological Society ureteroscopy global study. Eur Urol. 2014;66(1):102–9. https://doi.org/10.1016/j.eururo.2014.01.011. Epub 2014 Jan 23
22. McIntyre JF, Eifel PJ, Levenback C, Oswald MJ. Ureteral stricture as a late complication of radiotherapy for stage IB carcinoma of the uterine cervix. Cancer. 1995;75(3):836–43. https://doi.org/10.1002/1097-0142(19950201)75:3<836::aid-cncr2820750315>3.0.co;2-a.
23. Fokdal L, Tanderup K, Pötter R, Sturdza A, Kirchheiner K, Chargari C, Jürgenliemk-Schulz IM, Segedin B, Tan LT, Hoskin P, Mahantshetty U, Bruheim K, Rai B, Kirisits C, Lindegaard JC, EMBRACE Collaborative Group. Risk factors for ureteral stricture after radiochemotherapy including image guided adaptive brachytherapy in cervical cancer: results from the EMBRACE studies. Int J Radiat Oncol Biol Phys. 2019;103(4):887–94. https://doi.org/10.1016/j.ijrobp.2018.11.006. Epub 2018 Nov 10
24. Raglianti V, Rossi GM, Vaglio A. Idiopathic retroperitoneal fibrosis: an update for nephrologists. Nephrol Dial Transplant. 2021;36(10):1773–81. https://doi.org/10.1093/ndt/gfaa083.
25. Zahran MH, Osman Y, Soltan MA, Abolazm AE, Ghazy MK, Harraz AM, Shokeir AA, Abol-Enein H, Ali-El-Dein B. Idiopathic retroperitoneal fibrosis: clinical features and long-term renal function outcome. Int Urol Nephrol. 2017;49(8):1327–34. https://doi.org/10.1007/s11255-017-1608-9. Epub 2017 May 13
26. Vaglio A, Maritati F. Idiopathic retroperitoneal fibrosis. J Am Soc Nephrol. 2016;27(7):1880–9. https://doi.org/10.1681/ASN.2015101110. Epub 2016 Feb 9
27. Yachoui R, Sehgal R, Carmichael B. Idiopathic retroperitoneal fibrosis: clinicopathologic features and outcome analysis. Clin Rheumatol. 2016;35(2):401–7. https://doi.org/10.1007/s10067-015-3022-y. Epub 2015 Jul 25
28. Fernando A, Pattison J, Horsfield C, Bultitude M, D'Cruz D, O'Brien T. A lot of questions (and a few answers …) in retroperitoneal fibrosis. BJU Int. 2016;117(1):16–9. https://doi.org/10.1111/bju.13061. Epub 2015 May 23
29. Murphy DM, Fallon B, Lane V, O'Flynn JD. Tuberculous stricture of ureter. Urology. 1982;20(4):382–4. https://doi.org/10.1016/0090-4295(82)90460-5.
30. Mostbeck GH, Zontsich T, Turetschek K. Ultrasound of the kidney: obstruction and medical diseases. Eur Radiol. 2001;11(10):1878–89. https://doi.org/10.1007/s003300101011.

31. Lin WC, Wang JH, Wei CJ, Chang CY. Assessment of CT urography in the diagnosis of urinary tract abnormalities. J Chin Med Assoc. 2004;67(2):73–8.
32. Potenta SE, D'Agostino R, Sternberg KM, Tatsumi K, Perusse K. CT Urography for Evaluation of the Ureter. Radiographics. 2015;35(3):709–26. https://doi.org/10.1148/rg.2015140209. Epub 2015 Mar 27
33. Nolte-Ernsting CC, Bücker A, Adam GB, Neuerburg JM, Jung P, Hunter DW, Jakse G, Günther RW. Gadolinium-enhanced excretory MR urography after low-dose diuretic injection: comparison with conventional excretory urography. Radiology. 1998;209(1):147–57. https://doi.org/10.1148/radiology.209.1.9769826.
34. Arlen AM, Kirsch AJ, Cuda SP, Little SB, Jones RA, Grattan-Smith JD, Cerwinka WH. Magnetic resonance urography for diagnosis of pediatric ureteral stricture. J Pediatr Urol. 2014;10(5):792–8. https://doi.org/10.1016/j.jpurol.2014.01.004. Epub 2014 Jan 31
35. Rohrschneider WK, Haufe S, Wiesel M, Tönshoff B, Wunsch R, Darge K, Clorius JH, Tröger J. Functional and morphologic evaluation of congenital urinary tract dilatation by using combined static-dynamic MR urography: findings in kidneys with a single collecting system. Radiology. 2002;224(3):683–94. https://doi.org/10.1148/radiol.2243011207.
36. Thoeny HC, Binser T, Roth B, Kessler TM, Vermathen P. Noninvasive assessment of acute ureteral obstruction with diffusion-weighted MR imaging: a prospective study. Radiology. 2009;252(3):721–8. https://doi.org/10.1148/radiol.2523082090.
37. Zhou JY, Wang YC, Zeng CH, Ju SH. Renal Functional MRI and Its Application. J Magn Reson Imaging. 2018;48(4):863–81. https://doi.org/10.1002/jmri.26180. Epub 2018 Aug 13
38. Roy C, Ohana M, Host P, et al. MR urography (MRU) of non-dilated ureter with diuretic administration: Static fluid 2D FSE T2-weighted versus 3D gadolinium T1-weighted GE excretory MR. Eur J Radiol Open. 2014;1:6–13. https://doi.org/10.1016/j.ejro.2014.08.001.
39. Tartaglione G, Townsend DM, Bassi PF, Delgado Bolton RC, Giammarile F, Rubello D. Diuresis renography in equivocal urinary tract obstruction. A historical perspective. Biomed Pharmacother. 2019;116:108981. https://doi.org/10.1016/j.biopha.2019.108981. Epub 2019 May 25
40. Wolf JS Jr, Elashry OM, Clayman RV. Long-term results of endoureterotomy for benign ureteral and ureteroenteric strictures. J Urol. 1997;158(3 Pt 1):759–64. https://doi.org/10.1097/00005392-199709000-00016.
41. Grasso M, Li S, Liu JB, Beaghler M, Newman R, Bagley DH. Examining the obstructed ureter with intraluminal sonography. J Urol. 1999;162(4):1286–90.
42. Kagadis GC, Siablis D, Liatsikos EN, Petsas T, Nikiforidis GC. Virtual endoscopy of the urinary tract. Asian J Androl. 2006;8(1):31–8. https://doi.org/10.1111/j.1745-7262.2006.00096.x.
43. Chung SY, Stein RJ, Landsittel D, Davies BJ, Cuellar DC, Hrebinko RL, Tarin T, Averch TD. 15-year experience with the management of extrinsic ureteral obstruction with indwelling ureteral stents. J Urol. 2004;172(2):592–5. https://doi.org/10.1097/01.ju.0000130510.28768.f5.
44. Kachrilas S, Bourdoumis A, Karaolides T, Nikitopoulou S, Papadopoulos G, Buchholz N, Masood J. Current status of minimally invasive endoscopic management of ureteric strictures. Ther Adv Urol. 2013;5(6):354–65. https://doi.org/10.1177/1756287213505671.
45. Reus C, Brehmer M. Minimally invasive management of ureteral strictures: a 5-year retrospective study. World J Urol. 2019;37:1733–8. https://doi.org/10.1007/s00345-018-2539-5.
46. Lucas JW, Ghiraldi E, Ellis J, Friedlander JI. Endoscopic management of ureteral strictures: an update. Curr Urol Rep. 2018;19(4):24. https://doi.org/10.1007/s11934-018-0773-4.
47. Razdan S, Silberstein IK, Bagley DH. Ureteroscopic endoureterotomy. BJU Int. 2005;95(Suppl 2):94–101. https://doi.org/10.1111/j.1464-410X.2005.05207.x.
48. Forbes C, Scotland KB, Lange D, Chew BH. Innovations in ureteral stent technology. Urol Clin North Am. 2019;46(2):245–55. https://doi.org/10.1016/j.ucl.2018.12.013. Epub 2019 Mar 4

49. Wang HJ, Lee TY, Luo HL, Chen CH, Shen YC, Chuang YC, Chiang PH. Application of resonance metallic stents for ureteral obstruction. BJU Int. 2011;108(3):428–32. https://doi.org/10.1111/j.1464-410X.2010.09842.x. Epub 2010 Nov 9
50. Wenzler DL, Kim SP, Rosevear HM, Faerber GJ, Roberts WW, Wolf JS Jr. Success of ureteral stents for intrinsic ureteral obstruction. J Endourol. 2008;22(2):295–9. https://doi.org/10.1089/end.2007.0201.
51. Yossepowitch O, Lifshitz DA, Dekel Y, Gross M, Keidar DM, Neuman M, Livne PM, Baniel J. Predicting the success of retrograde stenting for managing ureteral obstruction. J Urol. 2001;166(5):1746–9.
52. Sali GM, Joshi HB. Ureteric stents: overview of current clinical applications and economic implications. Int J Urol. 2020;27(1):7–15. https://doi.org/10.1111/iju.14119. Epub 2019 Sep 23
53. Das K, Ordones F, Welikumbura S, et al. Ureteroiliac artery fistula caused by a metallic memokath ureteral stent in a radiation-induced ureteral stricture. J Endourol Case Rep. 2016;2:162–5.
54. Lynch MF, Anson KM, Patel U. Percutaneous nephrostomy and ureteric stent insertion for acute renal deobstruction consensus based guidance. Br J Med Surg Urol. 2008;1(3):120–5. https://doi.org/10.1016/j.bjmsu.2008.09.002.
55. Hausegger KA, Portugaller HR. Percutaneous nephrostomy and antegrade ureteral stenting: technique-indications-complications. Eur Radiol. 2006;16(9):2016–30. https://doi.org/10.1007/s00330-005-0136-7. Epub 2006 Mar 18
56. Fernández-Cacho LM, Ayesa-Arriola R. Quality of life, pain and anxiety in patients with nephrostomy tubes. Rev Lat Am Enfermagem. 2019;27:e3191. https://doi.org/10.1590/1518-8345.3039.3191.
57. Fontaine AB, Nijjar A, Rangaraj R. Update on the use of percutaneous nephrostomy/balloon dilation for the treatment of renal transplant leak/obstruction. J Vasc Interv Radiol. 1997;8(4):649–53. https://doi.org/10.1016/s1051-0443(97)70625-0.
58. Richter F, Irwin RJ, Watson RA, Lang EK. Endourologic management of benign ureteral strictures with and without compromised vascular supply. Urology. 2000;55(5):652–7. https://doi.org/10.1016/s0090-4295(00)00484-2.
59. Kristo B, Phelan MW, Gritsch HA, Schulam PG. Treatment of renal transplant ureterovesical anastomotic strictures using antegrade balloon dilation with or without holmium:YAG laser endoureterotomy. Urology. 2003;62(5):831–4. https://doi.org/10.1016/s0090-4295(03)00655-1.
60. Kuntz NJ, Neisius A, Tsivian M, Ghaffar M, Patel N, Ferrandino MN, Sur RL, Preminger GM, Lipkin ME. Balloon dilation of the ureter: a contemporary review of outcomes and complications. J Urol. 2015;194(2):413–7. https://doi.org/10.1016/j.juro.2015.02.2917. Epub 2015 Feb 26
61. Koukouras D, Petsas T, Liatsikos E, Kallidonis P, Sdralis EK, Adonakis G, Panagopoulos C, Al-Aown A, Decavalas G, Perimenis P, Siablis D, Karnabatidis D. Percutaneous minimally invasive management of iatrogenic ureteral injuries. J Endourol. 2010;24(12):1921–7. https://doi.org/10.1089/end.2010.0153. Epub 2010 Oct 21
62. Christman MS, Kasturi S, Lambert SM, Kovell RC, Casale P. Endoscopic management and the role of double stenting for primary obstructive megaureters. J Urol. 2012;187(3):1018–22. https://doi.org/10.1016/j.juro.2011.10.168. Epub 2012 Jan 20
63. Docimo SG, Dewolf WC. High failure rate of indwelling ureteral stents in patients with extrinsic obstruction: experience at 2 institutions. J Urol. 1989;142(2 Pt 1):277–9. https://doi.org/10.1016/s0022-5347(17)38729-3.
64. Abourbih S, Baldwin DD. Chapter 52: Endoscopic management of mid-ureteral obstruction. In: Smith AD, Preminger GM, Kavoussi LR, et al., editors. Smith's textbook of endourology. 4th ed. Hoboken, NJ: John Wiley & Sons Ltd.; 2019.
65. Cohen TD, Gross MB, Preminger GM. Long-term follow-up of Acucise incision of ureteropelvic junction obstruction and ureteral strictures. Urology. 1996;47(3):317–23. https://doi.org/10.1016/S0090-4295(99)80445-2.

66. Nakada SY. Acucise endopyelotomy. Urology. 2000;55(2):277–82. https://doi.org/10.1016/s0090-4295(99)00393-3.
67. Schwartz BF, Chatham JR, Bretan P, Goharderakhshan R, Stoller ML. Treatment of refractory kidney transplant ureteral strictures using balloon cautery endoureterotomy. Urology. 2001;58(4):536–9. https://doi.org/10.1016/s0090-4295(01)01275-4.
68. Davis DM, Strong GH, Drake WM. Intubated ureterotomy; experimental work and clinical results. J Urol. 1948;59(5):851–62. https://doi.org/10.1016/s0022-5347(17)69449-7.
69. Vasudevan VP, Johnson EU, Wong K, et al. Contemporary management of ureteral strictures. J Clin Urol. 2019;12(1):20–31. https://doi.org/10.1177/2051415813772218.
70. Polyakov N, Keshishev N, Kachmazov A, et al. Surgical treatment of the stricture of the lower third of ureter after radiation therapy of pelvic organs. Cancer Urol. 2016;12:68–73. https://doi.org/10.17650/1726-9776-2016-12-3-68-73.
71. Meretyk S, Albala DM, Clayman RV, Denstedt JD, Kavoussi LR. Endoureterotomy for treatment of ureteral strictures. J Urol. 1992;147(6):1502–6. https://doi.org/10.1016/s0022-5347(17)37608-5.
72. Shao Y-H, Wu S-T, Tang S-T, et al. Endoureterotomy for Ureteral stricture: a retrospective study of holmium versus thulium lasers. Int Surg. 2017;102(11–12):496–503. https://doi.org/10.9738/INTSURG-D-17-00096.1.
73. Lich R Jr, Howerton LW, Davis LA. Childhood urosepsis. J Ky Med Assoc. 1961;59:1177–9.
74. Konnak JW, Herwig KR, Turcotte JG. External ureteroneocystostomy in renal transplantation. J Urol. 1972;108(3):380–1. https://doi.org/10.1016/s0022-5347(17)60747-x.
75. Shanfield I. New experimental methods for implantation of the ureter in bladder and conduit. Transplant Proc. 1972;4(4):637–8.
76. Politano VA, Leadbetter WF. An operative technique for the correction of vesicoureteral reflux. J Urol. 1958;79(6):932–41. https://doi.org/10.1016/s0022-5347(17)66369-9.
77. Png JC, Chapple CR. Principles of ureteric reconstruction. Curr Opin Urol. 2000;10(3):207–12. https://doi.org/10.1097/00042307-200005000-00004.
78. Stefanović KB, Bukurov NS, Marinković JM. Non-antireflux versus antireflux ureteroneocystostomy in adults. Br J Urol. 1991;67(3):263–6. https://doi.org/10.1111/j.1464-410x.1991.tb15131.x.
79. Debruyne FM, Wijdeveld PG, Koene RA, Chafik ML, Moonen WA, Renders GA. Uretero-neo-cystostomy in renal transplantation. Is an antireflux mechanism mandatory? Br J Urol. 1978;50(6):378–82. https://doi.org/10.1111/j.1464-410x.1978.tb04214.x.
80. Sung J, Skoog S. Surgical management of vesicoureteral reflux in children. Pediatr Nephrol. 2012;27(4):551–61. https://doi.org/10.1007/s00467-011-1933-7.
81. Warwick RT, Worth PH. The psoas bladder-hitch procedure for the replacement of the lower third of the ureter. Br J Urol. 1969;41(6):701–9. https://doi.org/10.1111/j.1464-410x.1969.tb09981.x.
82. Riedmiller H, Becht E, Hertle L, Jacobi G, Hohenfellner R. Psoas-hitch ureteroneocystostomy: experience with 181 cases. Eur Urol. 1984;10(3):145–50. https://doi.org/10.1159/000463777.
83. Stein R, Rubenwolf P, Ziesel C, Kamal MM, Thüroff JW. Psoas hitch and Boari flap ureteroneocystostomy. BJU Int. 2013;112(1):137–55. https://doi.org/10.1111/bju.12103.
84. Boari A. L'urétéro-cystonostomie. Étude clinique et expérimentale. Ann Mal Org Gen Urin. 1899;14:1059–88. 141–70.
85. Kimchi D, Wiesenfeld A. Injuries to the lower third of ureter treated by bladder flap plasty: Boari-Kuss technique; report of two cases. J Urol. 1963;89:800–3. https://doi.org/10.1016/s0022-5347(17)64650-0.
86. Hofer MD, Aguilar-Cruz HJ, Singla N, Cordon BH, Scott JM, Morey AF. Expanding applications of renal mobilization and downward nephropexy in ureteral reconstruction. Urology. 2016;94:232–6. https://doi.org/10.1016/j.urology.2016.04.008. Epub 2016 Apr 22
87. Wenske S, Olsson CA, Benson MC. Outcomes of distal ureteral reconstruction through reimplantation with psoas hitch, Boari flap, or ureteroneocystostomy for benign or malignant ureteral obstruction or injury. Urology. 2013;82(1):231–6. https://doi.org/10.1016/j.urology.2013.02.046. Epub 2013 May 2

88. Groen VH, Lock MTWT, de Angst IB, et al. Psoas hitch procedure in 166 adult patients: The largest cohort study before the laparoscopic era. BJUI Compass. 2021;2:331–7. https://doi.org/10.1111/bco2.85.
89. Rassweiler JJ, Gözen AS, Erdogru T, Sugiono M, Teber D. Ureteral reimplantation for management of ureteral strictures: a retrospective comparison of laparoscopic and open techniques. Eur Urol. 2007;51(2):512–22. https://doi.org/10.1016/j.eururo.2006.08.004. Epub 2006 Aug 17. discussion 522-3
90. Ding G, Cheng S, Li X, et al. Experience managing distal ureteral strictures with Boari flap-psoas hitch and comparison of open and laparoscopic procedures. Transl Androl Urol. 2021;10(1):56–65. https://doi.org/10.21037/tau-20-789.
91. Drain A, Jun MS, Zhao LC. Robotic ureteral reconstruction. Urol Clin North Am. 2021;48(1):91–101. https://doi.org/10.1016/j.ucl.2020.09.001. Epub 2020 Nov 5
92. Singh I, Kader K, Hemal AK. Robotic distal ureterectomy with reimplantation in malignancy: technical nuances. Can J Urol. 2009;16(3):4671–6.
93. Yang C, Jones L, Rivera ME, Verlee GT, Deane LA. Robotic-assisted ureteral reimplantation with Boari flap and psoas hitch: a single-institution experience. J Laparoendosc Adv Surg Tech A. 2011;21(9):829–33. https://doi.org/10.1089/lap.2011.0028. Epub 2011 Aug 22
94. White C, Stifelman M. Ureteral Reimplantation, Psoas Hitch, and Boari Flap. J Endourol. 2020;34(S1):S25–30. https://doi.org/10.1089/end.2018.0750.
95. Stolzenburg JU, Rai BP, Do M, Dietel A, Liatsikos E, Ganzer R, Qazi H, Meneses AD, Kallidonis P. Robot-assisted technique for Boari flap ureteric reimplantation: replicating the techniques of open surgery in robotics. BJU Int. 2016;118(3):482–4. https://doi.org/10.1111/bju.13502. Epub 2016 May 17
96. Higgins C. Transureteroureteral anastomosis: report of a clinical case. J Urol. 1935;34:349.
97. Hodges CV, Moore RJ, Lehman TH, Benham AM. Clinical experiences with transureteroureterostomy. J Urol. 1963;90:552.
98. Hendren WH, Hensle TW. Transureteroureterostomy: experience with 75 cases. J Urol. 1980;123(6):826–33. https://doi.org/10.1016/s0022-5347(17)56151-0.
99. Strup SE, Sindelar WF, Walther MM. The use of transureteroureterostomy in the management of complex ureteral problems. J Urol. 1996;155(5):1572–4.
100. Noble IG, Lee KT, Mundy AR. Transuretero-ureterostomy: a review of 253 cases. Br J Urol. 1997;79(1):20–3. https://doi.org/10.1046/j.1464-410x.1997.02794.x.
101. Manjunath DA, Radhakrishna V, Vepakomma D. Transureteroureterostomy in children: a retrospective study. Am J Clin Exp Urol. 2021;9(2):163–9.
102. Ehrlich RM, Skinner DG. Complications of transureteroureterostomy. J Urol. 1975;113(4):467–73. https://doi.org/10.1016/s0022-5347(17)59502-6.
103. Sandoz IL, Paull DP, MacFarlane CA. Complications with transureteroureterostomy. J Urol. 1977;117(1):39–42. https://doi.org/10.1016/s0022-5347(17)58329-9.
104. Stief CG, Jonas U, Petry KU, Sohn C, Bektas H, Klempnauer J, Chavan A, Galanski M, Montorsi F. Ureteric reconstruction. BJU Int. 2003;91(2):138–42. https://doi.org/10.1046/j.1464-410x.2003.03060.x.
105. Sugarbaker PH, Gutman M, Verghese M. Transureteroureterostomy: an adjunct to the management of advanced primary and recurrent pelvic malignancy. Int J Color Dis. 2003;18(1):40–4. https://doi.org/10.1007/s00384-002-0399-2. Epub 2002 May 8
106. Iwaszko MR, Krambeck AE, Chow GK, Gettman MT. Transureteroureterostomy revisited: long-term surgical outcomes. J Urol. 2010;183(3):1055–9. https://doi.org/10.1016/j.juro.2009.11.031. Epub 2010 Jan 21
107. Hardy JD. High ureteral injuries. Management by autotransplantation of the kidney. JAMA. 1963;184:97–101. https://doi.org/10.1001/jama.1963.03700150051008.
108. Bodie B, Novick AC, Rose M, Straffon RA. Long-term results with renal autotransplantation for ureteral replacement. J Urol. 1986;136(6):1187–9. https://doi.org/10.1016/s0022-5347(17)45278-5.
109. Meng MV, Freise CE, Stoller ML. Expanded experience with laparoscopic nephrectomy and autotransplantation for severe ureteral injury. J Urol. 2003;169(4):1363–7. https://doi.org/10.1097/01.ju.0000054927.18678.5e.

110. Ali-El-Dein B, Osman Y, Shehab El-Din AB, El-Diasty T, Mansour O, Ghoneim MA. Anterior and posterior nutcracker syndrome: a report on 11 cases. Transplant Proc. 2003;35(2):851–3. https://doi.org/10.1016/s0041-1345(02)04026-5.
111. Cowan NG, Banerji JS, Johnston RB, Duty BD, Bakken B, Hedges JC, Kozlowski PM, Hefty TR, Barry JM. Renal autotransplantation: 27-year experience at 2 institutions. J Urol. 2015;194(5):1357–61. https://doi.org/10.1016/j.juro.2015.05.088. Epub 2015 Jun 6
112. Janssen MWW, Linxweiler J, Philipps I, et al. Kidney autotransplantation after nephrectomy and work bench surgery as an ultimate approach to nephron-sparing surgery. World J Surg Onc. 2018;16:35. https://doi.org/10.1186/s12957-018-1338-1.
113. Passerini-Glazel G, Meneghini A, Aragona F, Oliva G, Milani C, Pagano F. Technical options in complex ureteral lesions: 'ureter-sparing' surgery. Eur Urol. 1994;25(4):273–80. https://doi.org/10.1159/000475301.
114. Vrakas G, Sullivan M. Current review of renal autotransplantation in the UK. Curr Urol Rep. 2020;21:33. https://doi.org/10.1007/s11934-020-00986-z.
115. Zhao LC, Weinberg AC, Lee Z, et al. Robotic ureteral reconstruction using buccal mucosa grafts: a multi-institutional experience. Eur Urol. 2018;73:419–26.
116. Xiong S, Wang J, Zhu W, et al. Onlay repair technique for the management of ureteral strictures: a comprehensive review. Biomed Res Int. 2020;2020:6178286.
117. Zhao LC, Yamaguchi Y, Bryk DJ, Adelstein SA, Stifelman MD. Robot-assisted ureteral reconstruction using buccal mucosa. Urology. 2015;86(3):634–8.
118. Lee Z, Waldorf BT, Cho EY, Liu JC, Metro MJ, Eun DD. Robotic ureteroplasty with buccal mucosa graft for the management of complex ureteral strictures. J Urol. 2017;198(6):1430–5.
119. Somerville JJ, Naude JH. Segmental ureteric replacement: an animal study using a free non pedicled graft. Urol Res. 1984;12(2):115–9.
120. Naude JH. Buccal mucosal grafts in the treatment of ureteric lesions. BJU Int. 1999;83(7):751–4.
121. Barbagli G, Lazzeri M. Urethral reconstruction. Curr Opin Urol. 2006;16(6):391–5.
122. Badawy AA, Abolyosr A, Saleem MD, et al. Buccal mucosa graft for ureteral stricture substitution: initial experience. Urology. 2010;76:971–5. discussion 975
123. Fahmy O, Schubert T, Khairul-Asri MG, Stenzl A, Gakis G. Total proximal ureter substitution using buccal mucosa. Int J Urol. 2017;24(4):320–3.
124. Patterson JM, Chapple CR. Surgical techniques in substitution urethroplasty using buccal mucosa for the treatment of anterior urethral strictures. Eur Urol. 2008;53(6):1162–71.
125. Lee Z, Keehn AY, Sterling ME, et al. A review of buccal mucosa graft ureteroplasty. Curr Urol Rep. 2018;19:23.
126. Sanders AR, Schein CJ. The epithelial morphology of autogenous grafts when utilized as ureteral and vesical substitutes in the experimental animal: a collective review. J Urol. 1956;75:659–63.
127. Rosenberg ML, Dahlen GA. Autogenous vein grafts and venous valves in ureteral surgery: an experimental study. J Urol. 1953;70:434–7.
128. Calef C. Ureteral Replacement. Ann Ital di Chir. 1938;17:153–6. (abstracted in Zischr F Urol Chir 44: 185, 1938-1939).
129. Bettman AG. Ureteral replacement with subcutaneous skin tube. Plast Reconstruct Surg. 1947;2:80–3.
130. Lord JW, Stefko PL, Stevens AR. On bridging a gap in the ureter by means of a free fascial transplant over a straight vitallium tube: an experimental study. J Urol. 1943;49:249–51.
131. Horton CE, Politano VA. Ureteral reconstruction with splitt thickness grafts: an experimental study. Plast Reconstruct Surg. 1955;15:261–4.
132. Keshin JG, Fitzpatrick TJ. A new technique for urinary diversion using a full thickness skin tube as a conduit. J Urol. 1962;88:631–5.
133. Harvard BM, Camilleri JA, Nadig PW, Glenn JF. Experimental transplantation of freeze-dried homologous and autologous ureteral segments. J Urol. 1961;86:385–9. https://doi.org/10.1016/s0022-5347(17)65185-1.

134. Greenberg R, Coleman JW, Quiguyan CC, et al. Bladder mucosal grafts: experimental use as a ureteral substitute and observation of certain physical properties. J Urol. 1983;129(3):634–6. https://doi.org/10.1016/s0022-5347(17)52268-5.
135. Lord JW, Eckel JH. The use of vitallium tubes in the urinary tract of the dog. J Urol. 1942;48:412–5.
136. TULLOCH WS. Restoration of the continuity of the ureter by means of polythene tubing. Br J Urol. 1952;24(1):42–5.
137. ULM AH, KRAUSS L. Total unilateral teflon ureteral substitutes in the dog. J Urol. 1960;83:575–82. https://doi.org/10.1016/s0022-5347(17)65761-6.
138. Lewis HY, Sherwood NS, Pierce JM Jr. Experimental and clinical use of a ureteral prosthesis. J Urol. 1966;95(5):700–5. https://doi.org/10.1016/s0022-5347(17)63521-3.
139. Griffith DP, Mosely WG, Beach PD. Experimental studies in ureteral substitution. Investig Urol. 1973;11(3):239–43.
140. Desgrandchamps F, Paulhac P, Fornairon S, De Kerviller E, Duboust A, Teillac P, Le Duc A. Artificial ureteral replacement for ureteral necrosis after renal transplantation: report of 3 cases. J Urol. 1998;159(6):1830–2.
141. Smith TG, Gettman M, Lindberg G, et al. Ureteral replacement using porcine small intestine submucosa in a porcine model. Urology. 2002;60(5):931–4. https://doi.org/10.1016/S0090-4295(02)01890-3.
142. Sofer M, Rowe E, Forder DM, Denstedt JD. Ureteral segmental replacement using multilayer porcine small-intestinal submucosa. J Endourol. 2002;16(1):27–31. https://doi.org/10.1089/089277902753483682.
143. El-Assmy A, Hafez AT, El-Sherbiny MT, et al. Use of single layer small intestinal submucosa for long segment ureteral replacement: A pilot study. J Urol. 2004;171:1939–42.
144. Probst M, Dahiya R, Carrier S, Tanagho EA. Reproduction of functional smooth muscle tissue and partial bladder replacement. Br J Urol. 1997;79(4):505–15. https://doi.org/10.1046/j.1464-410x.1997.00103.x.
145. Atala A. Future perspectives in reconstructive surgery using tissue engineering. Urol Clin North Am. 1999;26(1):157–65., ix-x. https://doi.org/10.1016/s0094-0143(99)80013-5.
146. Xiong S, Wang J, Zhu W, Yang K, Ding G, Li X, Eun DD. Onlay repair technique for the management of ureteral strictures: a comprehensive review. Biomed Res Int. 2020;2020:6178286. https://doi.org/10.1155/2020/6178286.
147. Tachibana M, Nagamatsu GR, Addonizio JC. Ureteral replacement using collagen sponge tube grafts. J Urol. 1985;133(5):866–9. https://doi.org/10.1016/s0022-5347(17)49268-8.
148. Melinkoff AE. *Sur le remplacement de* l'uretère *par une anse isolée de* l'intestin *grêle*. Rev Clin Urol. 1912;1:601–9.
149. Richter F, Stock JA, Hanna MK. The appendix as right ureteral substitute in children. J Urol. 2000;163(6):1908–12.
150. Schein CJ, Sanders AR, Hurwitt ES. Experimental reconstruction of ureters: substitution with autogenous pedicled fallopian tube grafts. AMA Arch Surg. 1956;73(1):47–53.
151. Thompson IM. Repair of ureteropelvic junction and upper ureteral injury with renal capsule flaps. Urol Clin North Am. 1977;4(1):51–7.
152. Fiorelli C, Selli C, Nicita G, Turini D. Experimental ureteral replacement with a vascularized gastric tubule. Eur Urol. 1979;5(4):278–80. https://doi.org/10.1159/000473130.
153. Gil-Vernet JM Jr. The ileocolic segment in urologic surgery. J Urol. 1965;94(4):418–26. https://doi.org/10.1016/s0022-5347(17)63641-3.
154. Takeuchi M, Masumori N, Tsukamoto T. Ureteral reconstruction with bowel segments: experience with eight patients in a single institute. Korean J Urol. 2014;55(11):742–9. https://doi.org/10.4111/kju.2014.55.11.742.
155. Moore EV, Weber R, Woodward ER, Moore JG, Goodwin WE. Isolated ileal loops for ureteral repair. Surg Gynecol Obstet. 1956;102(1):87–97.
156. Shoemaker GE. VIII. Removal of the Ureter with a Tuberculous Kidney. Ann Surg. 1911;53(5):696–8. https://doi.org/10.1097/00000658-191105000-00008.

157. Goodwin WE, Winter CC, Turner RD. Replacement of the ureter by small intestine: clinical application and results of the ileal ureter. J Urol. 1959;81(3):406–18. https://doi.org/10.1016/s0022-5347(17)66035-x.
158. Ghoneim MA, Shoukry I. The use of ileum for correction of advanced or complicated bilharzial lesions of the urinary tract. Int Urol Nephrol. 1972;4(1):25–33. https://doi.org/10.1007/BF02081890.
159. Bonfig R, Gerharz EW, Riedmiller H. Ileal ureteric replacement in complex reconstruction of the urinary tract. BJU Int. 2004;93(4):575–80. https://doi.org/10.1111/j.1464-410x.2003.04672.x.
160. Tsivian A. Reconstruction of extensive upper ureteral damage. J Urol. 2004;171(1):329–30. https://doi.org/10.1097/01.ju.0000101260.82927.5d.
161. Goodwin WE, Cockett AT. Surgical treatment of multiple, recurrent, branched, renal (staghorn) calculi by pyelonephro-ileo-vesical anastomosis. J Urol. 1961;85:214–22. https://doi.org/10.1016/s0022-5347(17)65310-2.
162. Tveter KJ, Bloom DA, Goodwin WE. Ileal ureter: current status. Eur Urol. 1980;6(6):321–7. https://doi.org/10.1159/000473365.
163. Fontana I, Arcuri V, Verrina E, Basile G, Tommasi GV, Casolino V, Stubinski R, Podesta E, Gusmano R, Valente U. Tapered bowel segment for ureteral replacement in renal transplantation. Transplant Proc. 1994;26(1):117–8.
164. El-Mekresh M, Osman Y, Ali-El-Dein B, El-Diasty T, Ghoneim MA. Urological complications after living-donor renal transplantation. BJU Int. 2001;87:295–306.
165. Mattos RM, Smith JJ 3rd. Ileal ureter. Urol Clin North Am. 1997;24(4):813–25. https://doi.org/10.1016/s0094-0143(05)70422-5.
166. Launer BM, Redger KD, Koslov DS, Sax-Bolder AN, Higuchi TT, Windsperger AP, Flynn BJ. Long-term follow up of ileal ureteral replacement for complex ureteral strictures: single institution study. Urology. 2021;157:257–62. https://doi.org/10.1016/j.urology.2021.07.012. Epub 2021 Jul 24
167. Zhong W, Hong P, Ding G, et al. Technical considerations and outcomes for ileal ureter replacement: a retrospective study in China. BMC Surg. 2019;19:9. https://doi.org/10.1186/s12893-019-0472-1.
168. Xiong S, Zhu W, Li X, Zhang P, Wang H, Li X. Intestinal interposition for complex ureteral reconstruction: a comprehensive review. Int J Urol. 2020;27(5):377–86. https://doi.org/10.1111/iju.14222. Epub 2020 Mar 18
169. Verduyckt FJ, Heesakkers JP, Debruyne FM. Long-term results of ileum interposition for ureteral obstruction. Eur Urol. 2002;42(2):181–7. https://doi.org/10.1016/s0302-2838(02)00266-x.
170. Gomez-Avraham I, Nguyen T, Drach GW. Ileal patch ureteroplasty for repair of ureteral strictures: clinical application and results in 4 patients. J Urol. 1994;152(6 Pt 1):2000–4. https://doi.org/10.1016/s0022-5347(17)32290-5.
171. Gerharz EW, Turner WH, Kälble T, Woodhouse CR. Metabolic and functional consequences of urinary reconstruction with bowel. BJU Int. 2003;91(2):143–9. https://doi.org/10.1046/j.1464-410x.2003.04000.x.
172. Bazeed MA, El-Rakhawy M, Ashamallah A, El-Kappany H, El-Hammady S. Ileal replacement of the ureter: is it worthwhile? J Urol. 1983;130:245–7.
173. Ali-El-Dein B, El-Tabey N, Abdel-Latif M, Abdel-Rahim M, El-Bahnasawy MS. Late uro-ileal cancer after incorporation of ileum into the urinary tract. J Urol. 2002;167(1):84–8.
174. Van Helsdingen PJ. Ureter replacement by collagen and seromuscular parts of the large bowel in dogs. Eur Urol. 1984;10(4):276–81. https://doi.org/10.1159/000463807.
175. Zou L, Mao S, Liu S, Zhang L, Yang T, Hu Y, Ding Q, Jiang H. Ureteral reconstruction using a tapered non-vascularized bladder graft: an experimental study in a canine animal model. BMC Urol. 2017;17(1):97. https://doi.org/10.1186/s12894-017-0287-2.

176. Ordorica R, Wiegand LR, Webster JC, Lockhart JL. Ureteral replacement and onlay repair with reconfigured intestinal segments. J Urol. 2014;191(5):1301–6. https://doi.org/10.1016/j.juro.2013.11.027. Epub 2013 Nov 18
177. Shokeir AA, Ghoneim MA. Further experience with the modified ileal ureter. J Urol. 1995;154(1):45–8.
178. Prout GR Jr, Stuart WT, Witus WS. Utilization of ileal segments to substitute for extensive ureteral loss. J Urol. 1963;90:541–51.
179. Richie JP, Skinner DG, Waisman J. The effect of reflux on the development of pyelonephritis in urinary diversion: an experimental study. J Surg Res. 1974;16(3):256–61. https://doi.org/10.1016/0022-4804(74)90040-7.
180. Hendren WH. Tapered bowel segment for ureteral replacement. Urol Clin North Am. 1978;5(3):607–16.
181. Kristjánsson A, Bajc M, Wallin L, Willner J, Månsson W. Renal function up to 16 years after conduit (refluxing or anti-reflux anastomosis) or continent urinary diversion. 2. Renal scarring and location of bacteriuria. Br J Urol. 1995;76(5):546–50. https://doi.org/10.1111/j.1464-410x.1995.tb07776.x.
182. Fujisawa M, Isotani S, Ishimura T, Yamanaka K, Arakawa S, Kamidono S. A novel antireflux uretero-ileal anastomosis for urinary diversion: an experimental study. BJU Int. 2000;86(9):1064–7. https://doi.org/10.1046/j.1464-410x.2000.00946.x.
183. Gosalbez R Jr, Gousse AE. Reconstruction and undiversion of the short or severely dilated ureter: the antireflux ileal nipple revisited. J Urol. 1998;159(2):530–4. https://doi.org/10.1016/s0022-5347(01)63978-8.
184. Kato H, Abol-Enein H, Ogawa A, Ghoneim MA. The ileopsoas tunnel, a new antireflux technique for ureteroileal reimplantation: an experimental study in dogs. Urol Res. 1996;24(2):113–7.; discussion 117-8. https://doi.org/10.1007/BF00431089.
185. Nabizadeh I, Reid RE, Henderson JL. Simplified nonrefluxing ileovesical anastomosis. Experimental study and clinical application. Urology. 1981;18(1):11–4. https://doi.org/10.1016/0090-4295(81)90487-8.
186. Le Duc A, Camey M, Teillac P. An original antireflux ureteroileal implantation technique: long-term followup. J Urol. 1987;137(6):1156–8. https://doi.org/10.1016/s0022-5347(17)44433-8.
187. Yang WH. Yang needle tunneling technique in creating antireflux and continent mechanisms. J Urol. 1993;150(3):830–4. https://doi.org/10.1016/s0022-5347(17)35625-2.
188. Heaney JA, Althausen AF, Parkhurst EC. Ileal conduit undiversion: experience with tunneled vesical implantation of tapered conduit. J Urol. 1980;124(3):329–33. https://doi.org/10.1016/s0022-5347(17)55433-6.
189. Waters WB, Whitmore WF 3rd, Lage AL, Gittes RF. Segmental replacement of the ureter using tapered and nontapered ileum. Investig Urol. 1981;18(4):258–61.
190. Charghi A. Ureteral replacement using a new variation of the tailored ileal segment. J Urol. 1979;121(5):598–601. https://doi.org/10.1016/s0022-5347(17)56895-0.
191. Waldner M, Hertle L, Roth S. Ileal ureteral substitution in reconstructive urological surgery: is an antireflux procedure necessary? J Urol. 1999;162(2):323–6.
192. Boxer RJ, Fritzsche P, Skinner DG, Kaufman JJ, Belt E, Smith RB, Goodwin WE. Replacement of the ureter by small intestine: clinical application and results of the ileal ureter in 89 patients. J Urol. 1979;121(6):728–31. https://doi.org/10.1016/s0022-5347(17)56972-4.
193. Fritzsche P, Skinner DG, Craven JD, Cahill P, Goodwin WE. Long-term radiographic changes of the kidney following the ileal ureter operation. J Urol. 1975;114(6):843–7. https://doi.org/10.1016/s0022-5347(17)67157-x.
194. Vatandaslar F, Reid RE, Freed SZ, Smey P, Kogan SJ, Goldsmith D, Bernstein R, Levitt SB. Ileal segment replacement of ureter. I. Effects on kidney of refluxing vs nonrefluxing ileovesical anastomosis. Urology. 1984;23(6):549–58. https://doi.org/10.1016/0090-4295(84)90069-4.
195. Chung BI, Hamawy KJ, Zinman LN, Libertino JA. The use of bowel for ureteral replacement for complex ureteral reconstruction: long-term results. J Urol. 2006;175(1):179–83.; discussion 183-4. https://doi.org/10.1016/S0022-5347(05)00061-3.

196. Monti PR, Lara RC, Dutra MA, de Carvalho JR. New techniques for construction of efferent conduits based on the Mitrofanoff principle. Urology. 1997;49(1):112–5. https://doi.org/10.1016/S0090-4295(96)00503-1.
197. Pope J, Koch MO. Ureteral replacement with reconfigured colon substitute. J Urol. 1996;155(5):1693–5.
198. Kato H, Igawa Y, Nishizawa O. Transverse colon pouch with total replacement of the ureter by reconfigured colon segment. J Urol. 1999;161(6):1902–3.
199. Ubrig B, Waldner M, Roth S. Reconstruction of ureter with transverse retubularized colon segments. J Urol. 2001;166(3):973–6.
200. D'Elia G, Ali-El-Dein B, Thuroff J, El-Mekresh M, El-Baz M, Ghoneim MA. Reconfigured anti-reflux ileal ureter: a novel surgical technique. BJU Int. 2001;88(Suppl):75.
201. Ali-El-Dein B, Ghoneim MA. Bridging long ureteral defects using the Yang-Monti principle. J Urol. 2003;169(3):1074–7. https://doi.org/10.1097/01.ju.0000050151.66653.cc.
202. Rodríguez Alonso A, González Blanco A, Suárez Pascual G, Bonelli Martín C, Lorenzo Franco J, Cuerpo Pérez MA. Partial substitution of the ureter using a short segment of the ileum following the Monti procedure. Actas Urol Esp. 2005;29(6):607–10.
203. Castellan M, Gosalbez R. Ureteral replacement using the Yang-Monti principle: long-term follow-up. Urology. 2006;67(3):476–9.
204. Kamat NN, Khandelwal P. Laparoscopy-assisted reconstruction of a long-segment ureteral stricture using reconfigured ileal segment: application of the Yang Monti principle. J Endourol. 2007;21(12):1455–60.
205. Peeker R. Ureteric reconstruction and replacement. Curr Opin Urol. 2009;19:563–70.
206. Kim A, Nam W, Song SH, Jeong IG, Hong B. Use of the ileum for ureteral stricture and obstruction in bilateral, unilateral, and single-kidney cases. Urology. 2018;111:203–7.
207. Bao JS, He Q, Li Y, Shi W, Wu G, Yue Z. Yang-Monti principle in bridging long ureteral defects: cases report and a systemic review. Urol J. 2017;14(4):4055–61.
208. Ali-El-Dein B, El-Hefnawy AS, D'Elia G, El-Mekresh MM, Shokeir AA, Gad H, Bazeed MA. Long-term outcome of yang-monti ileal replacement of the ureter: a technique suitable for mild, moderate loss of kidney function and solitary kidney. Urology. 2021;152:153–9. https://doi.org/10.1016/j.urology.2020.09.061. Epub 2021 Jan 14
209. Ghoneim MA, Ali-El-Dein B. Replacing the ureter by an ileal tube, using the Yang-Monti procedure. BJU Int. 2005;95(3):455–70. https://doi.org/10.1111/j.1464-410X.2005.05369.x.
210. Maigaard T, Kirkeby HJ. Yang-Monti ileal ureter reconstruction. Scand J Urol. 2015;49(4):313–8. https://doi.org/10.3109/21681805.2014.882980. Epub 2015 Feb 11
211. Esmat M, Abdelaal A, Mostafa D. Application of Yang-Monti principle in ileal ureter substitution: is it a beneficial modification? Int Braz J Urol. 2012;38(6):779–85.; discussion 785-7. https://doi.org/10.1590/1677-553820133806779.
212. Wagner JR, Schimpf MO, Cohen JL. Robot-assisted laparoscopic ileal ureter. JSLS. 2008;12(3):306–9.
213. Brandao LF, Autorino R, Zargar H, Laydner H, Krishnan J, Samarasekera D, Haber GP, Kaouk JH, Chalikonda S, Stein RJ. Robotic ileal ureter: a completely intracorporeal technique. Urology. 2014;83(4):951–4. https://doi.org/10.1016/j.urology.2013.11.035. Epub 2014 Feb 8
214. Chopra S, Metcalfe C, Satkunasivam R, Nagaraj S, Becker C, de Castro Abreu AL, Azhar RA, Gill I, Desai M, Aron M, Berger A. Initial series of four-arm robotic completely intracorporeal ileal ureter. J Endourol. 2016;30(4):395–9. https://doi.org/10.1089/end.2015.0674. Epub 2016 Feb 9
215. Koenig JF, Rensing A, Austin PF, Vricella G. First-ever reported obstructing ureteral nephrogenic adenoma in a child and subsequent robotic-assisted laparoscopic ileal ureter. Urology. 2016;94:221–3. https://doi.org/10.1016/j.urology.2016.03.013. Epub 2016 Mar 18
216. Liu D, Zhou H, Hao X, Cao H, Ma L, Zhou X, Tao T, Cheng W, Feng Z. Laparoscopic Yang-Monti ureteral reconstruction in children. Urology. 2018;118:177–82. https://doi.org/10.1016/j.urology.2018.04.034. Epub 2018 May 8

217. Pamecha Y, Shelke U, Patil B, Patwardhan S, Kini S. Use of ileum for complex ureteric reconstruction: assessment of long-term outcome, complications, and impact on renal function. Urol Ann. 2018;10:369–74.
218. Wolff B, Chartier-Kastler E, Mozer P, Haertig A, Bitker M-O, Rouprêt M. Long-term functional outcomes after ileal ureter substitution: a single-center experience. Urology. 2011;78:692–5.
219. Ponnatapura J, Dyer RB. The "maiden waist" sign of the ureters. Abdom Radiol (NY). 2019;44(5):1940–1. https://doi.org/10.1007/s00261-018-01890-4.
220. Jadhav KK, Kumar V, Punatar CB, Joshi VS, Sagade SN. Retroperitoneal fibrosis-clinical presentation and outcome analysis from urological perspective. Investig Clin Urol. 2017;58(5):371–7. https://doi.org/10.4111/icu.2017.58.5.371. Epub 2017 Aug 4
221. Khosroshahi A, Stone JH. A clinical overview of IgG4-related systemic disease. Curr Opin Rheumatol. 2011;23(1):57–66. https://doi.org/10.1097/BOR.0b013e3283418057.
222. Srinivasan AK, Richstone L, Permpongkosol S, Kavoussi LR. Comparison of laparoscopic with open approach for ureterolysis in patients with retroperitoneal fibrosis. J Urol. 2008;179(5):1875–8. https://doi.org/10.1016/j.juro.2008.01.030. Epub 2008 Mar 18
223. Stein RJ, Patel NS, Quinn K, Berger M, Koff W, Shah G, Aron M, Berger AK. Laparoscopic ureterolysis with omental wrap for idiopathic retroperitoneal fibrosis. BJU Int. 2010;106(5):703–7. https://doi.org/10.1111/j.1464-410X.2009.09186.x.

Chapter 16
Ureteral Tumors

Stefan Aufderklamm, Moritz Maas, and Arnulf Stenzl

Abstract In non-muscle invasive, low-risk upper urinary tract urothelial carcinoma (UTUC), kidney-sparing surgery (KSS) is becoming more common. However, radical nephroureterectomy (RNU) remains the gold standard in larger or advanced tumors.

It is necessary to distinguish between imperative and elective indications in the case of kidney sparing. Additionally, pre-operative diagnostics such as imaging and endoscopic evaluation, as well as patient-related risk variables such as urine cytology, tumor localization, tumor size, and histopathology, have a major impact on therapy selection. New technical devices and biomarkers can improve pathological staging's restricted capabilities. The therapy can be done endoscopically, percutaneously, or by segmental ureter excision, depending on the risk classification.

KSS is recommended for low-risk malignancies, according to EAU recommendations. Organ preservation can be done in high-risk diseases in some circumstances and when necessary. All techniques necessitate a thorough tumor excision. A strict follow-up with regular radiographic, cytological, and endoscopic studies is required following KSS.

Keywords Upper tract urothelial carcinoma · Biomarkers · Nephron-sparing surgery · Endoscopy · Ureterorenoscopy · Percutaneous approach · Uretero-ureterostomy · Ureteroneocystostomy · Ileal interposition · Ileal ureter · Immunotherapy

Test your learning and check your understanding of this book's contents: use the "Springer Nature Flashcards" app to access questions. To use the app, please follow the instructions in chapter 1.

S. Aufderklamm (✉) · M. Maas · A. Stenzl
Department of Urology, Eberhard Karls University, Tübingen, Germany
e-mail: Stefan.aufderklamm@med.uni-tuebingen.de

M. Abdel-Gawad et al. (eds.), *The Ureter*,
https://doi.org/10.1007/978-3-031-36212-5_16

Abbreviations

CIS	Carcinoma in situ
CSM	Cancer specific mortality
KSS	Kidney sparing surgery
LND	Lymph node dissection
NSS	Nephron sparing surgery
RNU	Radical nephroureterectomy
UTUC	Upper urinary tract urothelial carcinoma
UTVH	Upper urinary tract tumors with variant histology
SCC	Squamous cell carcinoma
SEER	Surveillance, Epidemiology and End results database
OS	Overall survival
PFS	progression-free survival
CSS	Cancer-specific survival
EAU	European association of urology
CT	Computed tomography scan
PDD	Photodynamic diagnostics
cfDNA	Cell-free DNA
UUT	Upper urinary tract
NPV	Negative prognostic value
COX-2	Cyclooxygenase 2
NLR	Neutrophil-lymphocyte ratio
AGR	Albumin-globulin ratio
WBC	White blood cell count
HR	Hazard ratio
Hb	Hemoglobin
miRNA	MicroRNA
MSI	Microsatellite instability
PD-1	Programmed cell death protein 1
PD-L1	Programmed death ligand 1

Learning Objectives
After reading this chapter, the readers will be able to:

- Describe the pathological definition of non-muscle invasive UTUC.
- Describe challenges of pre-operative tissue sampling and staging, biomarkers in UTUC, and clinical and pathological risk stratification of the non-metastatic UTUC.
- Discuss imperative and elective indications for nephron sparing surgery, surgical treatment algorithm in KSS, oncological principles in minimal invasive RNU, adjuvant instillation therapy, the role of immunotherapy in UTUC, and follow-up regime.

16.1 Introduction: Tumors of the Upper Urinary Tract

Tumors of the upper urinary tract are rare, with urothelial carcinomas of the upper urinary tract (UTUC) being the most prevalent histologic entity showing an incidence of approximately 2:100,000 cases within western countries [1]. Within urothelial malignancies, this corresponds to a proportion of 5–10% [2].

The low incidence of these tumors leads to limited evidence compared to the 'bigger sibling' urothelial carcinoma of the bladder. However, the number of available studies for UTUC can be described as high compared to those focusing on histological variants of upper tract tumors. This results in limited evidence-based knowledge for tumors of variant histology, although it seems reasonable to assume a concordance in the characteristics of variable histology in the bladder and the upper urinary tract.

Malignant tumors of the upper urinary tract with variant histology (UTVH) include squamous cell carcinomas (SCC), adenocarcinomas, neuroendocrine carcinomas, and sarcomatoid carcinomas [3, 4]. In a recent analysis of 11,809 upper urinary tract tumor patients in the Surveillance, Epidemiology and End Results database (SEER), UTUC account for 97.3% of all upper urinary tract tumors, whereas histologic variants represent 2.7% of the tumors [4]. While tumors of pure histological variants are rare, cases with partially variant histology in an otherwise urothelial carcinoma are considerably more frequent [5].

Interestingly, no apparent differences are seen in terms of localization within the upper urinary tract when comparing UTUC and UTVH [4]. Both are commonly found in the renal pelvis, for UTUC this localization is twice as frequent as in the ureter [4, 6]. Within the ureter, the distal parts are more frequently affected by UTUCs than the intermediate and proximal ureter [7]. An intriguing deviation of the distribution pattern is found for neuroendocrine tumors, where approximately two-thirds of the cases are located in the ureter, whereas one-third is found in the renal pelvis [4].

Compared to UTUC, patients with UTVH are diagnosed more frequently in advanced T-stages (T3-4) or metastatic stages [4]. This also becomes evident in prognostic analyses: patients with UTVH show a shorter overall survival (OS), progression-free survival (PFS), and cancer-specific survival (CSS) and reciprocally have higher cancer-specific mortality (CSM) compared to UTUC patients [4, 8, 9].

According to EAU guidelines, therapy of upper urinary tract tumors should consider nephron-sparing surgery (NSS) in all low-risk malignancies regardless of the opposite kidney. Beyond that, it can be used in well-chosen patients with severe renal insufficiency or solitary kidneys with high-risk conditions to avoid the morbidity of radical nephroureterectomy (RNU). NSS can be done endoscopically, percutaneously, or by segmental ureter excision, depending on the risk classification of the tumor [10, 11]. When used in well-selected cases, no substantial impairment of oncological prognosis was identified compared to NSS and RNU.

Nevertheless, RNU remains the mainstay for surgical interventions of UTUCs that are bigger, invasive, multifocal, or show high-risk characteristics [10]. In this context, it is important to emphasize that already partially present variant histology leads to the classification of the tumor as a high-risk tumor [11]. The necessity of a thorough tumor excision is common to all surgical techniques. Especially for patients treated with NSS, a strict guideline-based follow-up with regular radiographic, cytological, and endoscopic studies is required.

In the following chapter, we focus on the diagnosis, therapy, and follow-up of patients with UTUC, given its prevalence compared to the histological variants.

16.2 Diagnostics and Imaging of Tumors of the Upper Urinary Tract

Excretory urography has lost its usefulness in the diagnosis of UTUC with the development of advanced computer tomography [12]. However, it is still a standard diagnostic instrument in clinical practice. Due to the obvious possibility of cystoscopic evaluation, retrograde ureteropyelography is broadly adopted to examine the upper urinary system. Furthermore, a urine sample from the ureter and renal pelvis can be collected for cytological investigation. CT imaging is the approach with the highest predictive accuracy for UTUC, with a sensitivity of 67–100% and a specificity of 93–99% [13]. For an accurate diagnosis, a urography phase should be performed 10–15 min after the contrast medium is applied. The benefit of CT scan over excretory urography in terms of diagnosis is the ability to detect a contrast-enhanced change of the renal pelvis or ureteral wall in the arterial or portal-venous stage in the absence of a urographically suspicious lesion [14]. Magnetic resonance urography and retrograde uretero-pyelography are diagnostic options in cases of contrast agent allergy or impaired renal function. The sensitivity of magnetic resonance urography is roughly 75% for UTUC below 2 cm in size [15]. However, because Gadolinium carries the potential risk of renal sclerosis in patients with severe kidney dysfunction or a glomerular filtration rate of less than 30 mL/min [16], the renal function of these patients should be taken into account for magnetic resonance imaging with contrast agents.

16.3 Tumor Biopsy in UTUC

The diagnostic semirigid or flexible ureterorenoscopy with the option of taking a biopsy is the preferred method for evaluating UTUC. Tumor diagnosis and differentiation by biopsy are accurate in 90% of patients, with a low false-negative rate [17]. However, due to the limited size of biopsies, undergrading and understaging are common. The anatomical features of the upper urinary tract and the manner of taking the biopsy make a significant discrimination of invasive and non-invasive tumors challenging. When preoperative and postoperative specimens following final surgery were analyzed, histopathological upgrading was observed in up to 51% of patients, highlighting the requirement for extended endoscopic tissue collection in the kidney-sparing surgery [18]. Although still preliminary, investigations on filter-based endoscopic methods report encouraging evidence, particularly for the endoscopic assessment of flat lesions of the urinary tract [19]. The wavelength of white light is lowered in narrow-band imaging (415–540 nm). Fine microstructures in the urothelial mucosa can be identified more consistently. Specific parts of the color spectrum are amplified by color tone shifting with the SPIES SPECTRA™ software, making blood vessels better visible. A few authors have investigated the use of photodynamic diagnostics (PDD) in the upper urinary system. The preoperative examination of upper tract tumors and the identification of CIS was reported as practically achievable by percutaneous instillation of 5-aminolevulinic acid (5-ALA) in the urinary system by nephrostomy or ureteral stent [20]. However, the limited volume of the renal pelvis and ureter and the limited time of local exposure should be considered a disadvantage.

16.4 Biomarkers in Upper Tract Urothelial Cancer

Although histologically similar to urothelial bladder cancer, upper tract urothelial cancer (UTUC) has several molecular, biological, and clinical characteristics that are distinct from bladder urothelial cancer, leading to the term "disparate twins" in the comparison of bladder urothelial cancer and UTUC features [21]. An example of this inequality is the existing evidence regarding the use and potential of biomarkers, which shows an imbalance in favour of lower urinary tract tumors. A major reason for this is the low incidence of UTUC, leading to a lack of prospective data. Despite the inadequate evidence in the direct comparison, guideline recommendations on the appropriate use of biomarkers have also been established for the UTUC. These guideline recommendations focus primarily on conventional biomarkers such as urine cytology and laboratory parameters. Beyond these parameters, however, research is increasingly focusing on "next-generation biomarkers"using genetic, epigenetic, and molecular assays to enable molecular characterization of the disease. Therefore, the following subchapter aims to provide an overview of current guideline recommendations, available biomarkers, and the potential of recent developments in genetic biomarkers. Conventional biomarkers are described first; these are divided into urine-based, blood-based and tissue-based markers based on their acquisition. Secondly, "next-generation biomarkers" are outlined and categorized into epigenetic markers, cfDNA and genotype markers. Figure 16.1 provides an overview of the described biomarkers.

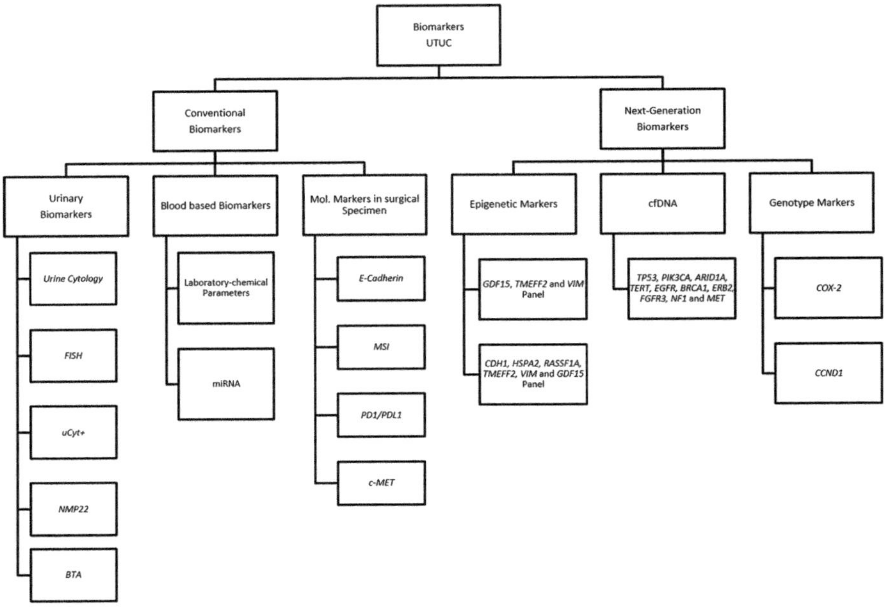

Fig. 16.1 Overview of Biomarkers in upper tract urothelial cancer (UTUC)

16.4.1 Conventional Biomarkers

16.4.1.1 Urinary Biomarkers

All urinary biomarkers used to diagnose bladder cancer can also be utilized to detect UTUC in urine (see Table 16.1 for an overview of urinary biomarkers). However, due to the different origins of the evaluated samples, several limitations should be addressed. In particular, the high impact of instrumented sampling of upper urinary tract (UUT) urine has to be considered. In current guidelines, the only recommended urine marker for diagnosis and follow-up in patients with UTUC is the evaluation of urinary cytology according to the Paris system 2015, which has recently been modified to harmonize the evaluation system [36]. Table 16.2 shows potential cytological findings and their therapeutic implications [37, 38].

Abnormal cytology may indicate a high-grade UTUC after cystoscopic exclusion of a bladder tumor [36]. The sensitivity of urinary cytology is lower for upper tract tumors than for bladder tumors. One reason for this seems to be that the smaller size of UTUC lesions resulting in a lower risk of cancer cell shedding compared to bladder tumors [22]. The morphology of both physiological urothelium and the malignant findings differ slightly but visibly between the upper urinary tract and the bladder. As such, the physiological, cytological specimens of the upper urinary tract show a higher proportion of basal cells, most likely due to the lower number of urothelial layers in the upper urinary tract. For the malignant findings, the

Table 16.1 Urinary biomarkers for upper tract urothelial cancer

Assay Name	Setting	Specimen	Evaluation of	Assay Type	Sensitivity (%)	Specificity (%)	Reference
Urine cytology	Diagnosis	Lower urinary tract urine	Morphology	Staining/ Microscopy	50–71	56–100	[22–25]
	Diagnosis	Upper urinary tract urine	Morphology	Staining/Microscopy	64–82	66–100	[22–25]
FISH	Diagnosis	Lower urinary tract urine	Aneuploidy of chromosomes 3,7, 17, loss of 9p21	Multitarget FISH	50–100	78–99.3	[23, 26–31]
	Diagnosis	Upper urinary tract urine	Aneuploidy of chromosomes 3,7, 17, loss of 9p21	Multitarget FISH	79	50.7	[23]
uCyt+	Diagnosis	Lower urinary tract urine	Tumour-associated cellular antigens	Immunofluorescence	50–75	69.8–95	[23, 24]
	Diagnosis	Upper urinary tract urine	Tumour-associated cellular antigens	Immunofluorescence	91–100	66.7–100	[23, 24]
NMP22	Diagnosis	Lower urinary tract urine	Nuclear matrix protein	Expression Level, Sandwich ELISA	44–62.5	31.3–98	[23, 32]
	Diagnosis	Upper urinary tract urine	Nuclear matrix protein	Expression Level, Sandwich ELISA	100	5.9	[23]
ADXBLADDER	Diagnosis	Lower urinary tract urine	MCM5 protein	ELISA	53–100	70–73	[33]
BTA stat	Diagnosis	Lower urinary tract urine	hCFHrp	Dipstick immunoassay	61.1–82	80–89	[34, 35]

Table 16.2 Paris system: Potential findings in urinary cytology

Cytology Findings	Unsatisfactory	Negative for high-grade urothelial carcinoma	Atypical urothelial cells	Low-grade urothelial neoplasm (LGUN) Suspicious for high-grade urothelial carcinoma (HGUC) High-grade urothelial carcinoma (HGUC) Other malignancy
Management	Repetition of urinary cytology	Pursuit of clinical follow-up	Elimination of potential influencing factors (e.g. infection) Repetition of urinary cytology after 1 month	Perform evaluation of bladder and upper urinary tract (e.g. cycstoscopy, biopsy, CT-urography)

commonly known morphological criteria of bladder tumors also apply to UTUC, although the extent of these criteria is lower in UTUC. Furthermore, the polymorphism of individual cells in UTUC is less distinctive than in bladder cancer. Since the introduction of the Paris system, this issue has garnered considerable attention, and it might lead to discrepancies in cytological diagnosis of UUT samples [37]

Since the sensitivity of cytology detecting UTUC is significantly higher in urine samples obtained from the upper urinary tract than in bladder-derived urine samples, it is suggested to acquire cytology selectively from the upper urinary tract [22].

However, manipulation during upper tract sampling may cause morphological alterations in urothelial cells, potentially leading to a lower specificity of upper tract samples compared to voided urine [22]. Overall sensitivity for urine cytology in UTUC patients collected from the lower urinary tract ranges from 50% to 71%, whereas urine from the upper urothelial tract ranges from 64% to 82% [22, 39, 40]. For bladder-derived urine, specificity ranges from 56% to 100%, and for UUT urine, from 66% to 100% [39, 40]. The tumor grade has a direct influence on the sensitivity: Low-grade tumors have lower sensitivity in both bladder urine (0–18.2%) and UUT urine (0–72.1%) than high grade tumors (bladder-derived urine 56–100%, UUT urine 71–92.3%) [22, 39, 40]. Urine cytology should be collected prior to applying larger amounts of contrast agent in retrograde urography since this may cause cytological specimens to deteriorate [22, 36]. A carefully obtained barbotage cytology may increase the sensitivity of urine cytology [39].

Based on the sensitivity and specificity rates of urine cytology in UTUC, a treatment decision between RNU vs. endoscopic, kidney-preserving therapy should not be based on cytology alone but rather on the combination of biopsy and cytology [22, 39, 41]. The addition of radiological examinations can further improve the accuracy of the diagnosis and thus minimize the risk of both under and over treatment [36, 40].

The **UroVysion® FISH (fluorescence in-situ hybridization)** assay can identify numeric chromosomal aberrations linked to urothelial carcinoma (aneuploidy of chromosomes 3, 7, 17 and loss of 9p21) (Fig. 16.2).

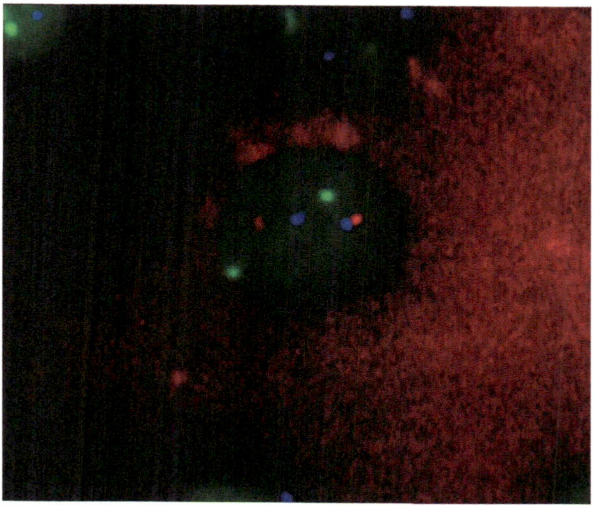

Fig. 16.2 Exemplary illustration for FISH: Physiological findings with diploidy of chromosomes 3 (red), 7 (green), 17 (blue). No gold fluorescence, indicating Locus 9p21 not present. An accurate result requires 25 morphologically abnormal cells. At least 4 cells with an increase of ≥2 chromosomes (3, 7 or 17) or at least 12 cells with no detectable 9p21 signal are required to diagnose a positive result

Due to the low sensitivity for molecular aberrations in UTUC, which is around 50%, the guidelines do not recommend its use for UTUC in clinical practice [26–28, 36]. FISH sensitivity is even lower for low-grade tumors, which is a major limitation, particularly in the follow-up after kidney preservation therapy [26]. However, other studies suggest a higher sensitivity for FISH in the diagnosis and follow-up of UTUC, contrary to the results of the studies referenced in the guideline. The algorithm for the FISH analysis seems to have a significant influence on the results: Overall sensitivities reported varied from 77% to 100% [29–31]. As in conventional cytology, the location of the sample acquisition has a relevant influence: In a recent study, upper urinary tract samples outperformed bladder samples, with a sensitivity of 79% and a specificity of 51% [23]. In studies evaluating sensitivity by tumour grade, HG tumors have higher sensitivity values (LG 28.6–73.3%, HG 86.4–100.0%) [23, 29]. Apart from the wide heterogeneity of the determined sensitivity and specificity rates, the implementation of the FISH assay in daily clinical practice is difficult due to high material and personal expenses. Hybridization and microscopic analysis take time and require specialized equipment and staff. Cell analysis automation may lower the influence of these elements in the future.

Fluorescent-labeled antibodies against sulfated mucin glycoproteins and carcinoembryonic antigens (CEA) as tumor-associated antigens are used in the **uCyt + assay**, which is a combination of cytology and immunostaining (Fig. 16.3).

The combination of urine cytology and uCyt+ improves sensitivity compared to cytology alone while preserving high specificity. The location of urine collection affects reported sensitivity. It ranges from 50% to 75% in voided urine samples to 91%–100% in upper urothelial tract samples [23, 24]. Urine cytology and uCyt+ combined achieved an 87% sensitivity [24]. For bladder-derived urine, specificity varies from 69.8% to 95% and 66.7–100% for UUT urine [23, 24]. In

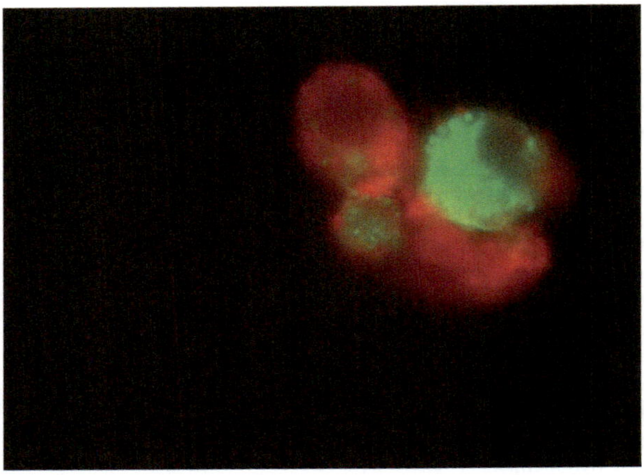

Fig. 16.3 Exemplary illustration for uCyt+. Antibodies against mucin glycoproteins and CEA stain basal cells green and orange. Suspicious findings require only 1 positive cell in combination with urine cytology

both bladder-derived and UUT-derived urine, sensitivity for HG tumors is higher than for LG tumors (66.7–100%) [23, 24]. Like FISH, uCyt+ has limitations in daily use due to the need for specialized laboratories, time to prepare specimens, and experience in sample assessment. Conditions including benign prostatic disease, hematuria, inflammations, urolithiasis, and mechanical stress due to instrumented sampling may further impact the result. The uCyt+ test is no longer commercially available.

The **NMP22** test is another potential urine biomarker from bladder cancer patients and can be used in UTUC. Although it is FDA-approved, its application in routine diagnosis is not recommended, neither for BC nor for UTUC [36, 42]. Higher levels of NMP22 are a correlate of more extensive cell apoptosis, resulting in increased sensitivity in HG tumors. The reported sensitivity for NMP22 in UTUC patients varies from 44% to 100% (upper and lower urinary tract) and 5.9–98% for specificity [23, 32]. Extrinsic variables such as hematuria, infections, prior BCG therapy, and ureteral or nephrostomy stents can affect NMP22 as it is a protein-based assay [43]. Another influencing factor leading to an impairment of specificity is the manipulative extraction of UUT urine. Consequently, the NMP22 assay as an urinary marker for UTUC is not recommended.

The **MCM5-ELISA** (ADXBLADDER®, Arquer) test may be a cytology-independent alternative in upper urinary tract diagnosis. The assay detects MCM5, a cell-cycle-associated protein and part of the helicase system. It is thereby an indicator of the cell cycle status. A recent study in 865 patients found an overall sensitivity of 73% and 100% for pT2 tumors at NPV 100%. It is not affected by benign illnesses and conditions like urinary tract infections or hematuria. However, some studies suggest that prostatitis may influence test performance due to epithelial damage, resulting in false positive MCM5 results [33]. The influence of instrumented acquisition of UUT urine on the assay's performance has not yet been investigated in detail.

The **BTA test** targets hCFHrp, a variant of human complement factor H. hCFHrp is an element of the complement cascade. It may be produced and excreted into the urine by urothelial cancer cells. It is assumed that the production of hCFHrp is a growth factor advantage for urothelial cancer cells and shelters them from the host's immune system [34]. The BTA test has a reported sensitivity in UTUC from 61.1–82% and a specificity from 80% to 89% [34, 35]. The BTA test is susceptible to blood contamination in the analyzed samples. False-positive tests are likely to be diagnosed in patients with macroscopic hematuria, benign inflammation, and ureteral or nephrostomy stents. Also, prior BCG therapy may influence test results. Therefore, the vulnerability of these factors is an important limitation of the BTA test [44].

Several studies have linked aberrant urine concentrations of cytokeratins 8, 18, and 19 to urothelial cancer Cytokeratins. Cytokeratins are cytoskeletal proteins of cells of epithelial origin that can be discovered in urine after cell death. Calculi, infections, or prior BCG treatments might cause false-positive results. Several cytokeratin assays are available and currently being studied. CYFRA 21.1 uses monoclonal antibodies to assess CK19 fragments. The UBC-ELISA targets CK8 and CK18. Most research on these biomarkers has focused on bladder cancer patients [45, 46].

16.4.1.2 Blood-based Biomarkers

In addition to the urine-based biomarkers several blood-based biomarkers can be used for UTUC (Table 16.3). While traditional laboratory biochemical parameters have their advantage primarily in their broad availability and applicability, "next-generation" biomarkers provide further information about the molecular characteristics of tumours.

Laboratory-chemical Markers

According to the guidelines, blood-based biomarkers can be used as prognostic markers and thus can help in clinical decisions and patient advice [36, 50]. In particular, the guidelines recommend the preoperative use of neutrophil-lymphocyte ratio and albumin as prognostic markers [36, 48]. In addition, several systemic inflammatory response markers have been evaluated for their prognostic potential.

The addressed markers quantify tumor-associated inflammation. Advanced tumors cause increased systemic inflammation markers by activating the intrinsic and extrinsic pathways [47]. Activation of associated factors leads to higher levels of inflammation mediators and cyclooxygenase 2 (COX-2) and promote tumour progression [51, 52]. A recent meta-analysis of 52 studies with 22,513 patients found a correlation between several inflammation-associated preoperative blood-based biomarkers and CSS: High preoperative neutrophil-lymphocyte ratio (NLR) was associated with a shorter CSS (HR 1.66), as were platelet-lymphocyte ratio (PLR, HR 1.68), albumin-globulin ratio (AGR, HR 3.00), white blood cell count (WBC, HR 1.58) and fibrinogen (HR 2.23) [47].

A further correlation could be found for hemoglobin (Hb, HR 1.51): Apart from low Hb caused by chronic inflammation, a further relation to the hypoxia pathway

Table 16.3 Prognostic blood based biomarkers in upper tract urothelial cancer

Analyzed Marker	Clinical Setting	Specimen	Assay Type	HR	95% CI	Reference
neutrophil-lymphocyte ratio (NLR)	Prognosis	Blood	Laboratory chemical analysis	1.66	1.34–2.06	[47]
Albumin	Prognosis	Blood	Laboratory chemical analysis	1.88	1.33–2.45	[48]
platelet-lymphocyte ratio (PLR)	Prognosis	Blood	Laboratory chemical analysis	1.68	1.30–2.17	[47]
albumin-globulin ratio (AGR)	Prognosis	Blood	Laboratory chemical analysis	3.0	1.87–4.84	[47]
white blood cell count (WBC)	Prognosis	Blood	Laboratory chemical analysis	1.58	1.02–2.46	[47]
fibrinogen	Prognosis	Blood	Laboratory chemical analysis	2.23	1.86–2.68	[47]
hemoglobin (HB)	Prognosis	Blood	Laboratory chemical analysis	1.51	1.22–1.87	[47]
miRNA (miR-151b)	Prognosis	Blood/pathological specimen	qRT-PCR	0.25	N/A	[49]

(essential for tumour survival, proliferation and progression) may be a rationale for that [53].

Although the meta-analysis mentions additional potential prognostic biomarkers, the only recommended guideline biomarkers are albumin and NLR. The meta-analysis has relevant limitations which need to be considered: These limitations are different cut-off values of the evaluated markers, heterogeneity in the definition of NLR, WBC and Hb in the included studies, a high proportion of patients from areas with high aristolochic acid exposure and the retrospective nature of the study.

miRNA

MicroRNAs (miRNA) are emerging as new diagnostic and prognostic biomarkers for UTUC patients. They may be serum-derived or tissue-derived. MiRNAs are small, non-protein coding RNAs with a 20–25 nucleotide length, involved in posttranscriptional gene regulation by repressing gene translation and degrading mRNA. Several miRNAs are differentially expressed in various human cancers, including urothelial cancer [54]. miRNAs have both diagnostic and prognostic potential. In a study by Tao et al., 10 miRNAs were identified as being able to distinguish patients with UTUC from patients of the control group (miR-664a-3p, miR-431-5p, miR-423-5p, miR-191-5p, miR-33b-3p, miR-26a-5p, miR-22-3p, miR-16-5p, let-7b-5p and let-7c; AUC >0.8) [55]. MiR-151b was further found to be associated with tumour progression (HR = 0.33, $p < 0.001$) and CSS (HR = 0.25; $p < 0.001$) in UTUC patients, making it a potential prognostic biomarker [49]. In a study comparing miRNA signatures and their potential to differentiate between low- and high-grade UTUC, a sensitivity of 83% and a specificity of 85% in identifying high-grade UTUC were observed [56]. Further, the miRNA signatures showed prognostic value for OS and RFS. Although this data is promising, using miRNAs as biomarkers is still experimental and need further validation, which is expressed in the absence of a guideline recommendation.

Table 16.3 gives an overview of blood-based biomarkers.

16.4.1.3 Tissue-based Molecular Markers

The guidelines describe various molecular markers and their potential prognostic impact without specific recommendations concerning their use [36]. These biomarkers include cell adhesion markers (E-Cadherin, CD24), microsatellite instability (MSI), cell differentiation (HER2), angiogenesis, proliferation, epithelial-mesenchymal transition (EMT), mitosis, apoptosis, vascular invasion, PD-1/PDL-1 expression, and c-MET protein. In univariate but not multivariate analysis, lower E-cadherin expression was linked to worse RFS (univariate: $p < 0.001$; multivariate: $p = 0.74$) and CSS (univariate $p = 0.006$; multivariate $p = 0.84$) [57]. For MSI, both univariate ($p = 0.02$) and multivariate ($p < 0.05$) analysis showed a positive correlation between prognosis and level of MSI [58]. Overexpression of HER2 is associated with clinically and biologically aggressive tumors and with disease recurrence ($p = 0.04$), OS ($p = 0.02$) and CSS ($p = 0.02$) [59]. PD-1 expression was identified as a prognosticator for RFS in univariate analysis and for CSS and OS in univariate and multivariate analyses (CSS $p = 0.039$; OS $p = 0.029$) [60]. Although the above biomarkers have shown prognostic value in studies, their use in clinical practice is uncommon due to time and material-consuming requirements.

16.4.2 Next-Generation Biomarkers

In the last decade, high-throughput technologies have significantly improved the ability to analyze molecular tumour features. They allow rapid and comprehensive characterization of molecular aberrations, thus providing deeper insights into tumor biology. Given the development of "targeted therapies" these markers will gain increasing relevance [61]. Like "conventional" biomarkers, specimens can be derived from blood, urine, or tissue.

Cyclooxygenase 2 (COX2) is a key enzyme in converting arachidonic acid to prostaglandins and can be induced by growth factors, pro-inflammatory cytokines, carcinogens, endotoxins, or tumor promotors. Its expression in benign tissue is low to undetectable [62]. COX2 genotyping in peripheral blood samples shows significant differences in COX2 genotypes between UTUC patients and the healthy control group, COX2 expression was further upregulated in tissue samples [62, 63]. COX2 G-765C/intron 5 carrying GG/AT variants have an increased risk of developing UTUC ($OR = 4.83$), whereas CG/TT variants have a decreased risk ($OR = 0.26$) [63].

Cyclin D1 (CCND1) is a key regulator of G1-S cell cycle progression and is associated with early recurrence, tumor differentiation, and clinical outcome in bladder cancer. In an evaluation of CCND polymorphisms and UTUC, CCND1 GC or GC + CC genotypes were more common in the UTUC patient group than in the control group (p = *0.05 and 0.03*). The GC genotype increased the risk of UC by 1.6-fold ($p = 0.05$), whereas the GC + CC genotypes had a 1.68-fold risk of UC ($p = 0.03$), each compared to the GG genotype. There was no association between CCND1 genotype and tumor grade, survival, or recurrence [64].

Epigenetic biomarker assays from urine samples represent another possible future biomarker development: A panel analyzing methylation levels of GDF15, TMEFF2 and VIM showed higher levels in UTUC than in the control group ($p = 0.022$; $p < 0.001$; $p < 0.001$). It has 91% sensitivity and 100% specificity in identifying UTUC. Low VIM promoter methylation level further predicts poor disease-specific survival [65]. In patients with gross hematuria, promoter methylation of CDH1, HSPA2, RASSF1A, TMEFF2, VIM, and GDF15 identified UTUC with 82% sensitivity and 68% specificity [66].

Future research will further focus on circulating tumor DNA in blood samples. It provides the benefits of "classic" biomarkers plus real-time tumor genome insights at all disease stages. These insights are not only useful in predicting disease risk, but also in the development of personalized tumor therapies.

Single-nucleotide variants, indels, fusion or copy number amplifications and alterations of TP53, PIK3CA, ARID1A, TERT, EGFR, BRCA1, ERB2, FGFR3, NF-1 and MET are genetic alterations which were identified in blood samples of UTUC patients. In metastatic UTUC, the frequency of genetic alterations varies between circulating DNA and initial tumor tissue for TP53 and FGFR3 [67]. TP53 and RB1 mutations are more common in BC, while FGFR3 and HRAS mutations are more common in UTUC [68]. FGFR3 expression is of particular interest in front of the FDA-approved therapy with Erdafitinib, it correlates with a luminal-papillary molecular subtype [69].

16.5 Tumor Staging and Classification

UTUC and urothelial bladder cancer have comparable tumor stages and categorizations [70].Tumors can be classified as non-invasive papillary tumors, flat lesions (carcinoma in situ) and invasive tumors [71].

Table 16.4 shows the TNM categorization of upper tract urothelial carcinoma.

At the initial diagnosis, 60% of all UTUCs have progressed to an invasive tumor stage with infiltration of the muscularis propria (>T1) [72]. A worse prognosis was documented in this case, with 5-year survival rates of fewer than 50% in pT2 or pT3 UTUCs [73, 74]. Biopsy and histological evaluation of the upper urinary tract

Table 16.4 TNM classification 2017 for upper tract urothelial cell carcinoma [70]

T - Primary tumor	
TX	Primary tumor unable to assess
T0	No primary tumor
Ta	Papillary non-invasive tumor
Tis	Carcinoma in situ
T1	Invasion of subepithelial connective tissue
T2	Invasion of muscularis propria
T3	Invasion of peripelvic fat/renal parenchyma (renal pelvis) or periureteric fat (ureter)
T4	Invasion of adjacent organs or through the kidney into perinephric fat
N - Lymph nodes	
NX	Regional lymph nodes unable to assess
N0	No regional lymph node metastasis
N1	Metastasis in a single lymph node 2 cm or less in the greatest dimension
N2	Metastasis in a single lymph node > 2 cm or multiple lymph nodes
M - Metastasis	
M0	No distant metastasis
M1	Distant metastasis

lesions might be difficult, resulting in a high risk of understaging the tumor in up to 51% of instances. The structural conditions of the ureter and the renal pelvis, the tissue sampling technique, and the sample size are all contributing factors for this [7, 18]. This often results in an insufficient pathological examination and a more difficult distinction between invasive and non-invasive cancers and the depth of infiltration in those. When KSS is being considered, an extensive endourological biopsy is required [18].

16.6 Risk Stratification of Non-metastatic Urothelial Cancer of the Upper Urinary Tract

Due to restrictions in the endoscopic and histopathological examination, clinical diagnosis of tumor stage in UTUC is challenging. As a result, to identify individuals who might be more appropriate for KSS, a risk classification involving low-risk and high-risk malignancies must be used [75, 76], Table 16.5.

According to these characteristics, a clinical algorithm can be utilized to determine if KSS is possible (Fig. 16.4). It must be mentioned though, that this surgery only applies to patients who have normally structured and functioning contralateral kidneys, based on the most recent EAU criteria. Histopathological tumor stage and grade have a substantial predictive significance in UTUC in this setting [73, 74, 77]. CIS in the upper urinary tract and the bladder is linked to significantly increased recurrence rates and cancer-specific mortality [78, 79]. Furthermore, the localization of the primary lesion plays an important role. When the tumor stage is considered, ureteral and multifocal cancers have a worse oncological result than tumors

Table 16.5 Risk-stratification factors include clinical and pathological factors

Parameters	
Low risk[a]	Tumor size < 2 cm
	Unifocal tumor
	low-grade URS biopsy
	low-grade urin cytology
	No invasive aspect in imaging
	Compliance for FU
High risk[b]	Tumor size > 2 cm
	Multifocal lesions
	High-grade URS biopsy
	High-grade cytology
	Endoscopic treatment failure for "low-risk UTUC"
	Invasive aspect in imaging
	Hydronephrosis
	Previous bladder cancer and/or cystectomy

a All of these factors
b Any of these factors [71, 72]

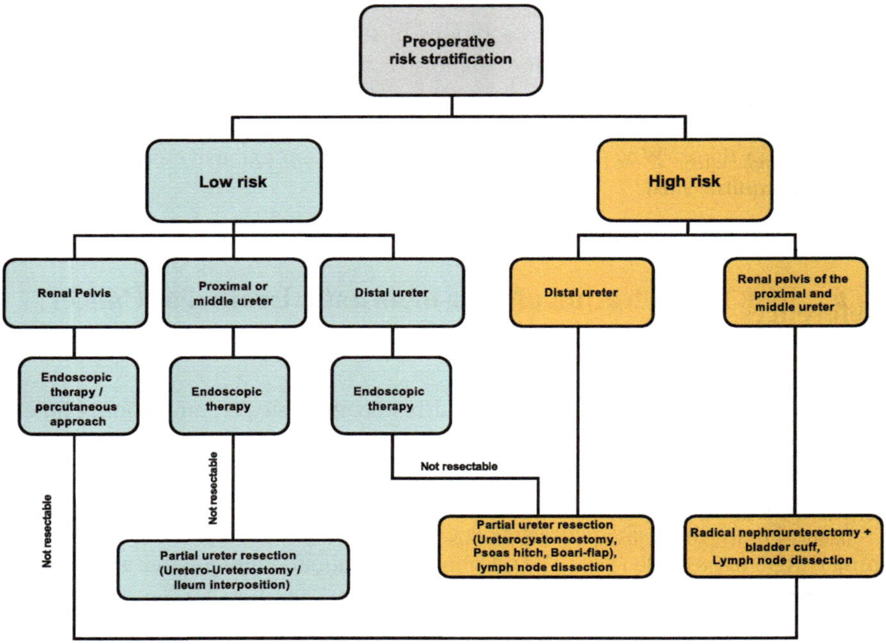

Fig. 16.4 Surgical treatment based on tumor location and risk classification [6]

that just affect the renal pelvis [80]. In addition, hydronephrosis is linked to a more invasive tumor and a worse prognosis [81–83]. Before surgery, other risk factors such as cigarette abuse, age, obesity, and comorbidities should be considered [84]. Clinical and pathological risk factors are summarized in Table 16.5.

16.7 Treatment

Radical nephroureterectomy (RNU) is still the recommended treatment for high-risk UTUC, independently of tumor site. Nonetheless, performance status or ASA classification (American Society of Anesthesiologists) of certain patients exclude radical surgery. Furthermore, also patients with a more advanced disease can benefit from palliative ureteroscopy and repeating treatments, with a 2-year overall survival rate of 45% [29].

In case of KSS, both mandatory (anatomical or functional single kidney, substantial nephropathy, or bilateral lesions) and optional (low-risk tumors and chosen cases of high-risk tumors) indications must be considered during the decision-making process [11]. Furthermore, other parameters such as risk classification (Table 16.5), tumor location, volume and ability for resection must be taken into account [10]. Surgical treatment can be performed endoscopically, percutaneously or by segmental ureter excision. Figure 16.4 depicts an organ preservation surgery algorithm.

Prior to surgery, patients must be advised about the importance of strict follow-up, including an early second-look ureterorenoscopy after 6–8 weeks and regular CT scans, as shown in Table 16.6 [85]. Despite this, due to limitations in diagnostics and biopsy-taking and the considerable potential of understaging, the risk of progression of the disease persists [86].

Table 16.6 Follow-up after NSS in UTUC, URS = Ureterorenoscopy [1]

	Modality	3 months	6 months	Year 1	Year 2	Year 3	Year 4	Year 5	After 5 years
Low risk	Cystoscopy	×	×	×	×	×	×	×	–
	CT Urography	×	×	×	×	×	×	×	–
	URS	×	–	–	–	–	–	–	–
High risk	Cystoscopy	×	×	×	×	×	×	×	Yearly
	Urinary cytology	×	×	×	×	×	×	×	Yearly
	CT Urography	×	×	×	×	×	×	×	Yearly
	Chest CT	×	×	×	×	×	×	×	Yearly
	URS	×	×	–	–	–	–	–	–
	Urinary cytology in situ	×	×	–	–	–	–	–	–

16.7.1 Radical Nephroureterectomy

16.7.1.1 Open Radical Nephroureterectomy

Independent of tumor site, open RNU with bladder cuff resection is the recommended gold-standard treatment for high-risk UTUC [72]. Oncological considerations must be followed when doing RNU to avoid tumor spreading [72].

16.7.1.2 Minimal Invasive Radical Nephroureterectomy

Performed by skilled surgeons who follow oncological considerations, laparoscopic RNU is a safe procedure. After laparoscopic or open RNU, there is a trend approaching similar oncological results [87, 88]. In a prospective randomized trial, laparoscopic RNU was inferior to open RNU for non-organ confined UTUC. But, because the trial was small (n = 80), it was probably underpowered [89]. Despite staging and surgical advancements, oncological success rates after RNU have not altered appreciably over the last three decades [90]. Recent findings demonstrate that a robot-assisted laparoscopic method is an oncologic equivalent to the other approaches [91, 92]. In rare cases, retroperitoneal metastatic spread and metastases along the trocar channel have been observed following the management of big tumors in a pneumoperitoneal setting [87]. Several measures should be taken to reduce the risk of tumor spillage:

- Avoid accidental opening of the urinary tract.
- Avoid direct instrumental contact with the tumor.
- Consider en bloc removal of the kidney, ureter, and bladder cuff.
- Advanced (T3/T4 and/or N+/M+) tumors are contraindications for minimal-invasive RNU since the result is worse than in the open approach [89].

16.7.1.3 Management of the Bladder Cuff

Because there is a high chance of tumor recurrence in this location and in the bladder, resection of the distal ureter and orifice should be accomplished [93–95]. The pluck technique, stripping, transurethral resection of the intramural ureter, and intussusception have all been proposed to make distal ureter resection easier. Neither of these methods has been found to be as effective as complete bladder cuff resection [95]

16.7.1.4 Lymph Node Dissection

The amount of lymph nodes eliminated is unlikely to have a higher influence on patient survival than using a lymph node dissection (LND) template [96]. Template-based lymph node dissection increases cancer-specific survival and lowers the probability of tumor recurrence in patients with muscle-invasive illness [97]. LND improves survival in clinically [98] and pathologically [99] node-negative individuals. The probability of lymph node metastasis rises as the tumor stage progresses [9]. Because of its minimal likelihood of metastasis in Ta and T1 UTUC, lymph node dissection seems redundant [100]. Nevertheless, pre-operative tumor staging may be erroneous. Thus, a template-based LND should be offered to patients eligible for RNU [101]

16.7.2 Endoscopic Nephron-sparing Treatment

In low-risk ureteral or renal pelvic cancer, endoscopic surgery of UTUC is recommended [102]. High-risk lesions of the renal pelvis (both solitary and resectable) can be treated endoscopically in some situations [76]. Surgical skill and technical devices, in combination with anatomical factors, play a central role in the control and therapy of UTUC [103]. A flexible ureterorenoscopy with an appropriate laser is required for renal surgery, particularly in cancers of the renal pelvicalyceal system, to ensure complete tumor removal or ablation [85, 104].

G1 tumors have superior cancer specific survival, recurrence-free upper urinary tract and bladder survival, and progression-free upper urinary tract survival than G3 cancers [102]. The 2-, 5-, and 10-year cancer-specific survival rates in patients with a low-grade UTUC managed with endoscopy were 98%, 87%, and 81%, respectively. Patients with low-grade malignancies managed by RNU had equivalent cancer-specific survival rates (97%, 87%, and 78%, respectively). Patients with high-grade UTUC, on the other hand, had 2-year overall survival rates of 54% after endoscopic KSS [105].

For endoscopic treatment of ureteral lesions, a rigid ureteral resectoscope or a surgical laser can be utilized [106, 107] (Fig. 16.5).

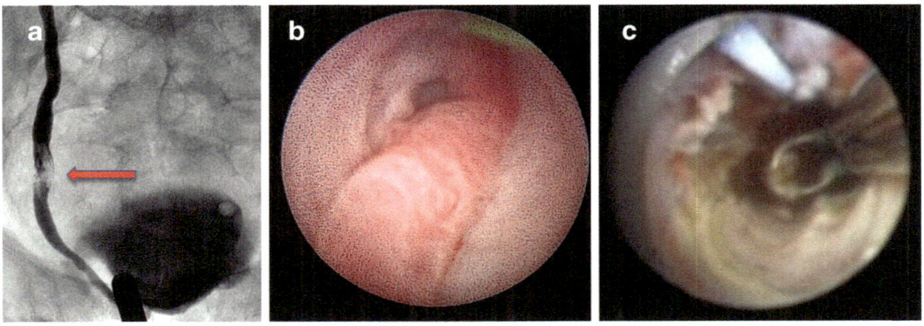

Fig. 16.5 (**a**, **b**) Distal ureter tumor with (**c**) transurethral endoscopic tumor resection with a rigid ureteral resectoscope (10 Charrière)

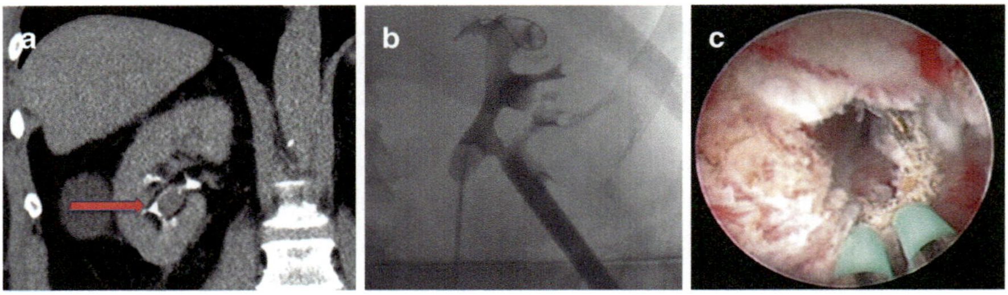

Fig. 16.6 Percutaneous resection of a UTUC of the lower calyx. (**a**) Retrograde urography with lower calyx tumor-localization, (**b**) percutaneous approach with resection with 16 charrière resectoscope (**c**)

16.7.3 Percutaneous Nephron-sparing Treatment

In low-risk UTUC of the renal pelvis, the transcutaneous technique could be used, particularly for the inferior renal calyx, which is not accessible by flexible ureterorenoscopy [108]. A resectoscope or a laser can be used to remove the lesion. A 16 Charrière device may be combined with a-20 or -22 Charrière Amplatz-shaft and a nephrostomy tube. Intraoperative problems such as acute blood loss and hematoma, tumor spilling, and harm to other anatomic structures such as the pleura or bowel are disadvantages of this surgical approach [109] (Fig. 16.6). Postoperatively, percutaneous antegrade chemo-instillation can be administered by the nephrostomy tube if required. Regarding surgical outcomes, a tumor recurrence rate of 41% was observed, with 74% of patients having their organs preserved [110]. Other researchers found that after percutaneous instillation therapy, 5-year cancer-specific survival rates were 79.5% [111 (Fig. 16.6)].

16.7.4 Ureteral Resection and Reconstruction

Preserving the ipsilateral kidney, partial ureterectomy provides acceptable surgical margins and pathological tissue for histopathological staging and grading [11]. In this context, partial resection of the ureter of the intermediate and proximal segment and distal ureter excision were found to be correlated with decreased oncological failure rates [94, 112].

16.7.4.1 Tumors of the Distal Ureter

A distal ureterectomy is recommended for distant low-risk lesions that cannot be entirely removed endoscopically or in distal high-risk tumors with an urgent need for KSS (single kidney or nephropathy) [94, 112]. Depending on the residual ureter length, ureteroneocystostomy (Fig. 16.7), psoas hitch, or Boari-flap could be performed for surgical reconstruction [94, 112], Figs. 16.8 and 16.9. Due to the

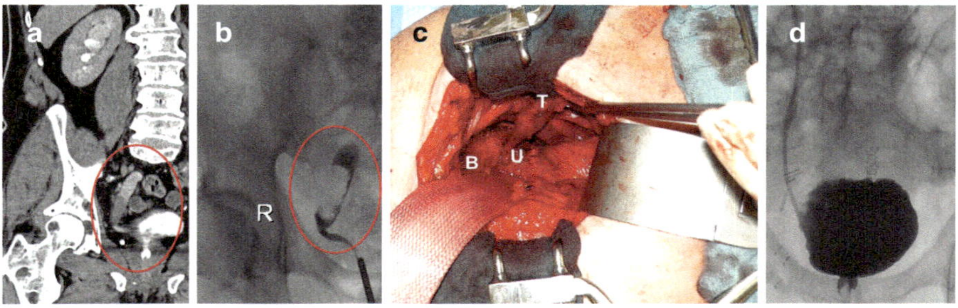

Fig. 16.7 Ureteral resection including bladder cuff and reconstruction with uretero-neocystostomy. CT scan of the initial tumor lesion in the distal ureter (red circle) **(a)**, Retrograde ureterography with distal tumor (red circle) **(b)**, intraoperative finding: (B = Bladder, U= Ureter, T = Tumor) **(c)**, cystography 7 days after surgery **(d)**

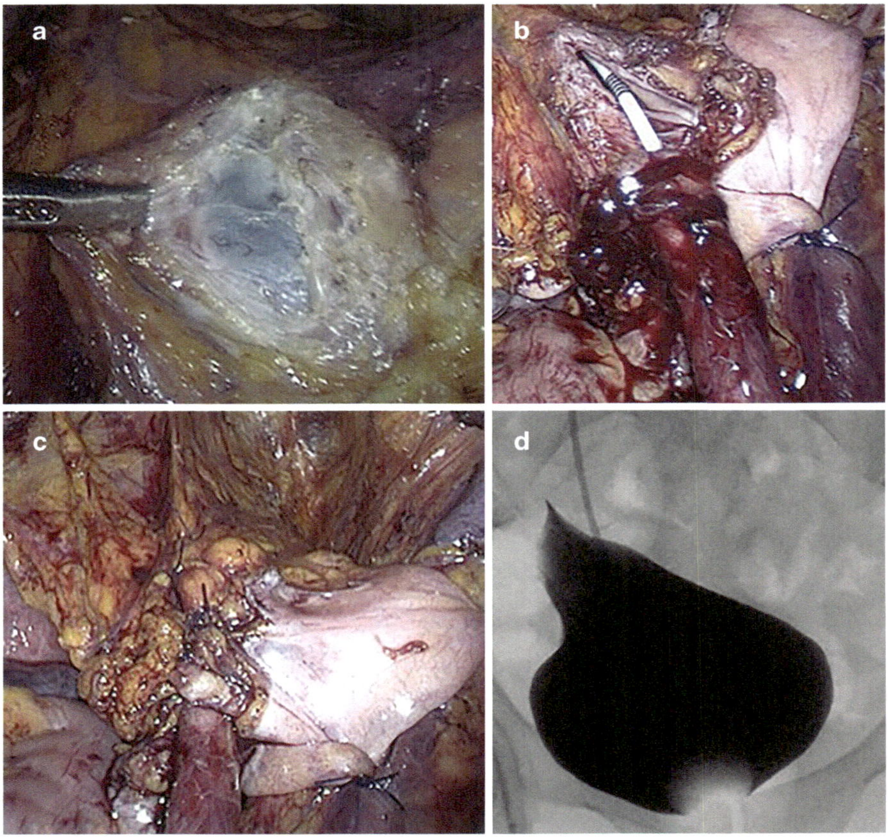

Fig. 16.8 Laparoscopic Psoas Hitch in a low grade distal right ureter tumor. Muscular tunnel after laparoscopic distal ureterectomy with bladder cuff (**a**). Psoas hitch sutures and ureteral anastomosis with Double J (**b**). Closure of the bladder and perivesical fat tissue (**c**). Cystogram after 7 days (**d**)

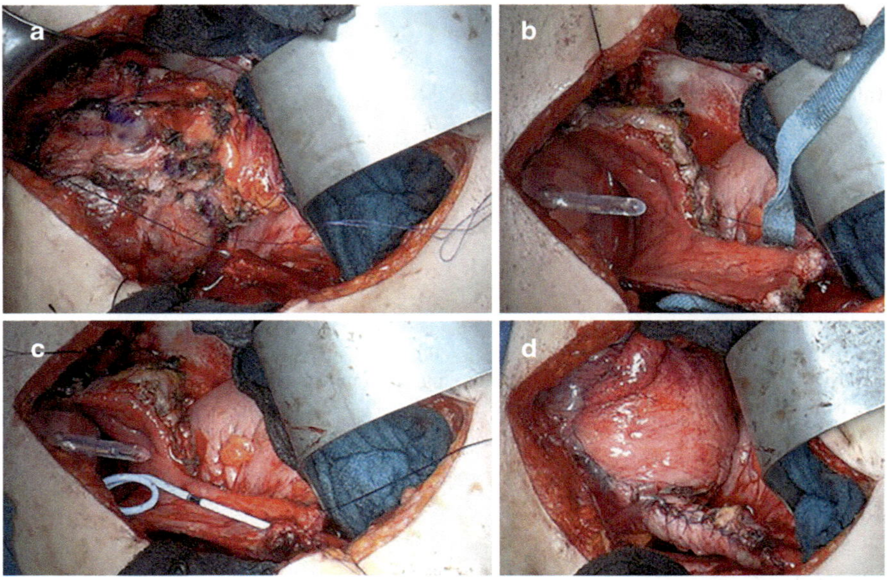

Fig. 16.9 Open Boari Flap after a low grade ureteral cancer of the middle part of the left ureter after open resection of the lower and middle ureter with bladder cuff. Marking the flap on the bladder (**a**). Incision of the necessary flap, 3 × 8 cm (**b**). Posterior ureteral anastomosis with Double J stent insertion (**c**). Closure of the bladder, 2 layers, running suture (**d**)

likelihood of tumor recurrence in the bladder, excision of the ureter orifice by resection of a bladder cuff is also strongly recommended [93, 95, 113].

In addition to RNU, in the case of KSS and partial ureteral resection, local lymphadenectomy must be considered. It is crucial to highlight that the risk of positive lymph nodes rises as the tumor stage progresses [114]. As a result, lymph node dissection appears less significant in Ta or T1 tumors [115, 116]. Given the challenging pre-operative staging of upper tract urothelial cancer, a template-based lymph node dissection should be done during partial ureterectomy [11].

16.7.4.2 Middle and Proximal Ureter Tumors

A partial excision and uretero-ureterostomy could be conducted in low-risk cancers of the middle and proximal ureter when endoscopic resection is not possible. This even applies to high-risk malignancies in patients with a strong need to preserve the kidney. In these cases, reconstruction of the ureter with a Psoas Hitch or Boari-flap can be performed with open or minimally invasive surgery [117], (Figs. 16.8 and 16.9).

Whenever ureteroureterostomy, Psoas Hitch, or Boari-flap is not possible due to tumor location (multifocality), interposition of an isoperistaltic ileal ureter (Fig. 16.10) could be implemented [118]. An appendix interposition can be utilized for reconstruction in exceptional situations, Fig. 16.11.

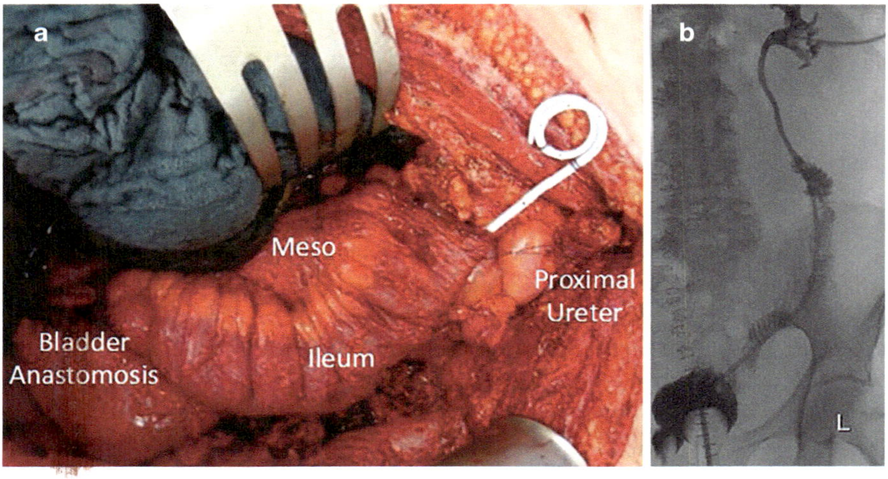

Fig. 16.10 Partial ureteral resection with ileum interposition. (**a**) Isoperistaltic ileal segment used for interposition; (**b**) antegrade and retrograde urography after 7 days

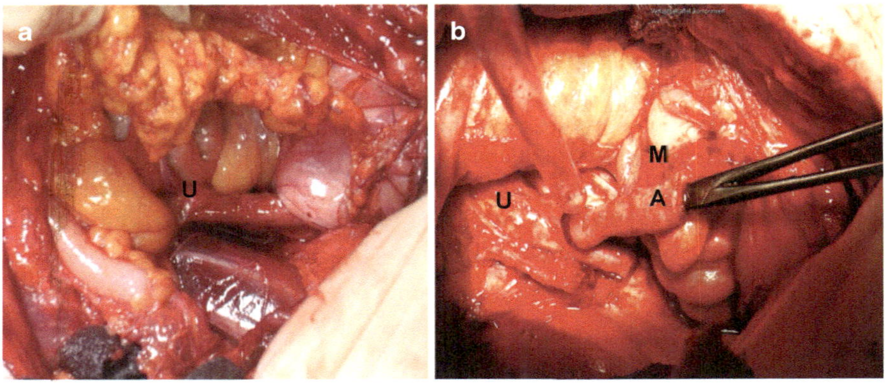

Fig. 16.11 Appendix interposition in a single kidney-patient, (**a**) intraoperative situs; (**b**) Appendix interposition A: Appendix, U: Ureter, M: Mesoappendix

16.7.5 Ureteral Metastases

In rare cases, metastases of other tumor entities can occur in the upper urinary tract, such as the ureter. However, there are few case reports on ureteral metastases in prostate cancer [119, 120]. Despite the lack of understanding about the process, ureteral metastases should be included in the differential diagnosis of prostate cancer patients with ureteral tumors.

16.7.6 Upper Urinary Tract Instillation of BCG or Mitomycin C

After KSS with complete tumor resection, upper urinary tract instillations can be used as an adjuvant therapy. The use of BCG (in the case of CIS or Ta-T1) or Mitomycin C (in the case of Ta-T1) instillation therapy by using an inlaying nephrostomy or ureteric stent (Mono J) has been studied [79, 121]. Various studies found no association in tumor recurrence, progression, cancer specific, or overall survival when the therapy was administered antegrade, retrograde or combination [122]. Conversely, in high-grade ureteral malignancies with persistent neoplasia or CIS, an antegrade percutaneous procedure should be used to avoid contact between the ureteral stent and the ureteral wall. Due to the apparent risk of toxic pyelovenous inflow or perirenal extravasation, instillation must only be used after confirming that the nephrostomy or ureteric stent is in the correct position (urography). An intravesical administration of BCG or Mitomycin C is no longer recommended in case of an inserted double J catheter. The consequent only little reflux has been demonstrated to be insufficient to reach the renal pelvis [123–125]. After RNU, a single injection (in certain circumstances up to 8 x weekly) of Mitomycin or Pirarubicin should be administered to prevent intravesical tumor recurrence [126, 127]. On the other hand, a similar impact for a subsequent intravesical single-dose instillation following KSS could not be demonstrated [36].

The success of adjuvant instillation therapy for the upper urinary tract urothelial carcinoma is unknown. In comparison to untreated individuals, some studies report equivalent recurrence rates. This is due to the continual urine output and ureteral peristalsis, which inhibits the instilled medication from being sufficiently retained [128]. As a result, therapies and instillation techniques should be investigated to validate and strengthen these findings [122].

16.7.7 Systemic Treatment in Advanced and Metastatic UTUC, EAU Guidelines 2021

16.7.7.1 Neoadjuvant Chemotherapy

Various retrospective studies examined the role of neoadjuvant chemotherapy in patients treated before RNU and have shown remarkable pathological downstaging and full success rates [129–131]. Furthermore, compared to RNU monotherapy, neoadjuvant chemotherapy has been found to reduce tumor recurrence and mortality rates without jeopardizing subsequent operative procedure [131–133]. Although no RCTs have been reported, prospective results from a phase II study demonstrated that neoadjuvant chemotherapy was linked to a 14% pathological complete response for high-grade upper tract urothelial cancer [134].

16.7.7.2 Adjuvant Chemotherapy

A phase III prospective randomized trial (n = 261) compared the advantage of adjuvant gemcitabine-platinum chemotherapy within 90 days after RNU versus surveillance in patients with pure urothelial cancer of the upper urinary tract. A significantly improved cancer-free survival was found in patients with pT2–pT4, N (any) or lymph node-positive (pT any, N+). Because this type of surgery may impair renal function, the fundamental restriction of adjuvant chemotherapy for advanced UTUC is the reduced ability to use a full dose cisplatin-based treatment following RNU [135, 136].

16.7.7.3 Systemic Treatments

First-line Therapy

Based on the bladder cancer data and single-center UTUC studies, platinum-based combination chemotherapy is used. Cisplatin seems to be effective as a first-line treatment for metastatic UTUC [137]. The benefit of immunotherapy with programmed death-1 (PD1) or programmed death-ligand 1 (PD-L1) inhibitors in the first-line scenario in metastatic patients, including those with UTUC, was further studied. In patients with the advanced or metastatic disease without progress or response to first-line chemotherapy, avelumab maintenance treatment after 4–6 cycles of gemcitabine plus cisplatin or carboplatin significantly improved OS compared to best supportive care [138].

In a single-arm phase II trial in cisplatin-ineligible metastatic UTUC disease (n = 119), atezolizumab was linked with a 39% response rate in 28% of the patients [139]. The median overall survival was 15.9 months, with acceptable toxicity.

Pembrolizumab was related to response rates of 22% in 69 (19%) cisplatin-unfit patients with metastatic UTUC in a single-arm phase II trial (n = 370) [140]. in the case of a PD-L1 expression of 10%, higher response rates were found. In patients with advanced urothelial bladder and upper urinary tract carcinoma, the combination of pembrolizumab and platinum-based chemotherapy did not have significant advantages regarding progression-free survival and overall survival compared to platinum-based chemotherapy monotherapy [141].

Second-line Therapy

Vinflunine was as beneficial in UTUC as in bladder cancer advancing after cisplatin-based treatment in a post-hoc subgroup study of locally progressed or metastatic urothelial cancer [142].

Further, a phase III RCT involving 542 patients who had obtained platinum-based chemotherapy for advanced urothelial cancer found that pembrolizumab reduced the risk of death by nearly half among those with UTUC (n = 75, 13.8%), but the data appeared marginally significant [143]. The collective response rate was 21.1%, with a median overall survival of 10.3 months.

Importantly, a single-arm phase II study proved that atezolizumab has enduring action related to PD-L1 expression on immune cells in patients with metastatic urothelial cancer [144], despite the fact that no subpopulation analysis was provided for UTUC patients (n = 65/21%). In the group of people who overexpress PD-L1, the response rate was 26%, compared to 15% in the general population. Although better safety characteristics, a phase III RCT involving 51 (21.8%) patients with UTUC found that it could not be related to a longer overall survival when matched to standard chemotherapy in patients expressing PD-L1 [145].

In patients with progress after platinum-based chemotherapy metastatic urothelial cancer, alternative immunotherapies like nivolumab [146], avelumab [147], and durvalumab [148] have exhibited response rates ranging from 17.8% to 19.6% and median overall survival from 7.7 months to 18.2 months. The amount of UTUC patients in these trials have only been mentioned for avelumab (n = 7/15.9%) [149], and there was no subgroup analysis based on initial tumor localization.

In phase I/II multicenter trial involving 78 patients with metastatic disease after platinum-based chemotherapy, the immunotherapy combination of nivolumab and ipilimumab showed considerable anti-tumor effectiveness, with an objective response rate of up to 38% [150].

Erdafitinib, a tyrosine kinase inhibitor of FGFR1–4, was linked with a 40% response rate in 99 patients with metastatic disease and FGFR mutations who progressed after first-line treatment recent phase II trial [151]. The response rate was 43% in this trial of 23 UTUC patients with visceral metastases.

16.8 Follow Up

Because ipsilateral tumor relapse in UTUC is prevalent after KSS, a detailed and intense follow-up with substantial patient compliance is essential [36]. Repeated radiographic and endoscopic examinations and urine cytology are part of the follow-up. Moreover, 6–8 weeks following KSS, a second look ureterorenoscopy should be conducted [85]. In addition, the development of metachronous bladder cancer should be considered. Table 16.6 shows the follow-up strategy. The use of ureterorenoscopy or urine cytology can be emphasized, particularly in high-risk cases [152, 153].

16.9 Conclusion

Kidney sparing surgery is becoming more popular for urothelial carcinoma of the upper urinary system since it is effective and preserves renal function. RNU plus bladder cuff excision, on the other hand, is the gold standard for high-risk UTUC treatment. As a result, specific oncologic and functional considerations should be considered while selecting whether or not to maintain the kidneys.

The diagnosis is usually made via endoscopy and simultaneous biopsy. However, small sample sizes make an accurate assessment difficult. Imaging techniques such as CT or MRI can provide significant support here. In addition, urine, blood-based or tissue-derived biomarkers have an important additive role in the diagnostic setting of upper tract urothelial cancer and can furthermore serve as prognostic indicators. Due to the low incidence of upper tract urothelial cancer, there is a lack of prospective randomized data, which is evident in the limited guideline recommendations. Currently recommended biomarkers are urine cytology, neutrophil-lymphocyte ratio, albumin, and various molecular pathological markers. "Next-generation biomarkers" are of future interest, as they can provide molecular genetic insights into tumors at different stages and therefore represent an approach toward personalized therapies.

Before doing kidney sparing surgery, it is critical to distinguish between imperative and elective causes. Another major consideration is the possibility of understaging upper tract cancers with endoscopic and histological evaluation. As a result, prior to organ preservation, it is essential to integrate a pre-operative risk assessment of the patient into the decision-making process. KSS includes endoscopic or percutaneous approaches and segmental ureteral resection in low-risk tumors based on localization and resectability. In the case of a high-risk tumor a partial ureter resection is considered only when the tumor is located in the distal ureter. Unless there is need for organ preservation, RNU is suggested for large, advanced disease, low-risk and invasive high-risk malignancies of the middle or proximal ureter and the renal pelvis. The available technological equipment and the surgeon's expertise determine the regimen to be used. The value of adjuvant instillation treatment with BCG or chemo instillation, as well as lymph node dissection as part of a segmental ureterectomy, has yet to be completely explored. Furthermore, it is unknown if novel biomarkers will have an impact on the KSS therapy protocol. A thorough follow-up with endoscopy, radiography, and urine cytology for at least 5 years is required to exclude the development of metachronous bladder cancer after kidney sparing procedures.

Questions

1. Please mark the **wrong** answer regarding tumors of the upper urinary tract:

(a) Tumors of the upper urinary tract are rare; within them urothelial carcinomas are most common.
(b) The endoscopically determined localization of a tumor within the upper urinary tract can be used to doubtlessly conclude its histology.
(c) Histologic variants of upper urinary tract tumors are associated with a worse prognosis.
(d) Already a partial histological variant within an urothelial carcinoma results in the classification of the tumor as high-risk tumor.

Answer: (b)

2. Please mark the **right** answer regarding diagnostic approaches for tumors of the upper urinary tract:

(a) Execratory urography is the approach with the highest accuracy for UTUC and shows a sensitivity of 67–100% and a specificity of 93–99%.
(b) CT-urography has no value in the diagnosis of upper urinary tract tumors.
(c) Undergrading and understaging are common in upper tract tumors, often caused by limited tissue collection during biopsies.
(d) Analogous to the bladder, PDD-assisted visualization represents the endoscopic standard in UTUC as well.

Answer: (c)

3. Please mark the **right** answer for the use of urinary biomarkers in UTUC:

(a) Urinary cytology remains the only recommended urine marker for diagnosis and follow-up in patients with UTUC.
(b) The method of obtaining urine specimens from the upper urinary tract has no effect on the evaluation of urine cytology.
(c) The decision between conducting nephron-sparing therapy and radical nephrectomy can be made based solely on the results of the cytologic analysis.
(d) NMP22 is an indispensable component of any diagnostic cascade in patients with upper urinary tract tumors.

Answer: (a)

4. Please mark the **wrong** answer regarding risk stratification of non-metastatic urothelial cancer of the upper urinary tract:

(a) The presence of a variant histology leads to the classification of the tumor as high-risk tumor.
(b) Multifocal tumors are always classified as high-risk tumors.
(c) A tumor size of 2.3 cm leads to a high-risk classification.
(d) A unifocal upper urinary tract tumor with a tumor size of 1.5 cm, a noninvasive aspect on CT, a low-grade URS biopsy, and a high-grade cytology is considered low risk.

Answer: (d)

5. Please mark the **right** answer regarding the treatment of upper urinary tract urothelial carcinomas:

(a) Endoscopic therapies are the only option to perform nephron-sparing surgery (NSS).
(b) Regardless of individual patient characteristics, patients with high-risk tumors must always be treated by radical nephroureterectomy (RNU).
(c) In laparoscopic RNU, the equally effective stripping technique can be used given the complicated technique of a complete bladder cuff.
(d) Lymph node dissection in clinically node-negative patients improves the survival.

Answer: (c)

6. Please mark the **wrong** answer regarding nephron-sparing surgery (NSS):

(a) A rigid ureteral resectoscope or a surgical laser are usually used methods for NSS.
(b) In patients with low-risk UTUC if the renal pelvis, a transcutaneous approach can be used, especially for tumors of the inferior renal calyx.
(c) A partial ureterectomy with adequate surgical margins is a acceptable surgical approach in low-risk tumors.
(d) Due to the always necessary ureteroureterostomy, the retention of a 1.5 cm pre-vesical ureteral stump is a prerequisite for NSS in distal ureteral tumors.

Answer: (d)

7. Please mark the **right** answer regarding the management of high-risk UTUC:

(a) Single post-operative intravesical instillation of chemotherapy has no effect on bladder cancer recurrence rate after high-risk.
(b) Adjuvant post-operative systemic platinum chemotherapy is recommended in platin-eligible patients with high-risk non-metastatic UTUC.
(c) In cisplatin-unfit patients, adjuvant immunotherapy is a guideline-recommended equivalent alternative.
(d) Laparoscopic radical nephroureterectomy (RNU) is the best surgical approach even in patients with non-organ confined UTUC.

Answer: (b)

8. Please mark the **wrong** answer regarding the management of high-risk UTUC:

(a) First-line treatment for cisplatin-eligible patients should be either a gemcitabine-cisplatin or a HD-MVAC regimen.
(b) In cisplatin-eligible patients first-line therapy should not use carboplatin instead of cisplatin.
(c) In cisplatin-unfit patients checkpoint inhibitors are options depending on PD-L1 status.
(d) FGFR-Inhibitors like Erdafitinib are no treatment option in patients with UTUC.

Answer: (d)

9. Please mark the **right** answer regarding the follow-up of UTUC:

(a) Ipsilateral tumor relapse after nephron-sparing surgery (NSS) is rare.
(b) Repeated radiographic and endoscopic examinations along with urine cytology are essential parts of the follow-up in patients after NSS.
(c) A second-look ureterorenoscopy (URS) is not necessary in patients with NSS.
(d) Patients after RNU need their first radiographic examination after 2–3 years.

Answer: (b)

References

1. Raman JD, Messer J, Sielatycki JA, Hollenbeak CS. Incidence and survival of patients with carcinoma of the ureter and renal pelvis in the USA, 1973-2005. BJU Int. 2011;107(7):1059–64.
2. Roupret M, Babjuk M, Burger M, Capoun O, Cohen D, Comperat EM, et al. European Association of Urology Guidelines on Upper Urinary Tract Urothelial Carcinoma: 2020 Update. Eur Urol. 2021;79(1):62–79.
3. Busby JE, Brown GA, Tamboli P, Kamat AM, Dinney CP, Grossman HB, et al. Upper urinary tract tumors with nontransitional histology: a single-center experience. Urology. 2006;67(3):518–23.
4. Deuker M, Stolzenbach LF, Colla Ruvolo C, Nocera L, Tian Z, Roos FC, et al. Upper urinary tract tumors: variant histology versus urothelial carcinoma. Clin Genitourin Cancer. 2021;19(2):117–24.
5. Mazzucchelli R, Scarpelli M, Galosi AB, Di Primio R, Lopez-Beltran A, Cheng L, et al. Pathology of upper tract urothelial carcinoma with emphasis on staging. Int J Immunopathol Pharmacol. 2014;27(4):509–16.
6. Lughezzani G, Burger M, Margulis V, Matin SF, Novara G, Roupret M, et al. Prognostic factors in upper urinary tract urothelial carcinomas: a comprehensive review of the current literature. Eur Urol. 2012;62(1):100–14.
7. Fang D, Liu P, Li X, Xiong G, Zhang L, Singla N, et al. Characteristics and treatment outcomes of pan-urothelial cell carcinoma: a descriptive analysis of 45 patients. Sci Rep. 2015;5:18014.
8. Hurand S, Jouan A, Feuillet-Palma C, Singh G, Biscaras J, Lesne E, et al. Field-effect control of superconductivity and Rashba spin-orbit coupling in top-gated LaAlO3/SrTiO3 devices. Sci Rep. 2015;5:12751.
9. Mori K, Janisch F, Parizi MK, Mostafaei H, Lysenko I, Kimura S, et al. Prognostic value of variant histology in upper tract urothelial carcinoma treated with nephroureterectomy: a systematic review and meta-analysis. J Urol. 2020;203(6):1075–84.
10. Rausch S, Gakis G, Bedke J, Stenzl A. [Elective organ and function preservation in ureter and renal pelvis tumors]. Urol A 2014;53(9):1284–94.
11. Seisen T, Peyronnet B, Dominguez-Escrig JL, Bruins HM, Yuan CY, Babjuk M, et al. Oncologic outcomes of kidney-sparing surgery versus radical nephroureterectomy for upper tract urothelial carcinoma: a systematic review by the EAU non-muscle invasive bladder cancer guidelines panel. Eur Urol. 2016;70(6):1052–68.
12. Roupret M, Babjuk M, Comperat E, Zigeuner R, Sylvester R, Burger M, et al. European guidelines on upper tract urothelial carcinomas: 2013 update. Eur Urol. 2013;63(6):1059–71.
13. Wang LJ, Wong YC, Chuang CK, Huang CC, Pang ST. Diagnostic accuracy of transitional cell carcinoma on multidetector computerized tomography urography in patients with gross hematuria. J Urol. 2009;181(2):524–31. discussion 31
14. Stacul F, van der Molen AJ, Reimer P, Webb JA, Thomsen HS, Morcos SK, et al. Contrast induced nephropathy: updated ESUR Contrast Media Safety Committee guidelines. Eur Radiol. 2011;21(12):2527–41.
15. Takahashi N, Glockner JF, Hartman RP, King BF, Leibovich BC, Stanley DW, et al. Gadolinium enhanced magnetic resonance urography for upper urinary tract malignancy. J Urol. 2010;183(4):1330–65.
16. Thomsen HS, Morcos SK, Almen T, Bellin MF, Bertolotto M, Bongartz G, et al. Nephrogenic systemic fibrosis and gadolinium-based contrast media: updated ESUR Contrast Medium Safety Committee guidelines. Eur Radiol. 2013;23(2):307–18.
17. Smith AK, Stephenson AJ, Lane BR, Larson BT, Thomas AA, Gong MC, et al. Inadequacy of biopsy for diagnosis of upper tract urothelial carcinoma: implications for conservative management. Urology. 2011;78(1):82–6.
18. Margolin EJ, Matulay JT, Li G, Meng X, Chao B, Vijay V, et al. Discordance between ureteroscopic biopsy and final pathology for upper tract urothelial carcinoma. J Urol. 2018;199(6):1440–5.

19. Traxer O, Geavlete B, de Medina SG, Sibony M, Al-Qahtani SM. Narrow-band imaging digital flexible ureteroscopy in detection of upper urinary tract transitional-cell carcinoma: initial experience. J Endourol. 2011;25(1):19–23.
20. Somani BK, Moseley H, Eljamel MS, Nabi G, Kata SG. Photodynamic diagnosis (PDD) for upper urinary tract transitional cell carcinoma (UT-TCC): evolution of a new technique. Photodiagn Photodyn Ther. 2010;7(1):39–43.
21. Green DA, Rink M, Xylinas E, Matin SF, Stenzl A, Roupret M, et al. Urothelial carcinoma of the bladder and the upper tract: disparate twins. J Urol. 2013;189(4):1214–21.
22. Messer J, Shariat SF, Brien JC, Herman MP, Ng CK, Scherr DS, et al. Urinary cytology has a poor performance for predicting invasive or high-grade upper-tract urothelial carcinoma. BJU Int. 2011;108(5):701–5.
23. Bier S, Hennenlotter J, Esser M, Mohrhardt S, Rausch S, Schwentner C, et al. Performance of urinary markers for detection of upper tract urothelial carcinoma: is upper tract urine more accurate than urine from the bladder? Dis Markers. 2018;2018:5823870.
24. Lodde M, Mian C, Wiener H, Haitel A, Pycha A, Marberger M Detection of upper urinary tract transitional cell carcinoma with ImmunoCyt: a preliminary report. Urology. 2001;58(3):362–6.
25. Jovanovic M, Soldatovic I, Janjic A, Vuksanovic A, Dzamic Z, Acimovic M, et al. Diagnostic value of the nuclear matrix protein 22 test and urine cytology in upper tract urothelial tumors. Urol Int. 2011;87(2):134–7.
26. Johannes JR, Nelson E, Bibbo M, Bagley DH. Voided urine fluorescence in situ hybridization testing for upper tract urothelial carcinoma surveillance. J Urol. 2010;184(3):879–82.
27. Chen AA, Grasso M. Is there a role for FISH in the management and surveillance of patients with upper tract transitional-cell carcinoma? J Endourol. 2008;22(6):1371–4.
28. McHale T, Ohori NP, Cieply KM, Sherer C, Bastacky SI. Comparison of urinary cytology and fluorescence in situ hybridization in the detection of urothelial neoplasia: an analysis of discordant results. Diagn Cytopathol. 2019;47(4):282–8.
29. Marin-Aguilera M, Mengual L, Ribal MJ, Musquera M, Ars E, Villavicencio H, et al. Utility of fluorescence in situ hybridization as a non-invasive technique in the diagnosis of upper urinary tract urothelial carcinoma. Eur Urol. 2007;51(2):409–15. discussion 15
30. Huang WT, Li LY, Pang J, Ruan XX, Sun QP, Yang WJ, et al. Fluorescence in situ hybridization assay detects upper urinary tract transitional cell carcinoma in patients with asymptomatic hematuria and negative urine cytology. Neoplasma. 2012;59(4):355–60.
31. Mian C, Mazzoleni G, Vikoler S, Martini T, Knuchel-Clark R, Zaak D, et al. Fluorescence in situ hybridisation in the diagnosis of upper urinary tract tumours. Eur Urol. 2010;58(2):288–92.
32. Coskuner E, Cevik I, Ozkan A, Dillioglugil O, Akdas A. In the cystoscopic follow-up of non-muscle-invasive transitional cell carcinoma, NMP-22 works for high grades, but unreliable in low grades and upper urinary tract tumors. Int Urol Nephrol. 2012;44(3):793–8.
33. Dudderidge T, Stockley J, Nabi G, Mom J, Umez-Eronini N, Hrouda D, et al. A novel, non-invasive test enabling bladder cancer detection in urine sediment of patients presenting with haematuria-a prospective multicentre performance evaluation of ADXBLADDER. Eur Urol Oncol. 2020;3(1):42–6.
34. Walsh IK, Keane PF, Ishak LM, Flessland KA. The BTA stat test: a tumor marker for the detection of upper tract transitional cell carcinoma. Urology. 2001;58(4):532–5.
35. Jovanovic M, Hadzi-Djokic J, Dzamic Z, Acimovic M. Evaluation of the Bard BTA-test in the diagnosis of upper urinary tract tumours. Acta Chir Iugosl. 2007;54(4):19–24.
36. Roupret M, Babjuk M, Comperat E, Zigeuner R, Sylvester RJ, Burger M, et al. European Association of Urology Guidelines on Upper Urinary Tract Urothelial Carcinoma: 2017 Update. Eur Urol. 2018;73(1):111–22.
37. Simon CT, Skala SL, Magers MJ, Weizer A, Kaffenberger SD, Chinnaiyan AM, et al. The utility of upper urinary tract urine cytology before and after application of the Paris system. Diagn Cytopathol. 2019;47(5):421–7.
38. Barkan GA, Wojcik EM, Nayar R, Savic-Prince S, Quek ML, Kurtycz DF, et al. The Paris system for reporting urinary cytology: the quest to develop a standardized terminology. Acta Cytol. 2016;60(3):185–97.

39. Williams SK, Denton KJ, Minervini A, Oxley J, Khastigir J, Timoney AG, et al. Correlation of upper-tract cytology, retrograde pyelography, ureteroscopic appearance, and ureteroscopic biopsy with histologic examination of upper-tract transitional cell carcinoma. J Endourol. 2008;22(1):71–6.
40. Brien JC, Shariat SF, Herman MP, Ng CK, Scherr DS, Scoll B, et al. Preoperative hydronephrosis, ureteroscopic biopsy grade and urinary cytology can improve prediction of advanced upper tract urothelial carcinoma. J Urol. 2010;184(1):69–73.
41. Renshaw AA. Comparison of ureteral washing and biopsy specimens in the community setting. Cancer. 2006;108(1):45–8.
42. Babjuk M, Burger M, Compérat EM, Gontero P, Mostafid AH, Palou J, et al. European Association of Urology Guidelines on Non-muscle-invasive Bladder Cancer (TaT1 and Carcinoma In Situ) - 2019 Update. Eur Urol. 2019;76(5):639–57.
43. Todenhöfer T, Hennenlotter J, Kühs U, Tews V, Gakis G, Aufderklamm S, et al. Influence of urinary tract instrumentation and inflammation on the performance of urine markers for the detection of bladder cancer. Urology. 2012;79(3):620–4.
44. Maas M, Walz S, Stühler V, Aufderklamm S, Rausch S, Bedke J, et al. Molecular markers in disease detection and follow-up of patients with non-muscle invasive bladder cancer. Expert Rev Mol Diagn. 2018;18(5):443–55.
45. Huang YL, Chen J, Yan W, Zang D, Qin Q, Deng AM. Diagnostic accuracy of cytokeratin-19 fragment (CYFRA 21-1) for bladder cancer: a systematic review and meta-analysis. Tumour Biol. 2015;36(5):3137–45.
46. Schmitz-Drager BJ, Droller M, Lokeshwar VB, Lotan Y, Hudson MA, van Rhijn BW, et al. Molecular markers for bladder cancer screening, early diagnosis, and surveillance: the WHO/ICUD consensus. Urol Int. 2015;94(1):1–24.
47. Mori K, Janisch F, Mostafaei H, Lysenko I, Kimura S, Egawa S, et al. Prognostic value of preoperative blood-based biomarkers in upper tract urothelial carcinoma treated with nephroureterectomy: a systematic review and meta-analysis. Urol Oncol. 2020;38(5):315–33.
48. Liu J, Wang F, Li S, Huang W, Jia Y, Wei C. The prognostic significance of preoperative serum albumin in urothelial carcinoma: a systematic review and meta-analysis. Biosci Rep. 2018;38(4):BSR20180214.
49. Montalbo R, Izquierdo L, Ingelmo-Torres M, Lozano JJ, Capitán D, Alcaraz A, et al. Prognostic value of circulating microRNAs in upper tract urinary carcinoma. Oncotarget. 2018;9(24):16691–700.
50. Mbeutcha A, Mathieu R, Rouprêt M, Gust KM, Briganti A, Karakiewicz PI, et al. Predictive models and prognostic factors for upper tract urothelial carcinoma: a comprehensive review of the literature. Transl Androl Urol. 2016;5(5):720–34.
51. Shariat SF, Matsumoto K, Kim J, Ayala GE, Zhou JH, Jian W, et al. Correlation of cyclooxygenase-2 expression with molecular markers, pathological features and clinical outcome of transitional cell carcinoma of the bladder. J Urol. 2003;170(3):985–9.
52. Lucca I, Hofbauer SL, Leitner CV, de Martino M, Özsoy M, Susani M, et al. Development of a preoperative nomogram incorporating biomarkers of systemic inflammatory response to predict nonorgan-confined urothelial carcinoma of the bladder at radical cystectomy. Urology. 2016;95:132–8.
53. Semenza GL. Hypoxia, clonal selection, and the role of HIF-1 in tumor progression. Crit Rev Biochem Mol Biol. 2000;35(2):71–103.
54. Huang X, Liang M, Dittmar R, Wang L. Extracellular microRNAs in urologic malignancies: chances and challenges. Int J Mol Sci. 2013;14(7):14785–99.
55. Tao J, Yang X, Li P, Wei J, Deng X, Cheng Y, et al. Identification of circulating microRNA signatures for upper tract urothelial carcinoma detection. Mol Med Rep. 2015;12(5):6752–60.
56. Browne BM, Stensland KD, Patel CK, Sullivan T, Burks EJ, Canes D, et al. MicroRNA expression profiles in upper tract urothelial carcinoma differentiate tumor grade, stage, and survival: implications for clinical decision-making. Urology. 2019;123:93–100.
57. Favaretto RL, Bahadori A, Mathieu R, Haitel A, Grubmuller B, Margulis V, et al. Prognostic role of decreased E-cadherin expression in patients with upper tract urothelial carcinoma: a multi-institutional study. World J Urol. 2017;35(1):113–20.

58. Rouprêt M, Fromont G, Azzouzi AR, Catto JW, Vallancien G, Hamdy FC, et al. Microsatellite instability as predictor of survival in patients with invasive upper urinary tract transitional cell carcinoma. Urology. 2005;65(6):1233–7.
59. Soria F, Moschini M, Haitel A, Wirth GJ, Karam JA, Wood CG, et al. HER2 overexpression is associated with worse outcomes in patients with upper tract urothelial carcinoma (UTUC). World J Urol. 2017;35(2):251–9.
60. Krabbe LM, Heitplatz B, Preuss S, Hutchinson RC, Woldu SL, Singla N, et al. Prognostic value of PD-1 and PD-L1 expression in patients with high grade upper tract urothelial carcinoma. J Urol. 2017;198(6):1253–62.
61. Tse J, Ghandour R, Singla N, Lotan Y. Molecular predictors of complete response following neoadjuvant chemotherapy in urothelial carcinoma of the bladder and upper tracts. Int J Mol Sci. 2019;20(4):793.
62. Ke HL, Tu HP, Lin HH, Chai CY, Chang LL, Li WM, et al. Cyclooxygenase-2 (COX-2) upregulation is a prognostic marker for poor clinical outcome of upper tract urothelial cancer. Anticancer Res. 2012;32(9):4111–6.
63. Chang WS, Liao CH, Hsu CM, Huang CY, Fang HY, Kao PY, et al. Significant association of cyclo-oxygenase 2 genotypes with upper tract urothelial cancer. Anticancer Res. 2015;35(5):2725–30.
64. Lin HH, Ke HL, Hsiao KH, Tsai CW, Wu WJ, Bau DT, et al. CCND1 1722 polymorphism and potential relevance to upper tract urothelial cancer. Anticancer Res. 2011;31(3):1043–7.
65. Monteiro-Reis S, Leça L, Almeida M, Antunes L, Monteiro P, Dias PC, et al. Accurate detection of upper tract urothelial carcinoma in tissue and urine by means of quantitative GDF15, TMEFF2 and VIM promoter methylation. Eur J Cancer. 2014;50(1):226–33.
66. Guo RQ, Xiong GY, Yang KW, Zhang L, He SM, Gong YQ, et al. Detection of urothelial carcinoma, upper tract urothelial carcinoma, bladder carcinoma, and urothelial carcinoma with gross hematuria using selected urine-DNA methylation biomarkers: a prospective, single-center study. Urol Oncol. 2018;36(7):342.e15–23.
67. Agarwal N, Pal SK, Hahn AW, Nussenzveig RH, Pond GR, Gupta SV, et al. Characterization of metastatic urothelial carcinoma via comprehensive genomic profiling of circulating tumor DNA. Cancer. 2018;124(10):2115–24.
68. Sfakianos JP, Cha EK, Iyer G, Scott SN, Zabor EC, Shah RH, et al. Genomic characterization of upper tract urothelial carcinoma. Eur Urol. 2015;68(6):970–7.
69. Robinson BD, Vlachostergios PJ, Bhinder B, Liu W, Li K, Moss TJ, et al. Upper tract urothelial carcinoma has a luminal-papillary T-cell depleted contexture and activated FGFR3 signaling. Nat Commun. 2019;10(1):2977.
70. Babjuk M, Bohle A, Burger M, Capoun O, Cohen D, Comperat EM, et al. EAU guidelines on non-muscle-invasive urothelial carcinoma of the bladder: update 2016. Eur Urol. 2017;71(3):447–61.
71. Soukup V, Capoun O, Cohen D, Hernandez V, Babjuk M, Burger M, et al. Prognostic performance and reproducibility of the 1973 and 2004/2016 World Health Organization grading classification systems in non-muscle-invasive bladder cancer: A European Association of Urology Non-muscle Invasive Bladder Cancer Guidelines Panel Systematic Review. Eur Urol. 2017;72(5):801–13.
72. Margulis V, Shariat SF, Matin SF, Kamat AM, Zigeuner R, Kikuchi E, et al. Outcomes of radical nephroureterectomy: a series from the Upper Tract Urothelial Carcinoma Collaboration. Cancer. 2009;115(6):1224–33.
73. Jeldres C, Sun M, Isbarn H, Lughezzani G, Budaus L, Alasker A, et al. A population-based assessment of perioperative mortality after nephroureterectomy for upper-tract urothelial carcinoma. Urology. 2010;75(2):315–20.
74. Abouassaly R, Alibhai SM, Shah N, Timilshina N, Fleshner N, Finelli A. Troubling outcomes from population-level analysis of surgery for upper tract urothelial carcinoma. Urology. 2010;76(4):895–901.
75. Roupret M, Colin P, Yates DR. A new proposal to risk stratify urothelial carcinomas of the upper urinary tract (UTUCs) in a predefinitive treatment setting: low-risk versus high-risk UTUCs. Eur Urol. 2014;66(2):181–3.

76. Seisen T, Colin P, Roupret M. Risk-adapted strategy for the kidney-sparing management of upper tract tumours. Nat Rev Urol. 2015;12(3):155–66.
77. Fajkovic H, Cha EK, Jeldres C, Donner G, Chromecki TF, Margulis V, et al. Prognostic value of extranodal extension and other lymph node parameters in patients with upper tract urothelial carcinoma. J Urol. 2012;187(3):845–51.
78. Wheat JC, Weizer AZ, Wolf JS Jr, Lotan Y, Remzi M, Margulis V, et al. Concomitant carcinoma in situ is a feature of aggressive disease in patients with organ confined urothelial carcinoma following radical nephroureterectomy. Urol Oncol. 2012;30(3):252–8.
79. Redrow GP, Guo CC, Brausi MA, Coleman JA, Fernandez MI, Kassouf W, et al. Upper urinary tract carcinoma in situ: current knowledge, future direction. J Urol. 2017;197(2):287–95.
80. Ouzzane A, Colin P, Xylinas E, Pignot G, Ariane MM, Saint F, et al. Ureteral and multifocal tumours have worse prognosis than renal pelvic tumours in urothelial carcinoma of the upper urinary tract treated by nephroureterectomy. Eur Urol. 2011;60(6):1258–65.
81. Ito Y, Kikuchi E, Tanaka N, Miyajima A, Mikami S, Jinzaki M, et al. Preoperative hydronephrosis grade independently predicts worse pathological outcomes in patients undergoing nephroureterectomy for upper tract urothelial carcinoma. J Urol. 2011;185(5):1621–6.
82. Verhoest G, Shariat SF, Chromecki TF, Raman JD, Margulis V, Novara G, et al. Predictive factors of recurrence and survival of upper tract urothelial carcinomas. World J Urol. 2011;29(4):495–501.
83. Messer JC, Terrell JD, Herman MP, Ng CK, Scherr DS, Scoll B, et al. Multi-institutional validation of the ability of preoperative hydronephrosis to predict advanced pathologic tumor stage in upper-tract urothelial carcinoma. Urol Oncol. 2013;31(6):904–8.
84. Hasan MN, Roupret M, Keeley F, Cracco C, Jones R, Straub M, et al. Consultation on UTUC, Stockholm 2018 aspects of risk stratification: long-term results and follow-up. World J Urol. 2019;37(11):2289–96.
85. Villa L, Cloutier J, Letendre J, Ploumidis A, Salonia A, Cornu JN, et al. Early repeated ureteroscopy within 6-8 weeks after a primary endoscopic treatment in patients with upper tract urothelial cell carcinoma: preliminary findings. World J Urol. 2016;34(9):1201–6.
86. Vemana G, Kim EH, Bhayani SB, Vetter JM, Strope SA. Survival comparison between endoscopic and surgical management for patients with upper tract urothelial cancer: a matched propensity score analysis using surveillance, epidemiology and end results-medicare data. Urology. 2016;95:115–20.
87. Roupret M, Smyth G, Irani J, Guy L, Davin JL, Saint F, et al. Oncological risk of laparoscopic surgery in urothelial carcinomas. World J Urol. 2009;27(1):81–8.
88. Ni S, Tao W, Chen Q, Liu L, Jiang H, Hu H, et al. Laparoscopic versus open nephroureterectomy for the treatment of upper urinary tract urothelial carcinoma: a systematic review and cumulative analysis of comparative studies. Eur Urol. 2012;61(6):1142–53.
89. Simone G, Papalia R, Guaglianone S, Ferriero M, Leonardo C, Forastiere E, et al. Laparoscopic versus open nephroureterectomy: perioperative and oncologic outcomes from a randomised prospective study. Eur Urol. 2009;56(3):520–6.
90. Adibi M, Youssef R, Shariat SF, Lotan Y, Wood CG, Sagalowsky AI, et al. Oncological outcomes after radical nephroureterectomy for upper tract urothelial carcinoma: comparison over the three decades. Int J Urol. 2012;19(12):1060–6.
91. Clements MB, Krupski TL, Culp SH. Robotic-assisted surgery for upper tract urothelial carcinoma: a comparative survival analysis. Ann Surg Oncol. 2018;25(9):2550–62.
92. Aboumohamed AA, Krane LS, Hemal AK. Oncologic outcomes following robot-assisted laparoscopic nephroureterectomy with bladder cuff excision for upper tract urothelial carcinoma. J Urol. 2015;194(6):1561–6.
93. Seisen T, Granger B, Colin P, Leon P, Utard G, Renard-Penna R, et al. A systematic review and meta-analysis of clinicopathologic factors linked to intravesical recurrence after radical nephroureterectomy to treat upper tract urothelial carcinoma. Eur Urol. 2015;67(6):1122–33.
94. Jeldres C, Lughezzani G, Sun M, Isbarn H, Shariat SF, Budaus L, et al. Segmental ureterectomy can safely be performed in patients with transitional cell carcinoma of the ureter. J Urol. 2010;183(4):1324–9.

95. Xylinas E, Kluth L, Passoni N, Trinh QD, Rieken M, Lee RK, et al. Prediction of intravesical recurrence after radical nephroureterectomy: development of a clinical decision-making tool. Eur Urol. 2014;65(3):650–8.
96. Kondo T, Hashimoto Y, Kobayashi H, Iizuka J, Nakazawa H, Ito F, et al. Template-based lymphadenectomy in urothelial carcinoma of the upper urinary tract: impact on patient survival. Int J Urol. 2010;17(10):848–54.
97. Dominguez-Escrig JL, Peyronnet B, Seisen T, Bruins HM, Yuan CY, Babjuk M, et al. Potential benefit of lymph node dissection during radical nephroureterectomy for upper tract urothelial carcinoma: a systematic review by the European Association of Urology guidelines panel on non-muscle-invasive bladder cancer. Eur Urol Focus. 2019;5(2):224–41.
98. Dong F, Xu T, Wang X, Shen Y, Zhang X, Chen S, et al. Lymph node dissection could bring survival benefits to patients diagnosed with clinically node-negative upper urinary tract urothelial cancer: a population-based, propensity score-matched study. Int J Clin Oncol. 2019;24(3):296–305.
99. Lenis AT, Donin NM, Faiena I, Salmasi A, Johnson DC, Drakaki A, et al. Role of surgical approach on lymph node dissection yield and survival in patients with upper tract urothelial carcinoma. Urol Oncol. 2018;36(1):9e1–9e.
100. Xylinas E, Rink M, Margulis V, Faison T, Comploj E, Novara G, et al. Prediction of true nodal status in patients with pathological lymph node negative upper tract urothelial carcinoma at radical nephroureterectomy. J Urol. 2013;189(2):468–73.
101. Matin SF, Sfakianos JP, Espiritu PN, Coleman JA, Spiess PE. Patterns of lymphatic metastases in upper tract urothelial carcinoma and proposed dissection templates. J Urol. 2015;194(6):1567–74.
102. Cutress ML, Stewart GD, Wells-Cole S, Phipps S, Thomas BG, Tolley DA. Long-term endoscopic management of upper tract urothelial carcinoma: 20-year single-centre experience. BJU Int. 2012;110(11):1608–17.
103. Herrmann TR, Liatsikos EN, Nagele U, Traxer O, Merseburger AS. Eau Guidelines Panel on Lasers T. EAU guidelines on laser technologies. Eur Urol. 2012;61(4):783–95.
104. Cornu JN, Roupret M, Carpentier X, Geavlete B, de Medina SG, Cussenot O, et al. Oncologic control obtained after exclusive flexible ureteroscopic management of upper urinary tract urothelial cell carcinoma. World J Urol. 2010;28(2):151–6.
105. Grasso M, Fishman AI, Cohen J, Alexander B. Ureteroscopic and extirpative treatment of upper urinary tract urothelial carcinoma: a 15-year comprehensive review of 160 consecutive patients. BJU Int. 2012;110(11):1618–26.
106. Musi G, Mistretta FA, Marenghi C, Russo A, Catellani M, Nazzani S, et al. Thulium laser treatment of upper urinary tract carcinoma: a multi-institutional analysis of surgical and oncological outcomes. J Endourol. 2018;32(3):257–63.
107. Kamijo T, Nutahara K, Homma Y, Minowada S, Higashihara E, Aso Y. Transurethral resection of papillary tumor in the lower end of the ureter: report of two cases. Hinyokika Kiyo. 1993;39(2):179–82.
108. Cutress ML, Stewart GD, Zakikhani P, Phipps S, Thomas BG, Tolley DA. Ureteroscopic and percutaneous management of upper tract urothelial carcinoma (UTUC): systematic review. BJU Int. 2012;110(5):614–28.
109. Argyropoulos AN, Tolley DA. Upper urinary tract transitional cell carcinoma: current treatment overview of minimally invasive approaches. BJU Int. 2007;99(5):982–7.
110. Palou J, Piovesan LF, Huguet J, Salvador J, Vicente J, Villavicencio H. Percutaneous nephroscopic management of upper urinary tract transitional cell carcinoma: recurrence and long-term followup. J Urol. 2004;172(1):66–9.
111. Roupret M, Traxer O, Tligui M, Conort P, Chartier-Kastler E, Richard F, et al. Upper urinary tract transitional cell carcinoma: recurrence rate after percutaneous endoscopic resection. Eur Urol. 2007;51(3):709–13. discussion 14
112. Colin P, Ouzzane A, Pignot G, Ravier E, Crouzet S, Ariane MM, et al. Comparison of oncological outcomes after segmental ureterectomy or radical nephroureterectomy in urothelial carcinomas of the upper urinary tract: results from a large French multicentre study. BJU Int. 2012;110(8):1134–41.

113. Phe V, Cussenot O, Bitker MO, Roupret M. Does the surgical technique for management of the distal ureter influence the outcome after nephroureterectomy? BJU Int. 2011;108(1):130–8.
114. Lughezzani G, Jeldres C, Isbarn H, Shariat SF, Sun M, Pharand D, et al. A critical appraisal of the value of lymph node dissection at nephroureterectomy for upper tract urothelial carcinoma. Urology. 2010;75(1):118–24.
115. Moschini M, Foerster B, Abufaraj M, Soria F, Seisen T, Roupret M, et al. Trends of lymphadenectomy in upper tract urothelial carcinoma (UTUC) patients treated with radical nephroureterectomy. World J Urol. 2017;35(10):1541–7.
116. Xylinas E, Kluth L, Rieken M, Roupret M, Hussein A, Al Awamlh B, Clozel T, et al. External validation of the pathological nodal staging score in upper tract urothelial carcinoma: A population-based study. Urol Oncol. 2017;35(1):33e21–6.
117. Armatys SA, Mellon MJ, Beck SD, Koch MO, Foster RS, Bihrle R. Use of ileum as ureteral replacement in urological reconstruction. J Urol. 2009;181(1):177–81.
118. Antonelli A, Zani D, Dotti P, Tralce L, Simeone C, Cunico SC. Use of the appendix as ureteral substitute in a patient with a single kidney affected by relapsing upper urinary tract carcinoma. ScientificWorldJournal. 2005;5:276–9.
119. Chausse G, Skinnider B, Crook J, Black P, Abikhzer G, Probst S. Ureteral metastasis from prostate cancer: a PSMA PET Pitfall. Clin Nucl Med. 2020;45(9):689–91.
120. Hongo H, Kosaka T, Yoshimine S, Oya M. Ureteral metastasis from prostate cancer. BMJ Case Rep. 2014;2014
121. Giannarini G, Kessler TM, Birkhauser FD, Thalmann GN, Studer UE. Antegrade perfusion with bacillus Calmette-Guerin in patients with non-muscle-invasive urothelial carcinoma of the upper urinary tract: who may benefit? Eur Urol. 2011;60(5):955–60.
122. Foerster B, D'Andrea D, Abufaraj M, Broenimann S, Karakiewicz PI, Roupret M, et al. Endocavitary treatment for upper tract urothelial carcinoma: a meta-analysis of the current literature. Urol Oncol. 2019;37(7):430–6.
123. Irie A, Iwamura M, Kadowaki K, Ohkawa A, Uchida T, Baba S. Intravesical instillation of bacillus Calmette-Guerin for carcinoma in situ of the urothelium involving the upper urinary tract using vesicoureteral reflux created by a double-pigtail catheter. Urology. 2002;59(1):53–7.
124. Horiguchi H, Yoneyama T, Hatakeyama S, Tokui N, Sato T, Fujita N, et al. Impact of bacillus Calmette-Guerin therapy of upper urinary tract carcinoma in situ: comparison of oncological outcomes with radical nephroureterectomy. Med Oncol. 2018;35(4):41.
125. Yossepowitch O, Lifshitz DA, Dekel Y, Ehrlich Y, Gur U, Margel D, et al. Assessment of vesicoureteral reflux in patients with self-retaining ureteral stents: implications for upper urinary tract instillation. J Urol. 2005;173(3):890–3.
126. O'Brien T, Ray E, Singh R, Coker B, Beard R. British Association of Urological Surgeons Section of O. Prevention of bladder tumours after nephroureterectomy for primary upper urinary tract urothelial carcinoma: a prospective, multicentre, randomised clinical trial of a single postoperative intravesical dose of mitomycin C (the ODMIT-C Trial). Eur Urol. 2011;60(4):703–10.
127. Ito A, Shintaku I, Satoh M, Ioritani N, Aizawa M, Tochigi T, et al. Prospective randomized phase II trial of a single early intravesical instillation of pirarubicin (THP) in the prevention of bladder recurrence after nephroureterectomy for upper urinary tract urothelial carcinoma: the THP Monotherapy Study Group Trial. J Clin Oncol. 2013;31(11):1422–7.
128. Donin NM, Strauss-Ayali D, Agmon-Gerstein Y, Malchi N, Lenis AT, Holden S, et al. Serial retrograde instillations of sustained release formulation of mitomycin C to the upper urinary tract of the Yorkshire swine using a thermosensitive polymer: Safety and feasibility. Urol Oncol. 2017;35(5):272–8.
129. Martini A, Daza J, Poltiyelova E, Gul Z, Heard JR, Ferket BS, et al. Pathological downstaging as a novel endpoint for the development of neoadjuvant chemotherapy for upper tract urothelial carcinoma. BJU Int. 2019;124(4):665–71.
130. Matin SF, Margulis V, Kamat A, Wood CG, Grossman HB, Brown GA, et al. Incidence of downstaging and complete remission after neoadjuvant chemotherapy for high-risk upper tract transitional cell carcinoma. Cancer. 2010;116(13):3127–34.

131. Meng X, Chao B, Vijay V, Silver H, Margolin EJ, Balar A, et al. High response rates to neoadjuvant chemotherapy in high-grade upper tract urothelial carcinoma. Urology. 2019;129:146–52.
132. Kubota Y, Hatakeyama S, Tanaka T, Fujita N, Iwamura H, Mikami J, et al. Oncological outcomes of neoadjuvant chemotherapy in patients with locally advanced upper tract urothelial carcinoma: a multicenter study. Oncotarget. 2017;8(60):101500–8.
133. Hosogoe S, Hatakeyama S, Kusaka A, Hamano I, Iwamura H, Fujita N, et al. Platinum-based neoadjuvant chemotherapy improves oncological outcomes in patients with locally advanced upper tract urothelial carcinoma. Eur Urol Focus. 2018;4(6):946–53.
134. Margulis V, Puligandla M, Trabulsi EJ, Plimack ER, Kessler ER, Matin SF, et al. Phase II trial of neoadjuvant systemic chemotherapy followed by extirpative surgery in patients with high grade upper tract urothelial carcinoma. J Urol. 2020;203(4):690–8.
135. Kaag MG, O'Malley RL, O'Malley P, Godoy G, Chen M, Smaldone MC, et al. Changes in renal function following nephroureterectomy may affect the use of perioperative chemotherapy. Eur Urol. 2010;58(4):581–7.
136. Lane BR, Smith AK, Larson BT, Gong MC, Campbell SC, Raghavan D, et al. Chronic kidney disease after nephroureterectomy for upper tract urothelial carcinoma and implications for the administration of perioperative chemotherapy. Cancer. 2010;116(12):2967–73.
137. Moschini M, Shariat SF, Roupret M, De Santis M, Bellmunt J, Sternberg CN, et al. Impact of primary tumor location on survival from the European organization for the research and treatment of cancer advanced urothelial cancer studies. J Urol. 2018;199(5):1149–57.
138. Powles T, Park SH, Voog E, Caserta C, Valderrama BP, Gurney H, et al. Avelumab maintenance therapy for advanced or metastatic urothelial carcinoma. N Engl J Med. 2020;383(13):1218–30.
139. Balar AV, Galsky MD, Rosenberg JE, Powles T, Petrylak DP, Bellmunt J, et al. Atezolizumab as first-line treatment in cisplatin-ineligible patients with locally advanced and metastatic urothelial carcinoma: a single-arm, multicentre, phase 2 trial. Lancet. 2017;389(10064):67–76.
140. Balar AV, Castellano D, O'Donnell PH, Grivas P, Vuky J, Powles T, et al. First-line pembrolizumab in cisplatin-ineligible patients with locally advanced and unresectable or metastatic urothelial cancer (KEYNOTE-052): a multicentre, single-arm, phase 2 study. Lancet Oncol. 2017;18(11):1483–92.
141. Alva AS, Mangat PK, Garrett-Mayer E, Halabi S, Hansra D, Calfa CJ, et al. Pembrolizumab in patients with metastatic breast cancer with high tumor mutational burden: results from the targeted agent and profiling utilization registry (TAPUR) study. J Clin Oncol. 2021;39(22):2443–51.
142. Heers H, DE Geeter P, Goebell PJ, Matz U, DE Schultz W, Edlich B, et al. Vinflunine in the treatment of upper tract urothelial carcinoma - subgroup analysis of an observational study. Anticancer Res. 2017;37(11):6437–42.
143. Bellmunt J, de Wit R, Vaughn DJ, Fradet Y, Lee JL, Fong L, et al. Pembrolizumab as second-line therapy for advanced urothelial carcinoma. N Engl J Med. 2017;376(11):1015–26.
144. Rosenberg JE, Hoffman-Censits J, Powles T, van der Heijden MS, Balar AV, Necchi A, et al. Atezolizumab in patients with locally advanced and metastatic urothelial carcinoma who have progressed following treatment with platinum-based chemotherapy: a single-arm, multicentre, phase 2 trial. Lancet. 2016;387(10031):1909–20.
145. Powles T, Duran I, van der Heijden MS, Loriot Y, Vogelzang NJ, De Giorgi U, et al. Atezolizumab versus chemotherapy in patients with platinum-treated locally advanced or metastatic urothelial carcinoma (IMvigor211): a multicentre, open-label, phase 3 randomised controlled trial. Lancet. 2018;391(10122):748–57.
146. Sharma P, Retz M, Siefker-Radtke A, Baron A, Necchi A, Bedke J, et al. Nivolumab in metastatic urothelial carcinoma after platinum therapy (CheckMate 275): a multicentre, single-arm, phase 2 trial. Lancet Oncol. 2017;18(3):312–22.
147. Patel MR, Ellerton J, Infante JR, Agrawal M, Gordon M, Aljumaily R, et al. Avelumab in metastatic urothelial carcinoma after platinum failure (JAVELIN Solid Tumor): pooled results from two expansion cohorts of an open-label, phase 1 trial. Lancet Oncol. 2018;19(1):51–64.

148. Powles T, O'Donnell PH, Massard C, Arkenau HT, Friedlander TW, Hoimes CJ, et al. Efficacy and safety of durvalumab in locally advanced or metastatic urothelial carcinoma: updated results from a phase 1/2 open-label study. JAMA Oncol. 2017;3(9):e172411.
149. Apolo AB, Infante JR, Balmanoukian A, Patel MR, Wang D, Kelly K, et al. Avelumab, an anti-programmed death-ligand 1 antibody, in patients with refractory metastatic urothelial carcinoma: results from a multicenter, Phase Ib study. J Clin Oncol. 2017;35(19):2117–24.
150. Sharma P, Siefker-Radtke A, de Braud F, Basso U, Calvo E, Bono P, et al. Nivolumab alone and with ipilimumab in previously treated metastatic urothelial carcinoma: CheckMate 032 nivolumab 1 mg/kg plus ipilimumab 3 mg/kg expansion cohort results. J Clin Oncol. 2019;37(19):1608–16.
151. Loriot Y, Necchi A, Park SH, Garcia-Donas J, Huddart R, Burgess E, et al. Erdafitinib in locally advanced or metastatic urothelial carcinoma. N Engl J Med. 2019;381(4):338–48.
152. Olgac S, Mazumdar M, Dalbagni G, Reuter VE. Urothelial carcinoma of the renal pelvis: a clinicopathologic study of 130 cases. Am J Surg Pathol. 2004;28(12):1545–52.
153. Locke JA, Hamidizadeh R, Kassouf W, Rendon RA, Bell D, Izawa J, et al. Surveillance guidelines based on recurrence patterns for upper tract urothelial carcinoma. Can Urol Assoc J. 2018;12(8):243–51.

Chapter 17
Fetal and Prenatal Ureter

Ahmed Abdelhalim and Ashraf T. Hafez

Abstract This book chapter will briefly review the normal embryologic development of the ureter. It will also demonstrate the pathophysiologic bases of some of the common ureteral anomalies and how these anomalies are suspected based on fetal imaging.

Keywords Ureter · Development · Embryology · Ureteric bud · Wolffian duct · Anomalies · Antenatal imaging · Hydroureter · Diagnosis · Management

Abbreviations

ANH	Antenatal hydronephrosis
MB	Metanephric blastema
PUV	Posterior urethral valve
RAS	Renin-angiotensin system
UB	Ureteral bud
UPJ	Ureteropelvic junction
UPJO	Ureteropelvic junction obstruction
UVJ	Ureterovesical junction
UVJO	Ureterovesical junction obstruction
VUR	Vesicoureteral reflux

Test your learning and check your understanding of this book's contents: use the "Springer Nature Flashcards" app to access questions. To use the app, please follow the instructions in chapter 1.

A. Abdelhalim (✉)
Mansoura Urology and Nephrology Center, Mansoura University, Mansoura, Egypt

West Virginia University, Morgantown, WV, USA

A. T. Hafez
Mansoura Urology and Nephrology Center, Mansoura University, Mansoura, Egypt

M. Abdel-Gawad et al. (eds.), *The Ureter*,
https://doi.org/10.1007/978-3-031-36212-5_17

17.1 Normal Ureteral Development

The ureter develops from the ureteral bud (UB), an outpouching from the distal end of the mesonephric (Wolffian) duct. The ureteral bud arises from the mesonephric duct in the fourth week of gestation as it bends ventrally to enter the cloaca. The distal segment of the Wolffian duct between the urogenital sinus and the take-off the UB is called the common excretory duct. Signals from the developing metanephric blastema (MB) induces the elongation of the ureteral bud and invasion of the metanephric blastema by the growing ureteral bud [1]. In fact, the UB grows straight in the direction of the MB, but little is known about the guidance mechanism. **Initial growth** of the emerging UB depends on the epithelial expression of FRAS1, a basement membrane protein that interacts with FREM1 and FREM2 to optimize the presentation of growth factors derived from the MB to UB and physically stabilize the UB/MB interaction by binding integrin α8 [2]; [3–5]. Lack of integrin α8 expression in mutant mice has resulted in arrest of UB progression [6]. TBX18 is a transcriptional factor that stimulates epithelial proliferation of the UB as evident by shorter ureteral length in mutant mice lacking this factor. **Further longitudinal growth** occurs irrespective of urine flow as evident in ureters of certain mutant embryos lacking kidneys. However, it is possible that urine contributes to optimize the differentiation of the growing UB [5].

Backflow of urine and solutes through the urothelium is prevented by plaques of uroplakin (UPK) protein. UPK is expressed early during urinary tract development and is present in the epithelial lining of the urogenital sinus. In mutant mice lacking UPK proteins, these plaques are disorganized and the urothelium is leaky. Lack of UPK also results in urinary tract anomalies with gaping ureteral orifices and dilated ureters subsequent to vesicoureteral reflux (VUR) or ureteral obstruction [7, 8].

17.2 Recanalization of the Ureter

At 28 days, the ureter is an epithelial tube surrounded by loose mesenchymal cells. Transient luminal obstruction occurs with subsequent recanalization during the seventh week [9, 10]. Recanalization process starts in the midureter and extends cranially and caudally in a bidirectional fashion. Chwalle's membrane is a two-layered cellular membrane that separates the developing ureter from the urogenital sinus. Subsequent dissolution of this membrane results in unimpeded urine flow from the kidney to the bladder [11].

The renin-angiotensin system (RAS) plays a key role in the development of the UB, its canalization and branching to form the renal pelvis and calyces. The angiotensin-converting enzyme converts angiotensin I to angiotensin II. Angiotensin II acts on AT1 and AT2 receptors and induces the production of glial-derived neurotrophic factor (GDNF) in the MB. By interacting with the RET receptor tyrosine kinase and glial cell-line derived neurotrophic factor receptor alpha (Gfralpha1), GDNF simulates cell proliferation at the tip of the UB, ureteral elongation, branching and invasion of the MB [12]. The role of RAS in ureteral development is supported by the high concentration of AT2 receptors in the mesenchymal cells around the UB at early development stages [13]. Also, knock-out mice for AT2 receptor gene demonstrate a high incidence of urinary tract anomalies including VUR and ureterovesical junction (UVJ) obstruction [14]. Pharmacological inhibition or mutations affecting the genes coding for components of the RAS result in a wide variety of congenital anomalies of the kidney and urinary tract including aberrant UB development, duplex kidneys, renal tubular dysgenesis, hydronephrosis, renal papillary hypoplasia, abnormal glomerulogenesis and renal vascular abnormalities [15]. Mutations resulting in the absence of GDNF, RET or Gfralpha1 will result in failure of UB growth and subsequently bilateral renal aplasia as shown in studies in mice [16, 17]. About 40% of cases of renal agenesis in humans are associated with RET mutations and 5–10% are associated with GDNF mutations [18]. Interestingly, experimental work has demonstrated that both the proximal and distal ends of the nascent ureter have the potential to branch and form and collecting duct tree [19]. Despite the available evidence, our understanding of the ureteral development remains incomplete.

17.3 Muscularization of the Ureter

Ureteral muscularization starts at 12 weeks of gestation. Smooth muscle differentiation is first observed at the ureterovesical junction (UVJ), then it ascends in a cranial direction. Initially, smooth muscle fibers are scanty and randomly arranged. Then, these fibers become more abundant and organized in three layers: inner longitudinal, middle circular and outer longitudinal layers. The epithelium attains a transitional configuration by 14 weeks [20, 21]. Ureteral epithelium stimulates the differentiation of the surrounding mesenchyme into smooth muscles by a paracrine effect. Several cellular mediators and transcriptional factors have been implicated in the differentiation of the peri-ureteral mesenchymal cells into smooth muscles including PTCH1, BMP4, TSHZ3, MYOCD and TSHZ3 [5].

After the shaft of the ureter becomes enveloped with smooth muscles, there seems to be a second wave of smooth muscle differentiation at the proximal end. This differentiation wave is mediated by calcineurin, the protein phosphatase and angiotensin II signaling. Disruption of these pathways during embryologic development results in hydronephrosis/hydroureter; because of the lack of ureteral peristalsis resulting in functional obstruction [22, 23]. It is also believed that fetal urine production by the kidney enhances the ureteric smooth differentiation and function. The mature ureter contains cholinergic, adrenergic, nitrergic and sensory nerve fibers that modify ureteral contractility [24].

The distal end of the mesonephric duct distal to the origin of the UB forms the common excretory duct. In the past, it was assumed that the trigone develops forms from the integration of the upper portion of the common excretory duct and the mesonephric ducts inferior to the UB origin into the bladder base. This assumption was later challenged by research that proposed an endodermal, rather than, mesodermal origin of the trigone [25]. This hypothesis is supported by molecular development and lineage tracing studies of the genetically labelled mesonephric duct cells. These

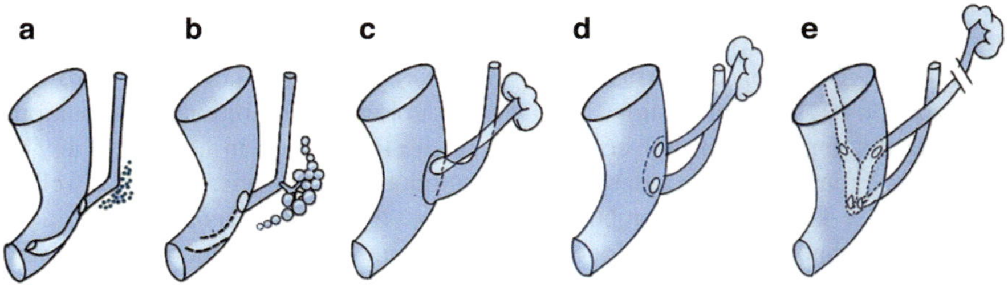

Fig. 17.1 (**a**, **b**) The ureteral bud originates from the distal part of the Wolffian duct and grows in the direction of the developing metanephric blastema. (**c**, **d**) The distal end of the Wolffian duct undergoes expansion and eventually absorption into the developing trigone or apoptosis and replacement by endoderm, resulting in separation of the openings of the ureter and the Wolffian duct (future vas deferens) in the corner of the trigone and urethra, respectively (**e**)

studies have shown that the most caudal part of the mesonephric duct undergoes apoptosis induced by signals from the developing bladder [26, 27]. After expansion and absorption of the common excretory duct into the bladder trigone or its involution by apoptosis and replacement by endoderm, the ureteral and Wolffian duct orifices become separate. The ureteral duct eventually enters the bladder at the lateral corner of the trigone, whereas the Wolffian duct opens at the verumontanum (seminal colliculus). Embryologic development of the ureter is summarized in Fig. 17.1.

17.4 Embryologic Basis of Some Ureteral Anomalies

17.4.1 Ureteral Atresia

Ureteral atresia is thought to occur due to relative or total ischemia of the UB during migration of the developing kidney as the ureter establishes regional blood supply. This assumption is derived from experimental studies on intestinal atresia [28]. In mice, mutations resulting in the absence or inactivation of the GDNF, RET or Gfralpha1 cause failure of the UB growth resulting in bilateral renal agenesis [29]. Failure of UB development or its elongation to reach the MB results in ipsilateral renal agenesis. Ureteral atresia and renal agenesis are associated with high incidence of Wolffian and Mullerian duct anomalies in males and females, respectively since the embryologic development of these structures is closely related.

17.4.2 Ureteral Duplication Anomalies

Ureteral duplication (or triplication) occurs if multiple ureteral buds arise from the Wolffian duct or if the UB divides prematurely before meeting the MB. Incomplete ureteral duplication occurs when the UB branches off prematurely after its takeoff from the Wolffian duct and before it reaches the MB. The anatomy can be greatly variable ranging from a mild form as bifid renal pelvis to complete ureteral duplication with separate ureteral orifices. The most superior cephalad bud interacts with the upper portion of the MB and forms the upper pole, while the lower bud induces the lower pole moiety. The site of interaction of the growing UB and the developing MB is crucial for normal kidney development. For instance, if one UB meets the center of the MB, the blastema would develop normally, whereas if the other UB meets one pole of the MB, the blastema might become dysplastic [30] (Fig. 17.2).

When both buds are close together and arise from acceptable position along the mesonephric duct, both ureters will have normally positioned orifices in the trigone. In this situation, ureteral duplication becomes merely a radiologic finding with little clinical significance. Conversely, when the buds are widely separated, one or both ureteral orifices will be ectopic. If the superior UB arises from an abnormally high position, caudal ectopia will result. If the take-off of the inferior bud is more caudal along the mesonephric duct, the distal part of the mesonephric duct will have longer time to become absorbed in the trigone and the ureteral orifice will become more lateral than usual, resulting in lateral ectopia. As such, ureteral duplication could be associated with upper moiety obstruction by ectopic ureteral insertion or ureterocele, and VUR into the lower moiety. This relationship, known as the Weigert-Meyer law, is usually consistent with extremely rare exceptions [31, 32].

17.4.3 *Ureteral Triplication*

Ureteral triplication is an exceedingly rare condition. Only small case series and case reports are available to describe this anomaly. Ureteral triplication arises from multiple ureteral buds originating from the mesonephric duct or division of one UB into three divisions. Ureteral triplication is more frequent in girls and on the left

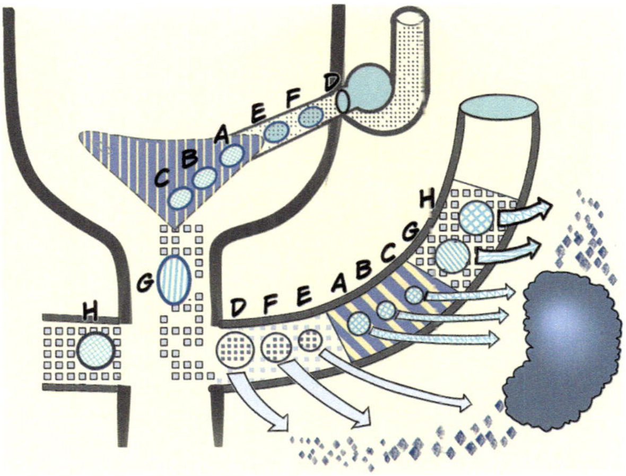

Fig. 17.2 Normal site of origin of the UB from the mesonephric duct is essential for normal renal-ureteral development (**a–c**). Abnormal take-off the UB from the mesonephric duct as in lateral (**d–f**) and caudal ectopia (**g**, **h**) is associated with renal dysplasia, as proposed by Mackie and Stephens [30]

more than the right side. It has been associated with ipsilateral or contralateral urinary tract anomalies including contralateral duplication, triplication, ureteral ectopia, ureterocele, VUR and renal dysplasia [33, 34]. It has also been reported in association with syndromes such as VACTERL [35]. Many cases of ureteral triplication are asymptomatic. However, patients may present with UTI, flank pain, incontinence or obstructive uropathy [35]. The diagnosis requires a high index of suspicion and relies on imaging studies such as ultrasound, voiding cystourethrogram, MRU, ureteropyelogram and renal scans. Symptomatic cases with preserved renal function may benefit from reconstruction. Patients with poorly functioning renal moieties may benefit from partial nephrectomy.

17.4.4 Ureteral Ectopia

Ureteral ectopia occurs when the ureteral orifice is located in a location other than the corner of the trigone. An ectopic ureter can drain within the bladder, urethra, male duct system, vestibule or female genital tract. Since an ectopic ureter drains above the urinary sphincter in males, urinary control is not affected in males with ureteral ectopia. On the other hand, ureteral ectopia can present with urinary incontinence in females if an ectopic ureter drains into the vestibule or Mullerian duct derivatives. Figure 17.3 depicts the possible sites of ectopic ureteral insertion in both males and females. Ureteral ectopia is commonly associated with ureteral duplication. Ectopic ureters can result from delay or absence of RET signaling. Fibroblast growth factors 7 and 10 and their receptor FGFR2 have also been implicated in the pathogenesis of ureteral ectopia [36]. Ureteral ectopia occurs as a result of abnormal take off the ureteral bud. Caudal ectopia results from abnormally high origin of the ureteral bud from the Wolffian duct. This abnormal origin allows less

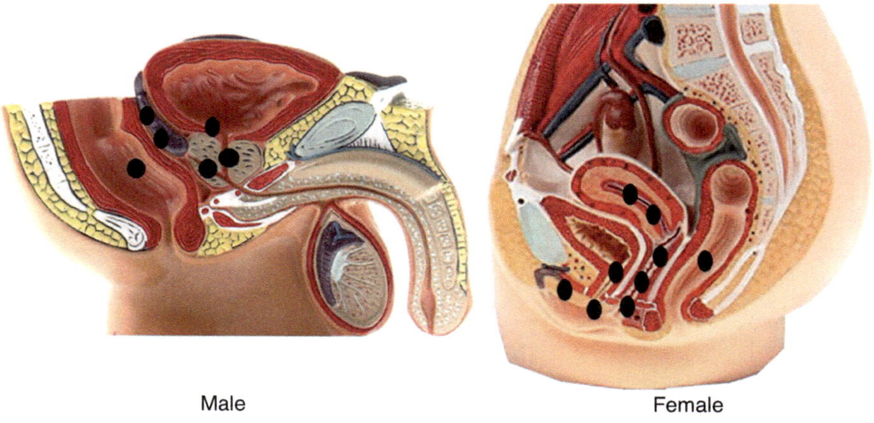

Fig. 17.3 Sites of ectopic ureteral insertion in both males and females

time for the orifice to be absorbed in the bladder, subsequently resulting in abnormal ureteral orifice location: medially in the trigone, in the urethra or along the path of Wolffian duct structures or remnants.

17.4.5 Congenital Ureteral Obstruction

Congenital ureteral obstruction occurs primarily at the ureteropelvic or ureterovesical junctions. Congenital obstruction can also occur where the ureter crosses the iliac vessels in the pelvis. Areas of obstruction are usually of normal caliber, but abnormally adynamic. On histologic examination, these segments are abnormally fibrous and lack smooth muscles, suggesting abnormal ureteral muscularization. As previously explained, mesenchymal differentiation into the ureteral musculature is induced by signals from the epithelium of the growing ureteral bud. It can be therefore assumed that congenital obstructive lesions, such as ureteropelvic junction obstruction (UPJO) and ureterovesical junction obstruction (UVJO), result from abnormal signaling (Sonic hedgehog signals) [37]. The following section will briefly discuss some of the common causes of congenital ureteral obstruction.

- **Ureteropelvic junction obstruction (UPJO)** is the commonest pathologic cause of antenatal hydronephrosis (ANH). It is suspected on antenatal ultrasound if there is dilation of the renal pelvis and collecting system with no associated ureteral dilation (Fig. 17.4). The clinical challenge lies in differentiating physiologic urinary tract dilation that can be safely observed without compromising renal function from obstruction that would require later surgical reconstruction. Increasing the severity of ANH is associated with increased likelihood of identifying obstruction on postnatal evaluation. However, there is no agreement on the

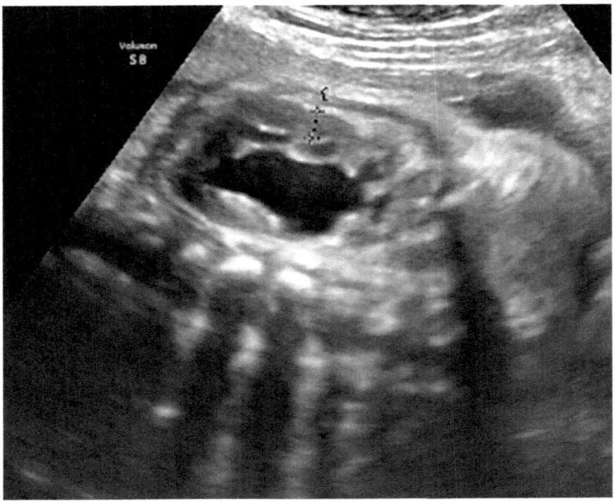

Fig. 17.4 Second trimester prenatal ultrasound showing right pyelectasis and caliectasis without associated hydroureter, suggestive of ureteropelvic junction obstruction, courtesy of Dr. Amal Mehna, MD

threshold of ANH that warrants postnatal evaluation [38]. There is little rationale for antenatal intervention or early delivery in cases of significant unilateral ANH. In rare situations, therapeutic aspiration has been recommended in cases of massive dilation to prevent dystocia and obstructed labor. Severe forms of UPJO may be associated with urinary ascites or perinephric urinomas which could predict poor split renal function [39].

- **Ureterovesical junction obstruction (UVJO):**
- UVJO is less common than UPJO and approximately represents 10% of ANH cases when evaluated postnatally. UVJO is distinguished from UPJO by ureteral dilation with variable degrees of renal pelvis and collecting system dilation. The ureter is best visualized at the bladder level, preferably in the transverse view. The differential diagnosis of ureteral dilation (hydroureter) includes primary obstruction at the UVJ, ectopic ureteral insertion into the bladder neck, ureterocele, high-grade VUR, prune belly syndrome or bladder outlet obstruction as in posterior urethral valve or urethral atresia (Fig. 17.5). The distinction between these conditions is typically made on postnatal evaluation [40].
- **Congenital ureteral stricture:**
- Congenital ureteral stricture is a rare condition. It is commonly seen at the upper and lower ends of the ureter, but it can also occur in the midureter. Associated contralateral renal anomalies have also been reported [41]. The histology of congenital ureteral stricture varies from hypertrophied smooth muscle layer to nearly absent muscle fibers, but these strictures are uniformly lined with transitional epithelium [42, 43]. The presentation depends on the severity of obstruction and the degree of renal function.

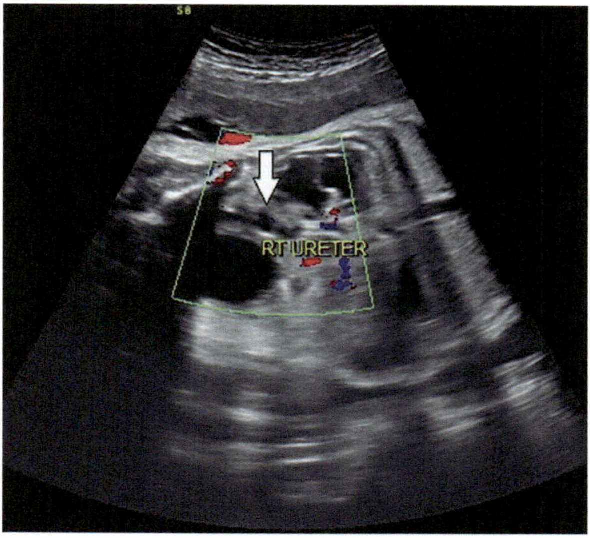

Fig. 17.5 Second trimester ultrasound showing right hydronephrosis and hydroureter (white arrow) in a male fetus that was diagnosed with posterior urethral valve on postnatal evaluation, courtesy of Dr. Amal Mehna, MD

Congenital ureteral strictures are usually discovered during the work-up for ANH. However, they are less amenable to conservative management when compared to other causes of antenatal hydronephrosis including UPJO and megarueter. Careful identification of the site and length of the stricture, usually by means of retrograde ureteropyelogram, is crucial for successful management [44]. Endoscopic management with dilatation and incision affords less favorable initial and long-term results relative to open repair. Surgical reconstruction involves excision of the affected segment with restoration of the ureteral continuity by open, laparoscopic or robotic approaches following the standard principles of ureteral reconstruction [45, 46].

- **Ureteral valves:**

  Ureteral valves are uncommon ureteral anomaly. They are thought to arise as a result of the abnormal persistence of the transverse folds (Ostling's folds) that arise as part of the normal ureteral development [45]. Ureteral valves are tissue folds covered with normal urothelium that project transversely into the ureteral lumen and block urine flow [45]. Ureteral folds are commonly seen in association with other ureteral anomalies including duplication, ureteral ectopia and VUR [47]. Coexisting ureteral strictures have also been reported [48]. Ureteral valves inhibit the antegrade but not the retrograde urine flow. Treatment of ureteral valves typically include resection and reconstruction with ureteroureterostomy, ureteropyelostomy or ureteroneocystotomy.
- **Ureteral polyps:**

  Fibroepithelial polyps are the most common benign ureteral neoplasms (Fig. 17.6) [49]. Although the exact etiology is unclear, it is believed that some polyps are congenital. Ureteral polyps could also arise secondary to acquired factors such as inflammation. These polyps have a fibrous core and covered by normal transitional epithelium [50]. Ureteral polyps are commonly diagnosed in adults than in children and in males than females [51]. The diagnosis is typically established with contrast-enhanced ureteral imaging: intravenous pyelogram,

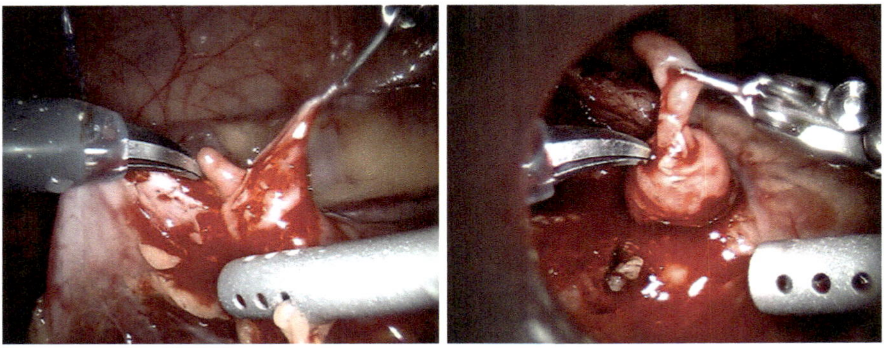

Fig. 17.6 Ureteral fibro-epithelial polyps discovered accidentally during robotic pyeloplasty

CTU, retrograde or antegrade ureteropyelogram [51]. The treatment entails endoscopic or open surgical resection. Open or laparoscopic polyp excision with ureteroureterostomy may be also required.

- **Retrocaval ureter:**

  Retrocaval ureter is a relatively rare ureteral anomaly with a reported incidence of 1 in 1000. It almost always involves the right ureter and is two to three times more common in males. Retrocaval ureter arises secondary to anomalous vascular development. Normally, most of the infrarenal portion of the inferior vena cava develops from supracardinal vein that lies dorsal to the ureter. The subcardinal lies ventral to the ureter and normally involutes. If the subcardinal vein persists, it becomes the infrarenal portion of the inferior vena cava resulting in retrocaval ureter (Fig. 17.7). The retrocaval segment of the ureter is often

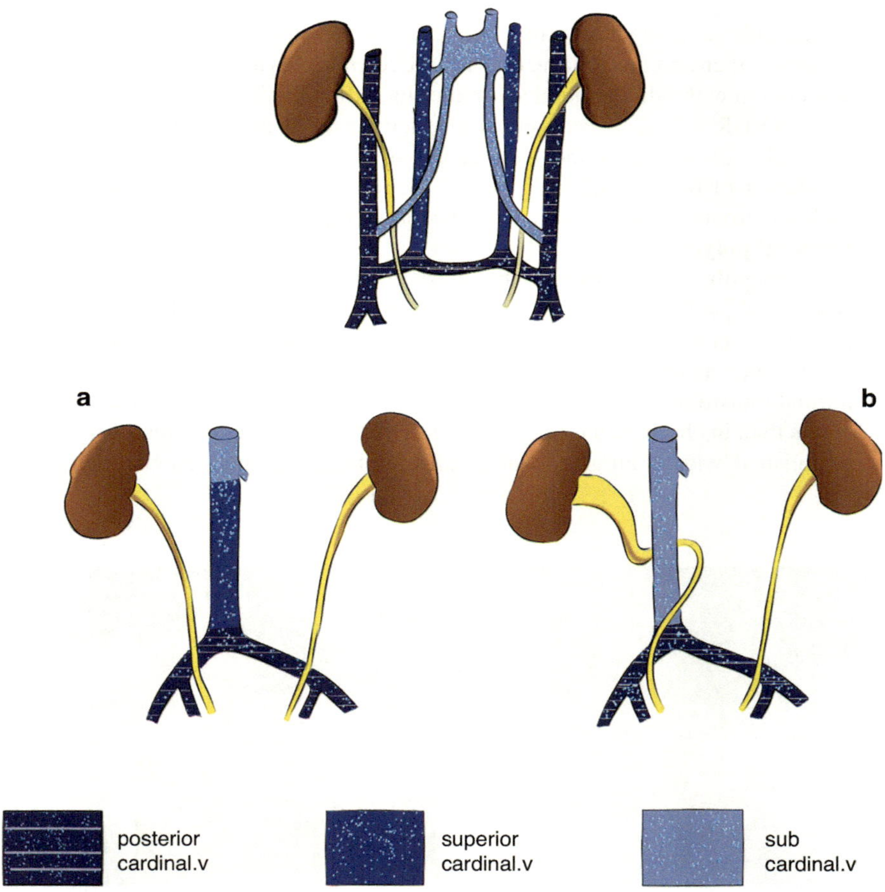

Fig. 17.7 Embryologic development of retrocaval ureter: (**a**) Normal development of the IVC and ureter, (**b**) development of retrocaval ureter

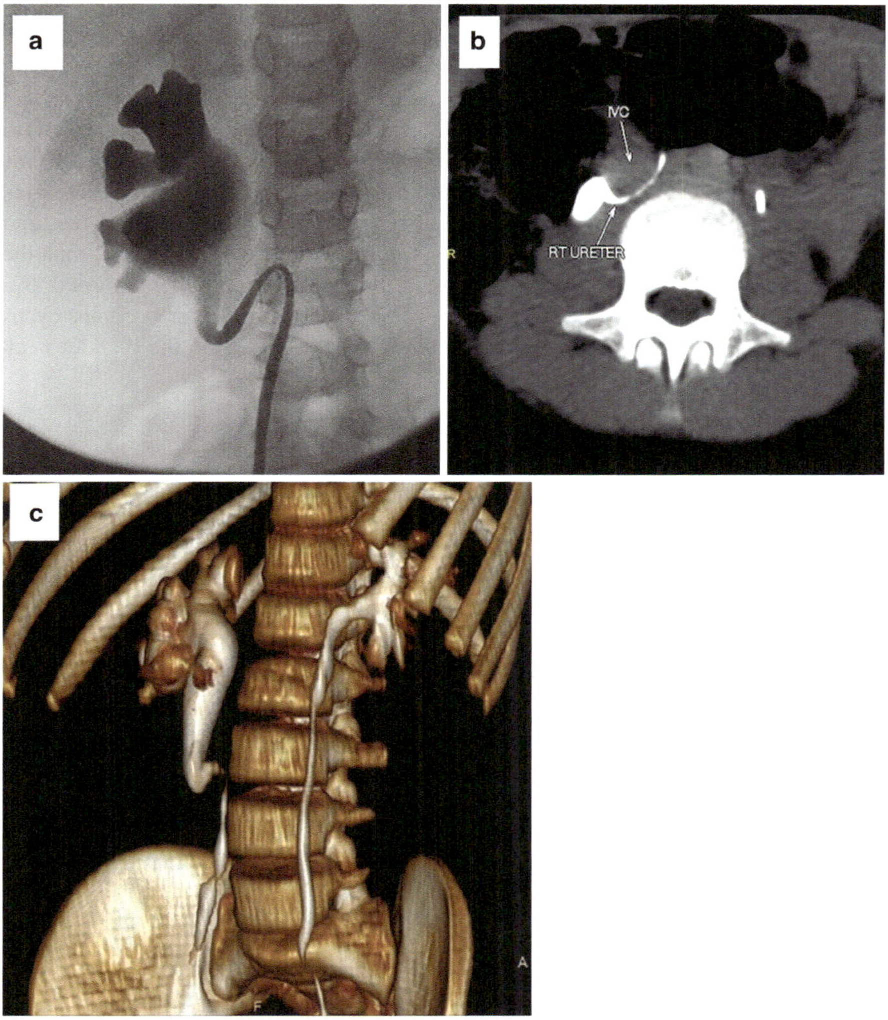

Fig. 17.8 (a) Retrograde ureteropyelogram of a patient with a retrocaval ureter showing the characteristic J-hooking appearance, (b) CT urogram of a right retrocaval ureter depicting the ureter crossing behind the inferior vena cava, (c) 3-D reconstruction of CT urogram with the characteristic J-hooking of the ureter

stenotic resulting in functional or anatomic obstruction [52]. The diagnosis is based on radiologic evaluation with excretory urograms or retrograde ureteropyelogram (Fig. 17.8). Treatment entails excision of the stenotic segment, transposition of the ureter anterior to the inferior vena cava and restoration of the ureter continuity.

- **Ectopic Ureteral Insertion**

  An ectopic ureter is a ureter that drains outside the trigonal area of the bladder. In females, it could enter into the bladder neck, urethra, perineum, Gartner's duct cyst (Wolffian duct remnant), vagina, uterus (Mullerian duct structure) or even the rectum. In males, it always drains above the external urethral sphincter into the bladder neck, prostatic urethra, seminal vesicles, ejaculatory ducts or vas deferens (Fig. 17.3). Ectopic ureter commonly occurs in association with duplex system, and is inevitably related to the upper pole ureter; because of its budding from the mesonephric duct later (more cephalad), a.k.a. caudal ectopia, than the lower pole ureter, as previously explained. Ureteroceles could be regarded as a version of the ectopic ureter when the distal aspect of the ureter becomes cystically dilated and is located within the bladder or extends into the bladder neck and urethra.

- **Ureteroceles**

  Ureteroceles are cystic dilations of the intramural ureter (Fig. 17.9). Several theories have been proposed to explain their origin. Popular theories explaining ureterocele origin include:

1. Persistence of the Chwalle's membrane, a two-layered membrane that separates the caudal end of the Wolffian duct from the urogenital sinus [11].
2. Abnormal muscular development of the terminal ureter resulting in ballooning of the distal ureter as a result of its muscular deficiency [53].
3. Abnormal widening of the mesonephric duct distal to the take-off the UB. This segment of the mesonephric duct (the common excretory duct) dilates after ureteral migration is complete and later undergoes apoptosis or absorption into the trigone. Proximal extension of this widening process could result in ureterocele formation [54].
4. Defective ureteral maturation affecting the UB detachment from the mesonephric duct. Abnormal UB origin from the mesonephric duct will result in abnormal interaction between the growing UB and MB and subsequently renal dysplasia that is commonly seen in association with duplex ureteroceles [27].

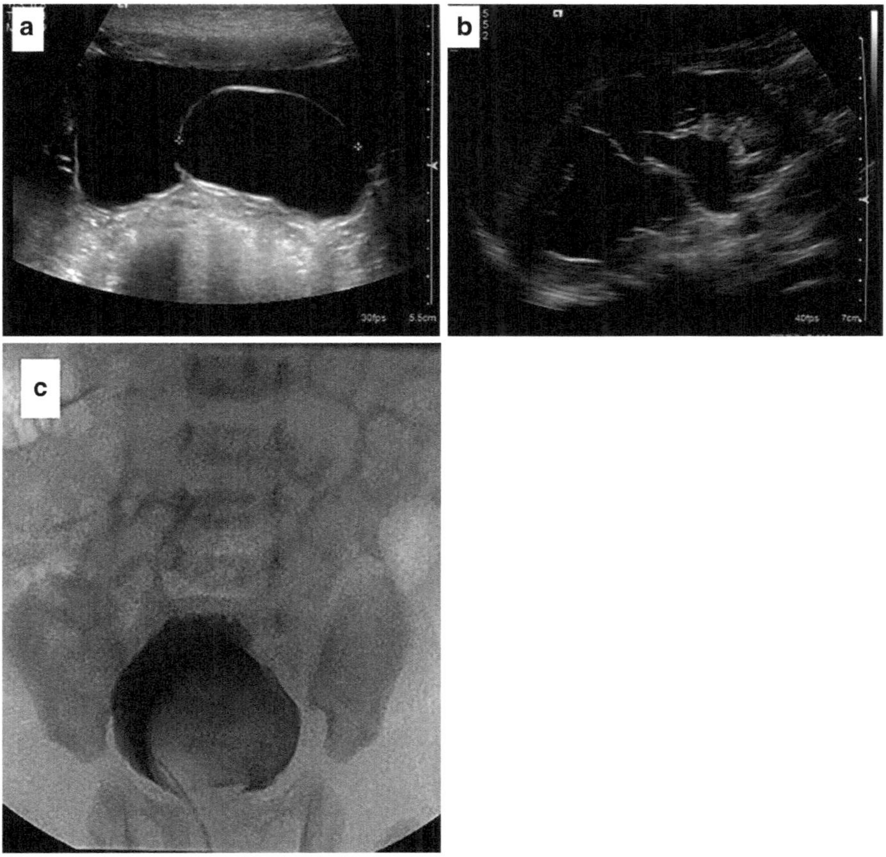

Fig. 17.9 Renal bladder ultrasound (**a**, **b**) and voiding cystourethrogram (**c**) images of a patient with left duplex system ureterocele and associated hydronephrosis of both upper and lower moieties

17.4.6 Vesicoureteral Reflux

Vesicoureteral reflux is retrograde flow of urine through the ureterovesical junction. Several passive and active mechanisms exist to prevent retrograde urine flow across the UVJ. Passive mechanisms include the obliquity of the intramural ureter course through the bladder wall, the length of the intramural ureter, adequate muscle backing and anchoring of the distal ureter to the bladder base to prevent lateral migration of the ureter and shortening of the intramural ureter with bladder filling [55, 56]. Although an anatomic vesicoureteral sphincter has not been identified, several studies have suggested that a "physiological sphincter" exists. Contraction of the longitudinal muscles of the UVJ during micturition provides the active component of anti-reflux mechanism by closing the meatus and submucosal tunnel [57].

Vesicoureteral reflux is thought to occur as a result of abnormal origin of the mesonephric duct at a point more caudal that normal. This allows longer time for migration of the ureteral orifice, resulting in a more lateral position than usual. The ureter will also have a shorter submucosal tunnel and an almost perpendicular course through the bladder wall. Patients with VUR have a smaller intramural tunnel length-to-width ratio compared to healthy controls [56]. Additionally, proper trigonal development is required to provide adequate muscular support to the ureters. The abnormal caudal takeoff of the UB from the mesonephric duct will result in a short common excretory duct, and subsequently poor trigonal development and poor muscular backing of the ureter. These anatomic changes will result in disruption of the passive component of the anti-reflux mechanism [58]. Also, the caudal origin of the UB and the shorter time for absorption of the common excretory duct into the bladder will give less time for the common mesenchyme to accumulate around the developing UB with deficient musculature of the intramural ureter and a patulous or gaping ureteral orifice. Histologic examination of the distal ureters in children with VUR has suggested that there may be dysplasia, atrophy and architectural derangement of the smooth muscle fibers of the distal ureters in children with VUR. Altered extracellular matrix deposition and deficient intramural ureter nerve supply are also additional histologic findings in patients with VUR [59, 60].

17.5 Imaging of the Ureter in Antenatal Life

The two modalities currently available to image the urinary tract during intrauterine life are ultrasound and MRI. Classic literature states that the fetal ureter is not normally visualized on antenatal ultrasound [61]. The cut-off for ureteral dilation depends on gestational age. Persistent visualization of the ureter on prenatal ultrasound is considered abnormal and warrants further evaluation. Megaureter is traditionally defined as ureteral diameter $\geq$ 7 mm in a fetus with gestational age of >30 weeks [40]. Hydroureter appears as a tortuous tubular structure communicating with the kidney, bladder or both. Observation of the bowel peristalsis can help to differentiate hydroureter from dilated bowel loops. Hydroureter is commonly found in association with renal pelvis and calyceal dilation. The presence of concomitant renal pelvis, calyceal or bladder dilation can help identify the underlying genitourinary anomaly.

With advances in the ultrasound technology, even normal non-dilated ureter can be visualized. In a study including 99 anatomically normal fetuses and 21 with isolated mild pyelectasis undergoing second trimester ultrasound, ureters were visualized in 62% of normal fetuses and 74% of the group with pyelectasis. Ureteral diameters ranged from 0.4 to 2.7 mm. More than half of the ureters were visualized at both the proximal and distal segments. Ureteral depiction is likely to reflect normal transient passage of urine associated with peristalsis and is not always a pathological finding [62].

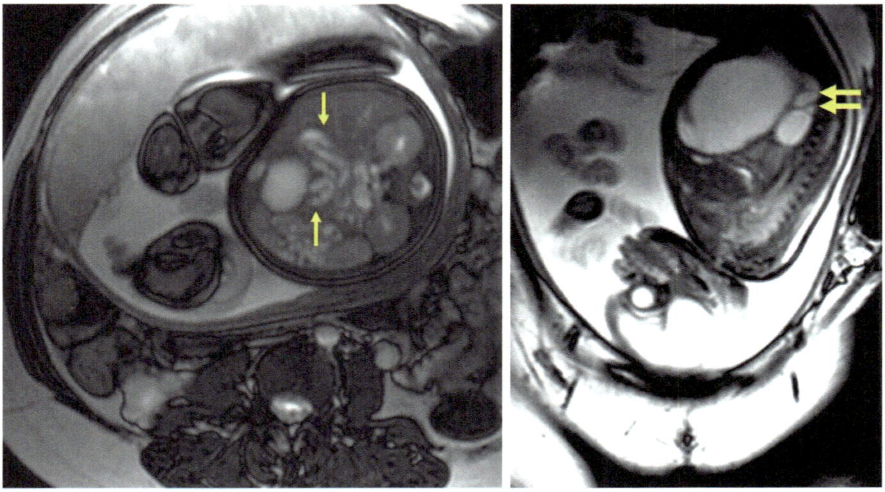

Fig. 17.10 Fetal MRI showing bilateral hydroureter (yellow arrows), hydronephrosis and megacystis in a male fetus suggestive of posterior urethral valve, courtesy of Dr. Zeinab A. Ramadan, MD from Mansoura University

Fetal ultrasound can be limited by maternal obesity, oligohydramnios, unfavorable fetal position and fetal movements [63]. In contrast, fetal MRI provides superior anatomic details with better visualization of the urinary tract anatomy without being affected by fetal position or amniotic fluid volume (Fig. 17.10) [64]. In a study by Pico et al., fetal MRI findings could accurately diagnose urinary tract anomalies in 97% of patients compared to 56% only with fetal ultrasound. Further, fetal MRI changed the perinatal care in 15% of patients included in that study [65]. In another study, fetal MRI diagnosed urinary tract anomalies with an overall diagnostic sensitivity of 96% versus 58% for fetal ultrasound and provided additional information in 37% of cases [66].

17.6 Fetal Hydroureter

Classic literature states that the normal fetal ureter should not visible. Ureteropelvic junction obstruction is characterized by varying degree of renal pelvis and calyceal dilation, but without associated hydroureter (Fig. 17.4). Fetal hydroureter is classically defined as ureteral diameter ≥7 mm in a fetus with gestational age of 30 weeks or more [40]. The differential diagnosis of hydroureter includes vesicoureteral reflux, megaureter, ectopic ureteral insertion, ureterocele, posterior urethral valve (PUV), urethral atresia and prune belly syndrome.

UPJO causes renal pelvic and calyceal dilation without associated hydroureter. UVJO causes hydroureter usually with associated hydronephrosis with a normal appearing bladder [67]. Fluctuation of the degree of the dilation of the ureter and renal pelvis could be suggestive of VUR. Bladder outlet obstruction should be suspected when there is bilateral hydroureter and hydronephrosis in the presence of a thick-walled, trabeculated and often non-cycling bladder (Figs. 17.5 and 17.10). Oligohydramnios can be seen in severe case of bladder outlet obstruction. The most common causes of bladder outlet obstruction are posterior urethral valves in males and urethral atresia in females [68]. It is crucial to establish the diagnosis of fetal bladder outlet obstruction since antenatal intervention, termination of pregnancy or induction of labor could be indicated in select cases, particularly in the presence of oligohydramnios. The classic triad of bilateral hydroureteronephrosis, megacystis and keyhole sign with or without oligohydramnios in a male fetus is suggestive of posterior urethral valve diagnosis. Antenatal ultrasound was reported to be 94% sensitive and 43% specific for diagnosing PUV. The low specificity of prenatal ultrasound in diagnosing PUV is explained by its limited ability in distinguishing PUV from other causes of fetal bladder outlet obstruction including urethral atresia and prune belly syndrome [69]. Fetal MRI can more reliably differentiate PUV from other causes of ANH in view of its superior anatomic details (Fig. 17.10) [65]. Other than causes of fetal bladder outlet obstruction, the differentiation between other etiologies of fetal hydroureter is less critical and is usually made on postnatal evaluation.

The long-term outcome of hydroureter depends on the underlying cause. The prognosis of primary megaureter is generally excellent. The majority of cases can be managed expectantly with spontaneous resolution occurring in almost three quarters of infants [70]. Infants with sever bladder outlet obstruction may suffer pulmonary hypoplasia, renal insufficiency or even perinatal mortality.

17.7 Conclusions

The ureter develops by budding from the mesonephric duct during the fourth week of gestation. The ureteric bud subsequently undergoes elongation, canalization and muscularization. Normal uretero-renal interaction is crucial for normal kidney development. Abnormal canalization or muscularization of the ureter results in a number of obstructive ureteral anomalies. Caudal or lateral ectopia results from abnormal take-off of the ureteral bud from the mesonephric duct and is usually associated with renal dysplasia. With advances in imaging technology, even normal ureters can be visualized on antenatal ultrasound in the majority of cases. Fetal MRI provides superior anatomic details and can more accurately diagnose congenital anomalies of the kidneys and urinary tract, compared to antenatal ultrasound. The prognosis of hydroureter depends on the underlying cause. Excellent outcome is expected in the majority of cases with primary megaureter, whereas patients with fetal bladder outlet obstruction may suffer renal insufficiency, pulmonary hypoplasia or even perinatal mortality.

Acknowledgement We acknowledge Dr. Heba Mahdi from Mansoura University for providing schematic illustrations for this chapter, Dr. Zeinab A. Ramadan and Dr. Amal Mehna for providing some of the figures included in the chapter.

Financial Disclosure The authors have no financial interests.

References

1. Grobstein C. Inductive epitheliomesenchymal interaction in cultured organ rudiments of the mouse. Science. 1953;118(3054):52–5. https://doi.org/10.1126/science.118.3054.52.
2. McGregor L, Makela V, Darling SM, Vrontou S, Chalepakis G, Roberts C, et al. Fraser syndrome and mouse blebbed phenotype caused by mutations in FRAS1/Fras1 encoding a putative extracellular matrix protein. Nat Genet. 2003;34(2):203–8. https://doi.org/10.1038/ng1142.
3. Pitera JE, Scambler PJ, Woolf AS. Fras1, a basement membrane-associated protein mutated in Fraser syndrome, mediates both the initiation of the mammalian kidney and the integrity of renal glomeruli. Hum Mol Genet. 2008;17(24):3953–64. https://doi.org/10.1093/hmg/ddn297.
4. Kiyozumi D, Osada A, Sugimoto N, Weber CN, Ono Y, Imai T, et al. Identification of a novel cell-adhesive protein spatiotemporally expressed in the basement membrane of mouse developing hair follicle. Exp Cell Res. 2005;306(1):9–23. https://doi.org/10.1016/j.yexcr.2005.01.020.
5. Woolf AS, Davies JA. Cell biology of ureter development. J Am Soc Nephrol. 2013;24(1):19–25. https://doi.org/10.1681/ASN.2012020127.
6. Muller U, Wang D, Denda S, Meneses JJ, Pedersen RA, Reichardt LF. Integrin alpha8beta1 is critically important for epithelial-mesenchymal interactions during kidney morphogenesis. Cell. 1997;88(5):603–13. https://doi.org/10.1016/s0092-8674(00)81903-0.
7. Hu P, Deng FM, Liang FX, Hu CM, Auerbach AB, Shapiro E, et al. Ablation of uroplakin III gene results in small urothelial plaques, urothelial leakage, and vesicoureteral reflux. J Cell Biol. 2000;151(5):961–72. https://doi.org/10.1083/jcb.151.5.961.
8. Kong XT, Deng FM, Hu P, Liang FX, Zhou G, Auerbach AB, et al. Roles of uroplakins in plaque formation, umbrella cell enlargement, and urinary tract diseases. J Cell Biol. 2004;167(6):1195–204. https://doi.org/10.1083/jcb.200406025.
9. Alcaraz A, Vinaixa F, Tejedo-Mateu A, Fores MM, Gotzens V, Mestres CA, et al. Obstruction and recanalization of the ureter during embryonic development. J Urol. 1991;145(2):410–6. https://doi.org/10.1016/s0022-5347(17)38354-4.
10. Ruano-Gil D, Coca-Payeras A, Tejedo-Mateu A. Obstruction and normal recanalization of the ureter in the human embryo. Its relation to congenital ureteric obstruction. Eur Urol. 1975;1(6):287–93.
11. Chwalle R. The process of formation of cystic dilatations of the vesical end of the ureter and of diverticula at the ureteral ostium. Urol Cutan Rev. 1927;31:499–504.
12. Yerkes E, Nishimura H, Miyazaki Y, Tsuchida S, Brock JW 3rd, Ichikawa I. Role of angiotensin in the congenital anomalies of the kidney and urinary tract in the mouse and the human. Kidney Int Suppl. 1998;67:S75–7. https://doi.org/10.1046/j.1523-1755.1998.06715.x.
13. Kakuchi J, Ichiki T, Kiyama S, Hogan BL, Fogo A, Inagami T, et al. Developmental expression of renal angiotensin II receptor genes in the mouse. Kidney Int. 1995;47(1):140–7. https://doi.org/10.1038/ki.1995.16.
14. Nishimura H, Yerkes E, Hohenfellner K, Miyazaki Y, Ma J, Hunley TE, et al. Role of the angiotensin type 2 receptor gene in congenital anomalies of the kidney and urinary tract, CAKUT, of mice and men. Mol Cell. 1999;3(1):1–10. https://doi.org/10.1016/s1097-2765(00)80169-0.
15. Yosypiv IV. A new role for the renin-angiotensin system in the development of the ureteric bud and renal collecting system. Keio J Med. 2008;57(4):184–9. https://doi.org/10.2302/kjm.57.184.

16. Schuchardt A, D'Agati V, Pachnis V, Costantini F. Renal agenesis and hypodysplasia in ret-k- mutant mice result from defects in ureteric bud development. Development. 1996;122(6):1919–29. https://doi.org/10.1242/dev.122.6.1919.
17. Shakya R, Watanabe T, Costantini F. The role of GDNF/Ret signaling in ureteric bud cell fate and branching morphogenesis. Dev Cell. 2005;8(1):65–74. https://doi.org/10.1016/j.devcel.2004.11.008.
18. Costantini F, Shakya R. GDNF/Ret signaling and the development of the kidney. BioEssays. 2006;28(2):117–27. https://doi.org/10.1002/bies.20357.
19. Sweeney D, Lindstrom N, Davies JA. Developmental plasticity and regenerative capacity in the renal ureteric bud/collecting duct system. Development. 2008;135(15):2505–10. https://doi.org/10.1242/dev.022145.
20. Baker LA, Gomez RA. Embryonic development of the ureter and bladder: acquisition of smooth muscle. J Urol. 1998;160(2):545–50.
21. Escala JM, Keating MA, Boyd G, Pierce A, Hutton JL, Lister J. Development of elastic fibres in the upper urinary tract. J Urol. 1989;141(4):969–73. https://doi.org/10.1016/s0022-5347(17)41080-9.
22. Chang CP, McDill BW, Neilson JR, Joist HE, Epstein JA, Crabtree GR, et al. Calcineurin is required in urinary tract mesenchyme for the development of the pyeloureteral peristaltic machinery. J Clin Invest. 2004;113(7):1051–8. https://doi.org/10.1172/JCI20049.
23. Miyazaki Y, Tsuchida S, Nishimura H, Pope JC, Harris RC, McKanna JM, et al. Angiotensin induces the urinary peristaltic machinery during the perinatal period. J Clin Invest. 1998;102(8):1489–97. https://doi.org/10.1172/JCI4401.
24. Canda AE, Turna B, Cinar GM, Nazli O. Physiology and pharmacology of the human ureter: basis for current and future treatments. Urol Int. 2007;78(4):289–98. https://doi.org/10.1159/000100830.
25. Tanaka ST, Ishii K, Demarco RT, Pope JC, Brock JW 3rd, Hayward SW. Endodermal origin of bladder trigone inferred from mesenchymal-epithelial interaction. J Urol. 2010;183(1):386–91. https://doi.org/10.1016/j.juro.2009.08.107.
26. Batourina E, Tsai S, Lambert S, Sprenkle P, Viana R, Dutta S, et al. Apoptosis induced by vitamin A signaling is crucial for connecting the ureters to the bladder. Nat Genet. 2005;37(10):1082–9. https://doi.org/10.1038/ng1645.
27. Mendelsohn C. Using mouse models to understand normal and abnormal urogenital tract development. Organogenesis. 2009;5(1):306–14. https://doi.org/10.4161/org.8173.
28. Louw JH, Barnard CN. Congenital intestinal atresia; observations on its origin. Lancet. 1955;269(6899):1065–7. https://doi.org/10.1016/s0140-6736(55)92852-x.
29. Rosenblum ND. Developmental biology of the human kidney. Semin Fetal Neonatal Med. 2008;13(3):125–32. https://doi.org/10.1016/j.siny.2007.10.005.
30. Mackie GG, Stephens FD. Duplex kidneys: a correlation of renal dysplasia with position of the ureteral orifice. J Urol. 1975;114(2):274–80. https://doi.org/10.1016/s0022-5347(17)67007-1.
31. Lund AJ. Uncrossed double ureter with rare intravesical orifice relationship; case report with review of literature. J Urol. 1949;62(1):22–9. https://doi.org/10.1016/s0022-5347(17)68880-3.
32. Meyer R. Normal and abnormal development of the ureter in the human embryo; a mechanistic consideration. Anat Rec. 1946;96(4):355–71. https://doi.org/10.1002/ar.1090960403.
33. Wahyudi I, Fahri M, Situmorang GR, Rodjani A. Bilateral ureteral triplication: a case report. Urol Case Rep. 2020;33:101406. https://doi.org/10.1016/j.eucr.2020.101406.
34. Shoda R, Ejiri S, Fujita T, Wada N. [A case of bilateral ureteral triplication]. Hinyokika Kiyo. 1985;31(3):475–81.
35. Kokabi N, Price N, Smith GH, Gibbons PJ, Holland AJ. Ureteral triplication: a rare anomaly with a variety of presentations. J Pediatr Urol. 2011;7(4):484–7. https://doi.org/10.1016/j.jpurol.2010.12.006.
36. Chia I, Grote D, Marcotte M, Batourina E, Mendelsohn C, Bouchard M. Nephric duct insertion is a crucial step in urinary tract maturation that is regulated by a Gata3-Raldh2-Ret molecular network in mice. Development. 2011;138(10):2089–97. https://doi.org/10.1242/dev.056838.

37. Yu J, Carroll TJ, McMahon AP. Sonic hedgehog regulates proliferation and differentiation of mesenchymal cells in the mouse metanephric kidney. Development. 2002;129(22):5301–12. https://doi.org/10.1242/dev.129.22.5301.
38. Nguyen HT, Benson CB, Bromley B, Campbell JB, Chow J, Coleman B, et al. Multidisciplinary consensus on the classification of prenatal and postnatal urinary tract dilation (UTD classification system). J Pediatr Urol. 2014;10(6):982–98. https://doi.org/10.1016/j.jpurol.2014.10.002.
39. Adorisio O, Silveri M, Colajacomo M, Bassani F, Rivosecchi M. The impact of perinatal urinoma formation on renal function: our experience and review of the literature. J Paediatr Child Health. 2011;47(4):217–22. https://doi.org/10.1111/j.1440-1754.2010.01927.x.
40. Farrugia MK, Hitchcock R, Radford A, Burki T, Robb A, Murphy F, et al. British Association of Paediatric Urologists consensus statement on the management of the primary obstructive megaureter. J Pediatr Urol. 2014;10(1):26–33. https://doi.org/10.1016/j.jpurol.2013.09.018.
41. Docimo SG, Lebowitz RL, Retik AB, Colodny AH, Bauer SB, Mandell J. Congenital midureteral obstruction. Urol Radiol. 1989;11(3):156–60. https://doi.org/10.1007/BF02926502.
42. Smith BG, Metwalli AR, Leach J, Cheng EY, Kropp BP. Congenital midureteral stricture in children diagnosed with antenatal hydronephrosis. Urology. 2004;64(5):1014–9. https://doi.org/10.1016/j.urology.2004.06.015.
43. Stephens FD, Smith ED, Hurson JM. Primary obstructed megaureter. In: Stephens FD, Smith ED, Hurson JM, editors. Congenital anomalies of the urinary and genital tracts. Oxford: Isis Medical Media; 2002. p. 212–21.
44. Hwang AH, McAleer IM, Shapiro E, Miller OF, Krous HF, Kaplan GW. Congenital mid ureteral strictures. J Urol. 2005;174(5):1999–2002. https://doi.org/10.1097/01.ju.0000176462.56473.0c.
45. Culp DA. Congenital anomalies of the ureter. In: Bergman H, editor. The ureter. New York: Springer; 1981. p. 625–47.
46. Thiel DD, Badger WJ, Winfield HN. Robot-assisted laparoscopic excision and ureteroureterostomy for congenital midureteral stricture. J Endourol. 2008;22(12):2667–9. https://doi.org/10.1089/end.2008.9692.
47. Rossi E, Salas JR, Aucatoma FC, Munoz MO, Fochs LM. Congenital ureteral valves: two new cases and a review of the literature. J Pediatr Urol. 2007;3(5):344–9. https://doi.org/10.1016/j.jpurol.2007.02.002.
48. Tartari F, Bezhani E, Rota T, Subashi S, Shehu M, Harito F, et al. Ureteral valves associated with ureteral stricture. Report of 4 cases. Eur Urol. 1998;33(4):412–3. https://doi.org/10.1159/000019627.
49. Cooper CS, Hawtrey CE. Fibroepithelial polyp of the ureter. Urology. 1997;50(2):280–1. https://doi.org/10.1016/S0090-4295(97)00221-5.
50. Adey GS, Vargas SO, Retik AB, Borer JG, Mandell J, Hendren WH, et al. Fibroepithelial polyps causing ureteropelvic junction obstruction in children. J Urol. 2003;169(5):1834–6. https://doi.org/10.1097/01.ju.0000061966.21966.94.
51. Kara C, Resorlu B, Oguz U, Unsal A. Incidentally detected ureteral fibroepithelial polyps in children: is endoscopic treatment of them really necessary? Int Urol Nephrol. 2010;42(1):1–5. https://doi.org/10.1007/s11255-009-9567-4.
52. Perimenis P, Gyftopoulos K, Athanasopoulos A, Pastromas V, Barbalias G. Retrocaval ureter and associated abnormalities. Int Urol Nephrol. 2002;33(1):19–22. https://doi.org/10.1023/a:1014436432109.
53. Tokunaka S, Gotoh T, Koyanagi T, Tsuji I. Morphological study of the ureterocele: a possible clue to its embryogenesis as evidenced by a locally arrested myogenesis. J Urol. 1981;126(6):726–9. https://doi.org/10.1016/s0022-5347(17)54721-7.
54. Tanagho EA. Embryologic basis for lower ureteral anomalies: a hypothesis. Urology. 1976;7(5):451–64. https://doi.org/10.1016/0090-4295(76)90179-5.
55. Noordzij JW, Dabhoiwala NF. A view on the anatomy of the ureterovesical junction. Scand J Urol Nephrol. 1993;27(3):371–80. https://doi.org/10.3109/00365599309180449.

56. Paquin AJ Jr. Ureterovesical anastomosis: the description and evaluation of a technique. J Urol. 1959;82:573–83. https://doi.org/10.1016/s0022-5347(17)65934-2.
57. Leung VY, Metreweli C, Yeung CK. The ureteric jet doppler waveform as an indicator of vesicoureteric sphincter function in adults and children. An observational study. Ultrasound Med Biol. 2002;28(7):865–72. https://doi.org/10.1016/s0301-5629(02)00537-9.
58. Stephens FD, Lenaghan D. The anatomical basis and dynamics of vesicoureteral reflux. J Urol. 1962;87:669–80. https://doi.org/10.1016/s0022-5347(17)65025-0.
59. Oswald J, Schwentner C, Brenner E, Deibl M, Fritsch H, Bartsch G, et al. Extracellular matrix degradation and reduced nerve supply in refluxing ureteral endings. J Urol. 2004;172(3):1099–102. https://doi.org/10.1097/01.ju.0000135673.28496.70.
60. Oswald J, Brenner E, Schwentner C, Deibl M, Bartsch G, Fritsch H, et al. The intravesical ureter in children with vesicoureteral reflux: a morphological and immunohistochemical characterization. J Urol. 2003;170(6 Pt 1):2423–7. https://doi.org/10.1097/01.ju.0000097146.26432.9a.
61. Feldman DM, DeCambre M, Kong E, Borgida A, Jamil M, McKenna P, et al. Evaluation and follow-up of fetal hydronephrosis. J Ultrasound Med. 2001;20(10):1065–9. https://doi.org/10.7863/jum.2001.20.10.1065.
62. Gokmen Karasu AF, Yuksel A, Kutuk MS, Keskin IG. Sonographic depiction of fetal ureters. J Mater Fetal Neonatal Med. 2016;29(14):2378–81. https://doi.org/10.3109/14767058.2015.1086330.
63. Robyr R, Benachi A, Daikha-Dahmane F, Martinovich J, Dumez Y, Ville Y. Correlation between ultrasound and anatomical findings in fetuses with lower urinary tract obstruction in the first half of pregnancy. Ultrasound Obstet Gynecol. 2005;25(5):478–82. https://doi.org/10.1002/uog.1878.
64. Abdelhalim A, Hafez AT. Antenatal and postnatal management of posterior urethral valves: where do we stand? Afr J Urol. 2021;27(1):140. https://doi.org/10.1186/s12301-021-00238-7.
65. Pico H, Dabadie A, Bourliere-Najean B, Philip N, Capelle M, Aschero A, et al. Contribution of the foetal uro-MRI in the prenatal diagnosis of uronephropathies. Diagn Interv Imaging. 2014;95(6):573–8. https://doi.org/10.1016/j.diii.2014.02.011.
66. Kajbafzadeh AM, Payabvash S, Sadeghi Z, Elmi A, Jamal A, Hantoshzadeh Z, et al. Comparison of magnetic resonance urography with ultrasound studies in detection of fetal urogenital anomalies. J Pediatr Urol. 2008;4(1):32–9. https://doi.org/10.1016/j.jpurol.2007.07.005.
67. Becker A, Baum M. Obstructive uropathy. Early Hum Dev. 2006;82(1):15–22. https://doi.org/10.1016/j.earlhumdev.2005.11.002.
68. Farrugia MK. Fetal bladder outlet obstruction: embryopathology, in utero intervention and outcome. J Pediatr Urol. 2016;12(5):296–303. https://doi.org/10.1016/j.jpurol.2016.05.047.
69. Bernardes LS, Aksnes G, Saada J, Masse V, Elie C, Dumez Y, et al. Keyhole sign: how specific is it for the diagnosis of posterior urethral valves? Ultrasound Obstet Gynecol. 2009;34(4):419–23. https://doi.org/10.1002/uog.6413.
70. Gimpel C, Masioniene L, Djakovic N, Schenk JP, Haberkorn U, Tonshoff B, et al. Complications and long-term outcome of primary obstructive megaureter in childhood. Pediatr Nephrol. 2010;25(9):1679–86. https://doi.org/10.1007/s00467-010-1523-0.

Chapter 18
Ureteral Pain

Yasin Yitgin and Kemal Sarica

Abstract Visceral pain is usually a vague and discomfort such as deep, squeezing, or colicky. Visceral pain comes from deep organs of the thorax, abdomen, or pelvis, is not as well localized as somatic pain.

Ureteral pain, which is a visceral pain, is a common problem and ureteric colic is one of the most intense pain conditions in clinic admissions. Pain relief is difficult and often leads to medical attention. Mechanoreceptors stimulated by pressure increase and chemoreceptors activated by ischemia or inflammation are the sensory receptors involved in the formation of this pain. Imaging methods play an important role to arrive at a correct diagnosis, and opiates, non-steroidal anti-inflammatory drugs, alpha-adrenergic blockers, calcium channel blockers and glucocorticoids are the approaches used to relieve ureteral pain.

Keywords Ureteral pain · Ureteral colic · Visseral pain · Somatic pain · Prostanoids · Nsaids · Corticosteroids · Calcium channel blockers · Alpha-adrenergic blockers

Learning Objectives

The learning objectives for this chapter are

- To describe the pathophysiology and clinical presentations of ureteral pain, and
- To describe the treatment of ureteral pain.

Test your learning and check your understanding of this book's contents: use the "Springer Nature Flashcards" app to access questions. To use the app, please follow the instructions in Chapter 1.

Y. Yitgin (✉)
Department of Urology, Istinye Universtiy Faculty of Medicine, Istanbul, Turkey

K. Sarica
Department of Urology, Biruni University, Medical School, Istanbul, Turkey
e-mail: kemalsarica@superonline.com

M. Abdel-Gawad et al. (eds.), *The Ureter*,
https://doi.org/10.1007/978-3-031-36212-5_18

18.1 Ureteral Pain

Pain can be divided into visceral and somatic pain according to origin. Visceral pain is complex and is one of the most common reasons for hospital admissions. Visceral pain is not related to injury. Cutting and injury of the ureter or kidney parenchyma are not sensitive to pain. There must be effective visceral stimuli such as distension, ischemia, and inflammation for pain response. Also, motor and autonomic reflexes accompany pain such as ureteral colic with nausea and vomiting, due to the fact that visceral afferents travel together with afferents of the autonomic nervous system [1–4].

The pain system consists of three order of neuron fibers. The first order neuron is afferent peripheral fibers and transmits the pain impulse to the second order neuron in the spinal dorsal horn. This neuron transmits information to the brain (third order neuron), where it is distributed to the supraspinal centers for processing. There is also a control system descending from the brain that modulates signals to the spinal cord [5, 6].

Ureteral visceral afferent fibers are unmyelinated C-fibers. These fibers have free nerve endings called nociceptors. These nociceptors respond to mechanical, thermal and chemical stimuli. The cell bodies of visceral afferent neurons are found in the dorsal root ganglia and typically terminate in the superficial laminae of the spinal dorsal horn. The afferent fibers travel in the spinothalamic tract to reach the thalamus and cortex. In addition, the spinothalamic and spinoreticular pathways have been shown to be two indirect pathways of pain transmission between the kidney and brainstem. These pathways have been reported to respond to cutaneous or muscle stimuli in addition to renal stimuli [7–10].

Renal pelvic pressure, normally between 0 and 10 mmHg, is under the control of α- and β-adrenoceptors in the smooth muscle cells of the renal pelvis and ureter. As it is known, while a-adrenergic agent promotes contraction, b-adrenergic agents cause relaxation of ureter and pelvis. The increase in renal pelvic pressure and tension in the wall cause pain, and as a result the renal afferent nerves transmit the signal to the spinal cord. Animal studies have shown that the ventrolateral medulla is affected after the activation of renal mechanics and chemoreceptors such as ureteric occlusions [11]. Also, the stimulation of cardiovascular reflexes after renal and ureteric mechanical stimuli is explained by these pathways [8–10].

Sensory receptors in the kidney are classified in two ways. The first are mechanoreceptors activated by increased renal pressure and the second are chemoreceptors activated by renal ischemia or changes in the chemical environment/inflammation. While chemoreceptors are thought to be present near the renal pelvic wall and throughout the renal vascular system, animal studies have shown that mechanoreceptors are additionally located in the renal parenchyma and ureter. Ureteral pain is a visceral pain that occurs in obstruction, inflammation, infectious disease and other visceral ailments and has a place in the diagnosis of the disease. Visceral pain differs from surface pain in that highly localized types of damage to internal organs rarely cause severe pain. On the other hand, any stimulus that causes widespread stimulation of pain nerve endings along the ureter can cause severe pain [12, 13].

The autonomic nerve supply of the proximal segment of the ureter is from the lower thoracic and lumbar plexus, and the distal and pelvic segment is from the sacral plexus. Preganglionic sympathetic fibers supply the ureter from the tenth thoracic to the second lumbar spinal segments. The postganglionic fibers originate from several ganglia located in the aorticorenal, superior, and inferior hypogastric (pelvic) autonomic plexuses. It is thought that the ureteric peristalsis is largely independent of its innervation and that a downward wave initiated in the collecting system is responsible for pushing the urine towards the bladder. An obstructive and inflammatory process can block this peristaltic activity and caused be pain [14–17]. Pain fibers leading to the ureter originate predominantly from the L1 and L2 segments. Nerve fibers are abundant in the distal ureteric segment and sparse in the proximal ureteric segment. The pain signals travel with sympathetic fibers and pain is felt in the segmental distribution of the ureter. Also, the pain is felt segmentally distributed of the subcostal, iliohypogastric, ilioinguinal, or genitofemoral nerve fibers [7, 18, 19].

The pain occurs with two possible mechanisms by the spasm of ureter. Firstly, it is the mechanical stimulation of pain nerve endings. Secondly, there are an increased metabolic need of the smooth muscle cells and decreased blood flow at the muscle. Also, formed in the tissue as a result of ischemia, acidic metabolic end products, tissue-degenerative products such as bradykinin, proteolytic enzymes cause ureteral pain by stimulating pain nerve endings. The cramping type pain seen in ureteral obstruction is due to periods of smooth muscle contraction. It is a cyclical continuation of this condition few minutes after a high degree of exacerbation of the pain and then reduction [20, 21].

18.2 A. Ureteral Colic

Ureteric colic, which is severe and sudden pain, is a condition frequently encountered in daily medical practice. The pain of ureteric colic resulted from acute upper urinary tract obstruction leading to distension and an increase of tension in the walls of the ureter and renal pelvis. The most common cause is the presence of stone in the collecting system. It may also be caused by urinary tract infection and urological neoplasm, or created by extrinsic compression such as retroperitoneal fibrosis, gynecological and enteric neoplasms. The patients are restless and try to find a position that will relieve their pain [22, 23]. In studies conducted to show the relationship of ureteral colic pain with the upper urinary tract, intra-pelvic pressure was measured by nephrostomy and noted that severe flank pain in patients with ureteric colic was associated with highly elevated pelvic pressures at the same time. In another study, it was observed that the rate of contrast instillation was a critical determinant during radiological examination with a nephrostomy tube in precipitating pain. Rapid infusion has been shown to cause pain, while a larger volume infused slowly has been shown to result in only mild awareness [24, 25].

18.3 Incidence

The prevalence of ureteral colic varies according to geographical distribution and has been reported between 5% and 15%. It is more common in the male population and there are recurrence rates of up to 50%. In a study conducted by Pearle et al., it has been reported that ureteral colic affects approximately 1.2 million people in the USA every year and constitutes approximately 1% of all hospital admissions [26]. It has been shown that urinary stone disease, which is the most common cause of ureteral colic, affects approximately 5–15% of the population in North America and Europe. Annual incidence is 0.5%, and lifetime incidence is 2–5%. The highest incidence in men is around 30 years old, while there are two peak incidence ages in women: 35 years and 55 years. Approximately 1–2% of the affected population in Western countries are children [27].

18.4 Pathophysiology

Colic pain is believed to be the result of an increase in upper urinary tract pressure causing pelvic wall tension. It occurs especially in conditions that cause acute ureteral obstruction such as ureteral stones. However, obstruction due to a stone less than the diameter of the ureter is thought to be the result of ureteral muscle spasm or mucosal edema [28, 29].

Some biochemical events occur as a result of an increase in renal pelvic pressure by ureteral obstruction. Phosphorylation of the N-methyl-Daspartate (NMDA) receptor resulting in influx of Ca^{2+} into the cell induces local mechanisms such as increased membrane excitability and formation of nitric oxide and prostanoids. Stimulation of local synthesis of prostanoids causes vasodilation. Also, prostanoids effect directly on the ureter to induce smooth muscle spasm. Subsequently, induction of diuresis further increases intrarenal pressure. As a result, ureteral colic ensures which causes acute, severe and unbearable pain. On the other hand, the result of an increase in upper tract pressure causing pelvic wall tension may occur nausea and vomiting, because of the common splanchnic innervation of the renal capsule and intestines [29, 30].

18.5 Location

The pain caused by renal capsule tension, which occurs with ureteral muscle spasm and increased renal pelvis pressure, starts from the hypochondrium and is felt in the lower anterior abdominal quadrant along the ureter. It may cause pain that is reflected to the testis and scrotum in male patients and to the vulva in female patients on the related side. Mid-ureteral pain typically produces pain on the lower quadrant and labia or testis. As a result, it can be confused with pain in diverticulitis, appendicitis or testicular disease. Likewise, lower ureteral obstruction can often cause symptoms of bladder irritability and suprapubic pain, which may radiate along the urethra and even the medial thigh [31, 32].

18.6 Diagnosis

The physical examination typically shows a patient writhing in distress and trying to find a comfortable position by leaning over the side area. Unlike acute abdomen with peritoneal irritation, the patient does not try to stay still to suppress the pain. The patient may have tenderness in the costovertebral angle or lower abdominal quadrant. If the patient has obstruction of the lower ureter, often experience symptoms of bladder irritability such as frequency or urgency. Some patients may also mention hematuria. In addition, signs of infection such as fever, weakness, nausea and vomiting may also be seen [33, 34]. After a routine history and clinical examination, the patient with suspected ureteral colic is required to perform laboratory workup such as urinalysis, complete blood count (CBC), creatinine, electrolytes and c-reactive protein (CRP), as well as radiological examinations such as plain radiograph of the kidney-ureter-bladder (KUB), ultrasound, intravenous urography or computed tomography. Pregnancy testing is recommended for all premenopausal women. Urinalysis demonstrating microscopic hematuria for urinary stone disease has a sensitivity 68.5–92.9% and specificity of 27.3–47.9% [35, 36].

A plain KUB is helpful in identifying radiopaque stones. KUB has sensitivity 29.4–59.0% and specificity of 70.8–77.0%. Its sensitivity varies depending on stone composition, location, size, and patient body habitus. Its accuracy is limited by false positive results such as pelvic phleboliths and intraabdominal calcifications [37].

Intravenous urography (IVU) begins with an intravenous injection of iodine-based contrast after straight KUB for the diagnosis of kidney and ureteral stones. It is usually completed with serial radiographs at 20 min and post-micturition. Before performing this imaging method, an allergic state to the contrast agent and renal failure should be excluded. In addition to contrast nephrotoxicity, it may lead to a 5–10% risk of allergic reaction and an anaphylactic reaction with a risk of 1/100,000 [38].

Ultrasonography (US) is an alternative imaging modality without disadvantage such as radiation and invasiveness in the ureteral colic. Advantages such as low cost and reproducibility have made it a widely used imaging modality. It has reported sensitivity 70.0–76.5% and specificity of 94.4–100% [39]. The sensitivity and specificity of US vary according to stone location. While the detection of stones located in the renal pelvis, renal calyx, ureteropelvic junction and ureterovesical junction is easier, ureteral stone detection is more challenging. Particularly, the diagnosis of middle ureteral stones is difficult as overshadowed of intestinal gas [40]. Ultrasonography also provides useful information about findings such as hydronephrosis, ureteral dilatation, and lack of ureteral jet flow due to obstruction. It has been mentioned that the chance of detecting ureteral stones can be increased with the combination of KUB and Doppler US. The twinkling sign, a sonographic artifact behind the stone detected using Doppler US, increases the detection rate of ureteral stones [41, 42]. US is used as the primary imaging modality in children and pregnant patients due to the lack of radiation exposure and contrast administration. In addition, it is the most commonly recommended imaging method evaluate the relief of obstruction and to follow-up of patients [40].

In recent years, computed tomography (CT) has been shown to be more sensitive and specific than IVU and US in detecting ureteral stones. Its sensitivity and specificity for detection of lithiasis ranges between 92% and 99% [42]. It is superior in detecting radiodense and radiolucent stones, as well as evaluating hydronephrosis, parenchymal tissue, perinephric and periureteric areas. It is also safe to perform in patients for whom the use of contrast agents is contraindicated. On the other hand, it has the disadvantage of a twofold increase in radiation compared to conventional IVU. A 2.5 mSv versus 4.7 mSv of radiation dose delivered with IVU and CT is reported in ureteral colic, respectively [34].

18.7 Treatment

The pain is often accompanied by nausea, vomiting, sweating, and changes in heart rate and blood pressure. This is due to the anatomical location of the autonomic nervous system and it is explained by the interaction between the visceral nerves [1]. The general approach is intravenous fluids, analgesia, and antiemetics. Acute pain management is the main expectation of patients suffering from severe and unbearable pain due to ureteral colic. Meta-analyses showed that non-steroidal anti-inflammatory drugs (NSAIDs) are more effective in relieving pain, causing less side effects, and are beneficial in stone removal by reducing ureteral inflammation. Due to the side effects of opiates such as nausea and vomiting, they are recommended to be used with caution. Particularly, pethidine, which causes more nausea, vomiting and dizziness, is advised to be avoided. Opiates can be used as an alternative to NSAIDs in patients with chronic renal failure and history of peptic ulcers [43]. In such cases, hydromorphine, pentazocine or tramadol are considered as second choice analgesics. It has also been mentioned that ketorolac and morphine combination therapy may be more effective than NSAIDs and opiates alone [44].

NSAIDs provide analgesia by acting directly on prostaglandin release, which is the main cause of pain. Although it has side effects such as kidney failure and gastrointestinal bleeding, there is no addiction risk like opiates. Previous studies have shown that opiates do not cause changes in ureteral tone. Moreover, opioids do not directly act on the cause of pain. NSAIDs suppress local edema and inflammation. They also reduce ureteral peristalsis and pressure by inhibiting the stimulation of ureteral smooth muscle. In addition to reducing pain of ureteral colic, NSAIDs can induce renal failure with pre-existing kidney disease by reducing renal blood flow.

NSAIDs have been reported to be more effective when administered intravenously. Also, it has been reported that there are significantly fewer episodes of colic compared to patients not treated with NSAIDs [45, 46]. Some side effect of NSAIDs has been also reported. These are myocardial infarction (MI), and therefore, the use of NSAIDs in patients with cardiovascular disease has been considered as a relative contraindication. A dose-related increase in cardiovascular events associated with the use of cyclooxygenase-2 (COX-2) inhibitors and diclofenac has also been reported in healthy individuals [47, 48].

Alternative analgesics have been studied and paracetamol (acetaminophen) has been compared with NSAIDs and opioids for efficacy and safety in the treatment of renal colic. It has been reported that there is no difference in treatment effect and treatment-related adverse events between NSAIDs and paracetamol. However, it has been reported that patients treated with NSAIDs needed less rescue analgesia compared to those treated with paracetamol. Additionally, some studies have concluded that paracetamol provides equal or better analgesia and has a better side-effect profile than opioids in the treatment of ureteral colic [49].

In the literature, it has been stated that there is no benefit of high-volume fluid therapy or diuretics to increase renal output and facilitate stone passage and elimination for patients with acute ureteral colic [27].

Medical expulsive therapy protocols have been developed to prevent the muscle spasm, local edema, inflammation and infection and to provide spontaneous stone removal. This protocols include corticosteroids to suppress inflammation and local edema, antibiotics to prevent or treat infection, calcium channel blockers and alpha-adrenergic blockers for ureteral spasm. Despite the probability of passing the stone varies according to the size and location of the stone, the spontaneous passage of ureteral stones smaller than 4 mm has been indicated approximately 50–95% as long as 40 days. Previous studies have shown that 50% of ureteral stones larger than 5 mm may require intervention [50].

COX enzymes induced by mucosal injury and stretching of the urinary tract affect ureteric contractility by increasing the release of prostanoids (prostaglandins and thromboxanes). NSAIDs are thought to be effective both in reducing colic pain and in facilitating stone passage by inhibiting COX enzymes. However, no increase in stone passage rates could be demonstrated in RCT [51, 52].

Studies have shown that the use of tamsulosin and nifedipine is not effective in reducing pain or hastened time to stone passage [22]. Also, it has been suggested that alpha-adrenergic blockers can be given together with analgesics to reduce recurrent renal colic attacks in patients with ureteral stones [53]. Alpha-adrenergic blockers and calcium channel blockers have been shown to reduce analgesic requirements for ureteral stones <10 mm and equally increase stone expulsion rates. However, due to the frequency of side effects of calcium channel blockers such as hypotension, palpitations and headache, alpha-adrenergic blockers are recommended for ureteral stones <10 mm [54, 55]. In a study comparing tamsulosin and nifedipine treatment, tamsulosin was found to be more effective in relieving renal colic pain and facilitating stone expulsion, and side effects were reported more in the nifedipine group [56].

On the other hand, corticosteroids have been tried in medical expulsive therapy. They can promote stone passage by reducing ureteral edema and inflammation with their anti-inflammatory effect. However, use of corticosteroids have been limited due to the inability to show its effect in stone passage and concerns about side effects and dosing [57, 58].

Questions

1. What are the differences between visceral pain and somatic pain?
   (a) Origin
   (b) Localized
   (c) autonomic reflexes accompany
   (d) underlying mechanism
   (e) *All of them*
2. Which plexuses provide the autonomic nerve supply of the ureter?
   (a) ninth thoracic and tenth thoracic
   (b) 10th and 11th thoracic
   (c) 12th thoracic
   (d) first and second lumbar
   (e) *B and D*
3. In which part of the kidney are chemoreceptors concentrated?
   (a) Gerota's fascia
   (b) Renal capsule
   (c) Renal pelvic wall
   (d) Renal vascular system
   (e) *C and D*
4. What is the prevalence of the ureteral colic?
   (a) 15–20%
   (b) 20–25%
   (c) 1–5%
   (d) 25–30%.
   (e) *5–15%*
5. In which segment is the possible ureteral obstruction in a patient who presents urgently with symptoms of bladder irritability and suprapubic pain in addition to ureteric colic?
   (a) Renal pelvis
   (b) Proximal ureter

(c) Mid ureter
(d) B and C
(e) *Distal ureter*

Competing Interests None

References

Ureteral Pain

1. Pedersen KV, Drewes AM, Frimodt-Møller PC, Osther PJ. Visceral pain originating from the upper urinary tract. Urol Res. 2010;38(5):345–55.
2. Cervero F, Laird JM. Visceral pain. Lancet. 1999;353(9170):2145–8.
3. Drewes AM. Visceral smerte. In: Jensen TS, Dahl JB, Arendt-Nielsen L, editors. Smerter–en lærebog. Copenhagen: Fadl's Forlag A/s; 2003. p. 153–69.
4. Arendt-Nielsen L, Laursen RJ, Drewes AM. Referred pain as an indicator for neural plasticity. Prog Brain Res. 2000;129:343–56.
5. Chernigovskii VN, Musiashichikova SS. Representation of afferent visceral systems in cerebral cortex in the cat. J Neurophysiol. 1966;29(3):565–82.
6. Ohara S, Lenz FA. Medial lateral extent of thermal and pain sensations evoked by microstimulation in somatic sensory nuclei of human thalamus. J Neurophysiol. 2003;90(4):2367–77.
7. Gebhart GF, Bielefeldt K. Physiology of visceral pain. Compr Physiol. 2016;6(4):1609–33.
8. Ammons WS. Primate spinothalamic cell responses to ureteral occlusion. Brain Res. 1989;496(1–2):124–30.
9. Ammons WS. Responses of spinoreticular cells to graded increases in renal venous pressure. Am J Phys. 1991;260(1 Pt 2):R27–31.
10. Ammons WS. Bowditch lecture. Renal afferent inputs to ascending spinal pathways. Am J Phys. 1992;262(2 Pt 2):R165–76.
11. Vizzard MA, Standish A, Ammons WS. Effects of renal receptor stimulation on neurons within the ventrolateral medulla of the cat. Am J Phys. 1993;265(2 Pt 2):R290–301.
12. Standish A, Vizzard MA, Ammons WS. Tonic descending modulation of spinal neuronal responses to activation of renal receptors. Am J Phys. 1993;265(6 Pt 2):R1291–303.
13. Sengupta JN, Gebhart GF. Mechanosensitive afferent fibers in the gastrointestinal and lower urinary tract. In: Gebhart GF, editor. Visceral pain. Progress in pain research and management; 1995. p. 75–98.
14. Soriano RM, Penfold D, Leslie SW. Anatomy. Kidneys: Abdomen and Pelvis; 2021.
15. Di Benedetto A, Arena S, Nicotina PA, Mucciardi G, Galì A, Magno C. Pacemakers in the upper urinary tract. Neurourol Urodyn. 2013;32(4):349–53.
16. Kuntz A. The autonomic nervous system. Philadelphia: Lea & Febiger; 1953.
17. Terry GC, Chopp TM. Functional anatomy of the shoulder. J Athl Train. 2000;35(3):248–55.
18. Mitchell GA. The innervation of the kidney, ureter, testicle and epididymis. J Anat. 1935;70(Pt 1):10–32. 15
19. Lescay HA, Jiang J, Tuma F. Anatomy, abdomen and pelvis, ureter. In: StatPearls [internet]. Treasure Island (FL): StatPearls; 2021.
20. Patti L, Leslie SW. Acute Renal Colic. In: StatPearls [internet]. Treasure Island (FL): StatPearls Publishing; 2021. p. 2021.
21. Zwergel U, Zwergel T, Ziegler M. Effects of prostaglandins and prostaglandin synthetase inhibitors on acutely obstructed kidneys in the dog. Urol Int. 1991;47(2):64–9.

A. Ureteral Colic

22. Pickard R, Starr K, MacLennan G, Lam T, Thomas R, Burr J, McPherson G, McDonald A, Anson K, N'Dow J, Burgess N, Clark T, Kilonzo M, Gillies K, Shearer K, Boachie C, Cameron S, Norrie J, McClinton S. Medical expulsive therapy in adults with ureteric colic: a multicentre, randomised, placebo-controlled trial. Lancet. 2015;386(9991):341–9.
23. Kiil F. The function of the ureter and renal pelvis. Philadelphia: WB Saunders Co.; 1957.
24. Bretland PM. Acute ureteric obstruction-clinical and radiological aspects. Proc R Soc Med. 1974;67(12 Pt 1):1215–7.
25. Michaelson G. Percutaneous puncture of the renal pelvis, intrapelvic pressure and the concentrating capacity of the kidney in hydronephrosis. Acta Med Scand. 1974;559:1.

Incidence

26. Pearle MS, Calhoun EA, Curhan GC. Urologic diseases in America project: urolithiasis. J Urol. 2005;173:848–57.
27. Worster AS, Bhanich SW. Fluids and diuretics for acute ureteric colic. Cochrane Database Syst Rev. 2012;2:CD004926.

Pathophysiology

28. Struthers NW, Constantinou CE. Ureteric physiology. Curr Opin Urol. 1992;2:310–3.
29. Travaglini F, Bartoletti R, Gacci M, Rizzo M. Pathophysiology of Reno-ureteral colic. Urol Int. 2004;72(suppl 1):20–3.
30. Shokeir AA. Renal colic: pathophysiology, diagnosis and treatment. Eur Urol. 2001;39:241–9.

Location

31. DeWolf WC, Fraley EE. Renal pain. Urology. 1975;6(4):403–8.
32. McAninch JW. Chapter 3. Symptoms of disorders of the genitourinary tract. In: JW MA, Lue TF, editors. Smith and Tanagho's general urology. 18th ed. McGraw Hill; 2013. Accessed 30 Oct 2021.

Diagnosis

33. Masarani M, Dinneen M. Ureteric colic: new trends in diagnosis and treatment. Postgrad Med J. 2007;83(981):469–72.
34. Denton ER, Mackenzie A, Greenwell T, Popert R, Rankin SC. Unenhanced helical CT for renal colic is the radiation dose justifiable? Clin Radiol. 1999;54(7):444–7.
35. Ripollés T, Errando J, Agramunt M, Martínez MJ. Ureteral colic: US versus CT. Abdom Imaging. 2004;29(2):263–6.
36. Argyropoulos A, Farmakis A, Doumas K, Lykourinas M. The presence of microscopic hematuria detected by urine dipstick test in the evaluations of patients with renal colic. Urol Res. 2004;32:294–7.
37. Jung SI, Kim YJ, Park HS, Jeon HJ, Park HK, Paick SH, Kim HG, Lho YS. Sensitivity of digital abdominal radiography for the detection of ureter stones by stone size and location. J Comput Assist Tomogr. 2010;34(6):879–82.

38. Fulgham PF, Assimos DG, Pearle MS, Preminger GM. Clinical effectiveness protocols for imaging in the management of ureteral calculous disease: AUA technology assessment. J Urol. 2013;189(4):1203–13.
39. Wong C, Teitge B, Ross M, Young P, Robertson HL, Lang E. The accuracy and prognostic value of point-of-care ultrasound for nephrolithiasis in the emergency department: a systematic review and meta-analysis. Acad Emerg Med. 2018;25(6):684–98.
40. Skolarikos A, Straub M, Knoll T, Sarica K, Seitz C, Petřík A, Türk C. Metabolic evaluation and recurrence prevention for urinary stone patients: EAU guidelines. Eur Urol. 2015;67(4):750–63.
41. Yilmaz S, Sindel T, Arslan G, Ozkaynak C, Karaali K, Kabaalioğlu A, Lüleci E. Renal colic:comparison of spiral CT, US and IVU in the detection of ureteral calculi. Eur Radiol. 1998;8(2):212–7.
42. Ripollés T, Martínez-Pérez MJ, Vizuete J, Miralles S, Delgado F, Pastor-Navarro T. Sonographic diagnosis of symptomatic ureteral calculi: usefulness of the twinkling artifact. Abdom Imaging. 2013;38(4):863–9.

Treatment

43. Afshar K, Jafari S, Marks AJ, Eftekhari A, MacNeily AE. Nonsteroidal anti-inflammatory drugs (NSAIDs) and non-opioids for acute renal colic. Cochrane Database Syst Rev. 2015;6:CD006027.
44. Safdar B, Degutis LC, Landry K, Vedere SR, Moscovitz HC, D'Onofrio G. Intravenous morphine plus ketorolac is superior to either drug alone for treatment of acute renal colic. Ann Emerg Med. 2006;48(2):173–81.
45. Tramèr MR, Williams JE, Carroll D, Wiffen PJ, Moore RA, McQuay HJ. Comparing analgesic efficacy of non-steroidal anti-inflammatory drugs given by different routes in acute and chronic pain: a qualitative systematic review. Acta Anaesthesiol Scand. 1998;42(1):71–9.
46. Laerum E, Ommundsen OE, Grønseth JE, Christiansen A, Fagertun HE. Oral diclofenac in the prophylactic treatment of recurrent renal colic. A double-blind comparison with placebo. Eur Urol. 1995;28(2):108–11.
47. Schjerning Olsen AM, Fosbøl EL, Lindhardsen J, Folke F, Charlot M, Selmer C, Lamberts M, Bjerring Olesen J, Køber L, Hansen PR, Torp-Pedersen C, Gislason GH. Duration of treatment with nonsteroidal anti-inflammatory drugs and impact on risk of death and recurrent myocardial infarction in patients with prior myocardial infarction: a nationwide cohort study. Circulation. 2011;123(20):2226–35.
48. Fosbøl EL, Gislason GH, Jacobsen S, Folke F, Hansen ML, Schramm TK, Sørensen R, Rasmussen JN, Andersen SS, Abildstrom SZ, Traerup J, Poulsen HE, Rasmussen S, Køber L, Torp-Pedersen C. Risk of myocardial infarction and death associated with the use of nonsteroidal anti-inflammatory drugs (NSAIDs) among healthy individuals: a nationwide cohort study. Clin Pharmacol Ther. 2009;85(2):190–7.
49. Pathan SA, Mitra B, Cameron PA. A systematic review and meta-analysis comparing the efficacy of nonsteroidal anti-inflammatory drugs, opioids, and paracetamol in the treatment of acute renal colic. Eur Urol. 2018;73(4):583–95.
50. Miller OF, Kane CJ. Time to stone passage for observed ureteral calculi: a guide for patient education. J Urol. 1999;162(3 Pt 1):688–90.
51. Mastrangelo D, Wisard M, Rohner S, Leisinger H, Iselin CE. Diclofenac and NS-398, a selective cyclooxygenase-2 inhibitor, decrease agonist-induced contractions of the pig isolated ureter. Urol Res. 2000;28(6):376–82.
52. Phillips E, Hinck B, Pedro R, Makhlouf A, Kriedberg C, Hendlin K, et al. Celecoxib in the management of acute renal colic: a randomized controlled clinical trial. Urology. 2009;74(5):994–9.
53. Dellabella M, Milanese G, Muzzonigro G. Randomized trial of the efficacy of tamsulosin, nifedipine and phloroglucinol in medical expulsive therapy for distal ureteral calculi. J Urol. 2005;174(1):167–72.

54. Amer T, Osman B, Johnstone A, Mariappan M, Gupta A, Brattis N, Jones G, Somani BK, Keeley FX Jr, Aboumarzouk OM. Medical expulsive therapy for ureteric stones: analysing the evidence from systematic reviews and meta-analysis of powered double-blinded randomised controlled trials. Arab J Urol. 2017;15(2):83–93.
55. Somani BK, Aboumarzouk O, Traxer O, Baard J, Kamphuis G, de la Rosette J. Medical expulsive therapy for ureteral stones: where do we go from here? Nat Rev Urol. 2016;13(10):608–12.
56. Ye Z, Yang H, Li H, Zhang X, Deng Y, Zeng G, Chen L, Cheng Y, Yang J, Mi Q, Zhang Y, Chen Z, Guo H, He W, Chen Z. A multicentre, prospective, randomized trial: comparative efficacy of tamsulosin and nifedipine in medical expulsive therapy for distal ureteric stones with renal colic. BJU Int. 2011;108(2):276–9.
57. Bandi G, Wilkinson EA, Cary-Coyle TL, Jerde TJ, Nakada SY. Third prize: effect of hydrocortisone on porcine ureteral contractility in vitro. J Endourol. 2008;22(6):1169–73.
58. Saita A, Bonaccorsi A, Marchese F, Condorelli SV, Motta M. Our experience with nifedipine and prednisolone as expulsive therapy for ureteral stones. Urol Int. 2004;72:43–5.

Chapter 19
Ureteral Stones

Fadl Hamouche, Leslie Charondo, and Marshall Stoller

Abstract Urolithiasis is a major health concern around the world, with renal colic being amongst the most common presentation. When a stone gets dislodged in the ureter, the resultant obstructive uropathy with the upstream backup of urine and increase in intrarenal pressure causes a stretch in the renal capsule, and the 'colicky pain' results. Despite the historical teaching that the ureter has three narrow points where stones can dislodge and obstruct the kidney, clinical studies have shown that most ureteral stones are distal on initial presentation. Multiple factors affect ureteral stone passage, mainly stone size, volume, location, and patient-related anatomical factors. Imaging is key to establishing a diagnosis of ureteral stone. While ultrasonography is an acceptable first line for upper tract stones, it is significantly less sensitive for distal ureteral stones, and non-contrast computed tomography is a superior alternative. Management of ureteral stones depends on the clinical presentation of the patient, with conservative management being an acceptable first line in the absence of infection or kidney injury, especially for smaller size stones. Other treatments include urinary diversion by a ureteral stent or a nephrostomy tube, shockwave lithotripsy, and ureteroscopy.

Keywords Ureter · Stone · Renal colic · Stone passage · Stone size · Ultrasonography · Lithotripsy

Test your learning and check your understanding of this book's contents: use the "Springer Nature Flashcards" app to access questions. To use the app, please follow the instructions in chapter 1.

F. Hamouche (✉)
Department of Urology, McGill University, Montreal, Quebec, Canada
e-mail: fadl.hamouche@mcgill.ca; Leslie.charondo@ucsf.edu; Marshall.stoller@ucsf.edu

L. Charondo · M. Stoller
Department of Urology, University of California San Francisco, San Francisco, CA, USA
e-mail: fadl.hamouche@mcgill.ca; Leslie.charondo@ucsf.edu; Marshall.stoller@ucsf.edu

M. Abdel-Gawad et al. (eds.), *The Ureter*,
https://doi.org/10.1007/978-3-031-36212-5_19

Abbreviations

AKI	Acute kidney injury
AQP	Aquaporin
CT	Computerized tomography
EHL	Electrohydraulic lithotripsy
IVU	Intravenous urogram
MET	Medical expulsive therapy
NSAIDs	Non-steroidal anti-inflammatory drugs
NT	Nephrostomy tube
PCNL	Percutaneous nephrolithotomy
RCT	Randomized controlled trial
SFR	Stone-free rate
SSP	Spontaneous stone passage
UAS	Ureteral access sheath
UPJ	Ureteropelvic junction
URS	Ureteroscopy
US	Ultrasonography
UVJ	Ureterovesical junction

Learning Objectives
After reading this chapter, the readers will be able to:

- Describe the epidemiology and pathophysiology of ureteral stones.
- Discuss the presentation of Ureteral stones.
- Analyse the diagnostic steps applied in the diagnosis of ureteral stones.
- Draw a plan for the management of Ureteral stones.

19.1 Introduction

In this chapter, a discussion of the epidemiology, pathophysiology, and process of ureteral stone formation is provided. In addition, the clinical manifestations, ways of diagnosis, and treatment are described.

19.2 Epidemiology

Kidney stones are a health concern around the world. Its increasing prevalence over the last decades has reached nearly 11% in industrialized countries like the United States [1]. The increasing incidence of nephrolithiasis worldwide reflects an increase in the economic burden on the healthcare system secondary to the emergency department (ED) presentations and overall management of kidney stones. A retrospective study on a single cohort from a stone clinic in the UK identified that a single patient costs the healthcare system up to 3 million £ over a 15-year follow-up period [2]. The socio-economic impact of kidney stones can be understood when considering its long-term nature and recurrence rate of symptomatic renal colic episodes. However, most literature does not differentiate between kidney and ureteral stones, which creates the assumption that the global incidence of upper tract nephrolithiasis, including ureteral stones, has increased over the last few decades.

19.3 Pathophysiology

Whether a renal stone can cause pain without obstruction is a dogma in modern Urology. However, it is accepted that when a stone gets dislodged in the ureter, the obstructive uropathy and the upstream backup of urine increase the intrarenal pressure and cause a stretch in the renal capsule contributing to the ‘colicky pain’. In fact, the physical stretching of nerve endings at the level of the renal capsule is the primary source of colicky pain [3]. This phenomenon is directly related to the ureteral obstruction that increases the intraluminal pressure in the collecting system and subsequently increases the wall tension. However, other physiological processes might participate in the manifestation of renal colic. For instance, ureteral obstruction by a stone can cause the activation of an inflammatory cascade and muscle ischemia from prolonged isotonic contraction that will eventually irritate nerve nociceptors and ultimately exacerbate the pain [4]. In addition, some in-vitro studies suggested that mucosal irritation and chemoreceptor activation contribute to pain, although they play a minor role [5].

According to Bretland, we can distinguish three phases in a renal colic attack: (1) onset, with continuous pain rising to its peak either slowly or quickly, sometimes with acute paroxysms; (2) plateau, with the constant pain of variable duration for up to 12 h, and (3) abatement phase, with pain that improves gradually and often spontaneously [6].

19.4 Ureteral Stone Formation

Kidney stone formation is a complex physiological process that includes a cascade of events starting with nucleation and ending with crystal growth and aggregation [7]. Although the detailed physiologic process of stone formation is beyond the intention of this chapter, it is worth noting that this process happens at the nephron level of the kidney. Previously, the supersaturation theory was based on the urine becoming supersaturated with stone-forming salts leading to the precipitation of crystals that can flow in the urine and lead to calculus formation. Recently, Stoller and colleagues hypothesized that the inciting event in the nephrolithiasis formation might be a vascular injury to the vasa recta near the renal papilla [8]. They also addressed the role of Randall plaques, <2 mm subepithelial calcification of the renal papilla, and their lithogenic potential in the process of stone formation [9]. Whether the initial step of stone formation is biochemical, vascular, or hypoxic in nature, it is believed that ureteral stones are formed in the kidney and migrate down to the ureter, with no stone formation occurring in situ at the level of the ureter.

19.5 Presentation and Location

The three narrowest points in the ureter are (1) the ureteropelvic junction (UPJ), (2) the point where the ureter crosses anterior to the external iliac vessels, and (3) the ureterovesical junction (UVJ). It has long been urological dogma that these three points are also the three most likely locations for ureteral stones to lodge [10, 11]. Despite these historical teachings, there is limited data to support this evidence. Furthermore, most of the historical data assessing the location of ureteral stones on presentation is based on outdated imaging modalities, such as the traditional excretory urography and plain abdominal X-ray, which are significantly less accurate than the computerized tomography (CT) widely used today.

To challenge these historical concepts, Eisner et al. performed a retrospective analysis of 94 consecutive patients presenting to the ED with a chief complaint of colic and computerized tomography showing a single unilateral ureteral calculus [12]. Axial, coronal, and 3-dimensional reformatted computerized tomography scans were evaluated, and stone position and size (maximal axial and coronal diameters) were recorded, as were the position of the ureteropelvic junction (UPJ), the iliac vessels (where the ureter crosses anterior to the iliac vessels), and the ureterovesical junction (UVJ). Interestingly, they found that two-thirds of the patients presented with a stone at the level of the UVJ. In fact, at the time of ED presentation for colic, the ureteral stone position was at the level of the UPJ in 10.6% of cases, between the UPJ and the iliac vessels in 23.4% of cases, where the ureter crosses anterior to the iliac vessels in 1.1% cases, between the iliac vessels and the UVJ in 4.3% cases, or at the UVJ in 60.6% cases (Fig. 19.1).

Similarly, Ordon et al. performed a retrospective analysis on 622 patients referred for shockwave lithotripsy (SWL) for the treatment of solitary ureteral stones [13]. Although the UPJ and the level where the ureter crosses anterior to the iliac vessels may be two of the three narrowest points of the ureter, stones are not typically lodged in those locations in patients who present with colic. Instead, they identified two peaks in stone location distribution around the proximal ureter and the UVJ.

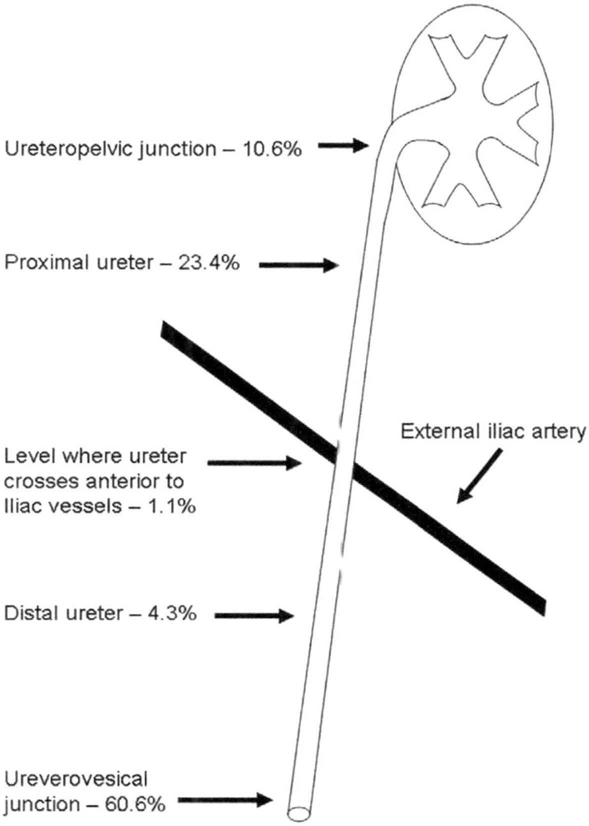

Fig. 19.1 Ureteral stone locations at emergency department presentation with colic

19.6 Ureteral Stone Size and Its Impact on Spontaneous Stone Passage

There is a strong correlation between stone size, location, and the likelihood of spontaneous stone passage [14]. It is generally observed that larger stones tend to be lodged more proximally in the ureter [12, 15].

Jendeberg et al. attempted to assess if the width and location of a ureteral stone can accurately predict the chance of spontaneous passage [16]. They retrospectively analyzed 392 consecutive patients with ureteric stones on Non-Enhanced CT, where they assessed stone size, location, hydronephrosis, and other factors until 26 weeks or stone expulsion. They found that the spontaneous passage rate in 20 weeks was 312 out of 392 stones, 98% in 0–2 mm, 98% in 3 mm, 81% in 4 mm, 65% in 5 mm, 33% in 6 mm, and 9% in ≥6.5 mm wide stones.

While most studies on ureteral stone size report the axial diameter and its relationship with stone passage or surgical outcomes, Kadihasanoglu et al. assessed the role of coronal diameter on stone passage [17]. They retrospectively analyzed 150 patients with ureteral stones and identified that in 75% of patients, the coronal diameter of the stone was larger than the axial diameter by an average of 1.2 mm. Furthermore, on their multivariate analysis, only coronal diameter, not axial, was found to affect spontaneous stone passage. Hence coronal diameter of the ureteral stone should not be overlooked and should be used in the clinical and surgical decision-making of patients with ureteral stones.

19.7 Role of Ureteral Stone Volume and Its Impact on Stone Passage

While the previously mentioned studies argue that stone passage rate depends on the stone's maximal diameter, whether axial or coronal, multiple studies have suggested that estimating the stone volume is a more accurate predictor [18]. In a recently published study, Abou Heidar et al. retrospectively assessed the role of a formula that estimates stone volume, to predict spontaneous stone passage (SSP).

They retrospectively analyzed 450 patients discharged from the ED on conservative treatment for ureteral stone (≤ 10 mm) and calculated ureteral stone volume using the ellipsoid formula ($V = \varpi * l * w * d * .167$). Then, they developed two models incorporating either estimated stone volume or maximal axial stone diameter and assessed its relationship with SSP. They found that more than half of the patients experienced SSP on medical therapy, and that stone volume was a better predictor factor for stone passage than maximal axial stone diameter. Furthermore, they identified that for every one mm^3 increase in stone volume, the risk of SSP failure increased by 2.5%.

Although using the same formula to calculate the stone volume for different stone types and shapes does not offer accurate volume estimation, it is reasonable to consider that stone volume, like stone size, affects spontaneous stone passage.

19.8 Imaging Diagnosis of Ureteral Stone

Patients presenting with renal colic are frequently evaluated with CT imaging. The use of unenhanced CT imaging to identify urolithiasis was first reported in 1995 and has now become the standard diagnostic tool to evaluate renal colic [19]. It offers the advantage over intravenous urogram (IVU) of avoiding contrast and being able

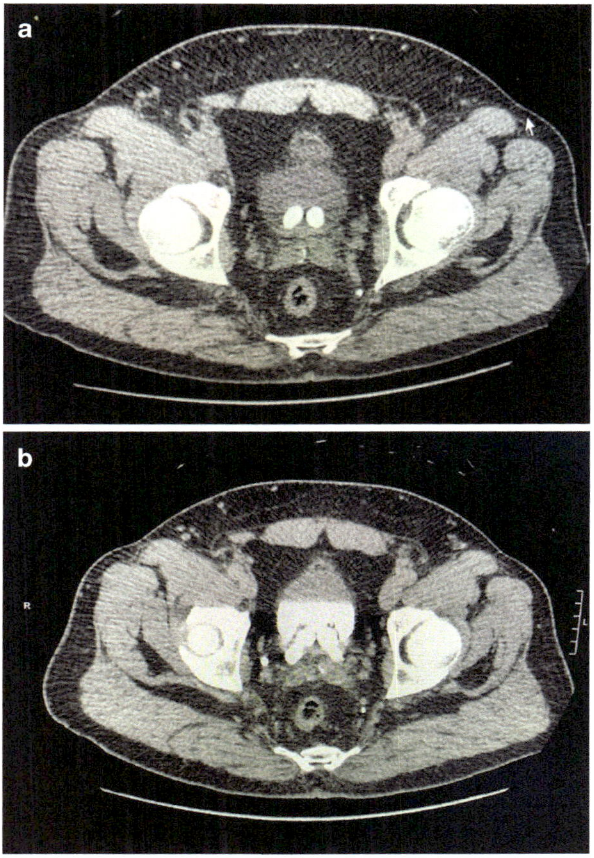

Fig. 19.2 CT shows bilateral intravesical ureteroceles with stones (**a**, **b**)

to diagnose other abdominal abnormalities that can also cause abdominal pain. Multidetector CT can readily diagnose radiolucent stones that may not have been seen on IVU and small stones even in the distal ureter. Except for some indinavir stones, all renal and ureteral stones can be detected on helical CT scan [20]. In the workup of urolithiasis, the unenhanced CT has a sensitivity ranging between 96% and 100% and a specificity ranging between 92% and 100% [21]. Stones in the distal ureter can be difficult to be differentiated from pelvic calcifications (Fig. 19.2). In these cases, the urologist needs to look for other signs of obstruction which may indicate the presence of a stone, including ureteral dilation, inflammatory changes in the perinephric fat, hydronephrosis, or a soft tissue rim surrounding the calcification within the ureter (Fig. 19.3). The latter represents irritation and edema in the ureteral wall [22].

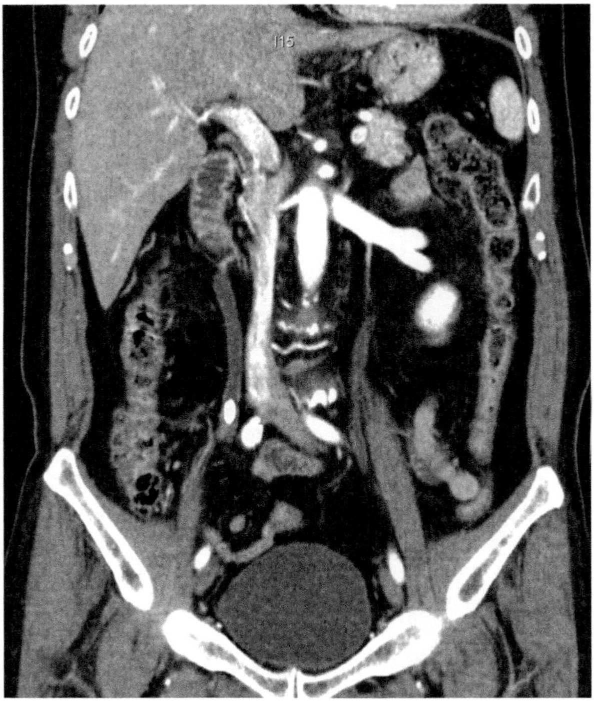

Fig. 19.3 CT shows right obstructive mid-ureteral stone causing upstream hydronephrosis

19.8.1 Role of Ultrasonography in Renal Colic Assessment

Although abdominal CT has become the most common initial imaging test for suspected nephrolithiasis because of its high sensitivity for the diagnosis of urinary stone disease, CT entails exposure to ionizing radiation with attendant long-term cancer risk and is associated with a high rate of incidental findings that can lead to inappropriate follow-up referrals and treatment [23].

Smith-Bindman et al. [24] conducted a multicenter, randomized trial comparing ultrasonography (US) with CT to assess the effect of diagnostic imaging techniques on patient outcomes. They randomized a total of 2759 patients presenting to the ED with renal colic to three imaging modalities: point-of-care US, radiology US, and CT scans. They identified no difference in high-risk diagnoses among the three groups. Furthermore, there was no difference in adverse events, return to ED visits, and hospitalizations, but there was a significant reduction of cumulative radiation exposure in both US groups compared to the CT scan group. Although the US was found to be adequate first-line imaging in the evaluation of renal colic and the detection of kidney stones, its role in the detection of ureteral stones remained questionable [25].

Kano et al. prospectively assessed the sensitivity and specificity of US to detect ureteral stones in 428 patients who underwent the US and a non-contrast-enhanced computed tomography (NCCT) on the same day [26]. They reported a sensitivity of 57.3% and a specificity of 97.5%. Stone sizes measured by the US correlated positively with those by CT. Interestingly, stone size and the presence of hydronephrosis were factors that independently affected ureteral stone detection by the US. To conclude, the US is an acceptable first-line imaging method in the evaluation and management of renal colic. However, its sensitivity for the detection of ureteral stones remains suboptimal to CT.

19.9 Management of Ureteral Stone

19.9.1 Conservative management of Ureteral Stone

Conservative management remains a reasonable first-line approach for most patients presenting with ureteral stones and renal colic. A 2010 meta-analysis of 37 studies showed that 38–71% of symptomatic ureteral stones <4 mm would pass spontaneously without any surgical intervention [27]. Similarly, the non-treatment arms of several large randomized controlled trials (RCTs) evaluating the efficacy of medical expulsive therapy (MET) noted spontaneous passage rates ranging from 40% to 80% for stones <10 mm [28]. Based on these spontaneous passage rates, an initial course of conservative management is an acceptable option for ureteral stones <10 mm.

19.9.2 Septic Stone Management

In the case of a "septic stone" or an "obstructed pyelonephritis" conservative management is not an option. With a sufficient index of suspicion, early goal-directed therapy, including blood and urine cultures, broad-spectrum intravenous antibiotics, resuscitation, and source control, is paramount [29]. Drainage of an obstructed pyelonephritis reduces mortality, and avoiding delays can prevent prolonged hospital admissions [30, 31]. Drainage of an obstructed kidney due to a ureteral stone can be done in a retrograde fashion with a ureteral stent or in an antegrade fashion with a percutaneous nephrostomy tube. The method of drainage should be tailored to the patient's clinical scenario and stone characteristics, as well as to the available resources at each center.

Both drainage methods are efficient and offer similar clinical outcomes. This concept was clarified in a prospective, randomized trial where patients presenting with a fever >38 °C, leukocytosis, and obstructing stone <15 mm were randomized to either a ureteric stent or a nephrostomy tube (NT) [32]. There were no differences in any clinical outcome evaluated, including time to defervescence, duration of hospital stay, and resolution of obstruction.

It is generally agreed that definitive treatment should not be undertaken until the obstructed system has been decompressed and the infection adequately treated [33]. Although there is no strong evidence of how long to wait after initial treatment, one study recommends a minimum of 7 days before definitive treatment [34].

19.9.3 Ureteral Stone and Acute Kidney Injury

An obstructed ureteral stone can alter kidney function by increasing the hydrostatic pressure in the collecting system and eventually decreasing the glomerular filtration rate [3]. Acute kidney injury (AKI) is present in approximately 6% of patients presenting with renal colic [35]. When significant renal impairment accompanies ureteral stones, early decompression or definitive therapy may mitigate further deterioration [29, 33, 36].

19.9.4 Ureteral Stone and Intractable Pain

Early intervention may also be warranted if the patient with a ureteral stone presents with intractable symptoms (pain, nausea, vomiting, etc.) or significant frailty/comorbidities that preclude observation. However, the data supporting early surgical intervention rather than a period of initial conservative therapy is limited. One RCT demonstrated that early ureteroscopy (URS) management (<12 h after ED admission) led to similar stone-free and complication rates but lower rates of post-operative stenting [37]. Similar results were found in two different RCTs looking at early SWL (<48 h) vs. delayed SWL (2–7 days). They demonstrated earlier time to stone-free status, fewer required treatments, and perhaps lower complications in the early SWL arms [38]. Importantly, the spontaneous stone passage rates in the delayed intervention arms of these RCTs were only 0–5.4%, which raises the question of a significant risk of selection bias.

19.9.5 Medical Management

1. *Medical expulsive therapy (MET)*

   Treatments that increase the likelihood of stone passage would be expected to benefit patients with ureteric colic because the need for an interventional procedure will be reduced. Medical expulsive therapy (MET) includes the use of smooth muscle relaxant drugs, tamsulosin (an α-adrenoceptor antagonist), and nifedipine (a calcium channel stabilizer) [39].

The role of MET has been questioned in recent years, with conflicting evidence about its clinical benefit. Multiple large RCTs failed to show improved stone passage rates or reduced analgesic requirements when using alpha-blockers for MET [28, 40, 41]. However, several published meta-analyses suggest the overall benefit of MET for ureteral stones [42, 43]. Subgroup analysis data suggests this benefit may be mainly for larger (5–10 mm) distal ureteral stones [43–45]. A Cochrane review of 67 studies analyzed all studies, specifically looking at lower- and higher-quality studies. The higher-quality, placebo-controlled studies showed a benefit with MET (relative risk [RR] 1.16, 95% confidence interval [CI] 1.07–1.25), a decrease in hospitalizations (RR 0.51, 95% CI 0.34–0.77), and no significant changes in the need for intervention [45, 46].

2. *Analgesia*

   Acute renal colic can be very painful and can cause significant distress. Hence why proper analgesia for pain control is paramount. Nonetheless, there remains uncertainty surrounding the optimal strategy for acute pain management in this population.

   In one study, 1645 adult acute care patients were randomized to intramuscular diclofenac, intravenous morphine, or intravenous paracetamol [47]. At 30 min, non-steroidal anti-inflammatories (NSAIDs) were more effective in reducing pain by 50% compared to morphine, with no adverse events. Patients randomized to IV morphine were more likely to suffer adverse events and require rescue analgesia than individuals in the other two groups.

   Another randomized trial showed that protocoled nonopioid analgesia could reduce opioid requirements during the initial presentation if first- and second-line interventions included NSAIDs and intravenous lidocaine. However, opioid-sparing approaches were associated with higher rates of repeat visits to the ED.

   Taken together, these data suggest that IM nonsteroidal anti-inflammatory medications should be considered as first-line analgesia in individuals presenting with renal colic. However, NSAIDs should not be used in patients with renal insufficiency because renal dysfunction can be exacerbated by the decrease in renal blood flow (RBF) induced by NSAIDs.

3. *Mechanism of action of anti-inflammatory in renal colic*

   NSAIDs cause a decrease in renal pelvic pressure in response to obstruction, which is thought to be mediated by a reduction in RBF [48]. NSAIDs were shown to induce a prompt reduction in both RBF and intrapelvic pressure in canines with unilateral ureteral obstruction [49]. Cyclooxygenase-2 (COX-2) inhibitors are a form of NSAID that block the synthesis of prostaglandins from arachidonic acid. It has previously been shown that COX-2 inhibitors can prevent prostaglandin E-mediated downregulation of aquaporin (AQP) channels and major sodium channels in response to obstruction. The resulting decrease in hydrostatic pressure within the tubules may provide an additional mechanism for the NSAID-mediated reduction in intrapelvic pressures [50].

19.9.6 Surgical Management

The urologist's armamentarium to surgically treat ureteral stones consists of four minimally invasive modalities, including SWL, URS, percutaneous nephrolithotomy (PCNL), and laparoscopic or robotic-assisted stone surgery. Open ureteral stone surgery is rarely performed when access to minimally invasive modalities exists and is often reserved for instances in which less invasive options have failed.

19.9.6.1 Shockwave Lithotripsy

Despite the progress in ureteroscopes and laser technologies over the last two decades, SWL remains a first-line treatment option for ureteral calculi. SWL outcomes can be directly influenced by case selection, surgical technique, and modifiable parameters to enhance safety and maximize successful outcomes. Most of the data for SWL outcomes is derived from patients with renal calculi and not ureteral calculi per se, but these findings could be generalizable to ureteric stones, particularly for those in the upper ureter, where renal parenchyma is included in the shockwave path [29, 33, 51]. Patient selection and surgeon's techniques, as well as stone characteristics, are all crucial to optimizing stone outcomes.

Technically speaking, dose escalation can improve stone fragmentation and reduce complications and renal injury. Gradually increasing SWL energy up to optimal dose allows for better patient accommodation to the sensation of treatment and, for upper ureteral stones, reduces renal injury by inducing renal vasoconstriction [52]. Alternatively, the surgeon can choose to pre-treat with a series of low-energy shocks, then pause treatment for a short period before resuming at higher-energy levels [53].

Another important factor is the rate of shockwave delivery to the stone. A slower rate might improve stone fragmentation. This was supported by multiple randomized trials that have indicated that a lower shock rate can improve stone fragmentation, particularly for stones larger than 1 cm. The optimal treatment rate is not specific and remains debatable. However, studies suggest that SWL at 60–90 shocks/min leads to better fragmentation than 120 shocks/min, particularly for larger stones [54, 55].

The ideal number of shocks has not been entirely determined. Although it is tempting to believe that a higher number of shocks will improve stone fragmentation, this needs to be balanced with the potential renal parenchymal injury, especially for proximal ureteral stones where the kidney is in the shock path. For upper ureteral stones, the recommended shock rate range is 2000–3500, but the manufacturer's guidelines should be carefully considered [56]. For mid to distal ureteric stones, where the renal parenchyma is not affected by SWL energy, treatment can safely be carried out with up to 4000 or more shocks (Fig. 19.4) [56, 57].

Multiple stone characteristics can decrease the success rate of SWL; for instance, some stone composition (pure calcium oxalate monohydrate, brushite, cystine

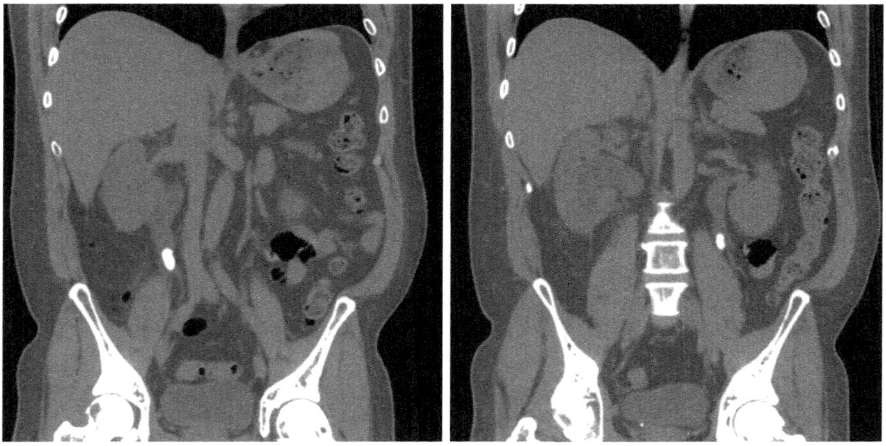

Fig. 19.4 NCCT shows bilateral obstructive ureteral stones

stones) can be resistant to shockwave [58]. Similarly, stone density (measured by HU on non-contrast CT scan) can affect the outcome of shockwave lithotripsy, with stones at a density higher than 1000 HU exhibiting difficult fragmentation and poor success rates [59]. Lastly, skin-to-stone distance (SSD) can also be a reasonable predictor of poor shockwave outcome, with multiple large series showing that a SSD >10-11 cm tends to decrease the success rate of SWL [60, 61].

Number of Treatments

If an initial SWL is unsuccessful, it can be repeated, but the benefit of more than two treatments for the same ureteric stone is small [62]. The optimal time interval between SWL treatments is unclear but can be short (2–3 days) for mid and distal ureteral stones [29, 33, 63].

19.9.6.2 Ureteroscopy

Modern URS has become a common modality in the surgical management of ureteral stones worldwide. As a result of advancements in technology in recent decades, URS can be safely performed with a high stone-free rate (SFR) and relatively low complications.

Different intraluminal lithotripsy devices have been historically used since the initial adoption of ureteroscopy for ureteral stone management. Electrohydraulic lithotripsy (EHL) is widely available worldwide and is cost-effective. However, its utilization decreased significantly after the development of laser lithotripsy. Fragmentation of calculi is produced by shock waves generated from an electric spark on the tip of the electrode [64]. Fragmentation of most calculi is good but can be less effective for more dense calculus compositions, such as cystine or calcium oxalate monohydrate. The small flexible EHL probes can be used with both rigid and flexible ureteroscopes. EHL can cause ureteral trauma because the energy is poorly focused. Although this rarely results in stricture formation, it can hinder visibility.

Another available lithotripsy modality is Pneumatic Lithotripsy which uses mechanical energy to fragment the stone, like a Jackhammer [65]. Despite its good fragmentation capacity, potential ureteral injury and stone retropulsion limited its wide adoption.

Laser lithotripsy was developed and replaced most of the available intraluminal lithotripters. Currently, the Holmium: YAG laser has become the intraluminal lithotripsy energy of choice. It has a wavelength of 2100 nm, which is absorbed in 3 mm of water, making it very safe for use in urology [66]. Fragmentation is produced by a photothermal reaction with the crystalline matrix of calculi and produces stone dust rather than fragments, effectively removing a moderate volume of the stone [67].

Another emerging laser lithotripsy source is the Thulium laser fiber (TFL). The TFL has a higher absorption coefficient and shorter optical penetration in water, and TFL has an ablation threshold of 4 times lower than the holmium laser. TFL is also a diode-pumped laser, unlike the flashlamp-pumped holmium laser. TFL allows greater control of pulse length and duration [68]. Furthermore, the TFL has been shown in vitro to have 5–10 times higher rates of stone vaporization than the holmium laser [69].

1. *Ureteroscopy technique*

   A detailed description of the surgical technique of ureteroscopy is beyond the scope of this chapter, but we will present the main surgical principles to consider during the endoscopic management of a ureteral stone. There are two main types of ureteroscopes: flexible and semirigid ureteroscopes.

   Flexible ureteroscopes are used for stones above the iliac vessels. Flexible ureteroscopes allow easy navigation of the upper tract and are the instrument of choice for calyceal stones. The flexible scopes need to be straight during the passage of a laser fiber to prevent damaging the working channel. During lithotripsy, maintaining clear visualization of the stone at all times prevents ureteral damage or perforation.

   Semirigid ureteroscopes are used for ureteral stones below the iliac vessels. Semirigid ureteroscopes have two working channels that permit better irrigation and improved visualization. Its more rigid nature allows easy manipulation inside the distal ureter and facilitates stone basketing.

   This distinction between the ureteroscopes facilitates surgical planning for ureteral stones and helps with equipment selection. However, it is important to note that in selected cases, a flexible ureteroscope can be used for a distal stone, and a semirigid ureteroscope can be used for proximal stones, especially in women.

2. *Ureteral access sheath (UAS)*

   Once retrograde access to the ureter is achieved, placing a ureteral access sheath (UAS) allows repeated entry to the intrarenal collecting system without reintubating the ureteral orifice with a wire at every passage. After placement under fluoroscopic guidance, the sheath facilitates stone fragment retrieval, enhances visibility, and allows for drainage and elimination of dust and stone fragments. In addition, the use of a UAS was shown to decrease intrapelvic pressure during URS, which can potentially reduce the risk of pyelovenous backflow and urosepsis [70].

UAS are available in different sizes—it is important to tailor the sheath to the patient's anatomy. Excessive force while advancing a ureteral access sheath should never be used to avoid ureteral perforation or avulsion.

Whether a UAS can improve URS outcomes and increase SFR is debatable. In a prospective cohort analysis of 2239 patients, no significant difference in SFR was seen whether a UAS was used or not during flexible URS (75.3% vs. 50.4%, $p = 0.604$). However, in a subgroup analysis of stones $\geq$10 mm, SFRs were significantly higher in the UAS group (84.9% vs. 81.5%, $p < 0.01$) [71].

Similarly, the use of UAS does not seem to increase ureteral complications. In a study of 2239 patients treated with flexible URS, no significant difference in ureteral injuries was reported in patients treated with UAS compared to those treated without UAS [71, 72]. Grades of ureteral injuries related to UAS were reported as low-grade injuries involving the mucosa in nearly half of the patients and high-grade lesions involving the smooth muscle layer in 15% of patients [73]. Endoscopically detected high-grade ureteral lesions following UAS insertion do not appear to increase stricture rates [74].

3. *Ureteral stenting*

Ureteral stent placement before or after a URS is part of the management of a ureteral stone. A ureteral stent impedes the peristalsis of the ureter hence allowing it to dilate. This is thought to improve postoperative drainage within and around the stent and prevents obstruction from postprocedural edema. It also maintains preoperative dilation if retrograde access to the ureter is not feasible.

Although pre-stenting facilitates the insertion of larger scopes or sheaths, whether this impacts surgical outcomes is unclear. Some studies have demonstrated no clear advantage in SFR nor complication rate with routine preoperative stenting [75, 76]. Others have shown that routine pre-URS stenting was associated with a higher SFR for larger stones [77]. The impact of post-URS stenting on SFR is also unclear; meta-analyses have shown conflicting results. One recent meta-analysis found that stenting did not improve SFR nor reduce late postoperative complications after routine URS [78]. Conversely, in another meta-analysis of 22 RCTs, the SFR was significantly better in the stented group (95% CI 0.34–0.89; $p = 0.01$) [79].

Regarding the impact on stricture rate, a meta-analysis of 14 trials and 1652 patients demonstrated that post-URS stenting likely does not reduce stricture rates at 90 days (RR 0.58, CI 0.23–1.47) [80]. Conversely, the use of a stent has been shown to reduce unplanned medical visits post-URS [81]. Following UAS use, routine ureteral stenting seems to be beneficial in reducing pain and unplanned medical visits [82]. However, there are instances where omitting a stent placement after a ureteroscopy is not advisable: suspected ureteric injury or

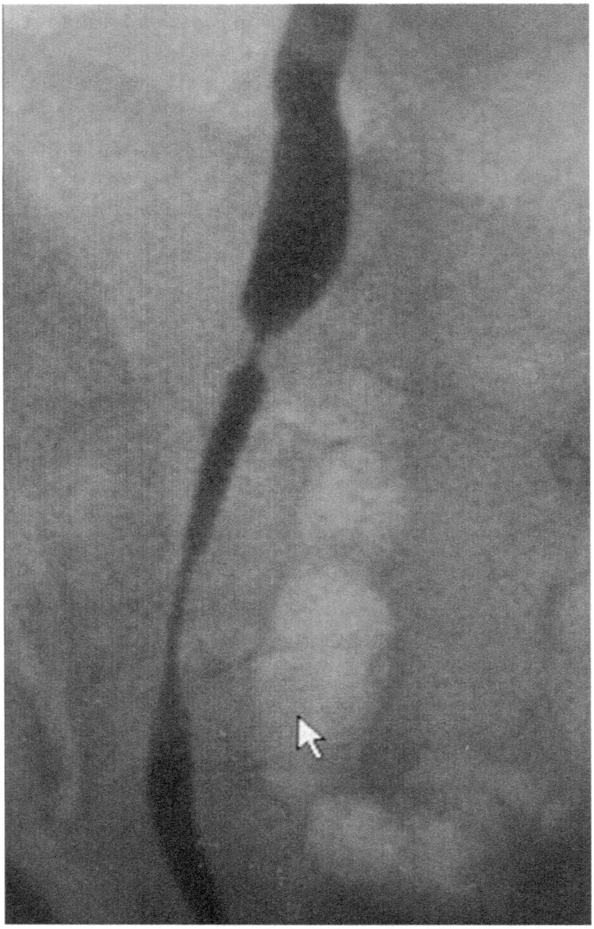

Fig. 19.5 Radiologic appearance of left ureteral stricture on retrograde pyelogram after treatment of an impacted ureteral stone

stricture, solitary kidney, and patient with renal impairment (Fig. 19.5). In these scenarios, a ureteral stent helps prevent serious potential complications, such as urosepsis or kidney injury. There is no consensus regarding the optimum duration of postoperative stenting. In an animal model, there were no histological ischemic changes in the ureteral wall 72 h post-UAS insertion, suggesting that 3 days may be sufficient [29, 33, 83, 84]. On the other hand, Paul et al. compared ureteral stent dwell times of three versus 7 days and found that removal at 3 days was linked to a higher probability of obstruction-related adverse events (23% vs. 3%) [29, 85, 86].

4. *Preoperative alpha-blockers*

 The use of alpha-blockers before URS appears to improve intraoperative outcomes and patient SFR. A recent systematic review and meta-analysis comprising 12 RCTs and 1352 patients evaluated alpha-blocker use before planned URS for the management of ureteral calculi. With a median preoperative use of 1 week, a 61% risk reduction in the need for ureteral dilatation was observed. Furthermore, the use of preoperative alpha-blockers significantly improved SFR (RR 1.18, 95% CI 1.11–1.24, $p < 0.0001$), reduced the operative time by an average of 6 min ($p = 0.004$), and decreased patient hospital stay ($p = 0.001$) [87].

5. *Percutaneous antegrade URS*

   Despite the advancement in URS techniques and the miniaturization of the devices, retrograde access can sometimes be unattainable, either due to anatomic characteristics (urinary diversion, ureteral stricture) or to stone characteristics (large proximal stone, imbedded or impacted stone). In either case, antegrade URS through percutaneous access can provide easier and more efficient access to the ureter. It can also facilitate the lithotripsy process through the anatomical funnel created by proximal hydronephrosis. A ureteral access sheath can also be advanced in an antegrade fashion to the level of the stone, which facilitates stone basketing and extraction. Therefore, an antegrade approach should be considered after a failed retrograde URS [29, 88].

19.9.6.3 Open Stone Surgery

Historically, most patients with symptomatic upper urinary tract calculi underwent open surgical lithotomy. Those patients with a small-to-moderate stone burden typically underwent pyelolithotomy, radial nephrolithotomy, or ureterolithotomy. This reality changed with the introduction of minimally invasive techniques like SWL and endoscopic approaches. Now, open stone surgery is rarely ever utilized. This dramatic decrease in stone surgery has been reported in multiple studies, with the current incidence ranging from 0.3% to 5.4% [89, 90].

Although ureterolithotomy has been a time-honored technique for many decades, it is seldom performed in the modern endourologic era. A meta-analysis undertaken for the American Urology Association (AUA) demonstrated median stone-free rates of 87% and 90% for stones in the distal ureter treated by open surgical removal and URS, respectively [51]. In the proximal ureter, the SFR for ureterolithotomy was 97% compared to 83% and 72% for SWL and URS, respectively. Although the results of open surgery in the proximal ureter in this historical analysis were somewhat better than those of minimally invasive techniques, the greater morbidity and longer hospitalization associated with open surgery favored a primary endourologic solution for ureteral stones. Further miniaturization of ureteroscopes, combined with the now widespread availability of the holmium: YAG laser, has increased the success rate for a ureteroscopic approach to proximal ureteral calculi. Open surgery for patients with ureteral stones is now indicated only as a salvage procedure when a planned abdominal operation coincides with a symptomatic ureteral stone episode or when another ureteral abnormality requires open surgical repair.

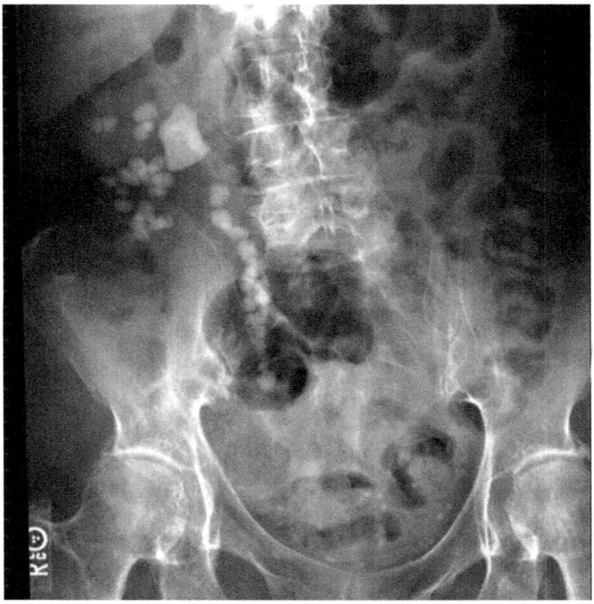

Fig. 19.6 Natural right-sided steinstrasse with large stone burden

19.9.6.4 Laparoscopic and Robotic Stone Removal

The development and widespread adoption of minimally invasive surgeries via laparoscopy and robotic surgeries add new tools to the armamentarium of urologists to tackle challenging stone cases. Any open lithotomy case can virtually be performed via a laparoscopic approach. However, the associated morbidity and longer hospital stay with this approach preclude it from being the initial treatment modality for ureteral stones.

There are few scenarios where a laparoscopic or robotic approach can be indicated: UPJ obstruction with a large renal pelvis stone where a pyeloplasty and a pyelolithotomy can be performed simultaneously; patients harboring stones in poorly functioning polar areas or with nonfunctioning kidneys where a nephrectomy can be the preferred management option; pelvic kidneys containing a large stone volume, in which laparoscopic techniques can be used to reflect overlying bowel, allowing pyelolithotomy or percutaneous stone removal; and ureterolithotomy for the extremely rare endoscopic failure or large/multiple impacted ureteral calculi (Fig. 19.6).

In current practice, the use of laparoscopy and robotics in the treatment of renal calculi continues to be limited; some reports suggest that the current incidence of this approach does not exceed 1%, with the most common indication being renal stones with a concomitant UPJ obstruction [91].

Questions

1. Pathophysiology of renal colic: A patient presented with renal colic to the emergency department. What is the most likely underlying pathophysiology to explain the pain? Select all that apply.

   (a) Stretching of the ureter at the site of the stone.
   (b) Activation of the inflammatory cascade and muscle ischemia from prolonged isotonic contractions.
   (c) Mucosal irritation.
   (d) Stretching of nerve endings at the level of the renal capsule.
   (e) Vasoconstriction of the renal artery of the affected side.

Answer: (b, c, d)

2. Location of ureteral stones in renal colic: what is the most common location of ureteral stones on presentation to the emergency department?

   (a) Renal pelvis & UVJ.
   (b) UPJ & UVJ.
   (c) Proximal Ureter & UVJ.
   (d) Level where ureter crosses anterior to iliac vessels & UVJ.
   (e) Proximal Ureter & Level where the ureter crosses anterior to iliac vessels.

Answer: (c)

3. Stone passage: Which stone size measurements were found to affect spontaneous stone passage?

   (a) Stone volume & coronal diameter.
   (b) Stone volume & axial diameter.
   (c) Stone volume only.
   (d) Coronal diameter & axial diameter.

Answer: (a)

4. Imaging: Which of the following modalities has the highest sensitivity for the detection of ureteral stones?

   (a) Xray.
   (b) Ultrasound (US).
   (c) Magnetic resonance imaging (MRI).
   (d) Computerized tomography (CT).

Answer: (d)

5. Conservative management: Although SWL remains a first-line treatment option for ureteral calculi, multiple stone characteristics can decrease its success rate.

Please select from the following choices the stone characteristics that decrease the SWL success rate.

(a) Pure calcium oxalate monohydrate stones.
(b) Uric acid stones.
(c) Ureteral stone location.
(d) Stone density > 1000 HU.
(e) Skin-to-stone distance >10 cm.

Answer: (a, d, e)

References

1. Sorokin I, Mamoulakis C, Miyazawa K, Rodgers A, Talati J, Lotan Y. Epidemiology of stone disease across the world. World J Urol. 2017;35(9):1301–20. https://doi.org/10.1007/s00345-017-2008-6. Epub 2017 Feb 17
2. Geraghty RM, Cook P, Walker V, Somani BK. Evaluation of the economic burden of kidney stone disease in the UK: a retrospective cohort study with a mean follow-up of 19 years. BJU Int. 2020;125(4):586–94. https://doi.org/10.1111/bju.14991. Epub 2020 Jan 24
3. Travaglini F, Bartoletti R, Gacci M, Rizzo M. Pathophysiology of reno-ureteral colic. Urol Int. 2004;72(Suppl 1):20–3. https://doi.org/10.1159/000076586.
4. Heid F, Jage J. The treatment of pain in urology. BJU Int. 2002;90(5):481–8. https://doi.org/10.1046/j.1464-410x.2002.02908.x.
5. Cervero F, Sann H. Mechanically evoked responses of afferent fibres innervating the guinea-pig's ureter: an in vitro study. J Physiol. 1989;412:245–66. https://doi.org/10.1113/jphysiol.1989.sp017613.
6. Bretland PM. Acute ureteric obstruction-clinical and radiological aspects. Proc R Soc Med. 1974;67(12 Pt 1):1215–7.
7. Ratkalkar VN, Kleinman JG. Mechanisms of stone formation. Clin Rev Bone Miner Metab. 2011;9(3–4):187–97. https://doi.org/10.1007/s12018-011-9104-8.
8. Stoller ML, Meng MV, Abrahams HM, Kane JP. The primary stone event: a new hypothesis involving a vascular etiology. J Urol. 2004;171(5):1920–4. https://doi.org/10.1097/01.ju.0000120291.90839.49.
9. Low RK, Stoller ML. Endoscopic mapping of renal papillae for Randall's plaques in patients with urinary stone disease. J Urol. 1997;158(6):2062–4. https://doi.org/10.1016/s0022-5347(01)68153-9.
10. Tanagho EA, McAninch JW. Smith's general urology. 16th ed. Columbus, Ohio: McGraw Hill; 2004. p. 727.
11. Brunicardi FC, Andersen DK, Billiar TR, Dunn DL, Hunter JG, Pollock RE. Schwartz's principles of surgery. Columbus: McGraw Hill; 2004. p. 2000.
12. Eisner BH, Reese A, Sheth S, Stoller ML. Ureteral stone location at emergency room presentation with colic. J Urol. 2009;182(1):165–8. https://doi.org/10.1016/j.juro.2009.02.131. Epub 2009 May 17.
13. Ordon M, Schuler TD, Ghiculete D, Pace KT, Honey RJ. Stones lodge at three sites of anatomic narrowing in the ureter: clinical fact or fiction? J Endourol. 2013;27(3):270–6. https://doi.org/10.1089/end.2012.0201. Epub 2012 Dec 26.
14. Ueno A, Kawamura T, Ogawa A, Takayasu H. Relation of spontaneous passage of ureteral calculi to size. Urology. 1977;10(6):544–6. https://doi.org/10.1016/0090-4295(77)90097-8.
15. Osorio L, Lima E, Soares J, Autorino R, Versos R, Lhamas A, Marcelo F. Emergency ureteroscopic management of ureteral stones: why not? Urology. 2007;69(1):27–31. https://doi.org/10.1016/j.urology.2006.08.1116. discussion 31–3.

16. Jendeberg J, Geijer H, Alshamari M, Cierzniak B, Lidén M. Size matters: the width and location of a ureteral stone accurately predict the chance of spontaneous passage. Eur Radiol. 2017;27(11):4775–85. https://doi.org/10.1007/s00330-017-4852-6. Epub 2017 Jun 7.
17. Kadihasanoglu M, Marien T, Miller NL. Ureteral stone diameter on computerized tomography coronal reconstructions is clinically important and under-reported. Urology. 2017;102:54–60. https://doi.org/10.1016/j.urology.2016.11.046. Epub 2017 Jan 12.
18. Cui HW, Tan TK, Christiansen FE, Osther PJS, Turney BW. The utility of automated volume analysis of renal stones before and after shockwave lithotripsy treatment. Urolithiasis. 2021;49(3):219–26. https://doi.org/10.1007/s00240-020-01212-8. Epub 2020 Sep 14.
19. Smith RC, Rosenfield AT, Choe KA, Essenmacher KR, Verga M, Glickman MG, Lange RC. Acute flank pain: comparison of non-contrast-enhanced CT and intravenous urography. Radiology. 1995;194(3):789–94. https://doi.org/10.1148/radiology.194.3.7862980.
20. Schwartz BF, Schenkman N, Armenakas NA, Stoller ML. Imaging characteristics of indinavir calculi. J Urol. 1999;161(4):1085–7.
21. Memarsadeghi M, Heinz-Peer G, Helbich TH, Schaefer-Prokop C, Kramer G, Scharitzer M, Prokop M. Unenhanced multi-detector row CT in patients suspected of having urinary stone disease: effect of section width on diagnosis. Radiology. 2005;235(2):530–6. https://doi.org/10.1148/radiol.2352040448. Epub 2005 Mar 9.
22. Heneghan JP, Dalrymple NC, Verga M, Rosenfield AT, Smith RC. Soft-tissue "rim" sign in the diagnosis of ureteral calculi with use of unenhanced helical CT. Radiology. 1997;202(3):709–11. https://doi.org/10.1148/radiology.202.3.9051021.
23. Lumbreras B, Donat L, Hernández-Aguado I. Incidental findings in imaging diagnostic tests: a systematic review. Br J Radiol. 2010;83(988):276–89. https://doi.org/10.1259/bjr/98067945.
24. Smith-Bindman R, Aubin C, Bailitz J, et al. Ultrasonography versus computed tomography for suspected nephrolithiasis. N Engl J Med. 2014;371:1100–10. https://doi.org/10.1056/NEJMoa1404446.
25. Kanno T, Kubota M, Sakamoto H, Nishiyama R, Okada T, Higashi Y, Yamada H. The efficacy of ultrasonography for the detection of renal stone. Urology. 2014;84(2):285–8. https://doi.org/10.1016/j.urology.2014.04.010. Epub 2014 Jun 5.
26. Kanno T, Kubota M, Sakamoto H, Nishiyama R, Okada T, Higashi Y, Yamada H. Determining the efficacy of ultrasonography for the detection of ureteral stone. Urology. 2014;84(3):533–7. https://doi.org/10.1016/j.urology.2014.04.047.
27. Skolarikos A, Laguna MP, Alivizatos G, Kural AR, de la Rosette JJ. The role for active monitoring in urinary stones: a systematic review. J Endourol. 2010;24(6):923–30. https://doi.org/10.1089/end.2009.0670.
28. Pickard R, Starr K, MacLennan G, et al. Medical expulsive therapy in adults with ureteric colic: a multicentre, randomised, placebo-controlled trial. Lancet. 2015;386(9991):341–9. https://doi.org/10.1016/S0140-6736(15)60933-3. Epub 2015 May 18.
29. Lee JY, Andonian S, Bhojani N, et al. Canadian urological association guideline: management of ureteral calculi-full-text. Can Urol Assoc J. 2021;15(12):E676–90. https://doi.org/10.5489/cuaj.7581.
30. Borofsky MS, Walter D, Shah O, Goldfarb DS, Mues AC, Makarov DV. Surgical decompression is associated with decreased mortality in patients with sepsis and ureteral calculi. J Urol. 2013;189(3):946–51. https://doi.org/10.1016/j.juro.2012.09.088. Epub 2012 Sep 24.
31. Haas CR, Smigelski M, Sebesta EM, Mobley D, Shah O. Implementation of a hospital-wide protocol reduces time to decompression and length of stay in patients with stone-related obstructive pyelonephritis with sepsis. J Endourol. 2021;35(1):77–83. https://doi.org/10.1089/end.2020.0626. Epub 2020 Sep 7.
32. Pearle MS, Pierce HL, Miller GL, et al. Optimal method of urgent decompression of the collecting system for obstruction and infection due to ureteral calculi. J Urol. 1998;160(4):1260–4.
33. Lee JY, Andonian S, Bhojani N, et al. Canadian urological association guideline: management of ureteral calculi-abridged version. Can Urol Assoc J. 2021;15(12):383–93. https://doi.org/10.5489/cuaj.7652.

34. Shi YF, Ju WL, Zhu YP, Xia SJ, Sun XW. The impact of ureteral stent indwelling time on the treatment of acute infection caused by ureteral calculi. Urolithiasis. 2017;45(6):579–83. https://doi.org/10.1007/s00240-017-0964-3. Epub 2017 Feb 22.
35. Kim HY, Choe HS, Lee DS, Yoo JM, Lee SJ. Transient renal impairment in the absence of pre-existing chronic kidney disease in patients with unilateral ureteric stone impaction. Urolithiasis. 2017;45(3):249–54. https://doi.org/10.1007/s00240-016-0904-7. Epub 2016 Jul 7.
36. Jiang P, Xie L, Arada R, Patel RM, Landman J, Clayman RV. Qualitative review of clinical guidelines for medical and surgical Management of Urolithiasis: consensus and controversy 2020. J Urol. 2021;205(4):999–1008. https://doi.org/10.1097/JU.0000000000001478. Epub 2020 Dec 7.
37. Guercio S, Ambu A, Mangione F, Mari M, Vacca F, Bellina M. Randomized prospective trial comparing immediate versus delayed ureteroscopy for patients with ureteral calculi and normal renal function who present to the emergency department. J Endourol. 2011;25(7):1137–41. https://doi.org/10.1089/end.2010.0554. Epub 2011 Jun 17.
38. Kumar A, Mohanty NK, Jain M, Prakash S, Arora RP. A prospective randomized comparison between early (<48 hours of onset of colicky pain) versus delayed shockwave lithotripsy for symptomatic upper ureteral calculi: a single center experience. J Endourol. 2010;24(12):2059–66. https://doi.org/10.1089/end.2010.0066. Epub 2010 Oct 25.
39. Hollingsworth JM, Rogers MA, Kaufman SR, Bradford TJ, Saint S, Wei JT, Hollenbeck BK. Medical therapy to facilitate urinary stone passage: a meta-analysis. Lancet. 2006;368(9542):1171–9. https://doi.org/10.1016/S0140-6736(06)69474-9.
40. Van Asseldonk B, Elterman DS. Medical expulsive therapy for ureteric colic: new hard evidence: commentary on: medical expulsive therapy in adults with ureteric colic: a multicentre, randomised, placebo-controlled trial. Urology. 2015;86(4):649–50. https://doi.org/10.1016/j.urology.2015.06.030.
41. Marchini GS, Vicentini FC, Mazzucchi E, Brito A, Ebaid G, Srougi M. Silent ureteral stones: impact on kidney function--can treatment of silent ureteral stones preserve kidney function? Urology. 2012;79(2):304–8. https://doi.org/10.1016/j.urology.2011.07.1436. Epub 2011 Nov 4.
42. Cui Y, Chen J, Zeng F, et al. Tamsulosin as a medical expulsive therapy for ureteral stones: a systematic review and meta-analysis of randomized controlled trials. J Urol. 2019;201(5):950–5. https://doi.org/10.1097/JU.0000000000000029.
43. Amer T, Osman B, Johnstone A, et al. Medical expulsive therapy for ureteric stones: analysing the evidence from systematic reviews and meta-analysis of powered double-blinded randomised controlled trials. Arab J Urol. 2017;15(2):83–93. https://doi.org/10.1016/j.aju.2017.03.005.
44. Sur RL, Shore N, L'Esperance J, et al. Silodosin to facilitate passage of ureteral stones: a multi-institutional, randomized, double-blinded, placebo-controlled trial. Eur Urol. 2015;67(5):959–64. https://doi.org/10.1016/j.eururo.2014.10.049. Epub 2014 Nov 20.
45. Campschroer T, Zhu X, Vernooij RWM, Lock TMTW. α-Blockers as medical expulsive therapy for ureteric stones: a Cochrane systematic review. BJU Int. 2018;122(6):932–45. https://doi.org/10.1111/bju.14454. Epub 2018 Aug 11.
46. Seitz C, Liatsikos E, Porpiglia F, Tiselius HG, Zwergel U. Medical therapy to facilitate the passage of stones: what is the evidence? Eur Urol. 2009;56(3):455–71. https://doi.org/10.1016/j.eururo.2009.06.012. Epub 2009 Jun 21.
47. Pathan SA, Mitra B, Straney LD, et al. Delivering safe and effective analgesia for management of renal colic in the emergency department: a double-blind, multigroup, randomized controlled trial. Lancet. 2016;387(10032):1999–2007. https://doi.org/10.1016/S0140-6736(16)00652-8. Epub 2016 Mar 16.
48. Perlmutter A, Miller L, Trimble LA, Marion DN, Vaughan ED Jr, Felsen D. Toradol, an NSAID used for renal colic, decreases renal perfusion and ureteral pressure in a canine model of unilateral ureteral obstruction. J Urol. 1993;149(4):926–30. https://doi.org/10.1016/s0022-5347(17)36261-4.

49. Jones JB, Dula DJ. The efficacy of sublingual hyoscyamine sulfate and intravenous ketorolac tromethamine in the relief of ureteral colic. Am J Emerg Med. 1998;16(6):557–9. https://doi.org/10.1016/s0735-6757(98)90217-0.
50. Nørregaard R, Jensen BL, Li C, et al. COX-2 inhibition prevents downregulation of key renal water and sodium transport proteins in response to bilateral ureteral obstruction. Am J Physiol Renal Physiol. 2005;289(2):F322–33. https://doi.org/10.1152/ajprenal.00061.2005. Epub 2005 Apr 19.
51. Segura JW, Preminger GM, Assimos DG, Dretler SP, Kahn RI, Lingeman JE, Macaluso JN Jr. Ureteral stones clinical guidelines panel summary report on the management of ureteral calculi. Am Urolog Assoc J Urol. 1997;158(5):1915–21. https://doi.org/10.1016/s0022-5347(01)64173-9.
52. Willis LR, Evan AP, Connors BA, Handa RK, Blomgren PM, Lingeman JE. Prevention of lithotripsy-induced renal injury by pretreating kidneys with low-energy shock waves. J Am Soc Nephrol. 2006;17(3):663–73. https://doi.org/10.1681/ASN.2005060634. Epub 2006 Feb 1.
53. McAteer JA, Evan AP, Williams JC Jr, Lingeman JE. Treatment protocols to reduce renal injury during shock wave lithotripsy. Curr Opin Urol. 2009;19(2):192–5. https://doi.org/10.1097/mou.0b013e32831e16e3.
54. Davenport K, Minervini A, Keoghane S, Parkin J, Keeley FX, Timoney AG. Does rate matter? The results of a randomized controlled trial of 60 versus 120 shocks per minute for shock wave lithotripsy of renal calculi. J Urol. 2006;176(5):2055–8. https://doi.org/10.1016/j.juro.2006.07.012. discussion 2058.
55. Pace KT, Ghiculete D, Harju M, Honey RJ. University of Toronto Lithotripsy associates. Shock wave lithotripsy at 60 or 120 shocks per minute: a randomized, double-blind trial. J Urol. 2005;174(2):595–9. https://doi.org/10.1097/01.ju.0000165156.90011.95.
56. Rassweiler JJ, Knoll T, Köhrmann KU, et al. Shock wave technology and application: an update. Eur Urol. 2011;59(5):784–96. https://doi.org/10.1016/j.eururo.2011.02.033. Epub 2011 Feb 23.
57. Elmansy HE, Lingeman JE. Recent advances in lithotripsy technology and treatment strategies: a systematic review update. Int J Surg. 2016;36(Pt D):676–80. https://doi.org/10.1016/j.ijsu.2016.11.097. Epub 2016 Nov 24.
58. Kallidonis P, Adamou C, Ntasiotis P, et al. The best treatment approach for lower calyceal stones ≤20 mm in maximal diameter: mini percutaneous nephrolithotripsy, retrograde intrarenal surgery or shock wave lithotripsy. A systematic review and meta-analysis of the literature conducted by the European section of Uro-technology and young academic urologists. Minerva Urol Nephrol. 2021;73(6):711–23. https://doi.org/10.23736/S2724-6051.21.04388-3. Epub 2021 Jun 22.
59. Gupta NP, Ansari MS, Kesarvani P, Kapoor A, Mukhopadhyay S. Role of computed tomography with no contrast medium enhancement in predicting the outcome of extracorporeal shock wave lithotripsy for urinary calculi. BJU Int. 2005;95(9):1285–8. https://doi.org/10.1111/j.1464-410X.2005.05520.x.
60. Wiesenthal JD, Ghiculete D, Ray AA, Honey RJ, Pace KT. A clinical nomogram to predict the successful shock wave lithotripsy of renal and ureteral calculi. J Urol. 2011;186(2):556–62. https://doi.org/10.1016/j.juro.2011.03.109.
61. Patel T, Kozakowski K, Hruby G, Gupta M. Skin-to-stone distance is an independent predictor of stone-free status following shockwave lithotripsy. J Endourol. 2009;23(9):1383–5. https://doi.org/10.1089/end.2009.0394.
62. Pace KT, Weir MJ, Tariq N, Honey RJ. Low success rate of repeat shock wave lithotripsy for ureteral stones after failed initial treatment. J Urol. 2000;164(6):1905–7.
63. Ordon M, Andonian S, Blew B, Schuler T, Chew B, Pace KT. CUA guideline: management of ureteral calculi. Can Urol Assoc J. 2015;9(11–12):E837–51. https://doi.org/10.5489/cuaj.3483. Epub 2015 Dec 14.
64. Denstedt JD, Clayman RV. Electrohydraulic lithotripsy of renal and ureteral calculi. J Urol. 1990;143(1):13–7. https://doi.org/10.1016/s0022-5347(17)39850-6.

65. Schulze H, Haupt G, Piergiovanni M, Wisard M, von Niederhausern W, Senge T. The Swiss Lithoclast: a new device for endoscopic stone disintegration. J Urol. 1993;149(1):15–8. https://doi.org/10.1016/s0022-5347(17)35985-2.
66. Blomley MJ, Nicholson DA, Bartal G, Bradley A, Myers M, Allison DJ. Penetration of the holmium:YAG laser through fluid. J Vasc Interv Radiol. 1995;6(6):903–10. https://doi.org/10.1016/s1051-0443(95)71210-6.
67. Zagone RL, Waldmann TM, Conlin MJ. Fragmentation of uric acid calculi with the holmium: YAG laser produces cyanide. Lasers Surg Med. 2002;31(4):230–2. https://doi.org/10.1002/lsm.10094.
68. Hutchens TC, Blackmon RL, Irby PB, Fried NM. Detachable fiber optic tips for use in thulium fiber laser lithotripsy. J Biomed Opt. 2013;18(3):038001. https://doi.org/10.1117/1.JBO.18.3.038001.
69. Blackmon RL, Irby PB, Fried NM. Holmium:YAG (lambda = 2,120 nm) versus thulium fiber (lambda = 1,908 nm) laser lithotripsy. Lasers Surg Med. 2010;42(3):232–6. https://doi.org/10.1002/lsm.20893.
70. Auge BK, Pietrow PK, Lallas CD, Raj GV, Santa-Cruz RW, Preminger GM. Ureteral access sheath provides protection against elevated renal pressures during routine flexible ureteroscopic stone manipulation. J Endourol. 2004;18(1):33–6. https://doi.org/10.1089/089277904322836631.
71. Traxer O, Wendt-Nordahl G, Sodha H, et al. Differences in renal stone treatment and outcomes for patients treated either with or without the support of a ureteral access sheath: the clinical research office of the endourological society ureteroscopy global study. World J Urol. 2015;33(12):2137–44. https://doi.org/10.1007/s00345-015-1582-8. Epub 2015 May 14.
72. Geraghty RM, Ishii H, Somani BK. Outcomes of flexible ureteroscopy and laser fragmentation for treatment of large renal stones with and without the use of ureteral access sheaths: results from a university hospital with a review of literature. Scand J Urol. 2016;50(3):216–9. https://doi.org/10.3109/21681805.2015.1121407. Epub 2016 Jan 12.
73. De Coninck V, Keller EX, Rodríguez-Monsalve M, Audouin M, Doizi S, Traxer O. Systematic review of ureteral access sheaths: facts and myths. BJU Int. 2018;122(6):959–69. https://doi.org/10.1111/bju.14389. Epub 2018 Jun 22.
74. Assimos DG. Re: a prospective study Analyzing the association between high-grade ureteral access sheath injuries and the formation of ureteral strictures. J Urol. 2019;202(3):454. https://doi.org/10.1097/01.JU.0000574492.77005.b6. Epub 2019 Aug 8.
75. Assimos D, Crisci A, Culkin D, Xue W, Roelofs A, Duvdevani M, Desai M. de la Rosette J; CROES URS global study group. preoperative JJ stent placement in ureteric and renal stone treatment: results from the clinical research office of endourological society (CROES) ureteroscopy (URS) global study. BJU Int. 2016;117(4):648–54. https://doi.org/10.1111/bju.13250. Epub 2015 Sep 6.
76. Jessen JP, Breda A, Brehmer M, et al. International collaboration in endourology: multicenter evaluation of prestenting for ureterorenoscopy. J Endourol. 2016;30(3):268–73. https://doi.org/10.1089/end.2015.0109. Epub 2015 Dec 22.
77. Netsch C, Knipper S, Bach T, Herrmann TR, Gross AJ. Impact of preoperative ureteral stenting on stone-free rates of ureteroscopy for nephroureterolithiasis: a matched-paired analysis of 286 patients. Urology. 2012;80(6):1214–9. https://doi.org/10.1016/j.urology.2012.06.064. Epub 2012 Oct 18.
78. Pengfei S, Yutao L, Jie Y, Wuran W, Yi D, Hao Z, Jia W. The results of ureteral stenting after ureteroscopic lithotripsy for ureteral calculi: a systematic review and meta-analysis. J Urol. 2011;186(5):1904–9. https://doi.org/10.1016/j.juro.2011.06.066. Epub 2011 Sep 23.
79. Wang H, Man L, Li G, Huang G, Liu N, Wang J. Meta-analysis of stenting versus non-stenting for the treatment of ureteral stones. PLoS One. 2017;12(1):e0167670. https://doi.org/10.1371/journal.pone.0167670.
80. Ordonez M, Hwang EC, Borofsky M, Bakker CJ, Gandhi S, Dahm P. Ureteral stent versus no ureteral stent for ureteroscopy in the management of renal and ureteral calculi. Cochrane Database Syst Rev. 2019;2(2):CD012703. https://doi.org/10.1002/14651858.CD012703.pub2.

81. Pais VM Jr, Smith RE, Stedina EA, Rissman CM. Does omission of ureteral stents increase risk of unplanned return visit? A systematic review and meta-analysis. J Urol. 2016;196(5):1458–66. https://doi.org/10.1016/j.juro.2016.05.109. Epub 2016 Jun 7.
82. Torricelli FC, De S, Hinck B, Noble M, Monga M. Flexible ureteroscopy with a ureteral access sheath: when to stent? Urology. 2014;83(2):278–81. https://doi.org/10.1016/j.urology.2013.10.002. Epub 2013 Nov 12.
83. Lallas CD, Auge BK, Raj GV, Santa-Cruz R, Madden JF, Preminger GM. Laser doppler flowmetric determination of ureteral blood flow after ureteral access sheath placement. J Endourol. 2002;16(8):583–90. https://doi.org/10.1089/089277902320913288.
84. Dushinski J. Both patient and stone factors determine "best" treatment for urolithiasis. Can Urol Assoc J. 2021;15(12):394. https://doi.org/10.5489/cuaj.7681.
85. Paul CJ, Brooks NA, Ghareeb GM, Tracy CR. Pilot study to determine optimal stent duration following ureteroscopy: three versus seven days. Curr Urol. 2018;11(2):97–102. https://doi.org/10.1159/000447201. Epub 2017 Dec 30.
86. Boyko AW, Merheb S, Hill S, et al. Ureteral stenting after routine ureteroscopy: is earlier stent removal feasible? Can J Urol. 2021;28(5):10865–70.
87. Alsaikhan B, Koziarz A, Lee JY, Pace KT. Preoperative alpha-blockers for ureteroscopy for ureteral stones: a systematic review and meta-analysis of randomized controlled trials. J Endourol. 2020;34(1):33–41. https://doi.org/10.1089/end.2019.0520. Epub 2019 Oct 9.
88. Sun X, Xia S, Lu J, Liu H, Han B, Li W. Treatment of large impacted proximal ureteral stones: randomized comparison of percutaneous antegrade ureterolithotripsy versus retrograde ureterolithotripsy. J Endourol. 2008;22(5):913–7. https://doi.org/10.1089/end.2007.0230.
89. Assimos DG, Boyce WH, Harrison LH, McCullough DL, Kroovand RL, Sweat KR. The role of open stone surgery since extracorporeal shock wave lithotripsy. J Urol. 1989;142(2 Pt 1):263–7. https://doi.org/10.1016/s0022-5347(17)38725-6.
90. Paik ML, Wainstein MA, Spirnak JP, Hampel N, Resnick MI. Current indications for open stone surgery in the treatment of renal and ureteral calculi. J Urol. 1998;159(2):374–8. https://doi.org/10.1016/s0022-5347(01)63922-3. discussion 378–9.
91. Desai RA, Assimos DG. Role of laparoscopic stone surgery. Urology. 2008;71(4):578–80. https://doi.org/10.1016/j.urology.2007.10.052.

Chapter 20
Management of Ureteral Stones

Muhammed Arif Ibis and Kemal Sarica

Abstract Evidence-based recommendations for the management of ureteral stones are provided. Ureteral stones less than 5 mm in diameter have a high chance of spontaneous passage. Medical expulsive therapy (MET) with alpha-blockers is effective for treating many patients with uncomplicated distal ureteral stones lass 10 mm in diameter. Extracorporeal shock wave lithotripsy (ESWL) is effective initial therapy for mid- and upper ureteral stones less than 10 mm in diameter. Routine double-J ureteral stenting before ESWL does not improve stone-free rates. Routine prophylactic antibiotics are not necessary. ESWL is not used during pregnancy because of potential harm to a fetus. Ureteroscopy and percutaneous antegrade ureterorenoscopy with laser lithotripsy are effective stone treatments. Routine double-J stenting is not necessary. In rare cases where ESWL and ureteroscopy are unsuccessful or unlikely to be successful, laparoscopic, hand-assisted laparoscopic, robotic-assisted laparoscopic, or open ureterolithotomy might be performed.

Keywords Extracorporeal shock wave lithotripsy · Laparoscopic · Laser · Medical expulsive therapy · Robotic · Spontaneous passage · Ureter · Ureteroscopy · Ureterolithotomy

Learning Objectives

The learning objectives for this chapter are

- To describe the treatment options for the management of ureteral stones,
- To describe the evaluation and treatment of early and late complications of the management of ureteral stones,

---

Test your learning and check your understanding of this book's contents: use the "Springer Nature Flashcards" app to access questions. To use the app, please follow the instructions in Chapter 1.

M. A. Ibis (✉)
Department of Urology, Ankara University School of Medicine, Ankara, Turkey

K. Sarica
Department of Urology, Biruni University, Medical School, Istanbul, Turkey

M. Abdel-Gawad et al. (eds.), *The Ureter*,
https://doi.org/10.1007/978-3-031-36212-5_20

- To gain the ability to choose the appropriate treatment for ureteral stones in clinical practice.

20.1 Introduction

Ureteral stone disease constitutes a common problem in clinical practice. The overall objectives of medical or surgical stone management are relieving patient discomfort and renal dysfunction associated with ureteral stones. Stone-related, patient-related, and technical factors shall be considered while determining the optimal treatment for patients with ureteral stones. The size, position, and composition/hardness of the stone constitute critical factors when choosing the optimal treatment. In addition, patient comorbidities such as concomitant infection, obesity, bleeding diathesis, or pregnancy influence the choice of therapy and constitute essential factors.

When intervention is required, these factors shall be considered to assist in selecting the treatment that will provide the patient with maximum stone clearance with minimal morbidity. In particular, in cases where more than one treatment option is considered appropriate, the final treatment decision shall be made in line with the patient's opinion. Existing kidney functions, treatment success, risk of complications, and quality of life in the early postoperative period constitute important issues that shall be discussed with patients while deciding on the surgery. Stone-free rates (SFRs) of the procedures and whether they might require additional treatment shall be discussed with the patient, and it shall be explained that practices with higher SFRs might have higher complication rates.

The epicenter of this chapter is the treatment of ureteral stones. Within this context, the topics are included: Medical expulsive therapy, Extracorporeal shock wave lithotripsy (ESWL), Ureteroscopic removal of the stones: Retrograde; antegrade; semirigid; flexible maneuvers, Laparoscopic and robotic ureterolithotomy, Open ureterolithotomy.

20.2 Medical Expulsive Therapy

Nephrolithiasis prevalence rates vary on a broader scale from 1% to 20%, depending on geographical, climatic, dietary, and genetic factors [1]. Patients often present to the emergency department with severe pain requiring analgesia. The choice of treatment modalities for urolithiasis shall be made depending on the size, location, composition of the stone, and the symptoms it causes. Even though the minimally invasive treatment options are considered effective in treating ureteral stones, the risk of complications and high costs are notable disadvantages of these treatments.

The rates of spontaneously stone passage vary among patients depending on the stone's size and location. For example, a recent meta-analysis expressed that 75%

of stones less than 5 mm pass spontaneously [2]. However, as well-known, the rate of spontaneous passage decreases as the stone size increases. For example, the spontaneous passage rate of ureter stones with a size of 6.5 mm and larger has been reported as 9% [3]. However, suppose the stone is expected to pass spontaneously within a reasonable time and the pain tolerable. In that case, the first approach shall be watchful waiting, with or without medical expulsive therapy (MET) [4].

The main objective of medical expulsive therapy is to increase the stone expulsion rate along the ureter and to eliminate the need for invasive intervention. Five pharmacological agents considered to affect ureteral motility and potentially increase the stone expulsion rate along the ureter are discussed in this section.

20.2.1 Non-steroidal Anti-inflammatory Drugs

Non-steroidal anti-inflammatory drugs (NSAIDs) inhibit the synthesis and the release of prostaglandins (PGH2, PGD2, PGE2, PGF2) from arachidonic acid, acting as non-selective inhibitors of cyclooxygenase (COX) enzymes, namely cyclooxygenase-1 (COX-1) and cyclooxygenase-2 (COX-2) isoforms [5]. While COX-1 is a constitutive form expressed in many tissues, COX-2 is an inducible form caused by various stimuli such as inflammatory mediators resulting from pathological events [6]; COX-2 expression is up-regulated in obstructed ureters as compared to unobstructed ureters [7]. The effect of PG release varies between obstructed and unobstructed ureters. It has been reported that PGF2α, PGD2, and TXA2 in vitro increase ureteral contraction, but PGE2 induces contraction in obstructed ureters while promoting relaxation in unobstructed ureters in porcine and human models [8].

Since prostaglandins promote ureteric contractility frequently, NSAIDs are considered to inhibit ureteric contractility. Non-selective COX inhibitors such as diclofenac and indomethacin and selective COX-2 inhibitors such as celecoxib are highly effective in preventing contractions of porcine and human ureters [9]. In addition, it is revealed that the selective COX-2 inhibitor NS-398 dose-dependently inhibits spontaneous rhythmic activity in humans and porcine [10]. Two randomized controlled trials demonstrated that patients using diclofenac and indomethacin do not experience improvement in stone passage rates or decreased time to passage. Additionally, it has been reported that COX inhibitors possess no impact on externally induced ureteric contractions in human and porcine ureters [11]. However, the effects of these drugs on ureteric contractility are still confusing. PG synthesis inhibition can lead to arteriolar vasoconstriction, potentially leading to acute renal failure. Therefore, whether they are appropriate pharmacological agents to induce spontaneous stone passage remains unclear.

It is well-known that increases are present in COX-2 expression and inflammatory prostaglandin production in the human ureter with acute ureteral obstruction. Since the alleged role of prostaglandins in increasing pain sensitivity, it is usual for NSAIDs to relieve renal colic in patients with urolithiasis. Consequently, NSAIDs are the recommended first-line treatment as they provide adequate analgesia in acute renal colic [4, 12]. However, since the primary purpose of medical expulsive therapy is to maintain spontaneous stone passage, using NSAIDs alone might be insufficient. A previous study revealed that these agents effectively reduce pain but still fail to alter the stone expulsion rate independently [13]. Nevertheless, patients presenting with renal colic might be offered NSAIDs in combination with α1-antagonists for pain relief and reduction of inflammation. As a result, the data we retrieved revealed that these drugs' impact is only to relieve pain.

20.2.2 α-Adrenoceptor Antagonists

α1-Adrenergic receptors (α1-ARs) are enabled by adrenaline and NA. Molecular clones have been isolated and characterized for three α1-subtypes as follows: α1A, α1B, and α1D. The α1B-subtype regulates blood pressure via contraction of the small resistance vessels, whereas α1A and α1D-subtype generally regulate smooth muscle tone in the ureter, prostate, and bladder neck. The three subtypes of α1-ARs are predominantly coupled by G-proteins of the Gq/11 family to activate the phospholipase C mechanism, stimulating smooth muscle contraction. Alpha-blockers shall be categorized as selective or non-selective based on their affinity for α1A and α1D receptors, which are abundant in the ureter [14]. The highest expression of α1D-adrenoceptors was observed in the ureter. However, the study of isolated human ureters reveals that the α1A adrenoceptor plays a more critical functional role in mediating contractile responses [14]. Several studies demonstrated that selective and non-selective alpha-blockers improve stone passage rates on distal ureter stones [15–17]. The mentioned studies suggest that these agents are effective in accelerating the passage of stones from the distal ureter and reducing attacks of renal colic. It is also reported that tamsulosin will facilitate the passage of stone fragments after shock wave lithotripsy and can be used as an additional medical treatment after SWL [18–20].

The SUSPEND trial published conflicting findings, a multicenter, randomized, placebo-controlled trial. One thousand and sixty-seven patients with a single ureteral stone smaller than 10 mm were randomly assigned to the study's placebo, nifedipine, or tamsulosin groups, which included 24 centers. No differences were present between the active treatment and placebo groups for up to 4 weeks or between the tamsulosin and nifedipine groups. No difference in pain score or time to stone passage was present [21]. Similar results were revealed in another randomized, double-blind, placebo-controlled, multicenter trial involving 403 patients. It was reported that tamsulosin has no overall benefit in patients with stones less than or equal to 10 mm in the distal ureter in terms of spontaneous passage, stone passage time, pain, or analgesia requirements. However, in the subgroup analysis of 5–10 mm stones, it was reported that tamsulosin increased the passage and should be considered [22]. These studies reported common side effects, including dizziness, hypotension, and retrograde ejaculation [23, 24].

Presently, there is an increase in interest in using the selective α1A-adrenoceptor antagonist silodosin. It has been reported that a significant increase is present in the stone expulsion rate. In a multi-institutional, randomized, double-blinded, placebo-controlled study investigating the efficacy of silodosin, no significant difference was present between the silodosin and placebo groups in terms of passage rate for all stones (52% vs. 44%). However, in the subgroup analysis, the distal ureteral stones passage rate was significantly higher with silodosin than with placebo (69% vs. 46%, respectively) [25].

In conclusion, current recommendations for medical expulsive therapy by the European Association of Urology are to use α-blockers as the most appropriate option for stones between 5 mm and 10 mm located in the distal ureter [4].

20.2.3 Calcium Channel Blockers

Calcium channel blockers constitute a group of medications that perform to inhibit either central or peripheral calcium channels. This inhibition results in decreased calcium influx and smooth muscle relaxation. Therefore, studies have been conducted on the issue of whether it might be utilized to encourage spontaneous passage while minimizing ureteral spasms and pain. For example, it was reported that calcium channel blockers such as nifedipine, verapamil, and diltiazem inhibit ureteric contraction in pigs and humans [26, 27].

It has been stated that nifedipine and verapamil inhibit fast-phase contractions while preserving slow-phase contractions. Thus, it has been reported to maintain normal peristalsis and prevent painful ureteral spasms [28]. However, in perhaps the first double-blind, placebo-controlled clinical study, it was stated that nifedipine was not significantly different from placebo in providing relief from acute renal colic [29].

Clinical studies have shown that nifedipine is highly effective in increasing stone passage when combined with corticosteroids. A randomized, double-blind study that compares the nifedipine versus placebo groups with methylprednisolone given to both groups included 86 patients, reveals the increased stone clearance rates (86% versus 65%) and a less mean time to passage (11.2 days vs. 16.5 days) in the nifedipine group compared to the placebo group [30]. In another study conducted in the following years, patients were divided into three groups: deflazacort + nifedipine, deflazacort + tamsulosin, and control group, and expulsion rates were reported as 80%, 85%, and 43%, respectively. Medical treatments with nifedipine and tamsulosin have been revealed to provide a reduced need for analgesic therapy with increasing expulsion rates [31]. Subsequent clinical studies investigating the clinical significance of nifedipine alone were shown to be effective in increasing the rate of excretion. However, it constitutes significantly lower efficacy compared to tamsulosin [21]. Furthermore, nifedipine is associated with side effects such as nausea, vomiting, headache, and drowsiness. Due to the requirement to be combined with steroid therapy and its lower effectiveness, it is one step behind the α-blockers today.

20.2.4 *β-Adrenoceptor Agonists*

In the lower urinary tract, β1-, β2- and β3-adrenoceptors cause relaxation of the detrusor muscle of the bladder. Normal bladder detrusors can express β1-, β2- and β3-adrenoceptors mRNAs, and selective β3-adrenoceptor agonists effectively relax the detrusor via both β1-adrenoceptor and β2-adrenoceptor [32, 33]. Mirabegron is the first β3-adrenoceptor agonist revealed to be clinically effective in reducing symptoms of overactive bladder. Its lower side-effect profile has rendered it a popular alternative over time.

Although a general functional predominance of α1-adrenoceptors in the ureter is present, the role of β-adrenoceptors in the ureter cannot be understated [34]. Human ureteral relaxation has been stated to be mediated by both β2- and β3 adrenoceptor stimulation. It has been emphasized that β3-adrenoceptor agonists have the potential to relax the human ureter, and clinical applications are expected in the treatment of ureteral stones [35].

Subsequent studies have shown varying mirabegron results in stone expulsion rates, stone expulsion time, and pain control [36, 37]. In addition, well-designed clinical trials are required regarding the utilization of mirabegron in MET.

20.2.5 *Phosphodiesterase (PDE) Inhibitors*

Phosphodiesterase 5 (PDE5) inhibitors such as sildenafil and tadalafil are mainly utilized to manage and endure conditions such as erectile dysfunction, pulmonary hypertension, and benign prostatic hyperplasia. PDE5 inhibitors catalyze the hydrolysis of second messengers and attenuate PDE enzyme function that usually suppresses intracellular cAMP or cGMP levels. In smooth muscle cells, these inhibitors increase cAMP/cGMP levels by preventing the degradation of second messengers by PDE, thereby enhancing the effects of nitric oxide (NO). In addition, nitric Oxide (NO) is an important inhibitory neurotransmitter in the lower urinary tract [38]. In addition, NO-mediated responses in smooth muscle have been revealed to be associated with increased formation of cGMP in the rabbit and pig urethra [39, 40]. Correspondingly, NO is an important inhibitory neurotransmitter in the ureter. In vitro, NO inhibits ureteral contractility in rats [41]. Based on axons that stain positively for NO synthase in the human ureter, it has been suggested that NO may play a role in ureteral relaxation [42]. Sildenafil, tadalafil, and vardenafil have also been shown to reduce KCl-induced tonic contractions in human isolated ureteral smooth muscle in vitro [43].

Even though there is evidence to support the use of PDE5 inhibitors for stone expulsion in physiological studies, there are currently few clinical studies recommending PDE5 inhibitors in medical expulsive therapy [44]. Although it has been reported that tadalafil is superior to tamsulosin in stone expulsion, this issue remains unclarified. For example, when tamsulosin vs. combined tamsulosin and tadalafil were compared, no significant difference in stone removal rate could be demonstrated [45]. However, due to these controversial issues, large-scale clinical studies are needed in the future.

Key Reading
Medical expulsive therapy with alpha-receptor antagonists potentially shortens the duration and increases the likelihood of spontaneous stone passage. Consideration should be given to offering it to patients with distal ureteral stones with a size of > 5 mm.

20.3 Extracorporeal Shock Wave Lithotripsy (ESWL)

20.3.1 History

Extracorporeal shock wave lithotripsy (ESWL) was developed in the early 1960s based on Claude Dornier's discovery. It has been revealed that raindrops might damage the wings of an airplane flying at the speed of sound and that the damage is not only caused by an external, pure blow but by shock waves transmitted inward by the water. This invention was the basis of the idea of treating kidney stones with the help of targeted shock waves in humans. The first standard lithotripter, "Human Model 3" (HM3), was genuinely developed in 1980 with the work of the Ludwig-Maximilians-University hospital in Germany. Even though ESWL has been an established treatment for urolithiasis [46], there are growing apprehensions about the effectiveness thereof compared to endoscopic techniques. Initially, spinal or general anesthesia was required for the applications performed with the HM3 system, depending on the patient's age. Another disadvantage is that the system cannot be used as versatile and multidisciplinary. In addition, it was challenging for the patient to maintain his position in the water pool. This system could not be used effectively in ureteral lower-end stones. Innovations in shock wave generation, focusing, and stone localization systems were carried out in the second generation stone crushing devices that were developed and marketed later. A water pad has been designed to discard the water pool in previous devices. Thus, patients were prevented from entering a completely water-filled pool, and the lower end stones of the ureter, which will be performed in the prone position, shall be easily managed. Nevertheless, the high level of initial effort, and especially the high cost of stone surgeries, conveyed technological advances. Although more advanced ESWL devices are used today, patients' demand to be completely stone-free in a single session has limited the use of ESWL in treating stones larger than 1 cm [47].

20.3.2 Fundamentals

Shock waves refer to acoustic impulses of high energy. These waves are produced at various energy levels using different (electro-hydraulic, electromagnetic, piezo-electric) techniques. Inside the body, the shock waves are transmitted through the aqueous tissues without being affected and can be focused on the intended treatment area. Despite many lithotripters, these devices are based on the same acoustic physics laws. The shock wave, consisting of a sharp peak in the positive wave followed by the negative withdrawal wave, is produced outside the body and passed through to fragment the stones [48].

20.3.2.1 Electrohydraulic Generator

Electrohydraulic Generator is the first electrohydraulic shock wave source utilized in the Dornier HM3. Shock waves are generated via a spark gap. High-voltage ignition creates rapid evaporation in the water and expands the surrounding liquid, resulting in the formation of a shock wave. The generator is positioned inside an ellipsoidal reflector, concentrating the reflecting shock waves in a second focal focus. Pressure values change significantly due to electrode burning (jitter effect). Accordingly, a maximum of 3000–4000 pulses might be produced with one electrode. The electroconductive system portrays a further technical development of electrohydraulic shock wave generation, and the electrode tips adapt after each shot. This technique minimizes the vibration effect and extends the service life of an electrode to 40,000 pulses.

20.3.2.2 Electromagnetic Generator

Electromagnetic shock wave devices have been used since 1985 and are the most widely used devices today. Shock waves in electromagnetic devices are generated when an electrical impulse moves a thin circular metallic membrane in the middle of the cylindrical shock tube. The shock wave passes through an acoustic lens and is directed to the first focal point. The shock wave reaches the body surface through the moving water pad and gel. Alternatively, the magnetic field generated as energy passes through the cylindrical coil pushes the cylindrical membrane to create a shock wave that can be focused on the parabolic reflector. The advantage of electromagnetic shock wave generation lies in its constant pressure values and long service life of about 1 million pulses.

20.3.2.3 Piezoelectric Generator

Piezoelectric shock wave generation is based on the simultaneous oscillation of spherically arranged piezoceramic elements. Only one of the original four systems is still in use today in a modified form. The piezoceramic elements tenderly come together to form a pulse of electrical energy. The sum of the simultaneous expansion of many piezoceramic elements aggregates into a high-energy shock wave directed towards the focal center at the center of the sphere. The shock wave propagates towards the small pool of water or the water-filled sac at the focal point. The spherical focusing mechanism of piezoelectric lithotriptors creates a wide shock wave entry point on the skin surface where patients may experience minimal discomfort.

However, it makes a narrow focal point with a bit of energy compared to other energy sources. The advantage of the piezoelectric system is the long service life with more than a million pulses, in addition to the low pain level.

20.3.3 Shockwave Focusing

The focal size and maximum shock wave pressure of a lithotripter depend primarily on the patency of the shock wave system and the energy emitted. A stone-specific adaptation of the focal size shall be helpful theoretically. This technique shall be applied in different ways. For example, with the Storz Modulith SLX-F2, the temporary lengthening of the shock wave pulse results in widening the focus area. At the same time, the Piezolith 3000 achieves to reach this by time-delayed activation of the two layers of the piezoceramic element. Recently, there has been an increasing interest in lithotripters with a broad focus and relatively low shock wave pressure.

On the one hand, this instance is based on stone fragmentation theories. In vitro studies show good disintegration efficiency of these systems in an animal model of stone with minimal kidney lesion [49]. Theoretically, the broad focus offers the advantage of applying sufficient shock wave energies with a relatively low energy density. On the other hand, however, there are no comparative clinical studies here either. Fluoroscopy and ultrasound ordinarily provide stone localization and focusing during the lithotripsy procedure. Fluoroscopy is a method familiar to the urologist and facilitates the utilization of contrast material to define the anatomy of the collecting system. However, it necessitates a larger area, bears the risk of ionizing radiation for the patient and healthcare team, and is unsuitable for radiolucent stones. Lithotripters utilizing sonography offer the advantage of stone localization with continuous monitoring. It demonstrates radiolucent stones without radiation risk.

Additionally, ultrasound has been proven effective in localizing smaller stone fragments [50]. The furthermost substantial disadvantage of stone localization with ultrasound is that urologists who perform this procedure might not have as much knowledge of ultrasound images as fluoroscopy. Despite this, it has been reported that urologists have recently commenced utilizing ultrasound appropriately in treating stones.

20.3.4 ESWL Therapy

As the standard, ESWL is performed in the supine position. Treatment in the prone position shall be chosen carefully, while stones cannot be reached by shock waves directly in the supine position. Routine use of JJ stents before ESWL does not improve SFRs, nor reduce the number of adjunctive therapies. However, it has been revealed to reduce the formation of steinstrasse [51, 52]. Patients with pacemakers can be treated with ESWL provided appropriate precautions are taken. For example, in patients with implanted cardioverter defibrillators, the firing mode shall be reprogrammed temporarily during ESWL therapy. However, this might not be necessitated in new generation ESWL devices [53]. No standard antibiotic prophylaxis before ESWL is recommended; however, prophylaxis is recommended in case of JJ stenting before ESWL and where the bacterial load may be high, such as an indwelling catheter, or nephrostomy tube, or infectious stones [54]. It has been reported that mechanical percussion and diuretic therapy shall significantly improve SFRs and accelerate stone passage after ESWL [55, 56].

More than 80% of urinary tract stones are suitable for SWL treatment. However, the success depends on the SWL device's effectiveness, the stone size, its localization, the skin to the stone distance, the stone type, and the anatomical features of the patient and ureter/kidney. Additionally, particular conditions such as the presence of obstruction, calyceal diverticula, abnormal kidneys, and the function of the contralateral kidney affect the ESWL success. One of the critical factors preventing success is the patient's body mass index (BMI). Most lithotripters have a focusing length of 15 cm. Excess fatty tissue prevents the energy from reaching the stone from the shock wave. In such patients, a stone-skin distance measured by non-contrast computed tomography is a better predictor than BMI [57]. The stone size is another factor affecting the success of ESWL. The EAU and AUA guidelines do not recommend ESWL as first-line therapy for stones larger than 2 cm. ESWL success is expected to be highly low in these stones, and alternative endourological methods should be preferred in these patients [4]. The variation in stone composition, which affects its fragmentation, creates differences in the ESWL response. For instance, uric acid and calcium oxalate dihydrate stones are more easily fragmented, but cystine, calcium oxalate monohydrate, and brushite stones are more difficult to fragment [58]. Another essential factor in a stone composition is the density of the stone. It is well-known that stones with a density of >1000 HU constitute a low probability of fragmentation with ESWL. A study investigating the efficacy of ESWL in upper ureteral stones stated that ureterorenoscopy (URS) was superior to ESWL in upper ureteral stones with a size of >10 mm. Still, no difference was found between ESWL and URS in stones with a size of <10 mm [59]. The success of ESWL was revealed to be 68.8% for upper ureteral stones and 72.7% for lower ureteral stones [60]. The EAU guidelines recommend URS as the first choice in treating upper ureteral stones >10 mm in size and ESWL or URS as the first choice in treating stones <10 mm. It has been reported that URS shall be the first choice for stones >10 mm in the lower ureter, and ESWL or URS may be chosen as the first choice for stones <10 mm [4].

In summary, the factors affecting the success of ESWL;

- The size of the stone,
- The content of the stone,
- The Hounsfield unit of the stone,
- Location of the stone,

- Anomalies of the kidney
- Anatomical differences in the location of the stone,
  - infundibulopelvic angle
  - infundibulum length and width
  - skin-to-stone distance
- The general physical condition of the patient,
- Patient compliance, and
- Type of device.

With medical expulsive therapy (MET) after ESWL, the rate of stone expulsion increases, and the need for NSAID use for pain decreases. Therefore, EAU guidelines recommend MET for treating residual fragments after ESWL. Within a systemic review made by Scolaricos et al., it has been revealed that the SFRs increased, and the time until stone resolution decreased with MET after ESWL [61].

20.3.5 Contraindications for SWL

Situations where ESWL is contraindicated are listed below:

- Urinary tract infection → risk of urosepsis.
- Impaired drainage distal to the stone → lack of passage capability
- Impaired hemostasis → risk of bleeding.
- Anticoagulation → risk of bleeding.
- Aneurysm in the target region or abdomen → risk of damage of aneurysm.
- Severe skeletal deformities and obesity → Difficult to focus
- Pregnancy → potential harm to the fetus

20.3.6 Complications

Although large series of studies demonstrate that ESWL is a safe and effective method, it is a fact that it possesses the potential for serious side effects and complications. Numerous studies are present regarding the direct traumatic impact of the shock wave on the kidney parenchyma. For example, in the renal parenchyma, the damage is initially observed in the medullary veins-arteries and tubules area (grade I lesion). Cortical arterioles are then ruptured (grade II/III lesion). Although the trauma mechanism is not yet fully understood, these lesions are dose-dependent [62]. Therefore, it is presumed that the pulling forces due to cavitation in the parenchyma and vessels fulfill a significant role [49].

Regarding the side effects associated with direct shock wave application, in addition to ecchymosis, which might occur in 5–35% of cases, shock wave-induced renal trauma might occur. Subcapsular hematoma rarely requires surgical intervention and appears in 4–5% of treatments [63]. Other complications caused by shock waves are rare: gastrointestinal bleeding up to colonic perforation and duodenal erosion were observed in 1.8% [64]. Rarely, spleen or liver hematoma might develop.

Early complications after ESWL are mainly based on problems with the stone expulsion. When the stone load is high, stone path formation might be observed. This instance might usually be managed with medical treatment. Ureteral JJ or percutaneous nephrostomy is required in 2–8% of cases, and endourological intervention is necessary for 2–10%. Although bacteremia is seen at a rate of 10–14%, the risk of urosepsis is less than 1%. Among the chronic effects of ESWL are decreased kidney function, scar development in the kidney, perirenal fibrosis, ureteral fibrosis, and ureterocolic fistula. In addition, a causal relationship between ESWL and the development of diabetes mellitus or hypertension has not been proven [65]. Risk factors that might cause complications shall be evaluated before the procedure, and short and long-term side effects of ESWL shall be well investigated and treated on time if necessary.

Key Reading
It might be the treatment method preferred in the first line, especially in adults with < 10 mm middle and upper ureteral stones. It should be known that the contraindications and its success are related to many factors related to the patient, stone, and equipment. Stone composition, stone density, and skin-to-stone distance should be used when possible to counsel patients regarding the success of ESWL treatment for patients presenting with ureteral stones. Known cystine, calcium oxalate monohydrate, and brushite stones are likely best treated with URS. Patients with ureteral stones with a density greater than 1000 HU or skin-to-stone distance greater than 10 cm are more likely to fail ESWL. Although it is the most minimally invasive treatment option, the complications that may arise and the need for additional treatment should be discussed with the patient.

20.4 Ureteroscopic Removal of the Stones: Retrograde; Antegrade; Semirigid; Flexible Maneuvers

20.4.1 History

The impact of endoscopic access in the field of urology shall not be overstated. Due to the miniaturization of endoscopic imaging and instruments since the early nineteenth century, open procedures have been completely replaced by endoscopic techniques. In the early 1960s, Marshall stated the first transurethral flexible ureteroscopy by inserting a 9 F flexible fiberoptic scope into a ureterotomy performed during open surgery to inspect for calculi. To visualize calculus, a 9 F flexible endoscope was passed through a 26 F McCarthy sheath into the ureter [66]. In later years, Goodman [67] and Lyon [68] utilized pediatric cystoscopes for distal ureteroscopy in women. Lyon subsequently used longer, juvenile cystoscopes in men [69]. But these tools were large, and techniques still had to be developed. In line with this purpose, urethral dilators, unguided interchangeable bougies, wire-guided bougies, and balloons were invented. Das performed the first transurethral ureteroscopic basket removal of a stone in 1981 [70]. Since the devices were not identified as flexible enough in those years, reaching the ureter proximal to the iliac vessels was impossible. In the 1980s, Olympus developed a flexible ureteroscope based on the pediatric bronchoscope. After these significant developments, the endoscopic systems with high technology we use today have been attained.

While specific notable differences are present, contemporary flexible ureteroscopes constitute similar features. Most flexible ureteroscopes have a 3.6 F working channel that allows passage of guidewires, stone baskets, laser fibers, and irrigation. The Richard Wolf Cobra vision ureteroscope is the only dual-channel ureteroscope with both 3.6 F and 2.4 F working channels. It allows simultaneous utilization of any binary combination of the instruments. Alternatively, irrigation might be achieved well by leaving one of the working channels empty. In flexible ureteroscopy, significant optical progress has been achieved in the last decade with the development of flexible digital ureteroscopes. Significant visual progress has been made in flexible ureteroscopy over the past decade. Flexible digital ureteroscopes provide significantly faster operating times and improvements in durability compared to fiberoptic flexible ureteroscope scopes [71, 72]. The tip size of reusable digital ureteroscopes ranges from 5.2 F to 8.4 F. Still, the more significant shaft size ranges from 8.5 F to 8.9 F for single-channel scopes and 9.9 F for dual-channel flexible ureteroscopes.

20.4.2 *Indication*

The European Association of Urology Guidelines has identified some indications for the active removal of ureteral stones. For example, stones that are unlikely to passage spontaneously, persistent pain despite adequate analgesic drug use, persistent obstruction, and renal dysfunction (kidney failure, bilateral obstruction, solitary kidney).

The EAU guidelines recommend URS as the first choice in treating upper ureteral stones >10 mm in size and ESWL or URS as the first choice in treating stones <10 mm. It has been reported that URS may be the first choice for stones >10 mm in the lower ureter, and ESWL or URS may be chosen as the first choice for stones <10 mm [4].

URS shall be performed during pregnancy only if a compulsive indication is present.

20.4.3 Ureteroscopy (Retrograde and Antegrade) for Ureter Stones

URSs are divided into two as follows: rigid and flexible. Rigid URS might be utilized for stones in any location in the ureter. Today, under optimum conditions, semirigid URS is recommended for distal ureter stones up to the iliac cross, and flexible URS is recommended for proximal stones thereon. The availability of digital scopes and technical advances support using flexible ureteroscopes in the ureter [73].

Rupel and Brown utilized a surgically established nephrostomy tract to remove an obstructing kidney stone [74]. About 15 years later, Goodwin et al. stated that a percutaneous nephrostomy tube was utilized to relieve obstruction and infection [75]. Percutaneous antegrade removal of ureteral stones can be applied in large (>15 mm), impacted proximal ureteral stones in the dilated renal collecting system [76, 77], or when the ureter is not amenable to retrograde manipulation [78, 79]. The procedure is performed in four consecutive steps, similar to percutaneous nephrolithotomy:

1. providing percutaneous access,
2. dilation of the tract
3. stone manipulation by fragmentation and extraction; and
4. drainage and tamponade of the tract after extraction.

Urinary tract infections shall be evaluated and treated before the procedure. Antibiotic prophylaxis shall be recommended in all patients before the endoscopic procedure. Even though it is possible to perform the operations under local or spinal anesthesia, most interventions are performed under general anesthesia conditions. Intravenous sedation might be applied in female patients with distal ureteral stones. Routine stenting before ureteroscopy is not recommended. Ureteroscopy might be performed in patients with bleeding disorders with a modest increase in complications [4].

20.4.3.1 Semirigid Ureteroscopy

The body of semirigid ureterorenoscopes enables a small amount of inclination, and the ends are generally conical (6–9 Fr). The proximal thickening provides both an increase in strength and a gradual dilatation as the ureteroscope progresses. The metal body comprises fiberoptic bundles (2.4–4 Fr) for light and vision outside the irrigation and working channel. Although the fiber optic system does not provide as good image quality as the rod lens system, it is favored today because of its thinning feature in the diameter of the ureteroscope. Today, digital semirigid ureterorenoscopes are developed with "Charge-coupled device (CCD) video chip technology.

Semirigid URS can be performed at certain times for renal pelvis and upper ureter stones. The procedure usually initiates with a diagnostic cystoscopy. Before semirigid instrument endoscopy of the ureter, a safety wire is placed in the renal pelvis under X-ray control. If pyuria occurs during the procedure, the procedure does not proceed, but a JJ stent is attached, and URS is performed in two stages [80].

Balloon and plastic dilators shall be available, if necessary. After reaching the stone, the stone is held in one piece with the stone basket, and the stone is removed so that the ureteral mucosa is not damaged. Therefore, it remains in the center of the endoscopic view. In particular cases of larger stones, firstly, the stone might be crushed and then the pieces removed. Extreme attention shall be given when removing sharp-edged parts. A size comparison can be made with the safety wire previously known to have a diameter of about 0.5–1 mm to determine the appropriate piece size that can be removed from the ureter without resistance. If the ureteroscope fails to advance through the ureter, the procedure is finished, and a JJ stent is placed. In the EAU guideline, stenting is not recommended in uncomplicated cases after URS. However, a stent shall be placed in all suspicious cases and cases with a high risk of complications such as ureteral trauma, residual stone fragments, bleeding, perforation, infection, or pregnancy. Alpha-blocker drugs can reduce stent-related symptoms [4].

20.4.3.2 Flexible Ureteroscopy

Working channels of flexible ureterorenoscopes vary between 2.5 and 5 Fr, usually 3.6 Fr. The tips vary between 5.2–8.4 Fr and widen as it approaches the proximal body parts. The tips of the flexible ureteroscope might deflect 160–275° in one direction and 130–250° in the other. During active utilization of the working channel (with laser, basket, etc.), the body of the ureterorenoscope begins more rigid. This feature reduces the deflection ability of the ureterorenoscope. Again, during the active utilization of the working channel, the irrigation flow decreases and might cause deterioration in image quality.

The imaging system in flexible ureterorenoscopes might be fiberoptic as well as digital systems based on complementary metal-oxide semiconductor (CMOS) or CCD technology. Due to the high repair and replacement costs of reusable flexible ureterorenoscopes, disposable flexible ureterorenoscopes have been developed. Certain types of these devices are fiberoptic, and some are digital. The advantages of disposable flexible URSs are that they are always ready for use, are permanently sterile, and have no traces of instrument wear. While these advantages protect from nosocomial infections, they reduce delays and waiting in operations. It also avoids sterilization and repair costs.

20.4.3.3 Other Instruments Used in Ureterorenoscopy

Guide Wires

Guidewires refer to wires used in ureteroscopic procedures to facilitate ureteral entry, guide instrumentation, and safety in highly curved ureters. Coating materials (PTFE, nitinol, hydrophilic polymer) and core materials (stainless steel, nitinol, triton) are accessible. They might be of a combined structure (such as hydrophilic tip and PTFE coated body). Various length (145–150 cm), diameter (0.025, 0.035 and 0.038) and tip configurations (straight or angled) are available.

Ureteral Dilators

Dilators might be needed in cases where ureteral access cannot be accessed, or the ureteral access sheath cannot be advanced, such as ureteral stricture, spasm, or narrow ureteral orifice. Ureteral balloon dilators are used when the ureteral access sheath cannot be advanced to the desired area. Balloon dilators have body diameters ranging from 3 F to 8 F; 30–150 cm long; having a lumen that allows the guidewire to pass through. These are the balloon catheters that, when inflated, reach a diameter of 12—30 F and a pressure of 20—30 atmospheres. Balloon dilatation is applied before ureteroscopy. It has side effects such as mucosal damage, ureteral extravasation, and temporary vesicoureteral reflux.

Ureteral Catheters

Ureteral catheters might be used for several functions, such as contrast agent infusion and ureteral dilation. It is mainly of polyurethane construction and is available in various lengths (70–135 cm), diameters (3–10 F), and tip (cone, olive, open, tube, spiral) configurations. The double lumen ones have a 0.038″ diameter guidewire channel and a 0.050″ diameter liquid, contrast material, or safety wire channel.

Basket Catheters, Graspers, and Forceps

Each instrument is ascertained by stone manipulation, the radial force it provides to open the ureter, and its ability to capture, hold, and, if necessary, release the stone. The first stone baskets were of Dornier design, with three or four helical steel wires and straight or filiform tips, and modifications are still used in semirigid URSs today. Segura-designed baskets consist of four flat stainless steel wires and might be opened widely in relatively small areas, thus collecting stones in the renal pelvis and calyces. However, its rigid structure prevents the deflection of flexible instruments and causes trauma in the minor calyces. The tipless design of the nitinol (nickel-titanium alloy) baskets and the flexibility of nitinol allow deflection of flexible devices while preventing papilla injury when collecting calyx stones. Reducing their size to 1.3 F diameter ensures minimal impact on irrigation, even with 7.5 F diameter flexible ureteroscopes.

Ureteral Stents

Ureteral stents dilate urinary strictures and remove kidney stones and temporary drainage. This type of stent might be made of polyurethane or silicone structure. Various lengths (14–32 cm), diameter (3–8 F), body, tip shapes (pigtail, double pigtail-JJ), and coating materials (carbon, hydrophilic, heparin) according to the purpose of utilization are present. Metal stents are also accessible for benign or malignant strictures.

Lithotripters

The most effective lithotripsy system is the Ho: YAG laser, which has become the gold standard for URS and flexible ureteroscopy due to its safety and effectiveness in all stone compositions. Compared to the electro-hydraulic lithotripter (EHL), Ho: YAG energy does not pose a risk of perforation even at short distances such as 0.5–0.9 mm to the ureteral wall, as the fluid well absorbs the energy. It also degrades and decomposes the stone by forming a vaporization bubble. The increase in laser probe diameter correlates with a decreased active deflection of the flexible nephroscope. However, the 365 μm laser probe is more durable and associated with higher lithotripsy rates. This deflection loss is 18–37% for the 365-μm probe and 7–16% for the 200-μm probe. The power of the holmium laser is set at 10–15 W to 0.5–1.2 J and 5–15 Hz. However, settings might vary depending on the lithotripsy method. When surgeons apply the dusting technique, they usually maintain power by increasing the speed and lowering the frequency.

Holmium YAG laser has some disadvantages, such as the retropulsion of stone fragments. To solve this problem, Lumenis has developed a technology called the Moses technology. In Moses technology, the current pulse is split into two adjacent peak pulses. The first peak beat separates the water and the second peak beat passes through the bubble formed by the separation of the water and proceeds towards the stone. Thus, less energy is lost, and the distance between the stone-laser cable becomes less critical. With Moses technology, less operation time and retropulsion might be achieved compared to the standard Ho: YAG laser. Currently, the cost is a significant problem. Thulium fiber laser (TFL) technology, in which a different element is used, is becoming popular daily. The TFL grants the advantages of having laser probes as small as 50 μm in stone crushing, pulse energy as low as 0.025 J, and super high pulse rates up to 2000 Hz. It is mentioned that with TFL, four times more ablation is achieved, stones might be divided into smaller pieces, and less retropulsion is present. It is also suggested that better deflection can be completed in devices with thin laser cable, a better image can be obtained with more irrigation fluid flow, and miniaturization devices provide better ergonomics. Since it is a new technology and clinical studies are scarce, more studies are needed to make it widespread in practical use.

20.4.4 Complications

Fever and urinary tract infections following ureteroscopy occur in up to 15% of cases [81]. Urosepsis occurs in up to 4% of patients following ureteroscopy. When they remain untreated, this complication might be fatal after ureteroscopy [82]. Mucosal ureteral erosions, false passages, submucosal tunneling, and ureteral perforations usually occur during lithotripsy, stone removal, ureteroscope ascending, or ureteral access sheath placement. The reported incidence of mucosal erosion and false passage after ureteroscopy is up to 10%, and perforation is up to 7% [83, 84]. Most authors recommend proceeding with intervention despite lesions and then retrograde or antegrade ureteral stenting. Ureteral strictures generally occur in up to 3% of patients after ureteroscopic procedures. Rarely these cases may require nephrectomy. A ureteral avulsion is one of the most devastating complications during ureteroscopy. It is relatively rare; moreover, an incidence of up to 0.4% has been revealed. An avulsion occurs more frequently in the proximal ureter because of the less prominent muscular wall [85]. Ureteral stent migration has a reported incidence of up to 4% [86]. Intraoperative bleeding frequently occurs during ureteroscopy. Blood transfusion is performed in up to 1% of ureteroscopic cases [85]. Rarely angiographic techniques are necessitated to treat life-threatening bleeding [87]. Rarely, urinoma, perirenal abscess, and subcapsular, perirenal, and retroperitoneal hematoma may occur during ureteroscopy due to high intrarenal pressure and iatrogenic trauma of the pelvicalyceal system. Rarely these cases may require nephrectomy.

Key Reading

Compared to SWL, URS is associated with higher SFRs. URS is associated with fewer needs for retreatment and secondary procedures, while higher complication rates and longer hospital stays. Patients should be informed that with URS, there is a better chance of achieving a stone-free state with a single procedure and that URS has higher complication rates than ESWL.

20.5 Laparoscopic and Robotic Ureterolithotomy

Due to developments in shock wave therapy, URS, and percutaneous interventions, minimally invasive interventions have largely replaced open surgery. The place of laparoscopic and open surgery in treating ureteral stones is finite today. Laparoscopic ureterolithotomy (LU) is indicated in patients with large, upper/middle/lower ureteral stones causing obstruction where other minimally invasive treatments have failed. Some randomized studies have reported a higher SFR (76–86% vs. 88–100%) in LU after the first procedure compared to endourological techniques. However, LU has some disadvantages regarding invasiveness, operative time, and complications. Consequently, LU should be considered second-line therapy for complex cases [88].

Laparoscopic stone treatment was first defined in 1994 [89]. Gaur's discovery of balloon dilation in the retroperitoneal space contributed significantly to the development of laparoscopy in urology [90]. Afterward, its efficacy has been demonstrated in numerous studies; the SFR has been revealed as 71–100%. The conversion rate to openness has been reported to be between 0% and 27% [91, 92]. Wang et al. summarized the results of PNL vs. LU in a 2013 meta-analysis. They found similarly reasonable success rates (>95%) after both procedures, advantages of PNL in terms of operative time and hospital stay, but disadvantages in terms of blood loss and occurrence of fever [93]. In a prospective study, ESWL, LU, and URS were compared in patients with stones larger than 1 cm, and the SFR was found to be higher in the LU group compared to URS and SWL (93% vs. 62% vs. 35%, respectively) [94]. In addition, LU and ureteroscopy were compared in the study, and a high SFR and short operation time were found in the LU group [95].

Technically, the basic surgical principles of the open surgical approach are also rational here. However, the most challenging part of the surgery is determining the stone's localization. Ureteral peristalsis helps determine the bulging stone localization created by the stone in the ureter. If available, intraoperative laparoscopic ultrasound or ICG (indocyanine green) are the other helpful techniques in determining the localization of the stone and ureter [96]. After the stone localization is selected, the stone is removed with a ureteral incision, and the ureter is sutured. Subsequent JJ stent placement is often preferred.

The most crucial advantage of LU is as follows: it provides 95% success in a single session without the need for additional intervention [97]. A complementary, flexible ureteroscopy might be performed through ports as part of laparoscopy. However, this has implications such as increased cost and processing time.

Even though it has been suggested that LU is a more practical approach for stones localized in the ureter segment between the lower border of the kidney and the common iliac vessels, it has been reported that LU has similar success rates in distal ureteral stones with laparoscopic experience [98]. LU is performed with a transperitoneal or retroperitoneal approach, depending on the surgeon's experience and preference. On the one hand, a risk is present regarding the contact of infected urine with the peritoneal cavity and organs in transperitoneal laparoscopic procedures for urinary system stones. On the other hand, studies report that no significant complications develop in transabdominal techniques [91, 99]. It has been shown that bowel motility is gained late with the transperitoneal approach, and the need for analgesics, ileus and hospital stay is more prolonged [100]. However, the transperitoneal approach also has advantages. These advantages incorporate larger space, familiar anatomical points, easy front access to the pelvis in horseshoe kidneys, and easy dissection to the lower levels of the ureter. In the first prospective nonrandomized study comparing the two methods in treating upper ureteral stones, the SFR rates of the two techniques were revealed to be similar. Total operative time, time to access the operative field, and time required for ureter suturing were shorter in the transperitoneal group [101]. In a prospective randomized study comparing transperitoneal and retroperitoneal approaches in patients with middle and upper ureteral stones, no significant difference was revealed between the groups regarding SFR rate, total operation time, intracorporeal suture time, and postoperative pain score. Morbidity and hospital stay were higher in the transperitoneal group [100].

The advantages of robot-assisted laparoscopy are due to the improved mobility of the instruments mainly. Suturing the kidneys, pyelocaliceal system, and ureters is much easier and faster, and also easier to grasp hard-to-reach concretes in the pyelocaliceal system without using a flexible ureteroscope. Therefore, it is not startling that the case series investigating the value of robotics in stone treatment has increased [102]. However, the increased costs, availability, and possibility of intraoperative fluoroscopy should be kept in mind.

Flexible ureteroscopy constitutes certain ergonomic shortcomings. The surgeon usually stands and controls the fluoroscopy and laser device with a foot pedal, fixing the position of the endoscope with one hand and deflecting/rotating it with the other. Placing the laser fiber or any accessory tool (basket, N-gage) is also challenging. In addition, certain researchers have developed newly developed robotic RIRS platforms (Robotic master-slave systems) for performing surgery by offering an ergonomic working position without increasing the risk of damaging the urogenital system.

Robotic master-slave systems include various robotic devices developed for neurosurgery, NOTES, interventional radiology, cardiology, and endourology [103–105]. In 2008, Desai et al. [106] stated a flexible robotic ureteroscopy using the Sensei-Magellan system (Hansen Medical, Mountain View, USA) designed initially for cardiology and angiography. Since 2010, ELMED (Ankara, Turkey) has been working on a robot named Roboflex Avicenna, which is specially designed for flexible ureteroscopy and provides the necessary functions for flexible URS [107]. Another platform is called the Monarch Platform. In March 2018, the Monarch Platform was used for the first time in a clinical case of robotic bronchoscopy. The system utilizes the standard endoscopy procedure to place a flexible robot in hard-to-reach places inside the human body.

Studies with the Avicenna Roboflex™ have revealed that it might safely and successfully implement all modern techniques and protocols of flexible URS, such as laser dusting, using the popcorn/Jacuzzi effect, and extraction of larger fragments [108]. A phase-3 study comparing robot-assisted and conventional flexible URS reported that treatment time and fragmentation time were similar, but the SFR was better in robot-assisted flexible URS (92.4% vs. 89.4%) [109].

The criticisms are present regarding the issue of utilizing the robot for flexible URS regarding unnecessary costs, robotic hype, and the eventual effectiveness of the device [110]. It should be noted that the most substantial aspect of these systems is that they provide ergonomics to the surgeon. Therefore, it shall not be startling to see similar SFRs with conventional flexible URS in future studies. Although no evidence exists, the absence of haptic sensation can cause unexpected complications.

Key Reading

Currently, laparoscopic or robotic ureterolithotomy has a narrow indication for managing ureteral stones. Laparoscopic or robotic ureterolithotomy may be considered when ureteroscopic procedures fail, or concomitant surgery is required.

20.6 Open Ureterolithotomy

Open surgical methods were considered the gold standard before using endoscopic techniques in the surgical treatment of ureteral stones. Due to the high invasiveness of open stone surgeries, and today almost every patient might be treated with a minimally invasive procedure, the rate of open surgeries has dropped sharply. Specific centers have reported that the share of open surgeries in urolithiasis is less than 1% [112]. Additionally, around 20,000 ESWL and endourological surgeries were performed in the UK during 2014/2015, but only 30 open surgeries were performed [113]. The ESWL and URS success rate decreases in treating upper and middle ureteral stones that are embedded or larger than 1 cm. 7% of ureteral stones treated with endourological methods require a second intervention. Approximately 1–10% of these patients may also require open surgery. Open surgery is indicated in the failure of other minimally invasive treatment modalities or the presence of pathologies requiring simultaneous open surgery. One of the indications for open surgery is impacted large-diameter ureteral stones. The importance of impacted stones is that they can result in up to 24% ureteral strictures in the postoperative period compared to some series [111].

The most significant advantage of open surgery is that it is stone free in a single session. Although open surgery has high success rates in proximal ureteral stones, its success in distal ureteral stones is similar to ESWL or URS. In open ureterolithotomy, the surgical incision is determined according to the localization of the stone in the ureter. Usually, a lumbotomy is performed for upper and middle ureteral stones, and a Gibson incision is performed for lower ureteral stones. Although some studies have shown that the open approach can achieve a higher SFR (PNL; 80–100% vs. 50–87%), it is associated with significantly higher morbidity and more prolonged healing [112]. In addition, LU has become a more minimally invasive alternative treatment method, as open surgery increases hospital stay and requires additional analgesic therapy for the patient. LU is superior to open surgery because its success rate is similar to open surgery, with less analgesic requirements, shorter hospital stay, faster recovery, and better cosmetic results [114].

Key Reading

Open ureterolithotomy may be considered when ureteroscopic procedures fail, or concomitant surgery is required. However, open ureterolithotomy has been replaced by laparoscopic ureterolithotomy as it is a more minimally invasive treatment option even in cases where endourological procedures fail.

Questions

1. According to EAU guidelines, which of the following is the first treatment option for upper ureteral stones >10 mm?

(a) Laparoscopic ureterolithotomy
(b) ESWL
(c) URS
(d) ESWL/URS

Answer: (d)

2. What is the preferred treatment opinion for a patient with a symptomatic 1.5-cm upper ureteral calculus and a coagulopathy?

(a) ESWL
(b) Indwelling ureteral stent
(c) PNL
(d) Flexible ureteroscopy

Answer: (d)

3. First-time stone former is diagnosed with a 5-mm mid-üreteral calculus. The best initial management is:

(a) Ureteral stent placement
(b) ESWL
(c) URS
(d) Expectant management

Answer: (d)

4. Which treatments are not acceptable for pregnant women with obstructive ureteral calculus?

(a) Placement of a JJ ureteral stent
(b) Placement of a nephrostomy tube
(c) Ureteroscopy
(d) ESWL

Answer: (d)

5. The management of a stone in a basket, with an avulsed ureter all in continuity and no safety guidewire in place, is:

(a) Nephrectomy
(b) Immediate ureteral reimplantation
(c) Placement of a JJ ureteral stent
(d) Placement of a nephrostomy drain

Answer: (d)

References

1. Trinchieri A. Epidemiology of urolithiasis: an update. Clin Cases Miner Bone Metab. 2008;5(2):101–6.
2. Yallappa S, Amer T, Jones P, Greco F, Tailly T, Somani BK, et al. Natural history of conservatively managed ureteral stones: analysis of 6600 patients. J Endourol. 2018;32(5):371–9.
3. Jendeberg J, Geijer H, Alshamari M, Cierzniak B, Lidén M. Size matters: the width and location of a ureteral stone accurately predict the chance of spontaneous passage. Eur Radiol. 2017;27(11):4775–85.
4. Türk C, Neisius A, Petřík A, Seitz C, Skolarikos A, Somani B, et al. EAU guidelines on urolithiasis. Urol: Eur. Assoc; 2021.
5. Gierse JK, Hauser SD, Creely DP, Koboldt C, Rangwala SH, Isakson PC, et al. Expression and selective inhibition of the constitutive and inducible forms of human cyclooxygenase. Biochem J. 1995;305(2):479–84.
6. Hawkey C. COX-1 and COX-2 inhibitors. Best Pract Res Clin Gastroenterol. 2001;15(5):801–20.
7. Nakada SY, Jerde TJ, Jacobson LM, Saban R, Bjorling DE, Hullett DA. Cyclooxygenase-2 expression is up-regulated in obstructed human ureter. J Urol. 2002;168(3):1226–9.
8. Ankem MK, Jerde TJ, Wilkinson ER, Nakada SY. Third prize: prostaglandin E2-3 receptor is involved in ureteral contractility in obstruction. J Endourol. 2005;19(9):1088–91.
9. Mastrangelo D, Wisard M, Rohner S, Leisinger H, Iselin CE. Diclofenac and NS-398, a selective cyclooxygenase-2 inhibitor, decrease agonist-induced contractions of the pig isolated ureter. Urol Res. 2000;28(6):376–82.
10. Nakada SY, Jerde TJ, Bjorling DE, Saban R. Selective cyclooxygenase-2 inhibitors reduce ureteral contraction in vitro: a better alternative for renal colic? J Urol. 2000;163(2):607–12.
11. Chaignat V, Danuser H, Stoffel MH, Z'Brun S, Studer U, Mevissen M. Effects of a non-selective COX inhibitor and selective COX-2 inhibitors on contractility of human and porcine ureters in vitro and in vivo. Br J Pharmacol. 2008;154(6):1297–307.
12. Pathan SA, Mitra B, Straney LD, Afzal MS, Anjum S, Shukla D, et al. Delivering safe and effective analgesia for management of renal colic in the emergency department: a double-blind, multigroup, randomised controlled trial. Lancet. 2016;387(10032):1999–2007.
13. Lv JL, Tang QL. Comparative evaluation of efficacy of use of naftopidil and/or celecoxib for medical treatment of distal ureteral stones. Urolithiasis. 2014;42(6) 541–7.
14. Karabacak OR, Yilmazer D, Ozturk U, Sener NC, Saltas H, Karabacak Y, et al. The presence and distribution of alpha adrenergic receptors in human renal pelvis and calyces. Urolithiasis. 2013;41(5):385–8.
15. Yu B, Zheng X, Sun Z, Cao P, Zhang J, Gao Z, et al. The safety and efficacy of doxazosin in medical expulsion therapy for distal ureteric calculi: a meta-analysis. PLoS One. 2021;16(1):e0245741.
16. Kaneko T, Matsushima H, Morimoto H, Tsuzaka Y, Homma Y. Efficacy of low dose tamsulosin in medical expulsive therapy for ureteral stones in Japanese male patients: a randomized controlled study. Int J Urol. 2010;17(5):462–5.
17. Morúa AG, García JDG, Montelongo RM, Guerra LSG. Use of alfuzosin for expulsion of stones in the distal third of ureter. Actas Urol Esp. 2009;33(9):1005–10.
18. Küpeli B, Irkilata L, Gürocak S, Tunç L, Kiraç M, Karaoğlan Ü, et al. Does tamsulosin enhance lower ureteral stone clearance with or without shock wave lithotripsy? Urology. 2004;64(6):1111–5.
19. Campschroer T, Zhu X, Vernooij RW, Lock MT. Alpha-blockers as medical expulsive therapy for ureteral stones. Cochrane Database Syst Rev. 2018;4(4):CD008509.
20. Oestreich MC, Vernooij RW, Sathianathen NJ, Hwang EC, Kuntz GM, Koziarz A, et al. Alpha-blockers after shock wave lithotripsy for renal or ureteral stones in adults. Cochrane Database Syst Rev. 2020;11:CD013393.

21. Pickard R, Starr K, MacLennan G, Lam T, Thomas R, Burr J, a. Medical expulsive therapy in adults with ureteric colic: a multicentre, randomised, placebo-controlled trial. Lancet. 2015;386(9991):341–9.
22. Furyk JS, Chu K, Banks C, Greenslade J, Keijzers G, Thom O, et al. Distal ureteric stones and tamsulosin: a double-blind, placebo-controlled, randomized, multicenter trial. Ann Emerg Med. 2016;67(1):86–95.e2.
23. Hollingsworth JM, Canales BK, Rogers MA, Sukumar S, Yan P, Kuntz GM, et al. Alpha blockers for treatment of ureteric stones: systematic review and meta-analysis. BMJ. 2016;355:i6112.
24. Liu C, Zeng G, Kang R, Wu W, Li J, Chen K, et al. Efficacy and safety of alfuzosin as medical expulsive therapy for ureteral stones: a systematic review and meta-analysis. PLoS One. 2015;10(8):e0134589.
25. Sur RL, Shore N, L'Esperance J, Knudsen B, Gupta M, Olsen S, et al. Silodosin to facilitate passage of ureteral stones: a multi-institutional, randomized, double-blinded, placebo-controlled trial. Eur Urol. 2015;67(5):959–64.
26. Andersson KE, Forman A. Effects of calcium channel blockers on urinary tract smooth muscle. Acta Pharmacol Toxicol. 1986;58(S2):193–200.
27. Forman A, Andersson KE, Henriksson L, Rud T, Ulmsten U. Effects of nifedipine on the smooth muscle of the human urinary tract in vitro and in vivo. Acta Pharmacol Toxicol. 1978;43(2):111–8.
28. Hertle L, Nawrath H. Calcium channel blockade in smooth muscle of the human upper urinary tract. I. Effects on depolarization-induced activation. J Urol. 1984;132(6):1265–9.
29. Caravati EM, Runge JW, Bossart PJ, Martinez JC, Hartsell SC, Williamson SG. Nifedipine for the relief of renal colic: a double-blind, placebo-controlled clinical trial. Ann Emerg Med. 1989;18(4):352–4.
30. Borghi L, Meschi T, Amato F, Novarini A, Giannini A, Quarantelli C, et al. Nifedipine and methylprednisolone in facilitating ureteral stone passage: a randomized, double-blind, placebo-controlled study. J Urol. 1994;152(4):1095–8.
31. Porpiglia F, Ghignone G, Fiori C, Fontana D, Scarpa RM. Nifedipine versus tamsulosin for the management of lower ureteral stones. J Urol. 2004;172(2):568–71.
32. Takeda M, Obara K, Mizusawa T, Tomita Y, Arai K, Tsutsui T, et al. Evidence for β3-adrenoceptor subtypes in relaxation of the human urinary bladder detrusor: analysis by molecular biological and pharmacological methods. J Pharmacol Exp Ther. 1999;288(3):1367–73.
33. Igawa Y, Yamazaki Y, Takeda H, Hayakawa K, Akahane M, Ajisawa Y, et al. Functional and molecular biological evidence for a possible β3-adrenoceptor in the human detrusor muscle. Br J Pharmacol. 1999;126(3):819–25.
34. Park Y-C, Tomiyama Y, Hayakawa K, Akahane M, Ajisawa Y, Miyatake R, et al. Existence of a β3-adrenoceptor and its functional role in the human ureter. J Urol. 2000;164(4):1364–70.
35. Matsumoto R, Otsuka A, Suzuki T, Shinbo H, Mizuno T, Kurita Y, et al. Expression and functional role of β3-adrenoceptors in the human ureter. Int J Urol. 2013;20(10):1007–14.
36. Bayar G, Yavuz A, Cakmak S, Ofluoglu Y, Kilinc MF, Kucuk E, et al. Efficacy of silodosin or mirabegron in medical expulsive therapy for ureteral stones: a prospective, randomized-controlled study. Int Urol Nephrol. 2020;52(5):835–40.
37. Solakhan M, Bayrak O, Bulut E. Efficacy of mirabegron in medical expulsive therapy. Urolithiasis. 2019;47(3):303–7.
38. Anderson K-E. Pharmacology of lower urinary tract smooth muscles and penile erectile tissues. Pharmacol Rev. 1993;45(3):253–308.
39. Persson K, Andersson K-E. Non-adrenergic, non-cholinergic relaxation and levels of cyclic nucleotides in rabbit lower urinary tract. Eur J Pharmacol Mol Pharmacol. 1994;268(2):159–67.
40. Schröder A, Hedlund P, Andersson K-E. Carbon monoxide relaxes the female pig urethra as effectively as nitric oxide in the presence of YC-1. J Urol. 2002;167(4):1892–6.

41. Iselin C, Alm P, Schaad N, Larsson B, Graber P, Andersson KE. Localization of nitric oxide synthase and haemoxygenase, and functional effects of nitric oxide and carbon monoxide in the pig and human intravesical ureter. Neurourol Urodyn. 1997;16(3):209–27.
42. Stief C, Ückert S, Truss M, Becker A, Machtens S, Jonas U. A possible role for nitric oxide in the regulation of human ureteral smooth muscle tone in vitro. Urol Res. 1996;24(6):333–7.
43. Gratzke C, Ückert S, Kedia G, Reich O, Schlenker B, Seitz M, et al. In vitro effects of PDE5 inhibitors sildenafil, vardenafil and tadalafil on isolated human ureteral smooth muscle: a basic research approach. Urol Res. 2007;35(1):49–54.
44. Kc HB, Shrestha A, Acharya GB, Basnet RB, Shah AK, Shrestha PM. Tamsulosin versus tadalafil as a medical expulsive therapy for distal ureteral stones: a prospective randomized study. Investig Clin Urol. 2016;57(5):351–6.
45. Kumar S, Jayant K, Agrawal S, Singh SK. Comparative efficacy of tamsulosin versus tamsulosin with tadalafil in combination with prednisolone for the medical expulsive therapy of lower ureteric stones: a randomized trial. Korean J Urol. 2014;55(3):196–200.
46. Fuchs G, Miller K, Rassweiler J, Eisenberger F. Extracorporeal shock-wave lithotripsy: one-year experience with the Dornier lithotripter. Eur Urol. 1985;11:145–9.
47. Hein S, Miernik A, Wilhelm K, Adams F, Schlager D, Herrmann TR, et al. Clinical significance of residual fragments in 2015: impact, detection, and how to avoid them. World J Urol. 2016;34(6):771–8.
48. Weizer A, Zhong P, Preminger G. Shock wave lithotripsy: current technology and evolving concepts. AUA Update Series. 2005;24:313–24.
49. Rassweiler JJ, Fritsche H-M, Tailly G, Klein J, Laguna P, Chaussy C. Shock wave lithotripsy in the year 2012. Clinical Management of Urolithiasis. Springer; 2013. p. 51–75.
50. Karlin G, Marino C, Badlani G, Smith A. Benefits of an ultrasound-guided ESWL unit. Arch Esp Urol. 1990;43(5):579–81.
51. Pengfei S, Min J, Jie Y, Xiong L, Yutao L, Wuran W, et al. Use of ureteral stent in extracorporeal shock wave lithotripsy for upper urinary calculi: a systematic review and meta-analysis. J Urol. 2011;186(4):1328–35.
52. Wang H, Man L, Li G, Huang G, Liu N, Wang J. Meta-analysis of stenting versus non-stenting for the treatment of ureteral stones. PLoS One. 2017;12(1):e0167670.
53. Platonov MA, Gillis AM, Kavanagh KM. Pacemakers, implantable cardioverter/defibrillators, and extracorporeal shockwave lithotripsy: evidence-based guidelines for the modern era. J Endourol. 2008;22(2):243–8.
54. Lu Y, Tianyong F, Ping H, Liangren L, Haichao Y, Qiang W. Antibiotic prophylaxis for shock wave lithotripsy in patients with sterile urine before treatment may be unnecessary: a systematic review and meta-analysis. J Urol. 2012;188(2):441–8.
55. Liu LR, Li QJ, Wei Q, Liu ZH, Xu Y. Percussion, diuresis, and inversion therapy for the passage of lower pole kidney stones following shock wave lithotripsy. Cochrane Database Syst Rev. 2013;12:CD008569.
56. Tao R-z, Tang Q-l, Zhou S, Jia C-p, Lv J-l. External physical vibration lithecbole facilitating the expulsion of upper ureteric stones 1.0–2.0 cm after extracorporeal shock wave lithotripsy: a prospective randomized trial. Urolithiasis. 2020;48(1):71–7.
57. Neisius A, Lipkin ME, Rassweiler JJ, Zhong P, Preminger GM, Knoll T. Shock wave lithotripsy: the new phoenix? World J Urol. 2015;33(2):213–21.
58. El-Nahas AR, El-Assmy AM, Mansour O, Sheir KZ. A prospective multivariate analysis of factors predicting stone disintegration by extracorporeal shock wave lithotripsy: the value of high-resolution noncontrast computed tomography. Eur Urol. 2007;51(6):1688–94.
59. Drake T, Grivas N, Dabestani S, Knoll T, Lam T, Maclennan S, et al. What are the benefits and harms of ureteroscopy compared with shock-wave lithotripsy in the treatment of upper ureteral stones? A systematic review. Eur Urol. 2017;72(5):772–86.
60. Yazici O, Tuncer M, Sahin C, Demirkol MK, Kafkasli A, Sarica K. Shock wave lithotripsy in ureteral stones: evaluation of patient and stone related predictive factors. Int Braz J Urol. 2015;41:676–82.

61. Skolarikos A, Grivas N, Kallidonis P, Mourmouris P, Rountos T, Fiamegos A, et al. The efficacy of medical expulsive therapy (MET) in improving stone-free rate and stone expulsion time, after extracorporeal shock wave lithotripsy (SWL) for upper urinary stones: a systematic review and meta-analysis. Urology. 2015;86(6):1057–64.
62. Rassweiler J, Köhrmann K, Back W, Fröhner S, Raab M, Weber A, et al. Experimental basis of shockwave-induced renal trauma in the model of the canine kidney. World J Urol. 1993;11(1):43–53.
63. Klein J, Netsch C, Sievert K, Miernik A, Westphal J, Leyh H, et al. Extrakorporale Stoßwellenlithotripsie. Urologe. 2018;57(4):463–73.
64. Maker V, Layke J. Gastrointestinal injury secondary to extracorporeal shock wave lithotripsy: a review of the literature since its inception. J Am Coll Surg. 2004;198(1):128–35.
65. Krambeck AE, Rule AD, Li X, Bergstralh EJ, Gettman MT, Lieske JC. Shock wave lithotripsy is not predictive of hypertension among community stone formers at long-term followup. J Urol. 2011;185(1):164–9.
66. Marshall VF. Fiber optics in urology. J Urol. 1964;91(1):110–4.
67. Goodman TM. Ureteroscopy with pediatric cystoscope in adults. Urology. 1977;9(4):394.
68. Lyon ES, Kyker JS, Schoenberg HW. Transurethral ureteroscopy in women: a ready addition to the urological armamentarium. J Urol. 1978;119(1):35–6.
69. Lyon ES, Banno JJ, Schoenberg HW. Transurethral ureteroscopy in men using juvenile cystoscopy equipment. J Urol. 1979;122(2):152–3.
70. Das S. Transurethral ureteroscopy and stone manipulation under direct vision. J Urol. 1981;125(1):112–3.
71. Somani BK, Al-Qahtani SM, de Medina SDG, Traxer O. Outcomes of flexible ureterorenoscopy and laser fragmentation for renal stones: comparison between digital and conventional ureteroscope. Urology. 2013;82(5):1017–9.
72. Multescu R, Geavlete B, Geavlete P. A new era: performance and limitations of the latest models of flexible ureteroscopes. Urology. 2013;82(6):1236–9.
73. Wendt-Nordahl G, Mut T, Krombach P, Michel MS, Knoll T. Do new generation flexible ureterorenoscopes offer a higher treatment success than their predecessors? Urol Res. 2011;39(3):185–8.
74. Rupel E, Brown R. Nephroscopy with removal of stone following nephrostomy for obstructive calculous anuria. J Urol. 1941;46(2):177–82.
75. Goodwin WE, Casey WC, Woolf W. Percutaneous trocar (needle) nephrostomy in hydronephrosis. J Am Med Assoc. 1955;157(11):891–4.
76. Wang Y, Zhong B, Yang X, Wang G, Hou P, Meng J. Comparison of the efficacy and safety of URSL, RPLU, and MPCNL for treatment of large upper impacted ureteral stones: a randomized controlled trial. BMC Urol. 2017;17(1):1–7.
77. Wu T, Duan X, Chen S, Yang X, Tang T, Cui S. Ureteroscopic lithotripsy versus laparoscopic ureterolithotomy or percutaneous nephrolithotomy in the management of large proximal ureteral stones: a systematic review and meta-analysis. Urol Int. 2017;99(3):308–19.
78. Topaloglu H, Karakoyunlu N, Sari S, Ozok HU, Sagnak L, Ersoy H. A comparison of antegrade percutaneous and laparoscopic approaches in the treatment of proximal ureteral stones. Biomed Res Int. 2014;2014:691946.
79. Moufid K, Abbaka N, Touiti D, Adermouch L, Amine M, Lezrek M. Large impacted upper ureteral calculi: a comparative study between retrograde ureterolithotripsy and percutaneous antegrade ureterolithotripsy in the modified lateral position. Urology Annals. 2013;5(3):140.
80. Rukin NJ, Somani BK, Patterson J, Grey BR, Finch W, McClinton S, et al. Tips and tricks of ureteroscopy: consensus statement part I. Basic ureteroscopy. Cent European J Urol. 2015;68(4):439.
81. Mandal S, Goel A, Singh MK, Kathpalia R, Nagathan DS, Sankhwar SN, et al. Clavien classification of semirigid ureteroscopy complications: a prospective study. Urology. 2012;80(5):995–1001.

82. Cindolo L, Castellan P, Primiceri G, Hoznek A, Cracco CM, Scoffone CM, et al. Life-threatening complications after ureteroscopy for urinary stones: survey and systematic literature review. Minerva Urol Nefrol. 2017;69(5):421–31.
83. Mursi K, Elsheemy MS, Morsi HA, Ghaleb A-KA, Abdel-Razzak OM. Semirigid ureteroscopy for ureteric and renal pelvic calculi: predictive factors for complications and success. Arab J Urol. 2013;11(2):136–41.
84. El-Nahas AR, El-Tabey NA, Eraky I, Shoma AM, El-Hefnawy AS, El-Assmy AM, et al. Semirigid ureteroscopy for ureteral stones: a multivariate analysis of unfavorable results. J Urol. 2009;181(3):1158–62.
85. Castro EP, Osther PJ, Jinga V, Razvi H, Stravodimos KG, Parikh K, et al. Differences in ureteroscopic stone treatment and outcomes for distal, mid-, proximal, or multiple ureteral locations: the clinical research office of the Endourological Society ureteroscopy global study. Eur Urol. 2014;66(1):102–9.
86. Cheung M, Lee F, Leung Y, Wong B, Chu S, Tam P. Outpatient ureteroscopy: predictive factors for postoperative events. Urology. 2001;58(6):914–8.
87. Somani B, Giusti G, Sun Y, Osther P, Frank M, De Sio M, et al. Complications associated with ureterorenoscopy (URS) related to treatment of urolithiasis: the clinical research office of Endourological society URS global study. World J Urol. 2017;35(4):675–81.
88. Borofsky MS, Lingeman JE. The role of open and laparoscopic stone surgery in the modern era of endourology. Nat Rev Urol. 2015;12(7):392–400.
89. Gaur D, Agarwal D, Purohit K, Darshane A. Retroperitoneal laparoscopic pyelolithotomy. J Urol. 1994;151(4):927–9.
90. Gaur D. Laparoscopic operative retroperitoneoscopy: use of a new device. J Urol. 1992;148(4):1137–9.
91. Nambirajan T, Jeschke S, Albqami N, Abukora F, Leeb K, Janetschek G. Role of laparoscopy in management of renal stones: single-center experience and review of literature. J Endourol. 2005;19(3):353–9.
92. Humphreys MR. The emerging role of robotics and laparoscopy in stone disease. Urol Clin. 2013;40(1):115–28.
93. Wang X, Li S, Liu T, Guo Y, Yang Z. Laparoscopic pyelolithotomy compared to percutaneous nephrolithotomy as surgical management for large renal pelvic calculi: a meta-analysis. J Urol. 2013;190(3):888–93.
94. Lopes Neto AC, Korkes F, Silva JL, Amarante RDM, Mattos MHE, Tobias-Machado M, et al. Prospective randomized study of treatment of large proximal ureteral stones: extracorporeal shock wave lithotripsy versus ureterolithotripsy versus laparoscopy. J Urol. 2012;187(1):164–8.
95. Fang Y-q, Qiu J-g, Wang D-j, Zhan H-l, Situ J. Comparative study on ureteroscopic lithotripsy and laparoscopic ureterolithotomy for treatment of unilateral upper ureteral stones. Acta Cir Bras. 2012;27:266–70.
96. Polom W, Markuszewski M, Rho YS, Matuszewski M. Use of invisible near infrared light fluorescence with indocyanine green and methylene blue in urology. Part 2. Cent European J Urol. 2014;67(3):310.
97. Kijvikai K, Patcharatrakul S. Laparoscopic ureterolithotomy: its role and some controversial technical considerations. Int J Urol. 2006;13(3):206–10.
98. Choi JD, Seo SI, Kwon J, Kim BS. Laparoscopic ureterolithotomy vs ureteroscopic lithotripsy for large ureteral stones. JSLS. 2019;23(2):e2019.00008.
99. Abuanz S, Gamé X, Roche J-B, Guillotreau J, Mouzin M, Sallusto F, et al. Laparoscopic pyeloplasty: comparison between retroperitoneoscopic and transperitoneal approach. Urology. 2010;76(4):877–81.
100. Singh V, Sinha RJ, Gupta DK, Kumar M, Akhtar A. Transperitoneal versus retroperitoneal laparoscopic ureterolithotomy: a prospective randomized comparison study. J Urol. 2013;189(3):940–5.

101. Bove P, Micali S, Miano R, Mirabile G, De Stafani S, Botteri E, et al. Laparoscopic ureterolithotomy: a comparison between the transperitoneal and the retroperitoneal approach during the learning curve. J Endourol. 2009;23(6):953–7.
102. Müller PF, Schlager D, Hein S, Bach C, Miernik A, Schoeb DS. Robotic stone surgery–current state and future prospects: a systematic review. Arab J Urol. 2018;16(3):357–64.
103. Sutherland GR, Maddahi Y, Gan LS, Lama S, Zareinia K. Robotics in the neurosurgical treatment of glioma. Surg Neurol Int. 2015;6(Suppl 1):S1.
104. Rassweiler J, Fiedler M, Charalampogiannis N, Kabakci AS, Saglam R, Klein J-T. Robot-assisted flexible ureteroscopy: an update. Urolithiasis. 2018;46(1):69–77.
105. Harris S, Arambula-Cosio F, Mei Q, Hibberd R, Davies B, Wickham J, et al. The Probot—an active robot for prostate resection. Proc Inst Mech Eng H J Eng Med. 1997;211(4):317–25.
106. Desai MM, Aron M, Gill IS, Pascal-Haber G, Ukimura O, Kaouk JH, et al. Flexible robotic retrograde renoscopy: description of novel robotic device and preliminary laboratory experience. Urology. 2008;72(1):42–6.
107. Saglam R, Muslumanoglu AY, Tokatlı Z, Çaşkurlu T, Sarica K, Taşçi Aİ, et al. A new robot for flexible ureteroscopy: development and early clinical results (IDEAL stage 1–2b). Eur Urol. 2014;66(6):1092–100.
108. Reichenspurner H, Damiano RJ, Mack M, Boehm DH, Gulbins H, Detter C, et al. Use of the voice-controlled and computer-assisted surgical system ZEUS for endoscopic coronary artery bypass grafting. J Thorac Cardiovasc Surg. 1999;118(1):11–6.
109. Geavlete P, Saglam R, Georgescu D, Mulţescu R, Iordache V, Kabakci AS, et al. Robotic flexible ureteroscopy versus classic flexible ureteroscopy in renal stones: the initial Romanian experience. Chirurgia (Bucur). 2016;111(4):326–9.
110. Hellawell G, Mutch S, Thevendran G, Wells E, Morgan R. Radiation exposure and the urologist: what are the risks? J Urol. 2005;174(3):948–52.
111. Roberts WW, Cadeddu JA, Micali S, Kavoussi LR, Moore RG. Ureteral stricture formation after removal of impacted calculi. J Urol. 1998;159(3):723–6.
112. Alivizatos G, Skolarikos A. Is there still a role for open surgery in the management of renal stones? Curr Opin Urol. 2006;16(2):106–11.
113. Heers H, Turney BW. Trends in urological stone disease: a 5-year update of hospital episode statistics. BJU international. 2016;118(5):785–9.
114. Wani MM, Durrani AM. Laparoscopic ureterolithotomy: experience of 60 cases from a developing world hospital. J Minim Access Surg. 2019;15(2):103.

Chapter 21
Ureteroscopy and Related Instruments

John Denstedt, Mario Basulto-Martínez, and Eduardo González-Cuenca

Abstract Ureteroscopy is one of the most significant advances in the field of endourology over the last decades, allowing urologists a minimally invasive approach to the upper urinary tract. Richard Wolf and Harold Horace Hopkins groundbreaking technological developments paved the way for ureteroscopy as we know it today. The invention of smaller caliber semi-rigid and flexible ureteroscopes made possible accessing the urinary tract with minimal morbidity. Ureteroscopy has become a standard diagnostic and treatment approach for upper urinary tract urothelial carcinoma as well as ureteric urinary stone treatment, among others. Specific and standardized clinical indications are described in the American and European guidelines. The continuous improvement of ureteroscopes, including ancillary tools and laser energy, has provided solutions to diseases that may have required a more invasive approach in the past. We aim to provide a brief description of indications, and step-by-step ureteroscopy, including ancillary equipment and future advancements.

Keywords Ureteroscopy · Semi-rigid ureteroscopy · Laser lithotripsy · Urolithiasis · Ancillary tools

Test your learning and check your understanding of this book's contents: use the "Springer Nature Flashcards" app to access questions. To use the app, please follow the instructions in chapter 1.

J. Denstedt (✉)
Professor of Urology Schulich School of Medicine and Dentistry, Western University, London, ON, Canada
e-mail: john.denstedt@sjhc.london.on.ca

M. Basulto-Martínez · E. González-Cuenca
Endourology, Laparoscopy, and Robotic Surgery Fellow, Schulich School of Medicine and Dentistry, Division of Urology, Western University, London, ON, Canada

M. Abdel-Gawad et al. (eds.), *The Ureter*,
https://doi.org/10.1007/978-3-031-36212-5_21

Learning Objectives
In this chapter, we aimed to:

- Describe the indications for ureteroscopy.
- Describe the technology of ureteroscopes and supplies utilized in the procedure.
- Describe the technique for ureteroscopy.
- Describe the complications and strategies for prevention.
- Describe the future direction of ureteroscopy.

21.1 Introduction

The development of the ureterorenoscopy (URS) has represented one of the most significant advances in endourology over the last several decades. Since the early twentieth century, physicians such as Howard A. Kelly had noted the need for light-guided devices to better inspect organs endoluminally and understand the afflicting pathologies [1, 2]. In 1964 Victor Marshall described the first use of a flexible endoscope to inspect the upper urinary tract. Ground-breaking progress led by researchers such as Richard Wolf and Harold Horace Hopkins paved the way for the first rigid ureteroscopic procedures described by Pérez-Castro Ellendt and Martinez-Penero in the early 1980s [3, 4]. Further refinements in the technology have enhanced vision, deflection, and irrigation flow rates while downsizing the overall instrument caliber. This has considerably improved the functionality of both rigid and flexible ureteroscopes and permitted routine access to the entire upper urinary tract for performance of a variety of diagnostic and therapeutic procedures. More recent evolution includes the development of high-quality disposable flexible ureteroscopes with performance measures equivalent to that of standard reusable instrumentation.

Concurrently, the development of a broad range of supplies such as guidewires, baskets, ureteral access sheaths (UAS), irrigation devices, anti-retropulsion devices, and a variety of energy sources including lasers, have evolved to facilitate the application of URS. As a result, URS-based procedures have assumed a central role in management of urinary calculi. Incorporation of the techniques into urology residency training programs, instructional courses, and the use of a variety of simulation-based training models have resulted in a rapid uptake of URS into day-to-day clinical practice by urologists globally. In this chapter we discuss the indications, required equipment and techniques for the performance of ureteroscopic procedures [1, 2].

21.2 Indications for Ureteroscopy

URS is indicated when visualization of the upper urinary tract is desired including for both diagnostic and therapeutic procedures. This includes disorders such as upper urinary tract strictures, fistulae, foreign bodies such as retained ureteral stents, tumors and most commonly ureteral and renal calculi [5–7].

Patients undergoing workup for upper tract urothelial cell carcinoma (UTUC) will commonly require URS as part of the diagnostic algorithm. This allows tumor visualization and biopsy, which can determine tumor grade in more than 90% of cases. Image-enhancing technologies such as narrow-band imaging may improve tumor visualization, especially in flat tumors. Furthermore, ablation treatments may also be delivered through URS and is recommended in patients with low-risk UTUC or in selected cases with high-risk UTUC, such as in patients with a solitary kidney or impaired renal function. Moreover, strictures of the upper tract can be assessed by URS, and same-session treatment may be delivered in the form of an endoscopic laser incision [8–10].

Urinary stone disease represents the main indication for URS. The American Urological Association (AUA) guidelines articulate that patients with uncomplicated ureteral stones ≤10 mm should be offered observation, and those with distal ureteral stones should be offered medical expulsive therapy (MET) with alpha-blockers. Noteworthy, complicated and obstructed patients with suspected infection must be diverted urgently whether by ureteral stenting or nephrostomy tube insertion. Furthermore, in patients who failed or are not candidates for MET, typically due to stone size, or if a recommendation for intervention has been made based on shared decision making, stone treatment is recommended. Extracorporeal shock-wave lithotripsy (ESWL) and URS are both feasible options, while the former has the least morbidity and lower complication rate, the latter is associated with a higher stone-free rate (SFR) in a single procedure. Hence, patients should be informed accordingly [11–13].

Some special considerations are worth emphasizing. In patients with middle or distal ureteral stones who failed or were not candidates for MET, URS is recommended as first-line therapy as the SFR is significantly higher than in ESWL in a single procedure. Similarly, in patients who failed MET and have suspected uric acid or cystine stones, URS is preferred over ESWL, as targeting these stones fluoroscopically for EWSL is challenging, and cystine stones are often ESWL resistant, making this treatment modality less effective [11, 12].

For patients with non-obstructing, asymptomatic calyceal stones, surveillance may be offered, whereas in those with a ≥ 20 mm stone burden, percutaneous nephrolithotomy (PCNL) is preferred as first-line treatment. Thus, either URS or ESWL is indicated as first line therapy for renal stones <20 mm in the renal pelvis and upper/middle calyces and for stones ≤10 mm in the lower pole. Some stone or patient variabilities have been demonstrated to impair ESWL outcomes, such as stone calcium oxalate monohydrate or brushite stone composition, stone density >1000 Hounsfield units, skin-to-stone distance >12 cm, infundibulopelvic angle <45°and a long lower pole calyx >10 mm and a narrow (<5 mm) and lengthy (>30 mm) infundibulum. Therefore, URS is often preferred if any of these parameters are encountered [11, 12, 14, 15].

For lower pole stones 10–20 mm with unfavorable factors for ESWL, either URS or PCNL, ideally through a miniaturized tract, are feasible options. Despite these well-reported stone burden cutoffs, current evidence has explored whether URS can be used for larger stones, and similar outcomes to miniaturized PCNL have been reported. Similarly, some patients are unwilling to undergo PCNL, or may not be good candidates due to increased risk of bleeding and complications. This includes anticoagulation therapy, high-risk for anesthesia, morbidly obese patients, and anatomic variant kidneys such as pelvic kidney. In these instances URS is often the safest and most effective option despite the stone burden, even as an staged procedure [16–18].

21.3 Ureteroscope Technology and Ancillary Equipment

21.3.1 Semi-Rigid Ureteroscopes

Semi-rigid URS is the preferred approach for lesions, including stones, in the distal ureter. Although semi-rigid instruments may be advanced further into the proximal ureter, particularly in female patients, surgeons should bear in mind the sharp end and stiffness of the instrument can injure the ureter and therefore flexible ureteroscopes are preferred for treating stones and other lesions above the iliac vessels. Semi-rigid ureteroscopes are available in a short and longer version; the former for most distal stones and female patients and the latter for male patients [19]. The commonly available semi-rigid ureteroscopes and their features are listed in Table 21.1.

Table 21.1 Characteristics of semi-rigid ureteroscopes available on the market

Manufacturer	Model	Size (cm)	Caliber (Fr)	Channel (Fr)	Eyepiece	View (°)
Olympus	OES pro	43 and 33 43	6.4/7.8 8.6/9.8	4.2 6.4	Straight/ angled	7
Karl Storz	27,000 L/K	34 and 43	6.5/9.9 (7)	4.8	Angled	6
	27,001 L/K	34 and 43	7/12 (8)	5	Angled	6
	27,002 L/K	34 and 43	8/12 (9.5)	6	Angled	6
	Michel	43	9/12 (9.5)	Dual: 2 and 3	Angled	6
	27,010 L/K	34 and 43	7/9.9 (7)	Dual: 3.4 and 1.4	Straight	6
	Gautier	41	7/13.5 (8)	5	Straight	6
	27002KP	25	7.3/9.9	3.6	Straight	6
Richard Wolf	Needle	31.5 and 43	4.5/6	3	Straight	5
	Ultrathin	33 and 43	6/7.5	4	Straight	5
	D.O.C.	33 and 43	6.5/8.5	Dual --	Angled	5
Stryker	SRU-6 SRU-6X	33 and 43	6.9/10	Dual --	Straight	--

21.3.2 Flexible Ureteroscopes

Flexible ureteroscopes are preferred for diagnostic and therapeutic procedures above the iliac vessels. The wide angle of deflection of the endoscope tip and movements allow navigation of the entire collecting system in most cases. Moreover, digital flexible ureteroscopes incorporate a CCD or CMOS chip in the tip as well as an LED light source, providing better image quality and are also lighter than fiberoptic ureteroscopes, as no camera head and light cord are needed. The weight of digital ureteroscopes is approximately 320 g whereas the fiberoptic counterparts are approximately 575 g. Nevertheless, fiberoptic scopes have smaller caliber (8.4–9.9 vs 5.3–8.7 Fr) [20–22].

The main shortcoming of flexible ureteroscope technology is the durability and expense associated with repairs of these fragile instruments. Damage to the deflection components, laser burns and perforation of the working channel may all result in a nonfunctional instrument and expensive repair costs. More recently, single-use ureteroscopes have advanced significantly in functionality and performance. The concept behind single use ureteroscopes is practicality. Not only are the devices lighter and display high-quality digital imaging, but there is no need for repairing, maintaining, sterilization and reprocessing and no fear of endoscope damage in challenging situations. The drawback of single use ureteroscopes is the cost per procedure; however, studies on cumulative cost are variable as when all in costs are considered the cumulative cost seems to be comparable. Most authors recommend the deployment of single-use ureteroscopes for the challenging cases where endoscope damage is anticipated such as stones in the lower pole and anatomically variant kidneys [20–25]. Another important concern is the environmental impact of single use ureteroscopes. Despite the paucity of evidence, it has been suggested that the carbon footprint is comparable for single use and reusable ureteroscopes; in fact a lower overall environmental impact is attributed to single use devices [26, 27].

Flexible ureteroscopes have important aspects that impact their performance, such as working channel size and position, shaft diameter and range of deflection. The features of commonly commercially available ureteroscopes are summarized in Table 21.2. In the case of lower pole stones and an acute angled calyx, a ureteroscope with a wider range of deflection may impact effectiveness. Similarly, the o'clock position of the working channel through which ancillary devices exit may facilitate effective lithotripsy. Studies suggest that a 3 o'clock working channel provides better access to the surface of a targeted stone located in right posterior and left anterior calyces than a 9 o'clock oriented channel. Conversely, a 9 o'clock position working channel provides better access to left posterior and right anterior calyces [28, 29].

Table 21.2 Characteristics of commonly commercialized flexible ureteroscopes

Manufacturer	Model	Up/Down deflection (°)	Caliber (Fr)	Working channel O'clock position	Working channel Size (Fr)	Type
Reusable						
Wolf	Viper	270/270	8.8	3	3.6	Digital
	Cobra vision EF	270/270	9.9	6/9	3.6/2.4[a]	Digital
	Boa EF	270/270	8.7	9	3.6	Digital
Karl Storz	Flex-XC	270/270	8.5	3	3.6	Digital
	Flex-X2	270/270	7.5	9	3.6	Fiberoptic
Olympus	URF-V	185/275	9.9	9	3.6	Digital
	URF-V2	275/275	8.4	9	3.6	Digital
	URF-P5	180/275	8.4	9	3.6	Fiberoptic
	URF-P6	275/275	7.95	9	3.6	Fiberoptic
Single-use						
Boston scientific	LithoVue	270/270	9.5	3	3.6	Digital
Pusen medical	Uscope	270/270	9.5	3	3.6	Digital
	Uscope mini	270/270	7.5	3	3.6	Digital
Karl Storz	Flex-XC1	270/270	9	3	3.5	Digital
Neoscope	NeoFlex	280/280	9	1	3.6	Digital
InnoMedicus	WiScope	275/275	8.6	12	3.6	Digital
Innovex	EU-scope	275/275	9.3	10	3.6	Digital

[a] Laser/irrigation channel, for fibers up to 365 μm

21.4 Guidewires

The guidewires commonly used in endoscopic surgery were firstly described for vascular procedures and have become an essential tool for accessing the ureter. The guidewires have two components, the inner core which gives the rigidity and flexibility (stainless steel or Nickel-titanium [Nitinol]) and the outer core which can be hydrophobic (polytetrafluoroethylene [PTFE]) or hydrophilic; the latter has a low-friction to bypass a ureteral obstruction but lack in stiffness [30, 31]. In the Table 21.3, we describe the most used guidewires to perform URS. In Fig. 21.1, we provide a photo comparing the tip of the three most commonly used guidewires.

Table 21.3 Common guidewires used in ureteroscopy

Guidewire	Brand	Material	Tip	Diameter	Length	Flexible tip	Taper length	Figures
Bentson	Cook medical	PTFE-coated stainless steel core	Straight	0.035”	145	6 cm	15	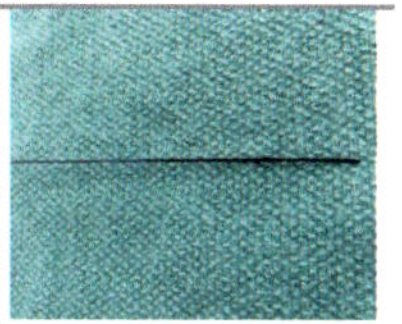
Sensor™	Boston scientific	PTFE-coated Nitinol core with hydrophilic tip	Straight/angled	0.035”	150	3 cm	5 cm hydro pass coating	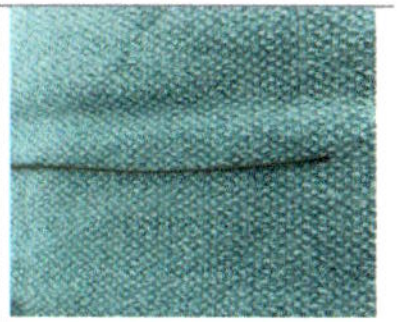
Terumo Glidewire®	Terumo I. systems	Nitinol core with hydrophilic coating	Straight/angled	0.038”	150	3 cm	–	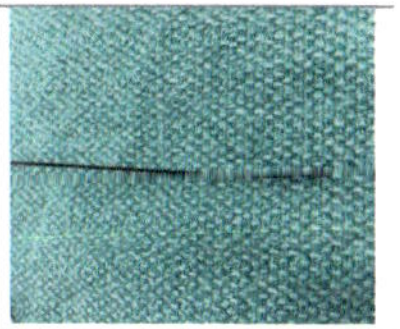

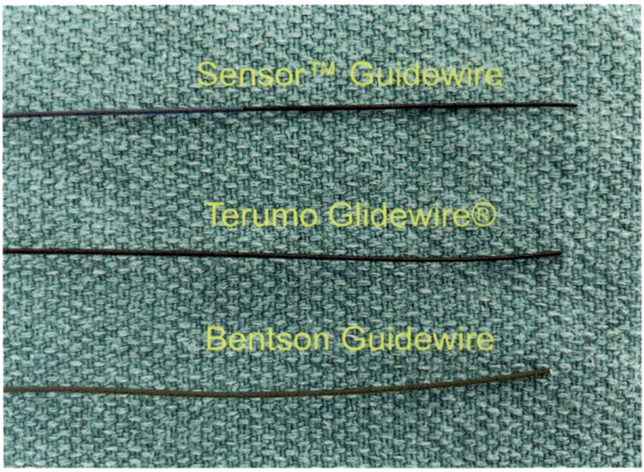

Fig. 21.1 Tip comparison of three different commonly used guidewires for endourologic procedures

21.5 Retrieval Devices (Baskets)

The stone retrieval devices are mostly useful for retrieving stone fragments following intracorporeal stone disruption with lithotripsy devices. There are numerous types of retrieval devices and each is differentiated by the force to open the ureter, capture and retain the stone. The most commonly used stone basket is the tipless four-wire nitinol basket [32]. A UAS may be used to facilitate the ureteroscope in-and-out access for basketing during flexible ureteroscopic procedures. [33].

21.6 Dilation Devices

Difficult passage or resistance to ureteroscope introduction can be met at the ureteric orifice. Cetti and colleagues estimated a difficult ureter will be encountered in 8% of patients undergoing URS [32, 34]. Dilation of the ureter can be performed in a passive or active fashion. Passive dilation refers to the placement of a ureteric stent and subsequent need for a staged procedure. Active dilation is performed via coaxial dilation or balloon dilation of the ureter/ureteric orifice. We use the Amplatz 8/10 Fr. set coaxial dilator (8/10 Dilator/Sheath Set, Boston Scientific) for dilation of the ureteric orifice under fluoroscopic vision and placement of a second wire through the 10 Fr. sheath. If resistance is still met, a balloon dilation can be performed with one of a number of available balloon dilators. We most commonly use a 10 cm 6 mm balloon for ureteral dilation. A study published by Kuntz et al., documented a 95% success rate of completing URS in a single-stage procedure and with low complication rates. [32, 35].

21.7 Ureteral Access Sheaths

Use of a UAS facilitates atraumatic and multiple entries to the mid and proximal ureter during flexible URS. The UAS is inserted over a working guidewire (with a safety guidewire in place) and inserted into the ureter under fluoroscopic vision, thus eliminating the risk of buckling the ureteroscope in the bladder during entry or re-entry [36]. The UAS consists of an inner part (dilator) and the outer sheath with a locking hub, there is a hydrophilic coating to minimize the friction during the introduction of the UAS [10]. The different diameters for UAS include 10/12 Fr, 11/13 Fr, and 12/14 Fr. with a length of 20–50 cm.

The benefits of the UAS are a decrease in intrarenal pressure during active irrigation, reduced operative time, improved visibility and decreased rates of postoperative sepsis. Whether improvement of stone-free rates is achieved by use of UAS is controversial. Reducing the intrarenal pressure may mitigate complications such as bleeding, hematoma, urinoma and sepsis. A 10/12 Fr or 12/14 Fr UAS will reduce intrarenal pressures to levels under 30 cm H_2O [37].

The drawbacks of using UAS are ureteral injury or perforation, ureteral ischemia and unknown long-term risk of stricture formation. The most common associated complications are bleeding and perforation, a prevalence of 5.9% was documented in an observational study for intraoperative complications [12]. A long indwelling time and resistance during the introduction of the UAS were associated with short-term formation of ureteral strictures in a porcine-model [38]. The use of UAS depends on the surgeon's preference according to the European Urological Association Guidelines [39].

21.8 Irrigation Devices

URS is performed under hydrodistension of the urinary tract and 0.9% saline is the preferred irrigation fluid. Rigid and flexible ureteroscopes both have an irrigation channel that permits the fluid inflow. Adequate irrigation is paramount for proper visualization of the urinary tract and there are many devices for enhanced irrigation. Nonetheless, working under high pressure may cause pyelovenous backflow increasing the risk of infection. The physiological pelvic pressure is 10 mmHg, and it has been demonstrated that pyelovenous backflow occurs when the 30–45 mmHg threshold is exceeded and forniceal ruptures can occur when exceeding 185 mmHg. Several studies have shown that renal pelvic pressure can reach up to more than 300 mmHg in some cases. Therefore, surgeons must always bear in mind that the goal is to get the best visualization achievable at the lowest pressure [40–42].

Standard gravity irrigation generates pelvic pressures of around 35 mmHg, nevertheless, features such as instrument caliber and height at which fluid bags are hung have their impact on the pelvic pressure. Gravity irrigation, however, is often solely not enough for optimal visualization during URS and therefore another irrigation option needs to be used. Some surgeons use bag pressure devices, by which the fluid bag can be pressurized at the desired pressured in order to optimize visualization [42]. Similarly, there are pump devices for fluid management, such as the Endoflow II® (Rocamed, Monaco), by which surgeons can set the desired pressure and temperature of the irrigation, keep it constant and altered as needed.

On-demand pressurization can be utilized as well. A simple 20 cc syringe may be used to increase the irrigation pressure by hand as necessary. There are some commercialized devices that can also be used for hand pressurization:

- Irri-Flo II (Olympus, Japan). Consists of a 10 cc syringe with a spring coiled around the plunge, hence, when the user releases the pressure from the plunge, the stretching of the spring will pull the air valve filling the syringe again. Depending on the force applied, this system may reach pressures over 145 cm H2O with an empty irrigation/working channel.
- SASP (Boston Scientific, USA). This device is a 10 cc syringe that utilizes a similar spring technology; however, the tip has a 3-way valve, one to the syringe, another allowing inflow from the fluid bag and the third with one-way valve for irrigation. This provides automatic refill while maintaining continuous irrigation.
- Cornwall (BD, USA). This device consists of a 10-cc syringe with a V-shaped plastic hand piece of which the base has openings that fit together with the plunger flange and barrel flange, resulting in a comfortable gun-shaped device. The inner vertex has a v-shaped metallic piece that keeps the hand piece open when no force is applied, permitting auto refill of the syringe. The tip has also a one-way valve.

21.9 Pressure Sensing Devices

As aforementioned, maintaining low-pressure during URS can reduce the risk of infectious complications. Therefore, some investigators have explored the use of pressure-sensing devices intraoperatively. A guidewire with a pressure-sensor is the most utilized device. The Pressure Wire (St. Jude Medical, Minnesota, USA) and the Comet™ II (Boston Scientific, Massachusetts, USA), are 0.014″ guidewires often in interventional cardiology, but have been used for pelvic pressure assessment [41, 43]. Similarly, other authors have developed prototypes of UAS with pressure sensor [44]. Recently, the LithoVue™ 2.0, a novel disposable URS with a built-in pressure sensor has been launched (Boston Scientific, Massachusetts, USA) and clinical trials are currently ongoing.

21.10 Intracorporeal Laser Lithotripsy

The use of "light amplification by stimulated emission of radiation" or the acronym "LASER" as a modality for intracorporeal lithotripsy was first described in the 1980s. The Holmium:yttrium-aluminium-garnet or Holmium:YAG laser (Ho:YAG) was first described for stone disease treatment in 1995 and is now considered as the standard for intracorporeal lithotripsy worldwide [45, 46].

The Ho:YAG laser results in stone disruption via two primary mechanisms: photo-acoustic (photo-mechanical) and photo-thermal. The photo-acoustic effect is related to the shockwave produced by the violent cavitation bubble collapse and the photo-thermal effect is the direct absorption of the laser energy by the stone and the absorption of this energy wavelength by the water molecules inside the stone (melting effect) [46–50].

The Ho:YAG laser and the newer Superpulsed Thulium Fiber Laser platforms operate at similar wavelengths; however there are physical and clinical differences. The Ho:YAG laser operates via a flashlamp-pumped solid-state configuration (YAG crystal chemically doped with Holmium ions) and has an infrared wavelength of 2210 nm. The laser has a pulsed mode, 0.2–6.0 J pulse energy, 250–1500 μs pulse duration, 5–80 Hz pulse rate and an average power up to 120 W. The Thulium Fiber Laser (TFL) operates via an electronic modulated diode-pumped configuration (Long 10–30 m silica fiber chemically doped with Thulium ions) and has an infrared wavelength of 1940 nm (closer to water absorption peak). The TFL has a 0.025–6.0 J pulse energy, 50–12,000 μs pulse duration, 1–2000 Hz pulse rate and an average power up to 60 W. Due to TFL water's absorption coefficient (four-fold higher) than the Ho:YAG laser, a higher ablation efficiency can be expected at equivalent pulse energies according to pre-clinical studies [50–52].

The Ho:YAG laser efficacy has demonstrated safety and effectiveness in multiple publications since its introduction as kidney stone lithotripter. In large series, the stone-free rates have exceeded 90% accompanied by low rates of complications (ureteral perforation). The Ho:YAG has proved to be an effective and versatile lithotrite for endoscopic treatment due to its ability to disrupt all composition of stones (including calcium oxalate monohydrate and cystine) [53, 54].

The "fragmentation technique" of stones uses higher energy settings (0.6–1 J) with a low frequency (6–15 Hz), so that the stone breaks down into smaller fragments to allow "basketing" or spontaneous passage of the pieces. The "dusting technique" uses lower energy settings (0.2–0.4 J) with a high frequency (50–80 Hz) and disrupts the stone into dust without the need for basketing, allowing spontaneous passage of the dust. The SFR for both techniques are 74.3% VS 58.2%, respectively [54, 55].

Prospective trials comparing the efficacy and SFR of Ho:YAG vs TFL are in development and no specific settings have been described for the new laser technology, the higher efficiency of TFL has been demonstrated in-vitro studies and

Table 21.4 Energy settings for laser lithotripsy in ureteroscopy

Technique	Laser settings	Pulse width
Fragmentation/basketing	Energy: 0.6–0.8 J	Short
	Frequency: 6–15 Hz	
Dusting	Energy: 0.2–0.4 J	Long
	Frequency: 40–80 Hz	

randomized clinical studies are still pending. The recommended laser settings for Ho:YAG laser in the ureter are summarized in Table 21.4.

21.11 Preoperative Care

Proper preoperative planning is paramount for a successful URS. This includes a comprehensive assessment of the patient's medical history for identifying any risk factors for complications. Thorough evaluation of the patient's imaging allows familiarization with the urinary tract anatomy and stone features. This enables the surgeon to anticipate most possible scenarios and plan accordingly.

Good communication and coordination of the operating room team is another key fundamental for a successful URS. This will allow surgeon to request the proper instruments and supplies streamlining operating time. Furthermore, a forethought of the operation with the anesthesia team grants adequate preparation and maintaining patient safety. It is also important to discuss baseline comorbidities with other physicians involved in the care of the patient. In addition, an efficient and informative conversation with the patient beforehand, reviewing patient's expectations, will assist with recovery and follow up.

Surgeons must always assess patients for any symptoms suggestive of preoperative urinary tract infections and a urine culture should be obtained. Every patient should undergo treatment for UTI or asymptomatic bacteriuria before surgery. Furthermore, single-dose antibiotic prophylaxis is mandatory for every patient undergoing URS. Antibiotics selection should be based on prior urine culture results when available, or otherwise by local guidelines. Most common regimens recommend second generation cephalosporins or fluoroquinolones [11, 56, 57].

21.12 Technique for Semi-Rigid and Flexible Ureteroscopy

In the following section, we will describe the step-by-step technique of URS for both diagnostic and therapeutic purposes. This includes room setup, patient positioning, necessary equipment, and tips and tricks. Our emphasis will be on URS as a treatment for urinary tract stone disease.

21.12.1 Operating Room Setup

The necessary equipment to perform a URS includes:

- Lithotomy drapes (cloth reusable drapes or disposable)
- Basic surgical instrumentation (snap clamp, Kelly clamp, field clamp)
- Cystoscope (rigid or flexible)
- Ureteroscope (semi-rigid, flexible, fiberoptic or digital)
- Endoscopic tower, camera and light cord
- Guidewires
- Ancillary equipment including ureteral catheters, coaxial dilator, stone basket, ureteral balloon dilator, ureteric stent
- Irrigation system (gravity or a variety of devices for delivering pressurized irrigation)
- 16 Fr. In-and-out catheter
- Lithotripsy devices (multiple technologies available, e.g , Ho:YAG laser, TFL, pneumatic lithotripter)
- C-arm or fixed fluoroscopy unit and ionizing radiation protective equipment (PPE)

The Fig. 21.2 provides a diagram of the configuration of the operating room for URS. Figs. 21.3 and 21.4 provides an example of the table set-up for ureteroscopy.

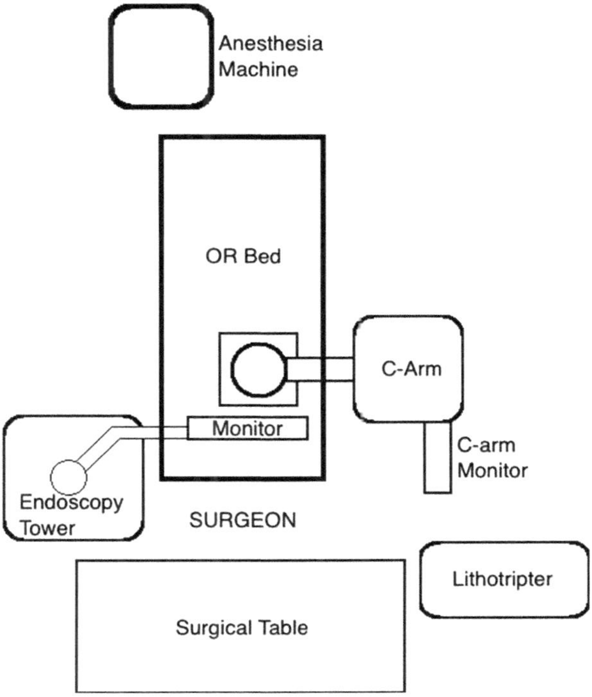

Fig. 21.2 Room setup for ureteroscopy

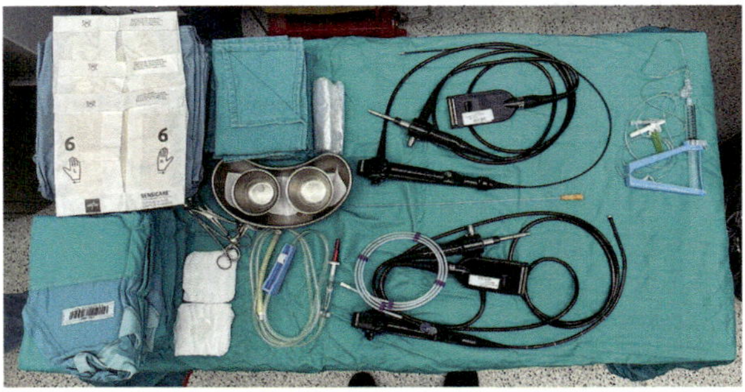

Fig. 21.3 Surgical table set-up for a ureteroscopy (*digital flexible ureteroscope*)

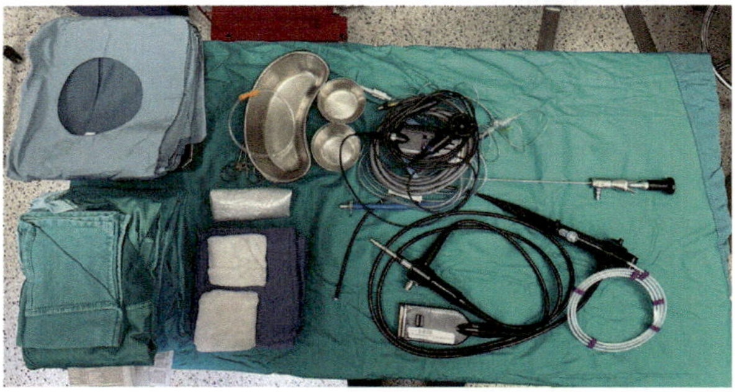

Fig. 21.4 Surgical table set-up for a ureteroscopy (*semi-rigid ureteroscope*)

21.12.2 Patient Positioning

After completing the required surgical safety checklist and antibiotic surgical prophylaxis, the patient is anesthetized with the appropriate general anesthetic (*laryngeal mask airway or endotracheal intubation*). The patient is placed in dorsal lithotomy position with padded stirrups (Yellowfin Apex Stirrups®). The patient can also be positioned with modified dorsal lithotomy (*slight extension and abduction of the treated side*) in performing semi-rigid URS [3]. The surgical bed is advanced towards the surgeon to allow the placement of fluoroscopy C-arm in the Kidney-ureters-bladder (KUB) field for assistance during the procedure.

21.12.3 Cystourethroscopy and Guidewire Placement

We generally perform a systematic cystoscopy with a flexible (16 Fr) or a rigid cystoscope (30° telescope and 17 or 22 Fr sheath), as an assessment of the lower urinary tract including urethra and bladder and configuration of the ureteric orifices. In the scenario of an enlarged prostate, prominent cystocele or stone in a distal ureter it is the preference of the authors to use a rigid cystoscope with a 22 Fr sheath. Once the desired ureteric orifice is identified, it is cannulated with a Teflon coated hydrophilic guidewire under endoscopic and fluoroscopy guidance up to the renal pelvis. If resistance is met due to an impacted ureteric stone, the guidewire is buttressed with a 5 Fr. open-end ureteral catheter. Other techniques for navigating an impacted ureteral stone include the deployment of angled hydrophilic wires and catheters.

21.12.4 Semi-Rigid Ureteroscopy

In most instances and when using contemporary semi rigid ureteroscopes of 7 Fr or smaller diameter dilation of the ureteral orifice is not required. When necessary, the ureteral orifice can be dilated with either a 10 Fr coaxial dilator over the guidewire or with a 6 mm diameter ureteral balloon dilator. The semi rigid ureteroscope is introduced under direct vision transurethrally and the ureteral orifice is identified. The safety guidewire can be utilized as a pathway to identify the orifice. Once the orifice is identified, an attempt is usually conducted to enter below the guidewire to take advantage of the tented ureteric orifice. The advancement of the ureteroscope is performed under direct visualization at all times of the ureteric lumen and being sure the ureteral lumen is always visible and the scope sliding freely along the ureteral wall. Access can also be facilitated with manual pressure irrigation such as with a handheld syringe or other device to open the orifice. In the case of a stone in a ureteral location we typically maintain a safety guidewire throughout the case.

The disruption of the stone is performed with the Ho:YAG laser lithotripter (272-micron straight-tip) until the stone is fragmented in small pieces and flushed out the ureter with manual irrigation. We inspect the ureter as proximal as possible depending on the anatomy of the ureter under direct and fluoroscopy vision. If no sizable stone pieces or migration of stone are documented, the ureteroscope is removed and a double pig-tail ureteric stent is placed under fluoroscopy over the safety guidewire.

21.12.5 Flexible Ureteroscopy

Once a guidewire is properly placed and the coaxial dilation of the intramural ureter is performed, in the case of mid and proximal ureteral stones, we advance a second guidewire (working guidewire) via a coaxial dilator up to the renal pelvis under fluoroscopic vision. If the target stone is in an intrarenal location, we do not deploy a second guidewire and the initial access wire is removed once the flexible endoscope is satisfactorily advanced to the renal pelvis. If the ureteroscope is unable to be advanced past the ureteral orifice formal dilation with a 6 mm balloon dilator is undertaken under fluoroscopic control or alternatively a semi rigid ureteroscope may be used to accomplish the dilation.

The bladder is emptied with an in-and-out catheter (16 Fr.) and the flexible ureteroscope (Digital 8.4 Fr. flexible, 3.6 Fr working channel) is introduced over the working guidewire. Under fluoroscopy vision, we advance the ureteroscope until the stone is reached. If resistance is met at the ureteric orifice or distal ureter, we performed a second coaxial dilation with the 8/10 Fr Amplatz dilator set or balloon dilation (18 Fr [6 mm] × 10 cm balloon dilator). A third option is to advance an optical flexible ureteroscope with a slimmer/thinner tip (Optical 7.9 Fr, flexible).

When the stone is visualized, the working guidewire is removed, and gravity or manual irrigation is utilized to provide a clear field of view. Disruption of the stone is performed with a Ho:YAG laser lithotripter (272-micron straight-tip) until the stone is dusted or fragmented in small pieces. We inspect the collecting system for migrated sizable stone fragments and inspect the ureter while the ureteroscope is removed. Once the ureteroscope is removed, a double pig-tail ureteric stent is placed under fluoroscopy over a guidewire.

21.13 Radiation Safety

The risks of radiation exposure can be divided into deterministic or stochastic effects. The deterministic effects are related to direct cell injury related to direct exposure of the biological tissue to high doses of radiation and has a radiation threshold. The stochastic effects are events that can occur by chance without relation to the threshold levels of radiation (no relation between severity and radiation dose). The greatest stochastic risks are hematologic and solid organ malignancies. As a urologist performing URS under fluoroscopy, we must adhere to the ALARA principles ("as low as reasonably achievable") which takes into account time, distance and shielding. Fluoroscopy time reduction could be achieved such as by digital fluoroscopy, "last imaging hold" technology, pulsed fluoroscopy (fewer frames per second) and keeping track of the time during the procedure. Shields should be used at all times during the procedure and the most common type of shield is protection lead. Lead-impregnated eyeglasses, gloves, thyroid shields, chest and pelvic aprons have shown to attenuate the radiation exposure by 96–99.5% (0.5 mm lead) [58].

Predictors of increased radiation during URS include obese patients, flexible URS, prolonged surgical time, postoperative stenting under fluoroscopy, balloon dilation and surgeon experience. Using "last image hold" and the surgeon controlling the foot-pedal, documented a reduction in radiation exposure of 40 times in a study performed by Bagley et. Al [59]. As previously mentioned, pulsed fluoroscopy at (4 frames per second) was associated with a decreased of 62.4% in fluoroscopy time [60].

Inoue and Matsuda conclude that simple methods to minimize occupational and patient radiation during URS are: controlling fluoroscopy time, collimating the images, pulsed fluoroscopy mode, maximized distance between the x-ray tube and the patient, using protective shielding and wearing a personal dosimeter to track the radiation dose exposure by the urologist [61]. Radiation safety measures should become a priority for urologists due to low-radiation risks exposure inherent to URS procedures.

21.14 Postoperative Care

URS can be routinely and safely conducted as a day procedure. Postoperative pain is usually well-tolerated and non-steroidal anti-inflammatory medications typically provide adequate patient comfort. Post-operative antibiotic therapy is still debatable and controversial. In various centers, prophylactic antibiotics are continued after the discharge in presence of a preoperative negative urine culture, and usually prescribed 3–5 days after the endoscopic procedure. Commonly used antibiotics are quinolones, cephalosporins and trimethoprim/sulfamethoxazole [62].

Urine drainage after URS can be impaired due to urothelial edema related to the mechanical trauma of the ureteroscope. There is no definitive consensus for patient selection and post-operative stent insertion, apart from a URS in transplanted kidney or a solitary kidney. Hollenbeck and colleagues reported an increased morbidity after URS in patients with a prior history of urolithiasis, recurrent urinary tract infections and an increased operative (>45 min) time with lithotripsy [63].

A meta-analysis documented that patients with no post-operative stent placement have a higher risk of unplanned visits to the emergency department in comparison to stented patients, even though, stented patients were more likely to complain of stent-related associated symptoms [64]. Additionally, the ideal duration of the post-operative stent is not well established, and it has been described that the vast majority of urologists remove the post-operative stent at 1–2 weeks and others up to 4–6 weeks after reviewing postoperative imaging; this could be related to different treatment techniques (fragmentation VS dusting) [39, 62, 63].

21.15 Complications

URS is a generally safe intervention; however, significant and even life-threating complications can occur. Certainly, a methodical and stepwise technique is paramount to prevent complications. Minor intraoperative complications are common and often underreported and are mostly found in the form of ureteral wall injury. These may arise from the passage of the scope or guidewires, UAS placement, off-target lasering and stone basketing. Endoscopic and postoperative classifications have been proposed and can be useful for reporting ureteral wall injuries. Whereas most minor intraoperative injuries require no further treatment, some might hinder the procedure, by causing bleeding impairing visualization or extravasation distorting fluoroscopic delimitation of the urinary tract. Ureteric avulsion is a catastrophic intraoperative complication that occurs in less than 0.5% of cases. Ureteric avulsion is commonly caused by exerting excessive force while engaging a large stone fragment with a basket. Therefore, avoiding basketing large fragments, especially in the proximal ureter is the best first step to avoid avulsions. Surgeons should downsize stone fragments before attempting any extraction maneuver. [65–67].

Infectious complications are usually encountered in the early postoperative period and adequate prophylaxis and baseline negative cultures are the most important steps for prevention. While some patients develop urinary tract infections or transient fever that are easy to manage, some patients will develop life-threating infection. Sepsis rate ranges from 1% to 10% and septic shock occurs in around 3% of URS cases but can be fatal if treatment is delayed; in fact, it is the most common cause of death in URS. Thus, early detection and timely onset of management are fundamental. The risk factors for sepsis after URS include stone size, irrigation pressure, prolonged stent indwelling time, prior sepsis as an indication for urgent stent insertion, preoperative positive urine culture, female gender, type 2 diabetes, and long surgical time. Aggressive fluid resuscitation, broad-spectrum antibiotics, urinary tract decompression and close monitoring are the most important aspects of sepsis management. The quick SOFA is an easy-to-use score to detect patients with risk of sepsis and the Surviving Sepsis Campaign guidelines properly outline the stepwise management for the septic patient [65, 68–71].

21.16 Future Perspectives

URS is a well "established" yet evolving intervention and an important component of day to day practice for most general urologists. Disposable instrumentation including pressure-sensing devices are likely to gain traction in the clinical setting soon, and clinical trials will assist in understanding the significance of intrarenal pressure means and how monitoring could help preventing complications, especially sepsis. Similarly, researchers have incorporated devices for stone fluorescence spectra recognition into lasers, which allows automatic discrimination between stones and tissue. This may facilitate prevention of off-target lasering and avoiding ureteral wall injuries [72, 73].

Although an in-depth analysis of laser technology is not within the scope of this chapter, it is worth emphasizing that the improvement and development of emerging energies such as the TFL may widen the stone burden amenable for retrograde URS [72, 74].

One of the more unique recent innovations is the use of robot-assisted URS. Although the main advantage of this technology is ergonomics, some improvements in precision can be expected. The Avicenna Roboflex™ (Elmed Medical, Ankara, Turkey) consists of a console where surgeons can be comfortably sitting, with armrest, and a control with joysticks used to manipulate the movements of the ureteroscope. Thus, surgeon in more comfortable and away from the radiation source. The console permits adjusting features as irrigation and laser fiber position which might have a positive impact on precision. Further refinements in the development of robot-assisted URS are anticipated in coming years.

Questions

1. According to the American Urological Association Guidelines, what would be the ideal treatment for a 45-year-old male, otherwise healthy, with a symptomatic 1.2 cm and 950 Hounsfield unit kidney stone in the right upper pole:
   (a) Surveillance
   (b) Percutaneous nephrolithotomy
   (c) Ureteroscopy with lithotripsy
   (d) Extracorporeal shockwave lithotripsy
   (e) Either Ureteroscopy with lithotripsy or Extracorporeal shockwave lithotripsy

Answer: (e)

2. Which characteristic of the Thulium Fiber Laser, provides its increased water absorption peak (four-fold) and higher stone ablation efficiency?
   (a) Wider pulse duration (50–12,000 μs)
   (b) Light source (Flashlamp Vs Diode configuration)
   (c) Water-cooled system to refrigerate the chemically-doped crystal
   (d) Infrared wavelength (1940 mm)
   (e) Lower pulse energy (0.025–6.0 J)

Answer: (d)

3. What does the photo-acoustic mechanism refer to? In relation to the mechanism for laser lithotripsy stone disruption.
   (a) "Partition of waters" via a primary short pulse emission
   (b) Absorption of laser energy in the water molecules inside the stone
   (c) Violent cavitation bubble collapse
   (d) Melting of the stone surface via absorption of laser energy
   (e) Moses effect

Answer: (c)

4. Sepsis is a life-threatening complication of ureteroscopy. Which of the following are key steps in preventing this complication?
   (a) Pre-stenting patients with obstructive stones
   (b) An empirical preoperative course of antibiotics
   (c) Adequate antibiotic prophylaxis

(d) Negative preoperative urine culture (or treated if positive) and adequate antibiotic prophylaxis
(e) Treating preoperative urinary tract infections

Answer: (d)

5. A worrisome consequence of a high intrarenal pressure in ureteroscopy, especially when exceeding 185 mmHg:

   (a) Pyelovenous backflow
   (b) Stone migration
   (c) Forniceal rupture
   (d) Extravasation
   (e) Pseudoaneurysm

Answer: (c)

References

1. Bagley DH, Calio B. The history of the development of ureteral endoscopy. In: Ureteroscopy. Cham: Springer International Publishing; 2020. p. 1–15.
2. Lyon ES. The birth of modern ureteroscopy: the Albona Jaybis story. J Endourol. 2004;18:525–6. https://doi.org/10.1089/end.2004.18.525.
3. Pérez-Castro Ellendt E, Martínez-Piñeiro JA. Transurethral ureteroscopy. A current urological procedure. Arch Esp Urol. 1980;33:445–60.
4. Marshall VF. Fiber optics in urology. J Urol. 1964;91:110–4. https://doi.org/10.1016/S0022-5347(17)64066-7.
5. Whitehurst LA, Somani BK. Semi-rigid ureteroscopy: indications, tips, and tricks. Urolithiasis. 2018;46:39–45. https://doi.org/10.1007/s00240-017-1025-7.
6. Doizi S, Traxer O. Flexible ureteroscopy: technique, tips and tricks. Urolithiasis. 2018;46:47–58. https://doi.org/10.1007/s00240-017-1030-x.
7. Giusti G, Proietti S, Peschechera R, et al. Sky is no limit for ureteroscopy: extending the indications and special circumstances. World J Urol. 2015;33:257–73. https://doi.org/10.1007/s00345-014-1345-y.
8. Territo A, Gallioli A, Meneghetti I, et al. Diagnostic ureteroscopy for upper tract urothelial carcinoma: friend or foe? Arab J Urol. 2021;19:46–58. https://doi.org/10.1080/2090598X.2021.1883810.
9. Rouprêt M, Babjuk M, Burger M, et al. European association of urology guidelines on upper urinary tract urothelial carcinoma: 2020 update. Eur Urol. 2021;79:62–79. https://doi.org/10.1016/j.eururo.2020.05.042.
10. Proietti S, Marchioni M, Eisner BH, et al. Conservative treatment of upper urinary tract carcinoma in patients with imperative indications. Minerva Urol Nephrol. 2021;73:245–52. https://doi.org/10.23736/S2724-6051.20.03710-8.
11. Assimos D, Krambeck A, Miller NL, et al. Surgical management of stones: American urological association/endourological society guideline, PART I. J Urol. 2016;196:1153–60. https://doi.org/10.1016/j.juro.2016.05.090.
12. Assimos D, Krambeck A, Miller NL, et al. Surgical management of stones: American urological association/endourological society guideline, PART II. J Urol. 2016;196:1161–9. https://doi.org/10.1016/j.juro.2016.05.091.

13. Pradère B, Doizi S, Proietti S, et al. Evaluation of guidelines for surgical management of urolithiasis. J Urol. 2018;199:1267–71. https://doi.org/10.1016/j.juro.2017.11.111.
14. Basulto-Martínez M, Klein I, Gutiérrez-Aceves J. The role of extracorporeal shock wave lithotripsy in the future of stone management. Curr Opin Urol. 2019;29:96–102. https://doi.org/10.1097/MOU.0000000000000584.
15. Kroczak T, Scotland KB, Chew B, Pace KT. Shockwave lithotripsy: techniques for improving outcomes. World J Urol. 2017;35:1341–6. https://doi.org/10.1007/s00345-017-2056-y.
16. Dorantes-Carrillo LA, Basulto-Martínez M, Suárez-Ibarrola R, et al. Retrograde intrarenal surgery versus miniaturized percutaneous nephrolithotomy for kidney stones >1 cm: a systematic review and meta-analysis of randomized trials. Eur Urol Focus. 2022;8:259–70. https://doi.org/10.1016/j.euf.2021.02.008.
17. Scotland KB, Rudnick B, Healy KA, et al. Retrograde ureteroscopic management of large renal calculi: a single institutional experience and concise literature review. J Endourol. 2018;32:603–7. https://doi.org/10.1089/end.2018.0069.
18. Pevzner M, Stisser BC, Luskin J, et al. Alternative management of complex renal stones. Int Urol Nephrol. 2011;43:631–8. https://doi.org/10.1007/s11255-010-9880-y.
19. Giusti G, Proietti S, Rodríguez-Socarrás ME, et al. Semirigid ureteroscopy: step by step. J Endourol. 2020;34:S13–6. https://doi.org/10.1089/end.2018.0286.
20. Scotland KB, Chan JYH, Chew BH. Single-use flexible ureteroscopes: how do they compare with reusable ureteroscopes? J Endourol. 2019;33:71–8. https://doi.org/10.1089/end.2018.0785.
21. Proietti S, Pavia MP, Rico L, et al. Disposable flexible ureteroscopes. In: Flexible ureteroscopy. Singapore: Springer Nature Singapore; 2022. p. 209–14.
22. Scotland KB, Lim JRZ, Chew BH. Flexible ureteroscope technology. In: Ureteroscopy. Cham: Springer International Publishing; 2020. p. 35–50.
23. Ventimiglia E, Somani BK, Traxer O. Flexible ureteroscopy: reuse? Or is single use the new direction? Curr Opin Urol. 2020;30:113–9. https://doi.org/10.1097/MOU.0000000000000700.
24. Yeow Y, Proietti S, Basulto-Martinez M, et al. Accessories, sterilization, and instrument care in flexible ureteroscopy. In: Flexible ureteroscopy. Singapore: Springer Nature Singapore; 2022. p. 41–52.
25. Hennessey DB, Fojecki GL, Papa NP, et al. Single-use disposable digital flexible ureteroscopes: an ex vivo assessment and cost analysis. BJU Int. 2018;121:55–61. https://doi.org/10.1111/bju.14235.
26. Davis NF, McGrath S, Quinlan M, et al. Carbon footprint in flexible ureteroscopy: a comparative study on the environmental impact of reusable and single-use ureteroscopes. J Endourol. 2018;32:214–7. https://doi.org/10.1089/end.2018.0001.
27. Hogan D, Rauf H, Kinnear N, Hennessey DB. The carbon footprint of single-use flexible cystoscopes compared with reusable cystoscopes. J Endourol. 2022;36:1460–4. https://doi.org/10.1089/end.2021.0891.
28. Giusti G, Proietti S, Villa L, et al. Current standard technique for modern flexible ureteroscopy: tips and tricks. Eur Urol. 2016;70:188–94. https://doi.org/10.1016/j.eururo.2016.03.035.
29. Villa L, Ventimiglia E, Proietti S, et al. Does working channel position influence the effectiveness of flexible ureteroscopy? Results from an in vitro study. BJU Int. 2020;125:449–56. https://doi.org/10.1111/bju.14923.
30. Clayman M, Uribe CA, Eichel L, et al. Comparison of guide wires in urology. Which, when and why? J Urol. 2004;171:2146–50. https://doi.org/10.1097/01.ju.0000124486.78866.a5.
31. De La Cerda J, Tseng TY. Access to the ureter. In: Smith's textbook of endourology. Chichester: John Wiley & Sons, Ltd; 2018. p. 514–20.
32. Pedro RN, Monga M. Ureteroscopy working instruments. In: Smith's textbook of endourology. Oxford: Wiley-Blackwell; 2012. p. 388–94.
33. Calvert RC. Devices for stone management. In: Ureteroscopy. Cham: Springer International Publishing; 2020. p. 85–99.

34. Cetti R, Biers S, Keoghane S. The difficult ureter: what is the incidence of pre-stenting? Ann R Coll Surg Engl. 2011;93:31–3. https://doi.org/10.1308/003588411X12851639106990.
35. Kuntz NJ, Neisius A, Tsivian M, et al. Balloon dilation of the ureter: a contemporary review of outcomes and complications. J Urol. 2015;194:413–7. https://doi.org/10.1016/j.juro.2015.02.2917.
36. Shah O, Silva MV. Access to the ureter. In: Smith's textbook of endourology. Chichester: John Wiley & Sons, Ltd; 2018. p. 521–31.
37. Rehman J, Monga M, Landman J, et al. Characterization of intrapelvic pressure during ureteropyeloscopy with ureteral access sheaths. Urology. 2003;61:713–8. https://doi.org/10.1016/S0090-4295(02)02440-8.
38. Alenezi H, Howlett CJ, El-Warrak AO, et al. PD23-09 is prolonged use of ureteral access sheath safe? J Urol. 2016;195:e509. https://doi.org/10.1016/j.juro.2016.02.1748.
39. Türk C, Petřík A, Sarica K, et al. EAU guidelines on interventional treatment for urolithiasis. Eur Urol. 2016;69:475–82. https://doi.org/10.1016/j.eururo.2015.07.041.
40. Lee MS, Connors BA, Agarwal DK, et al. Determining the threshold of acute renal parenchymal damage for intrarenal pressure during flexible ureteroscopy using an in vivo pig model. World J Urol. 2022;40:2675–81. https://doi.org/10.1007/s00345-022-04154-5.
41. Kottooran C, Twum-Ampofo J, Lee J, et al. Evaluation of fluid absorption during flexible ureteroscopy in an in vivo porcine model. BJU Int. 2022;131(2):213–8. https://doi.org/10.1111/bju.15858.
42. Jung H, Osther PJS. Intraluminal pressure profiles during flexible ureterorenoscopy. Springerplus. 2015;4:373. https://doi.org/10.1186/s40064-015-1114-4.
43. Doizi S, Letendre J, Cloutier J, et al. Continuous monitoring of intrapelvic pressure during flexible ureteroscopy using a sensor wire: a pilot study. World J Urol. 2021;39:555–61. https://doi.org/10.1007/s00345-020-03216-w.
44. Zhong Y, Xie D, Luo C, et al. Clinical application of flexible ureteroscopic sheath with controllable intraluminal pressure in treating ureteral stones. Asian J Urol. 2021;10(2):166–71. https://doi.org/10.1016/j.ajur.2021.08.007.
45. Denstedt JD, Razvi HA, Sales JL, Eberwein PM. Preliminary experience with holmium:YAG laser lithotripsy. J Endourol. 1995;9:255e8. https://doi.org/10.1089/end.1995.9.255.
46. Chan KF, Joshua Pfefer T, Teichman JMH, Welch AJ. A perspective on laser lithotripsy: the fragmentation processes. J Endourol. 2001;15:257–73. https://doi.org/10.1089/089277901750161737.
47. Pierre S, Preminger GM. Holmium laser for stone management. World J Urol. 2007;25:235–9. https://doi.org/10.1007/s00345-007-0162-y.
48. Jansen ED, Asshauer T, Frenz M, et al. Effect of pulse duration on bubble formation and laser-induced pressure waves during holmium laser ablation. Lasers Surg Med. 1996;18:278–93. https://doi.org/10.1002/(SICI)1096-9101(1996)18:3<278::AID-LSM10>3.0.CO;2-2.
49. Vassar GJ, Chan KF, Teichman JMH, et al. Holmium: YAG lithotripsy: photothermal mechanism. J Endourol. 1999;13:181–90. https://doi.org/10.1089/end.1999.13.181.
50. Traxer O, Keller EX. Thulium fiber laser: the new player for kidney stone treatment? A comparison with holmium:YAG laser. World J Urol. 2020;38:1883–94. https://doi.org/10.1007/s00345-019-02654-5.
51. Blackmon RL, Irby PB, Fried NM. Comparison of holmium:YAG and thulium fiber laser lithotripsy: ablation thresholds, ablation rates, and retropulsion effects. J Biomed Opt. 2011;16:071403. https://doi.org/10.1117/1.3564884.
52. Hardy LA, Vinnichenko V, Fried NM. High power holmium:YAG versus thulium fiber laser treatment of kidney stones in dusting mode: ablation rate and fragment size studies. Lasers Surg Med. 2019;51:522–30. https://doi.org/10.1002/lsm.23057.
53. Sofer M, Watterson JD, Wollin TA, et al. Holmium: Yag laser lithotripsy for upper urinary tract calculi in 598 patients. J Urol. 2002;167:31–4. https://doi.org/10.1016/S0022-5347(05)65376-1.

54. Sourial MW, Knudsen BE. Ho:YAG laser lithotripsy. In: Ureteroscopy. Cham: Springer International Publishing; 2020. p. 101–12.
55. Humphreys MR, Shah OD, Monga M, et al. Dusting versus basketing during ureteroscopy–which technique is more efficacious? A prospective multicenter trial from the EDGE research consortium. J Urol. 2018;199:1272–6. https://doi.org/10.1016/j.juro.2017.11.126.
56. Schnabel MJ, Wagenlehner FME, Schneidewind L. Perioperative antibiotic prophylaxis for stone therapy. Curr Opin Urol. 2019;29:89–95. https://doi.org/10.1097/MOU.0000000000000576.
57. Knopf H-J, Graff H-J, Schulze H. Perioperative antibiotic prophylaxis in ureteroscopic stone removal. Eur Urol. 2003;44:115–8. https://doi.org/10.1016/S0302-2838(03)00189-1.
58. Noureldin YA, Andonian S. Radiation safety during diagnosis and treatment. In: Smith's textbook of endourology. Chichester: John Wiley & Sons, Ltd; 2018. p. 14–37.
59. Bagley DH, Cubler-Goodman A. Radiation exposure during ureteroscopy. J Urol. 1990;144:1356–8. https://doi.org/10.1016/S0022-5347(17)39739-2.
60. Elkoushy MA, Shahrour W, Andonian S. Pulsed fluoroscopy in ureteroscopy and percutaneous nephrolithotomy. Urology. 2012;79:1230–5. https://doi.org/10.1016/j.urology.2012.01.027.
61. Inoue T, Matsuda T. Radiation safety during surgery for urolithiasis. In: Ureteroscopy. Cham: Springer International Publishing; 2020. p. 51–62.
62. Sabler IM, Katafygiotis I, Duvdevani M. Postoperative care of the ureteroscopy patient. In: Ureteroscopy. Cham: Springer International Publishing; 2020. p. 141–50.
63. Hollenbeck BK, Schuster TG, Seifman BD, et al. Identifying patients who are suitable for stentless ureteroscopy following treatment of urolithiasis. J Urol. 2003;170:103–6. https://doi.org/10.1097/01.ju.0000069546.53896.6a.
64. Pais VM, Smith RE, Stedina EA, Rissman CM. Does omission of ureteral stents increase risk of unplanned return visit? A systematic review and meta-analysis. J Urol. 2016;196:1458–66. https://doi.org/10.1016/j.juro.2016.05.109.
65. De Coninck V, Keller EX, Somani B, et al. Complications of ureteroscopy: a complete overview. World J Urol. 2020;38:2147–66. https://doi.org/10.1007/s00345-019-03012-1.
66. Traxer O, Thomas A. Prospective evaluation and classification of ureteral wall injuries resulting from insertion of a ureteral access sheath during retrograde intrarenal surgery. J Urol. 2013;189:580–4. https://doi.org/10.1016/j.juro.2012.08.197.
67. Schoenthaler M, Buchholz N, Farin E, et al. The post-ureteroscopic lesion scale (PULS): a multicenter video-based evaluation of inter-rater reliability. World J Urol. 2014;32:1033–40. https://doi.org/10.1007/s00345-013-1185-1.
68. Corrales M, Sierra A, Doizi S, Traxer O. Risk of sepsis in retrograde intrarenal surgery: a systematic review of the literature. Eur Urol Open Sci. 2022;44:84–91. https://doi.org/10.1016/j.euros.2022.08.008.
69. Rhodes A, Evans LE, Alhazzani W, et al. Surviving sepsis campaign: international guidelines for management of sepsis and septic shock: 2016. Intensive Care Med. 2017;43:304–77. https://doi.org/10.1007/s00134-017-4683-6.
70. Song J-U, Sin CK, Park HK, et al. Performance of the quick sequential (sepsis-related) organ failure assessment score as a prognostic tool in infected patients outside the intensive care unit: a systematic review and meta-analysis. Crit Care. 2018;22:28 https://doi.org/10.1186/s13054-018-1952-x.
71. Scotland K, Lange D. Prevention and management of urosepsis triggered by ureteroscopy. Res Reports Urol. 2018;10:43–9. https://doi.org/10.2147/RRU.S128071.
72. Secker A, Rassweiler J, Neisius A. Future perspectives of flexible ureteroscopy. Curr Opin Urol. 2019;29:113–7. https://doi.org/10.1097/MOU.0000000000000575.
73. Schlager D, Schulte A, Schütz J, et al. Laser-guided real-time automatic target identification for endoscopic stone lithotripsy: a two-arm in vivo porcine comparison study. World J Urol. 2021;39:2719–26. https://doi.org/10.1007/s00345-020-03452-0.
74. Kallidonis P, Vagionis A. The future of laser technology in kidney stones. Curr Opin Urol. 2022;32:411–4. https://doi.org/10.1097/MOU.0000000000001006.

Chapter 22
The Ureter and Urinary Diversion

Bedeir Ali-El-Dein

Abstract In this chapter, a short introduction on the types of urinary diversion is made. The methods of the uretero-enteric anastomosis in various types of urinary diversion are discussed. In addition, the current trends of uretero-enteric anastomosis, especially in low pressure reservoirs, are presented. Furthermore, a detailed discussion is provided on the main ureter-related complications, their causes, risk factors, incidence, diagnosis, and treatment. The most important of these complications, namely, uretero-enteric anastomotic stricture is critically described and analysed, together with its diagnostic methods, and treatment options. In the end of this chapter, a hint on the future perspective of urinary diversion is provided.

Keywords Alpha-adrenergic blockers · urinary diversion · Neobladder · Ileal loop conduit · Colon conduit · Continent cutaneous urinary diversion · Uretero-enteric anastomosis · Anti-reflux techniques · Direct anastomosis · Uretero-enteric anastomotic stricture · Open revision · Endourologic treatment · Minimally invasive approaches

Learning Objectives
The learning objectives for this chapter are

- To describe the various methods of urinary diversion and the techniques of ureteral implantation in each of them,
- To discuss the ureter-related complications after urinary diversion, and
- To describe the various techniques of treatment of these complications.

Test your learning and check your understanding of this book's contents: use the "Springer Nature Flashcards" app to access questions. To use the app, please follow the instructions in chapter 1.

B. Ali-El-Dein (✉)
Urology Department, Urology and Nephrology Center, Faculty of Medicine, Mansoura University, Mansoura, Egypt

M. Abdel-Gawad et al. (eds.), *The Ureter*,
https://doi.org/10.1007/978-3-031-36212-5_22

22.1 Introduction

Urinary diversion is the creation of a new pathway for the urine to be drained outside the body. Urinary diversion is performed in cases of inability to use the normal pathway of urine or when the bladder is functionless or dangerous, such as in bladder cancer; the latter is the commonest cause of urinary diversion.

There are two main types of urinary diversion: continent and incontinent and there are multiple methods to implant the ureter in urinary diversion. Ureter-related complications of urinary diversion range from mild complications requiring prolongation of catheter and stents to life threatening sepsis.

22.2 Classification of the Types of Urinary Diversion

In this discussion, a hint on the types of urinary diversion is given. The types of urinary diversion can be classified in different ways, namely continent and incontinent, heterotopic and orthotopic, internal and external or according to the duration into temporary and permanent, or according to the purpose into palliative and definitive.

One of the characteristics of an ideal urinary diversion is that it maintains or improves the kidney function and the upper urinary tract. Therefore, the method of ureteral implantation in the urinary diversion is of utmost importance.

The diagram in Fig. 22.1 demonstrates the various types of continent and incontinent urinary diversion.

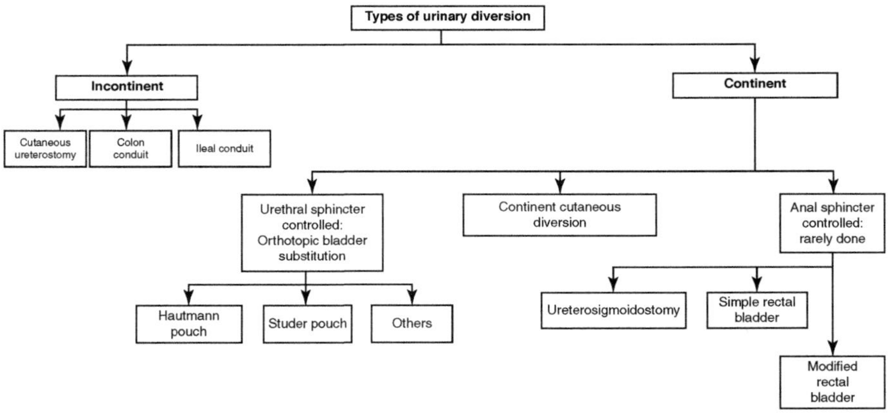

Fig. 22.1 A diagram showing the various types of continent and incontinent urinary diversion

22.3 Ureteral Anastomosis in the Common Urinary Diversion Techniques

John Simon was the first one to describe a urinary diversion technique in 1852, where bilateral ureterosigmoidostomy was performed in a 13-year old child suffering from bladder exstrophy [1]. Since then, the indications and techniques of urinary diversion have shown major expansion.

22.3.1 Historical Perspective

The basic mechanism associated with uretero-enteric anastomosis was first introduced by Coffey in 1911, where direct uretero-colic anastomosis resulted in severe pyelonephritis, sepsis and kidney function loss in dogs due to the marked increase of intrarectal pressure (more than 200 cm water) with subsequent passage of the fecal matter into the upper urinary tract [2]. Based on the conclusion of this experiment, it was conceived that an antireflux submucosal uretero-colic anastomosis is essential to protect the upper tract [3, 4]. Similarly, following the advent of the ileal conduit in the 1950s and the ileal conduit-related deterioration of the kidney function on the long term, the colon conduit with performance of an antireflux uretero-colic anastomosis was reported [5, 6].

Later on, the rectal diversion techniques and their modifications have become very rarely conducted, and currently the creation of continent low pressure reservoirs, either in the form of orthotopic or continent cutaneous pouches, and ileal conduit have become the most commonly performed techniques. With the low pressure reservoirs, performing an anti-reflux uretero-enteric anastomosis is no longer necessary, and it has been proven that the kidney function is maintained with direct ureteral anastomosis [7–12].

The first formal uretero-enteric anastomosis was reported by Bricker in 1956, where the ureteral adventia was connected to the intestinal segment serosa, followed by an incision in the intestinal wall, almost equal to the diameter of the cut ureter, and suturing of the ureter full thickness including the adventia to the intestinal mucosa using 5/0 sutures on a tapered needle [5].

Subsequently, after describing the Bricker technique as time consuming and tedious, Wallace reported on a different technique in 1966, with less sutures, faster to perform, and with fewer complications [13].

Thereafter, a variety of various techniques of uretero-intestinal anastomosis was reported, as will be detailed later in this chapter.

22.3.2 *General Principles*

A delicate manipulation of the ureter with preservation of the periureteral vascular network, avoidance of thermal dissection, a mucosa to mucosa water-tight anastomosis, avoidance of kinking, and tension free stented mucosa-to-mucosa anastomosis are important key elements. In addition, the ureteral length has to be as short as possible without compromising the principle of tension free anastomosis. If the ureter is short, the pouch or the conduit is brought to the ureter and not the reverse. Furthermore, fine absorbable sutures are used, and if possible the bowel is preferably fixed to the abdominal cavity and the ureter is kept in the retroperitoneum as much as possible.

22.3.3 *Ureteral Implantation in Different Urinary Diversion Techniques*

22.3.3.1 Incontinent Urinary Diversion

Cutaneous Ureterostomy

History

A primitive technique of cutaneous ureterostomy was first theorized by Gigon in 1856; thereafter, a report was introduced by Gluck and Zeller in 1881 in dogs, and other modifications were described [14–19]. The first cutaneous ureterostomy was reported by Hayes Agnew; the first bilateral cutaneous ureterostomy was reported by Papin in 1913, and novel technical modifications were advised by Chutte and Sallade in 1961, Eckstein in 1963, and Lusuardi et al. in 2005 [14–19].

Technique, Complications, Modifications

This technique is usually performed after radical cystectomy, where the distal ends of both ureters are spatulated and exteriorized through a hiatus made in the abdominal wall, and anastomosed to the skin (Fig. 22.2). It is the least complex, fastest, and simplest mode of urinary diversion; however, it has been attended with high rates of stricture and other complications that limited its use. Nevertheless, it is used nowadays in patients with severe comorbidities, in whom other methods of urinary diversion using the bowel are very difficult to conduct [20–23].

Recently, some modifications have been described to reduce the complications of cutaneous ureterostomy and to make this technique a valid option for patients unfit for other modes of urinary diversion [19, 20, 24].

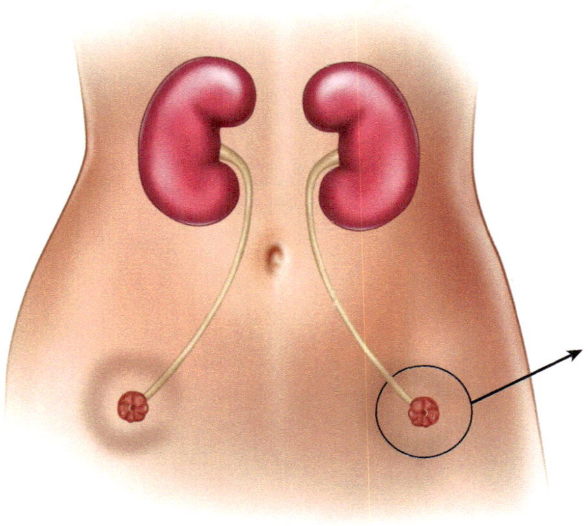

Fig. 22.2 A diagram demonstrating bilateral cutaneous ureterostomy. The arrow refers to the details of the technique provided in Fig. 22.3

Ileal Conduit (Bricker's Conduit)

In this technique, an isoperistaltic, 15–20-cm long segment of the ileum, 10–15 cm proximal to the ileocecal valve is isolated [25]. The ureters are then implanted into the proximal part of the isolated loop and the distal end of the loop is exteriorized through a hiatus in the anterior abdominal wall, followed by nippling of the distal end and ileo-cutaneous anastomosis (Fig. 22.4).

Methods of Uretero-Enteric Anastomosis in Ileal Loop Conduit

The direct refluxing Bricker and Wallace uretero-enteric anastomoses are the most commonly performed techniques in association with ileal loop conduit [5, 13]**.**

Bricker Technique

In his original description in the early 1950s, the Bricker technique was performed by spatulating the ureter and separate anastomosis of each ureter to the serosa of the isolated ileal loop [5]. A button hole is made in the side wall of the bowel with removal of a full thickness plug, the posterior line of the uretero-ileal anastomosis is conducted, a stent is placed, and the anterior line of the anstomosis is completed

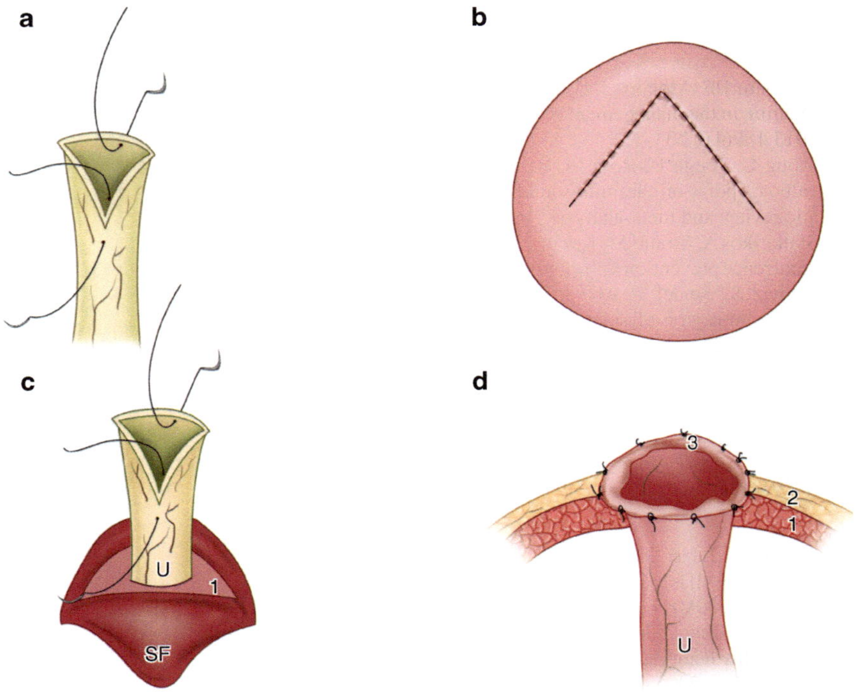

Fig. 22.3 Diagrammatic representation of the details of cutaneous ureterostomy. The ureter is dissected carefully and disconnected from the bladder, the distal end is spatulated (1.5 cm), and 2 stay sutures (5/0 absorbable) were used to hold the spatulated angle and the contralateral side (**a**). A V-shaped incision is made in the skin on either side, usually the iliac fossa; it is done as a modification to prevent stricture at the anstomotic site (**b**). A hiatus (1) is made in the peritoneum and anterior abdominal wall, wide enough to prevent stenosis, the spatulated ureter (U) is exteriorized without kinking, and the V-shaped skin flap (SF) is everted (**c**). (**d**) Shows the final shape of the ureterocutaneous anastomosis, where the ureter (U) is brought through the hiatus in the abdominal wall muscle (1) and subcutaneous tissue (2), and anastomosed at its distal end to the skin using interrupted absorbable sutures (3)

with 5/0 absorbable sutures, including the ureteral adventia and ileal serosa (Fig. 22.5). Several hundreds of ileal loop conduit diversions with this technique were carried out, with good outcome [26].

Wallace Technique

During the same era, radiotherapy had been adopted by European urologists as the standard of care for invasive bladder cancer [27]. At this time, the Wallace technique of uretero-enteric anastomosis was described in the early 1960s, and popularized, thereafter [28–30].

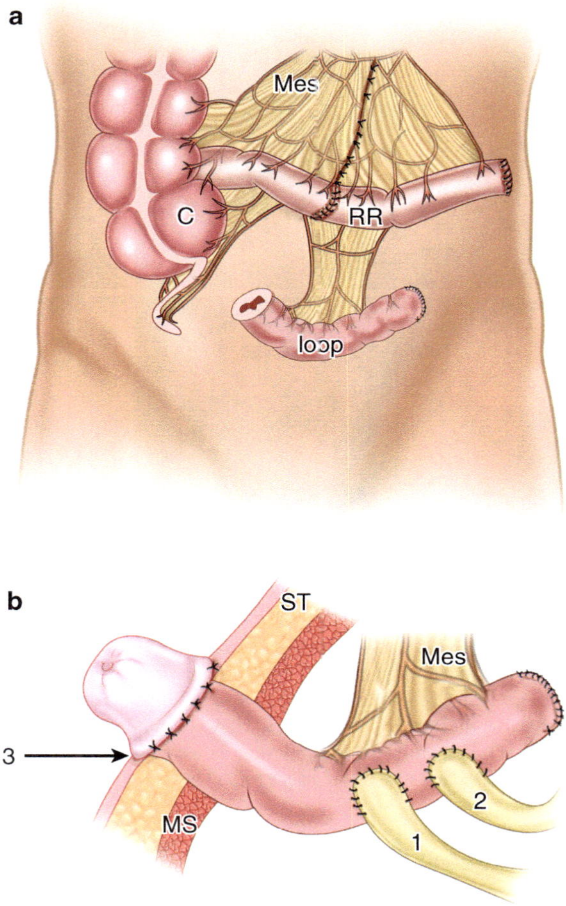

Fig. 22.4 Diagram demonstrating the technique of ileal loop (Bricker) conduit. (**a**) An isoperistaltic, 15–20-cm long segment of the ileum (loop), 10–15 cm proximal to the ileocecal valve is isolated, and followed by restoration of the continuity of the ileum (RR) and closure of the mesentery (Mes). C refers to the cecum. (**b**) The ureters (1&2) are then implanted into the proximal part of the isolated loop and the distal end of the loop is exteriorized through a hiatus in the anterior abdominal wall (muscles = Ms; subcutaneous tissue = ST), followed by nippling of the distal end and ileo-cutaneous anastomosis (3)

In the original description (Wallace 1), the two ureters are spatulated, then a side to side anastomosis, of the medial walls of the two ureters, is conducted, and the resulting common stem (lateral walls of both ureters) is then connected to the proximal part of the isolated bowel segment (Fig. 22.6) [13]. In the Wallace two procedure, the head-to-tail anastomotic modification was reported in 1969 (Fig. 22.6) [31]. In this technique, the vascularity of both ends of the ureters is preserved by anastomosing the apex of one ureter to the end of the second, followed by anastomosing the common stem (made of the ends of the lateral walls) to the wall of the isolated ileal (or bowel) segment.

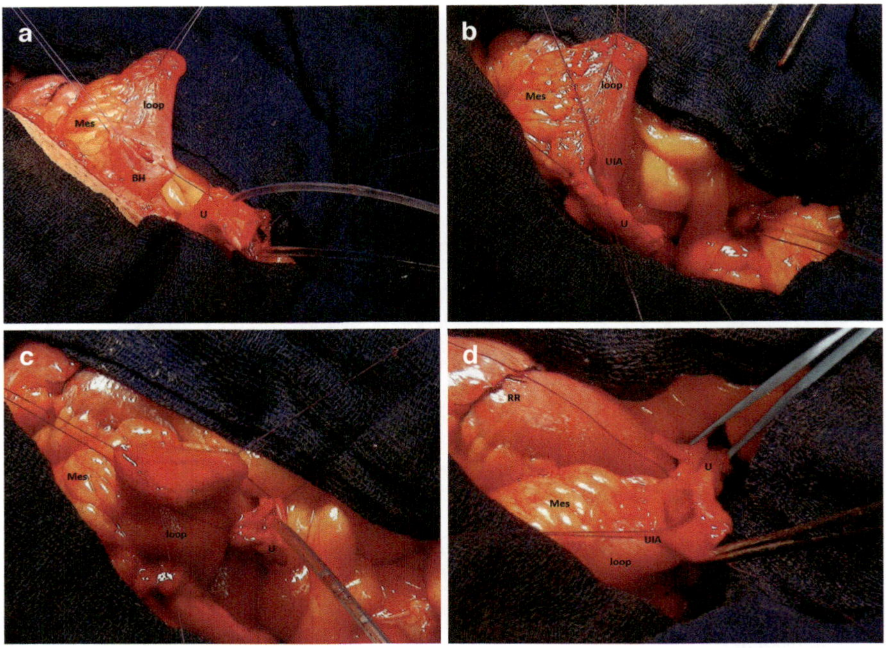

Fig. 22.5 Intra-operative photos showing the end-to-side and end-to-end uretero-ileal anastomosis (UIA). (**a**) The end of the right ureter (U) is spatulated, a button hole (BH) is made in the anterior wall of the loop (loop) and stay sutures are held. (**b**) The uretero-ileal anastomosis (UIA) is started, the posterior row of the UIA is completed, and a stent is seen. (**c**) The end of the left ureter (U) is spatulated, and stay sutures were taken to start the end-to-end uretero-ileal anastomosis. (**d**): The first row of the uretero-ileal anastomosis (UIA) is conducted, a stent is left

Bricker Versus Wallace Technique

The most important complication of the Bricker procedure is the high potential for anastomotic stricture [32]. On the other hand, the Wallace technique is criticized by the increased possibility of posing both kidneys at danger secondary to a possible bilateral ureteric obstruction at the anastomotic site, due to a possible faulty technique, recurrence of cancer, or bilateral stone disease [33].

There has been no significant difference between Bricker and Wallace techniques in the rates of complications, especially uretero-enteric anastomotic stricture [34, 35]. This conclusion is held true even in the presence of confounding factors, such as age, gender, history of irradiation, and duration of follow-up [34]. However, in the recent review of Krafft et al., a higher risk of bilateral uretero-enteric anastomotic stricture was suggested with the Wallace technique under consideration of the individual renal units [35].

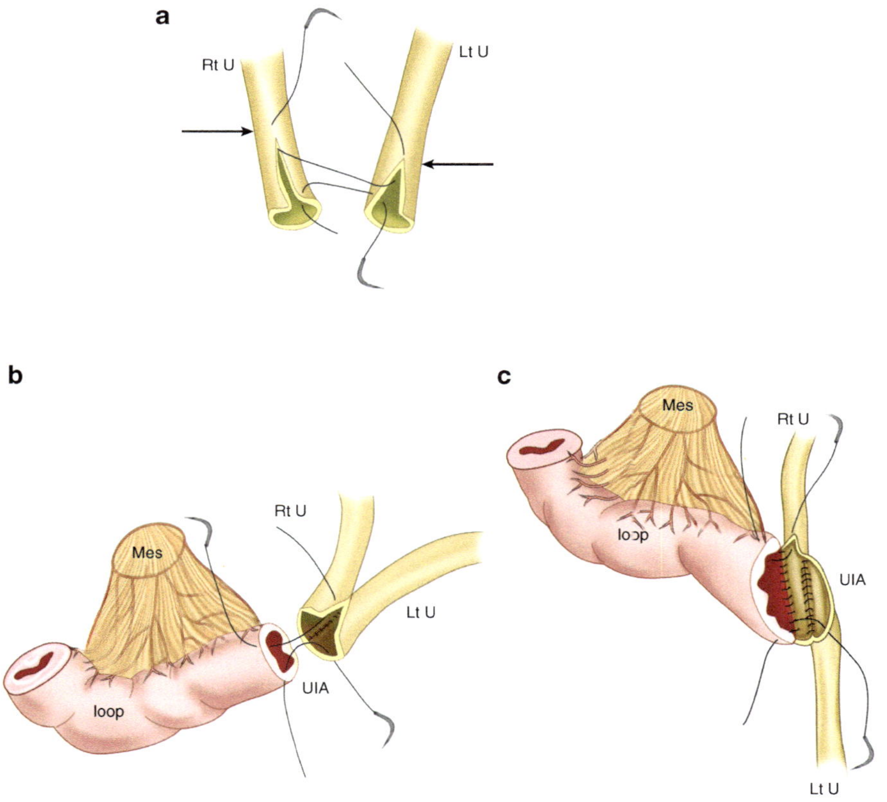

Fig. 22.6 Wallace technique is demonstrated. (**a**) In Wallace 1 uretero-ileal anastomosis (UIA), the two ureters (Rt U & Lt U) are spatulated, and a side to side anastomosis, of the medial walls of the two ureters, is conducted. (**b**) The resulting common stem (lateral walls of both ureters) is then connected to the proximal part of the isolated bowel segment (loop). (**c**) Diagram showing Wallace 2 uretero-ileal anstomosis (UIA), the head-to-tail anastomotic modification of Wallace 1. The apex of one ureter is anastomosed to the end of the second, followed by anastomosing the common stem (made of the ends of the lateral walls) to the wall of the isolated ileal segment (loop)

Modifications of Bricker and Wallace Techniques

Multiple modifications of Bricker and Wallace uretero-enteric anastomotic techniques were described to minimize the incidence of ureter-related complications, particularly stricture and leakage [36–39]. However, the original techniques are still conducted in the majority of large volume hospitals.

Anti-Refluxive Uretero-Ileal Anastomosis with Ileal Loop Conduit

An antireflux uretero-ileal anastomosis was proposed by Le Duc et al. (Le Duc technique), where an incision (3–5 cm) on the anti-mesenteric border of the proximal end of the isolated ileal loop is made, followed by creation of two longitudinal rents (incisions) in the ileal mucosa for 1–2 cm starting from the site of entry of each ureter, and the mucosa of the rents is raised [40]. A serosal hole is made at the distal end of the mucosal incision, through which the ureter is pulled. Thereafter, the ends of the ureters are spatulated, laid down in the mucosal troughs, and sutured to the mucosa of the ileum, using 4/0 or 5/0 absorbable sutures, without approximation of the ileal mucosa over the top of the ureter, but rather using few stitches to suture the mucosa to the side of the ureter (Fig. 22.7).

Overall, the type of the uretero-ileal anastomosis is decided based on surgeon expertise and preference, the length and width of both ureters, and the renal function. Both Bricker and Wallace procedures have passed the test of time; have been widely used, and associated with reasonable rates of uretero-enteric strictures [41].

Methods of Uretero-Enteric Anastomosis in Colon Conduit

Colon conduit is indicated in cases of history of irradiation to treat malignancy, *as a salvage procedure in cases of a previously failed diversion, such as ileal conduit or ureterosigmoidostomy, and when the ureter is too short for a Bricker conduit* [42–44]. The methods of uretero-colic anastomosis are the same as those used in ileal conduit, namely the direct refluxing Bricker and Wallace uretero-enteric anastomoses, and the Le Duc procedure [5, 13, 40].

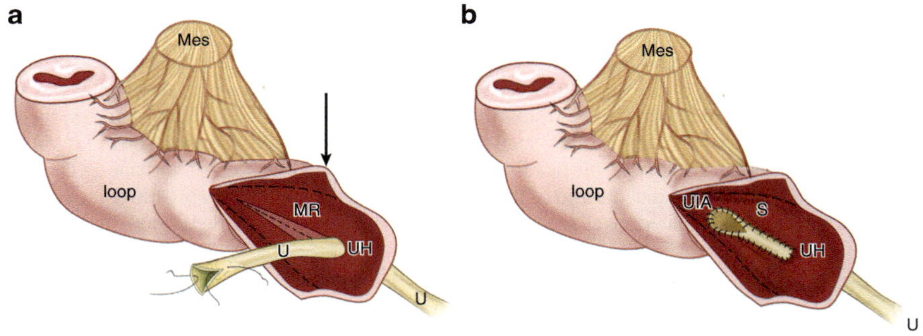

Fig. 22.7 Diagram showing Le Duc antirefluxive uretero-ileal anstomosis (UIA). (**a**) An incision (3–5 cm) on the anti-mesenteric border of the proximal end of the isolated ileal loop is made (arrow), followed by creation of a longitudinal rent (MR) in the ileal mucosa for 1–2 cm starting from the site of entry of the ureter, and the mucosa of the rent is raised. A serosal hole (UH) is made at the distal end of the mucosal incision, through which the ureter is pulled. Thereafter, the end of the ureter (U) is spatulated. (**b**) The spatulated ureter is laid down in the mucosal trough, and sutured to the mucosa of the ileum (UIA), using 4/0 or 5/0 absorbable sutures, without approximation of the ileal mucosa over the top of the ureter, but rather using few stitches (S) to suture the mucosa to the side of the ureter

22.3.3.2 Continent Urinary Diversion

This mode of diversion includes a wide variety of techniques.

22.3.3.3 Urethral Sphincter-Controlled Urinary Diversion (Orthotopic Bladder Substitution)

The term neobladder is often used as a synonym to orthotopic urinary diversion. There have been several types of neobladder, including but not limited to, the U-shaped neobladder of Camey I, Camey II, the Z-shaped of modified Camey II, the sagittally-folded U-shaped of the Kock, T-pouch, Studer, the W-shaped of Hautmann, Abol-Enein and Ghoneim modification, the circular neobladder of the vesica Ileale Padovana, the ileo-colonic (Mainz), and the sigmoid neobladder (Reddy) [45, 46]. Herein, the methods of ureteral implantation used in the most common neobladders are described.

The Urethral Hemi-Kock Pouch

The original Kock pouch was first described by Nils Kock as a continent cutaneous pouch, made of a reservoir and staple-held nipple valve as a continence mechanism [47]. Later on, it was subjected to multiple modifications and was used as an orthotopic bladder substitute (urethral hemi-Kock pouch) in both males and females [48–53]. *The anti-reflux uretero-ileal mechanism was performed by the staple-held nipple valve.* Skinner popularized this technique, and devised several modifications to decrease the nipple valve-associated problems [50, 51]. However, problems associated with the nipple valve, such as desusception, reflux, stone formation on the staples, ureteral obstruction, and the subsequent high re-operation rates have limited the use of the hemi-Kock pouch with time, until *it becomes historical nowadays* [47–54].

Studer Pouch

The technique of Studer pouch was first reported in 1989 [55, 56]. *Since that time, it has been widely used all over the world, as such or with some modifications* [57–59]. According to its original description, the Studer pouch is constructed from an ileal segment around 55-cm long, and 25-cm proximal to the ileo-cecal valve [55, 56]. Both ends of the isolated ileal segment are closed, followed by incision of the anti-mesenteric border of the distal 40–45 cm long segment of the ileum, and implantation of the two ureters into the ileum (Fig. 22.8).

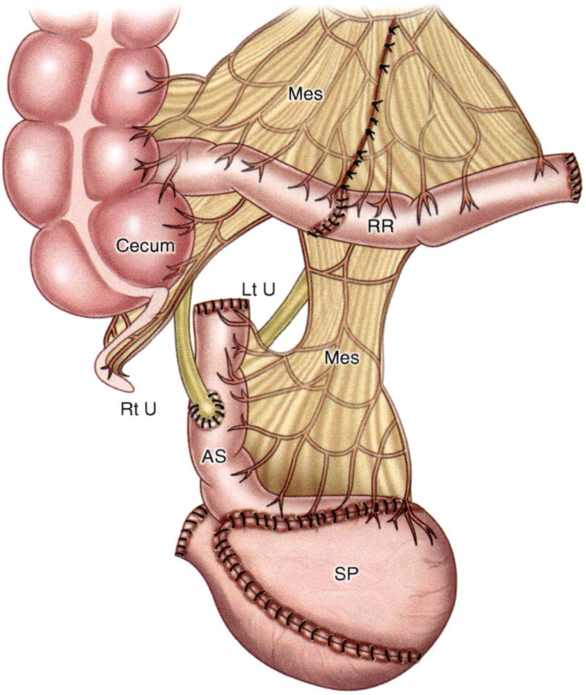

Fig. 22.8 Diagram showing Nesbit direct end-to-side uretero-ileal anstomosis in Studer pouch. The ileal segment for construction of the Studer pouch (SP) is isolated, as usual. The continuity of the ileum is restored by reanastomosis (RR), the mesenteric window (Mes) is closed, the pouch is fashioned as usual, and the right ureter (Rt U) and left ureter (Lt U) were implanted into the afferent tubular segment (AS) by Nesbit technique of direct, end-to-side ureteroileal anastomosis, using 4/0 or 5/0 absorbable sutures

Nesbit Uretero-Ileal Anstomosis

A direct end-to-side, and stented anastomosis of the two ureters to the paramedian anti-mesenteric border of the 12–15 cm long afferent tubular segment of the isolated ileum (chimney) is performed.

Hautmann Pouch (Ileal W Neobladder)

This pouch was originally described by Hatmann in 1985, where he constructed a reservoir from the ileum using the principles of detubularization and double folding [60, 61]. Sice then, the technique has gained wide acceptance among urologists, and has been effective, simple, and reproducible [62–65].

A Hint on the Technique

The technique starts with isolation of a 60-cm long ileal segment, 20–25 cm away from the ileocecal valve. A W-shaped configuration is made, leaving two chimneys; each is 2–3 cm long, on both sides of the “W”. Then the reservoir is fashioned after detubularization and double folding.

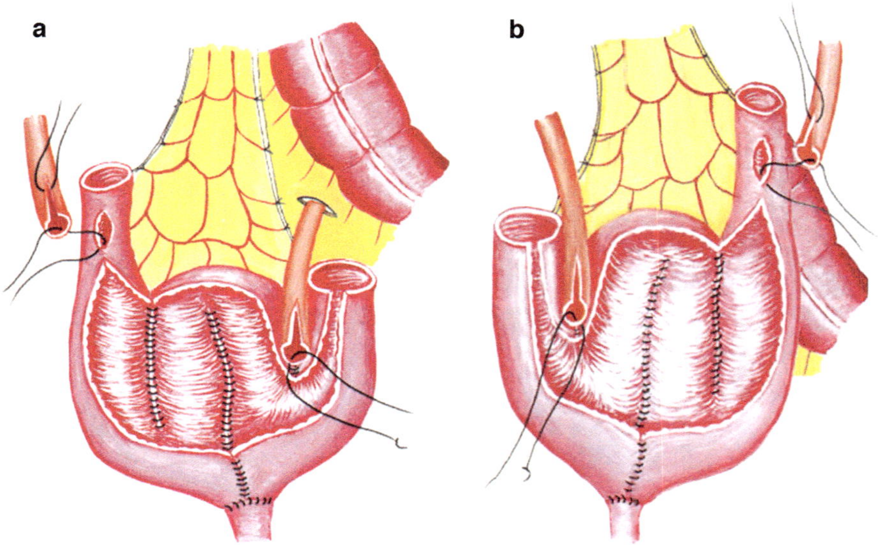

Fig. 22.9 Diagrammatic representation of two methods of implanting the ureter into ileal "W" neobladder: the right ureter is directly implanted into the chimney and the left is implanted by antireflux technique, using the serous-lined extramural tunnel, crossed behind the colon (**a**), the left ureter is direct, not crossed behind the colon and the right is antirefluxing (**b**). *Reproduced with permission from Shaaban et al.* [10]

Uretero-Ileal Anastomosis

- *Direct refluxing anastomosis*

  The ureters are spatulated over a distance of 1.5–2 cm and implanted into the chimneys by a direct refluxing anastomosis using the Wallace or Nesbit technique, as end-to-side (usually) or end-to-end procedure (Figs. 22.9 and 22.10).
- *Anti-reflux techniques in association with Hautmann (W) neobladder*

  In one of the anti-reflux techniques, the two ureters are implanted into the chimney-free ileal "W" neobladder by the *serous-lined extramural tunnel*, described by Abol-Enein and Ghoneim [66] as demonstrated in Fig. 22.9. Another anti-reflux technique is the *Camey-Le Duc* technique, which was initially used with the Hautmann pouch, and was found to be followed by a high uretero-ileal anastomotic stricture rate [67–69]. This technique was discussed before in the section of ileal loop conduit.

Vesica Ileale Padovana (VIP) Pouch

The VIP pouch is constructed from an ileal segment, around 40–50 cm long, and 15–20 cm proximal to the ileo-cecal valve, which is configured into a sideways "U", incised along its anti-mesenteric border, and the distal segment (3–4 cm) is funneled

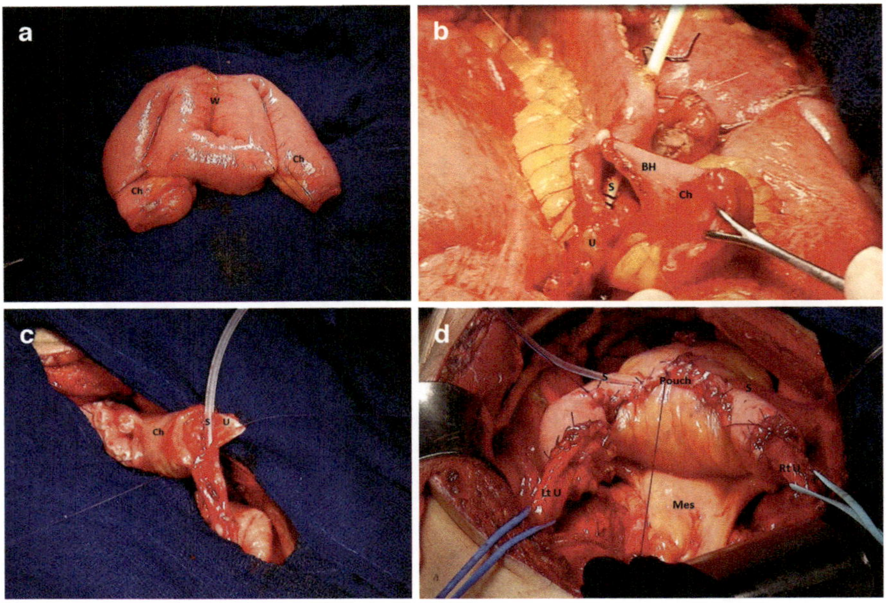

Fig. 22.10 Intra-operative photos demonstrating direct end-to-side and end-to-end uretero-ileal anastomosis with the chimney of Hautmann pouch.(**a**) The isolated ileal segment (50–60 cm) is configured into "W" with two chimneys (Ch), 3–5 cm each. (**b**) The ureter (U) is spatulated and a button hole (BH) is made in the side of the left chimney (Ch), and the posterior row of stitches (4/0 or 5/0 absorbable) between the ureter (U) and the button hole (BH) of the chimney (Ch) is completed. (**c**) The ureter (U) is spatulated, and the posterior row of stitches (4/0 or 5/0 absorbable), between the spatulated ureter (U) and the end of the chimney (Ch), is completed leaving a soft silastic stent (S). (**d**) The final scene is shown, where the nearly globular pouch is constructed, the right (Rt U), and the left ureter (Lt U) were anastomosed end-to-end to the chimney (Ch), and the two stents (S) are seen exiting the anterior pouch wall

to form the neobladder neck [70]. Then, the proximal segment is spirally configured, and the adjacent bowel walls are sutured together to make the posterior plate of the reservoir. Thereafter, a cephalad to caudad folding of the pouch is conducted.

Uretero-Ileal Anstomosis

The ureters are implanted into the upper part of the pouch by *a direct anastomosis* (Fig. 22.11).

Orthotopic Ileo-Cecal Neobladders

Maintz Pouch

The technique starts with isolation of the terminal 30 cm of the ileum and the first 10 cm of the cecum and ascending colon; this is followed by spatulated ileo-colonic (to ascending colon) anastomosis, and separation of the ileal segment into 20 cm

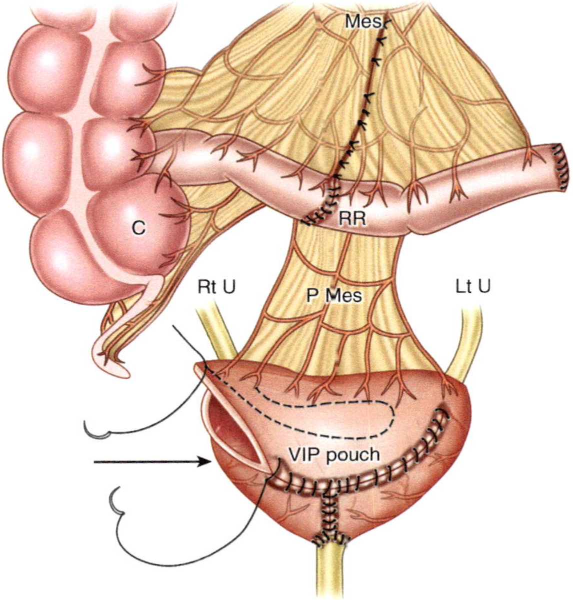

Fig. 22.11 Diagram showing direct uretero-ileal anstomosis in Vesica Ileale Padovana (VIP) pouch. The ileal segment for construction of the VIP pouch is isolated with its mesentery (P Mes), as usual. The continuity of the ileum is restored by reanastomosis (RR), the mesenteric window (Mes) is closed, and the pouch is fashioned and configured into a sideways "U" (arrow), as described in its original description. The right ureter (Rt U) and left ureter (Lt U) were implanted into the superior part of the pouch by direct ureteroileal anastomosis, using 4/0 or 5/0 absorbable sutures

proximal and 10-cm distal prevalvular segment [71, 72]. Then, the proximal 20 cm of the ileum is configured into U and incised along its anti-mesenteric border, the cecum and ascending colon are incised, in a similar way, at their anti-mesenteric tenia, and the pouch is fashioned by side-to-side anastomosis of the ileal and colonic segments posteriorly and then anteriorly.

Ureteral Implantation in Mainz Pouch

The *right ureter* is anastomosed by a stented *Nesbit technique (end-to-side)* to the prevalvular ileum. The *left ureter* is pulled through the mesentery, brought into the right retroperitoneum, and then, anastomosed by a stented *Wallace technique (end-to-end)* to the end of the prevalvular ileum (Fig. 22.12).

Le Bag Pouch

It is an ileo-colonic pouch [73]. In the colon part of the reservoir, *the ureters are implanted by the standard uretero-colic anastomosis, described by Goodwin* in uretero-sigmoidostomy [3]. The Goodwin technique will be described later in this chapter.

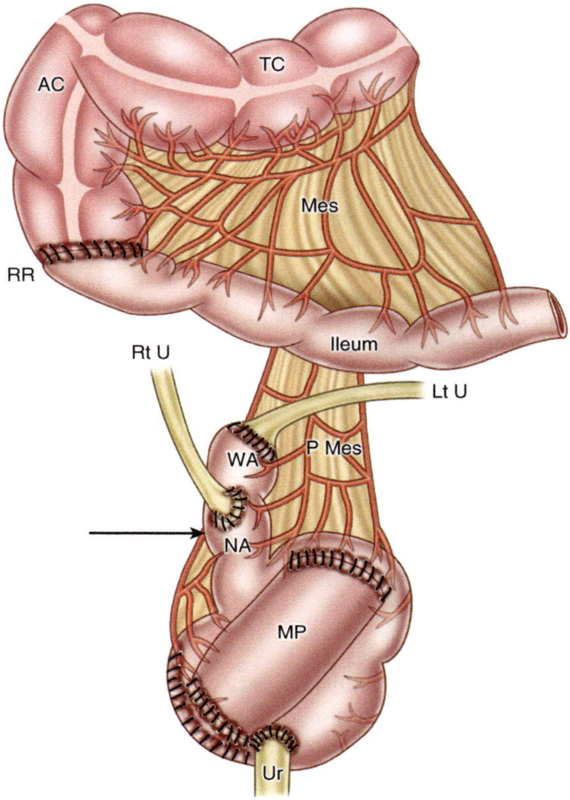

Fig. 22.12 Diagram showing Nesbit, end-to-side (NA) and Wallace, end-to-end (WA) uretero-ileal anstomosis of the right ureter (Rt U) and left ureter (Lt U), respectively, to the prevalvular ileal segment (arrow) in orthotopic Mainz pouch (MP). The ileo-cecal segment for construction of the Mainz pouch is isolated. The continuity of the bowel is restored by Ileo-ascendostomy (RR), the mesenteric window (dotted line) is closed, the pouch is fashioned as usual, and the urethra (Ur) is anastomosed to a button hole made in the deepest part of the pouch. P Mes, AC, and TC refer to pouch mesentery, ascending, and transverse colon, respectively

The Sigmoid (Reddy) Neobladder

The Reddy pouch is constructed from a segment of around 20–25 cm of the detubularized sigmoid, which is configured in a "U" or "J" shape, anastomosed to the urethra at its most dependent part [74]. *At each end of the loop, the right and left ureters are implanted by anti-reflux tunneled uretero-colonic anastomosis.*

Table 22.1 shows the common types of orthotopic neobladders, bowel segment used, and technique of uretero-enteric anastomosis.

22.3.3.4 Continent Cutaneous Urinary Diversion (Continent Cutaneos Stoma)

These reservoirs have been described as early as in the early 1950s, when Gilcrest and Merricks reported on their continent right colon pouch [75]. This is followed by the development of several reservoirs of varying characters, fashioned usually

Table 22.1 The common types of orthotopic neobladders, bowel segment used, and technique of uretero-enteric anastomosis

Type	Bowel segment	Technique of uretero-enteric anastomosis
The urethral hemi-Kock pouch	Ileum	Anti-reflux uretero-ileal anastomosis using the staple-held nipple valve
Studer pouch	Ileum	Nesbit direct uretero-ileal anstomosis to the afferent segment
Hautmann pouch (Ileal W neobladder)	Ileum	– Direct Wallace or Nesbit technique to the chimneys (the current trend) – Serus-lined extramural tunnel anti-reflux technique – Le Duc anti-reflux technique
Vesica Ileale Padovana (VIP) pouch	Ileum	Direct anastomosis
Mainz orthotopic pouch	Ileo-cecal	Nesbit and Wallace direct anastomosis
Le Bag pouch	Ileo-colonic	Standard Goodwin uretero-colic anastomosis
The sigmoid (Reddy) neobladder	Colonic	Anti-reflux tunneled uretero-colonic anastomosis

from the ileo-cecal region, and less frequently from purely ileal segments. The ideal principles for creation of continent catheterizable cutaneous pouch include construction of a spherical (or almost spherical), with low pressure and maximum capacity when filled, a trustable continent mechanism, easy intermittent catheterization through the stoma, and low complication rate, such as metabolic consequences [23].

Construction of the continence mechanism is the most vital part in the discussion of the varieties of these reservoirs. The continence mechanisms in the majority of these pouches can be grouped under three different types. An intussuscepted nipple valve is one of such continence mechanisms, where the ileal segments are telescoped and fixed, without the use of the ileo-cecal valve, such as in the Koch and T-pouch, or with the use of the ileo-cecal valve, as in Mainz pouch [76–79]. The second group of continence mechanism uses the reinforced ileocecal valve, such as in Indiana pouch [80]. The third type of continence mechanism relies on the Mitrofanoff principle, as in the Penn Pouch [81].

Ureteral Implantation in Continent Cutaneous Urinary Diversion

Kock Pouch

The ureters are implanted into the pouch by *antirefluxive intussuscepted ileal nipple valve* [76]. The use of nipple valve with staples has been obsolete nowadays.

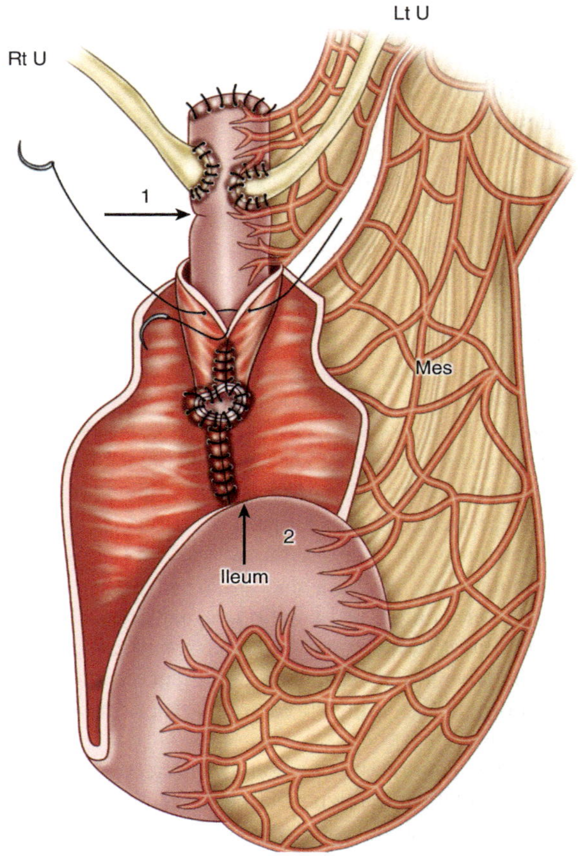

Fig. 22.13 Diagram showing the T-pouch. A tapered ileal tube (arrow 1) is used as anti-reflux mechanism, using the flap-valve technique of the serous-lined extramural tunnel (the 2 meeting arrows). The ureters (Rt U & Lt U) are implanted into this tube using the Nesbit technique

T-Pouch and Mansoura Pouch

A tapered ileal tube is used as anti-reflux mechanism, using the flap-valve technique of the serous-lined extramural tunnel (Figs. 22.13 and 22.14) [77, 78]. The ureters are implanted into this tube using the Nesbit technique.

Indiana Pouch

The ureters are implanted into the cecal part of the ileo-cecal pouch by a *tunneled anti-reflux anastomosis along the cecal tenia* (Fig. 22.15) [80].

Mainz Pouch as a Continent Cutaneous Reservoir

In this pouch, *the ureters are implanted into the colonic part using the open end technique and a 4–5 cm long submucosal tunnel* (Fig. 22.16) [79].

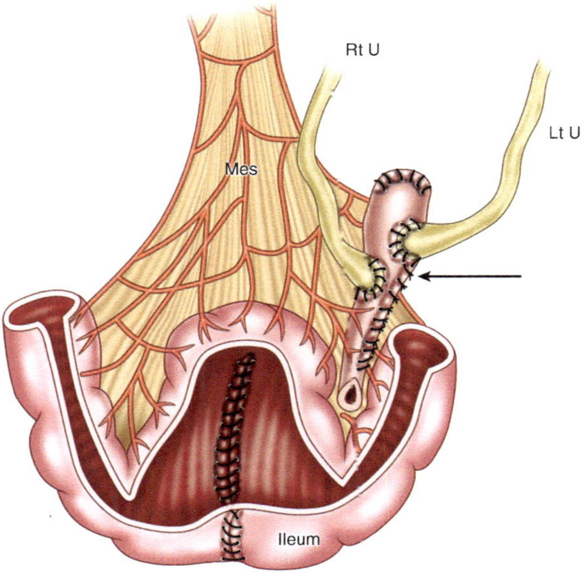

Fig. 22.14 Diagram showing the Mansoura pouch. The ileum is configured into "W". A tapered ileal tube (arrow) is used as anti-reflux mechanism, using the flap-valve technique of the serous-lined extramural tunnel. The ureters (Rt U & Lt U) are implanted into this tube using the Nesbit technique

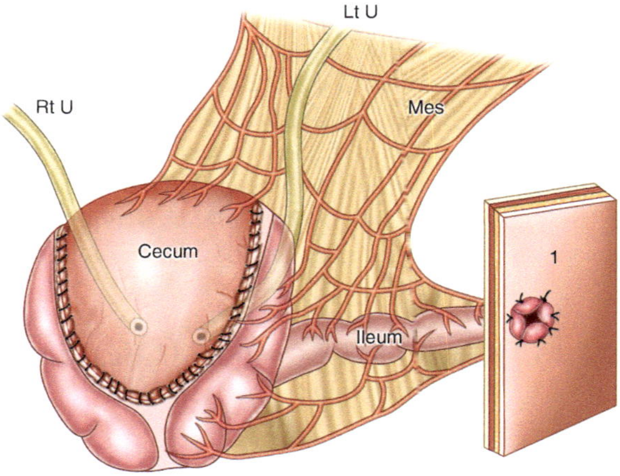

Fig. 22.15 Diagram demonstrationg Indiana pouch. The ureters (Rt U & Lt U) are implanted into the cecal part of the ileo-cecal pouch by a tunneled anti-reflux anastomosis along the cecal tenia. The continent cutaneous stoma is shown (1)

Penn Pouch

In this type of diversion, *which is the first continent cutaneous reservoir utilizing the Mitrofanoff principle* to achieve the continence mechanism, the appendix is tunneled and acts as a flap valve [81]. *The ureter is reimplanted into the colonic part of the reservoir.*

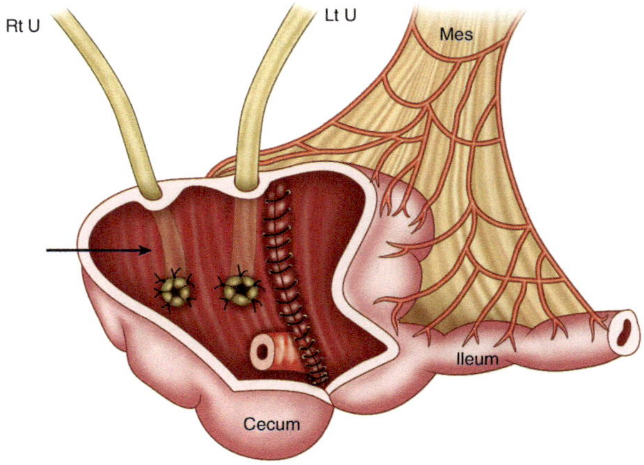

Fig. 22.16 Diagram demonstrationg Mainz continent cutaneous pouch. In this pouch, the ureters (Rt U & Lt U) are implanted into the colonic part using the open end technique and a 4–5 cm long submucosal tunnel (arrow)

Florida and Miami Pouch

The Florida pouch is mainly composed of the cecum and right colon, while the included 10–12 cm of the terminal ileum and the ileo-cecal valve act as the efferent continent limb after pliccation of the ileocecal valve [82]. *In the original description, uretero-colonic anastomosis was carried out using the antireflux LeDuc or the Goodwin technique, as previously mentioned* [3, 40]. *Later on, the uretero-colonic anstomosis was modified into a direct anastomosis.*

The Miami pouch is essentially composed of the same bowel segments, but the segments are incised at the antimesenteric border and configured into a "U" shape [83]. *The uretero-colonic anastomosis is performed using a non-tunneled technique.*

Table 22.2 demonstrates the common types of continent cutaneous pouches, bowel segment used, and technique of uretero-enteric anastomosis.

22.3.3.5 Anal Sphincter-Controlled Urinary Diversion (Continent Rectal Diversion)

Continent rectal diversion had accounted for the majority of urinary reservoirs in the era from 1852, when the first urinary diversion was described, till the 1950s, when the conduit urinary diversion techniques were introduced.

Table 22.2 The common types of continent cutaneous pouches, bowel segment used, and technique of uretero-enteric anastomosis

Type	Bowel segment	Technique of uretero-enteric anastomosis
The Kock pouch	Ileum	Anti-reflux uretero-ileal anastomosis using the staple-held nipple valve
T-pouch and Mansoura pouch	Ileum	Nesbit anstomosis to the tapered ileal tube implanted by the anti-reflux Serus-lined extramural tunnel
Indiana pouch	Ileo-cecal	Tunneled anti-reflux anastomosis along the cecal tenia
Mainz pouch as a continent cutaneous reservoir	Ileo-colonic	The ureters are implanted into the colonic part using the open end technique submucosal tunnel
Penn pouch	Ileo-cecal	The uretera are implanted into the colonic part of the reservoir
Florida pouch	Colonic	In the original description, the antireflux LeDuc or the Goodwin technique, was used. Later on, the uretero-colonic anstomosis was a direct anastomosis
Miami pouch	Colonic	A non-tunneled technique

Ureterosigmoidostomy

Ureterosigmoidostomy is the prototype of continent rectal diversions diversions, in which the ureters are directly implanted into the sigmoid colon to divert the urine with the fecal stream [84]. Because of the high mortality and morbidity, associated with ureterosigmoidostomy complications, such as peritonitis and pyelonephritis, the investigators recognized that reflux of fecal matter into the kidney was the cause of these serious complications. As a result, several surgical procedures were devised and introduced to achieve anti-reflux uretero-colic anastomosis.

The anti-reflux era started In 1911, when *Coffey* reported on the technique of tunneled uretero-colonic anastomosis, which has made ureterosigmoidostomy relatively safer and more effective [1, 2, 85]. In addition, *Goodwin, Petit-Leadbetter, and Strickler techniques for anti-refluxive uretero-enteric anastomosis* were later described (Fig. 22.17) [3, 4, 86]. Incontinence to urine and stool was another major problem after ureterosigmoidostomy, and was due to the high pressure inside the colon. To circumvent this problem, multiple techniques have been described, mainly entailing the principle of detubularization with the aim to increase the volume and to decrease the intrarectal pressure [87–89].

Currently, continent rectal diversions are very rarely conducted and have nearly become obsolete because of the potential increased risk to develop colonic malignancy at the urocolic anastomosis, metabolic acidosis, disturbance of electrolyte balance, fecal and urinary incontinence, and urinary stone formation [90, 91]. Nevertheless, the use of continent rectal reservoirs had not disappeared from the urologic literature, especially in children [92].

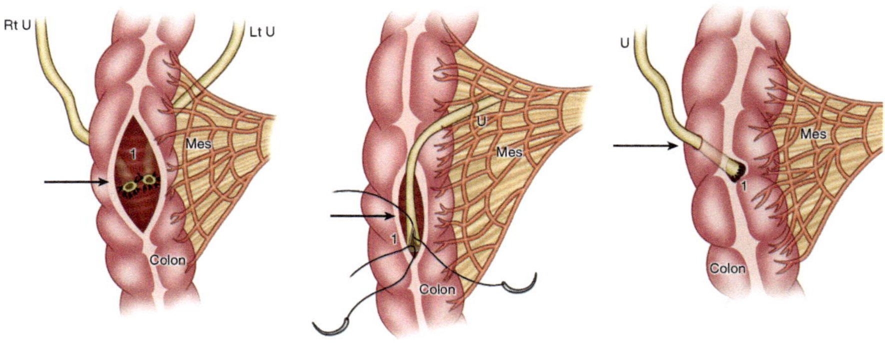

Fig. 22.17 Diagram demonstrationg three anti-reflux uretero-colonic anastomoses. (**a**) The Goodwin trans-colonic technique of ureterosigmoidostomy. The colon is incised anteriorly (arrow), a mucosal incision is made, and a 3–4 cm long submucosal tunnel (1) is made by elevation of the mucosa from the muscle layer with a mosquito clamp, which is advanced to make a rent in the serosa. The ureters (Rt U & Lt U) are pulled through the serosal rents and the submucosal tunnels, spatulated, and their openings are anastomosed into the holes of the colonic mucosa, with reinforcement of the anastomosis using some sutures in the muscle layer. The entry of the ureter in the serosa is reinforced by some fine absorbable stitches. (**b**) The Petit-Leadbetter extracolonic technique of ureterosigmoidostomy. A linear incision in the tenia of the colon is made (arrow); this is facilitated by submucosal injection of saline using needle, the tenia is raised and the underlying mucosa is identified. The ureter (U) is laid in the tunnel, and its spatulated end is anastomosed to a hole in the colonic mucosa (1). The seromuscular layed (tunnel) is then closed over the ureter. (**c**) The Strickler techniques for anti-refluxive uretero-enteric anastomosis. A small linear incision is perfomed in the tenia of the colon. The mucosa is dissected off the submucosa to make a submucosal tunnel, 3–4 cm long (arrow), with its lateral end exiting the serosa. Then, a button hole is made I the mucosa, the ureter (U) is laid in the tunnel, and its spatulated end is anastomosed to the hole in the colonic mucosa (1). The tenia is closed with interrupted fine absorbable sutures, and the entry of the ureter into the serosa is secured with a suture

22.4 Uretero-Enteric Anastomosis in Cases of Double Ureter

The ureters can be anastomosed side-to-side (Wallace technique) and the common stem is implanted into the bowel segments as previously detailed. Alternatively, the ureters are implanted as single ureter anastomosis.

22.5 Anti-refluxive Versus Direct Uretero-Enteric Anastomosis

In a recent meta-analysis, it has been found that the incidence of uretero-enteric anastomotic stricture was higher in anti-refluxive compared to direct uretero-enteric anastomosis, which can result in renal function deterioration and increased need to subsequent surgical interventions [12]. In addition, the lower incidence of anastomotic stricture seems to outweigh the postulated advantages of preventing reflux and the associated acute pyelonephritis, calculi formation, or azotemia [9]. Although the neobladder to ureter reflux was reported to be higher in direct compared to anti-refluxive uretero-enteric anastomosis, this was not directly related to deterioration of the kidney function [12].

Similarly, in other studies, uretero-enteric reflux has not been found to be associated with impairment of the renal function, either in low pressure neobladders, or in continent cutaneous reservoirs [8–11, 58, 69, 93–97]. In addition, the direct anastomotic techniques are simpler and less time consuming compared to the anti-reflux procedures.

Overall, according to the current guidelines, the recently published articles and systematic reviews and meta-analysis, direct uretero-enteric anastomosis is favored in low pressure reservoirs, including orthotopic neobladders and continent cutaneous diversions.

22.6 Ureter Related Complications in Urinary Diversion and their Treatment

To start with, the complications of urinary diversion include functional, surgical, and metabolic complications, which occur as early within 30 days, or late after 30 days and onwards. The early and late complications of urinary diversion are summarized in Table 22.3.

Of relevance to this chapter are the ureter related complications, which include urinary leakage/fistula, uretero-enteric anastomotic stricture (UEAS), reflux, and urinary tract infection/pyelonephritis.

Table 22.3 Early and late complications of urinary diversion

Parameter	
Early complications (within 30 days)	Urinary or fecal leakage/ fistula Urinary tract infection/ pyelonephritis Obstruction of the ureter Urethral or stomal obstruction/ stenosis Prolonged ileus Wound problems (infection or dehiscence) Stomal bleeding Stomal retraction, or ischemia Deep venous thrombosis (DVT)/ pulmonary embolism (PE)
Late complications (31 days onwards)	Urinary tract infection/ pyelonephritis Renal function deterioration Stone disease in the upper tract or reservoir Uretero-enteric anastomotic stricture (UEAS) Neocysto-ureteral reflux Intestinal obstruction Incisional or parastomal hernia Metabolic complications/ metabolic acidosis Functional complications; incontinence; chronic urinary retention (hypercontinence) Urethro-ileal or urethra-colonic anastomotic problems

22.6.1 Urinary Leakage/Fistula

The incidence of prolonged urinary leakage or urinary fistula at the uretero-enteric anastomosis after urinary diversion *is rare and is within the range of 1.9–5.7%*, and it is relatively rare when compared to leakage at the urethra-enteric anstomosis [98–103]. This complication usually manifests itself in the early post-operative period after diversion. If it presents late, we have to suspect recurrence of carcinoma at the ureter or uretero-enteric anastomosis [102]. The diagnosis is suspected when there is excessive drainage from the drains or from the wound, with or without fever, urinary tract infection, or wound problems. The diagnosis is confirmed by estimation of the creatinine level in the fluid collected from the drain or from the wound and its level is determined by ascending radiography of the pouch or loopogram, antegrade nephrostogram, and to a less extent by retrograde study, if the latter is possible [100].

The use of soft silastic stents has minimized the incidence of urinary fistula in the most recent reports.

Treatment is usually conservative, by prolongation of the catheter and stent duration, with or without decompression of the urinary tract by PCN. In the recent era, several minimally invasive approaches have been described to treat intractable urinary fistulas or those developing after advanced malignant recurrence. These include, but are not limited to, retrograde ureteral approach, antegrade stent exchange, percutaneous ureteral occlusion with platinum coils and Gelfoam, percutaneous transrenal balloon catheters, and bilateral ureteric occlusion using angioplasty balloon catheters [100, 103–105].

22.6.2 Uretero-Enteric Anastomotic Stricture (UEAS)

As previously mentioned, there have been several uretero-enteric anastomotic techniques in all types of urinary diversion, including direct and anti-reflux procedures. *One of the common complications of the uretero-enteric anastomosis is uretero-enteric anastomotic stricture (UEAS).* This is a serious complication that should be taken in consideration and should be anticipated. Therefore, the patients should be closely monitored after surgery. UEAS can lead to deterioration or even loss of the kidney function, if left untreated or if the diagnosis is delayed.

22.6.2.1 Incidence

As listed in Table 22.4, for all types of urinary diversion *UEAS develops in 1.3–17% of cases*, and the majority of these strictures develop in the first 24 months after the operation and *the majority are benign in nature* [10, 32, 34, 62, 66, 100, 106–121].

Table 22.4 The rates of uretero-enteric anastomotic stricture in various types of urinary diversion

Study	Type of diversion	Uretero-enteric anastomosis	Follow-up (months)	Stricture rate (%)	Notes
Abol-Enein & Ghoneim [66]	Hautmann with SLET	SLET	Mean 38	3.8	
Perimenis et al. [106]	ONB (Studer)	Direct Nesbit	Median 73	3.5 (obstruction)	
Shaaban et al. [10]	ONB (Hautmann; Hautmann with SLET)	Direct versus SLET	Mean 23	Direct: 1.7; SLET: 8.3	Higher rate of stricture with SLET
Ali-El-Dein et al. [100]	Females; Mainly ONB (Hautmann; Hautmann with SLET)	Direct; SLET; few cases ileal nipple valve	Mean 54	Overall 6.5%; SLET: 7.5%	
Studer et al. [107]	ONB (Studer)	Direct Nesbit	Median 32	2.7	
Yang et al. [108]	IC	Bricker or Nesbit	91	4	
Kouba et al. [32]	IC	Bricker or Wallace	Median 20.5–21.4	1.9	No strictures were found in the Wallace group
Katkoori et al. [109]	LC; ONB	Bricker	26; 28.5	1.3	
Hautmann et al. [62]	ONB (Hautmann)	Le Duc; Direct Wallace	3–160	11	UEAS was lower in the direct (5.4%) versus Le Duc technique (16.3%)
Shimko et al. [110]	IC; CC	Bricker	186	10	Mainly IC
Anderson et al. [110]	IC; ONB; CCUD	Bricker	Median 8.2	9.4	The rate was 8.5 for ORC; 12.6 for RARC
Large et al. [112]	IC; CC	Bricker	41 for interrupted; 29 for running sutures	8.5 for interrupted; 12.7 for running sutures	Higher rate of UEAS in the group with running sutures
Davis et al. [34]	IC	Bricker or Wallace	26,27	2.9 for Bricker; 1.9 for Wallace	No significant difference between Bricker and Wallace techniques

(continued)

Table 22.4 (continued)

Study	Type of diversion	Uretero-enteric anastomosis	Follow-up (months)	Stricture rate (%)	Notes
Shah et al. [113]	ONB; CCUD; IC	Direct Bricker anastomosis	Median 149	2.6	
Ahmed et al. [114]	IC	ND	Median 23	13%	All cases were performed by RARC
Hosseini et al. [115]	IC; ONB	Wallace, running sutures	Median 33	6.5	RARC with a totally intracorporeal urinary diversion; higher rate with ONB
Ericson et al. [116]	IC; CCUD; ONB; CC	Bricker	Median 11–22	11.3	ORC 9.3%;RARC (ECUD 11.3% or ICUD 13%)
Goh et al. [117]	Majority incontinent diversion	NA	More than 24	11.4 for ORC; 14.6 for RARC	Higher rates of UEAS in RARC versus ORC
Faraj et al. [118]	ONB (14.8%)	Bricker or Wallace	Median 55–71	8 for ORC; 9.6 for RARC (ECUD); 2.6 for RARC (ECUD)	
Magnusson et al. [119]	variable	variable	Median 23.5	8.9	Highest incidence of UEAS in the 1st 2 years
Reesink et al. [120]	IC; ONB	Bricker technique, running in RARC	Median 50	17%	Higher stricture rate in robot-assisted versus open cystectomy
Alonso Mediavilla et al. [121]	IC; ONB	Bricker, Wallace	12–72	27%	Higher stricture rate in laparoscopic, and robot-assisted versus open cystectomy

However, some UEASs may develop as late as 160 months after surgery [62]. In addition, it is worth noting that the exact incidence of UEAS is difficult to define, and usually under-estimated, because of the variations in the reporting studies [111]. These variations include variations in follow-up periods, methods of diagnosis of UEAS, imaging techniques, frequency of imaging, and necessity to do corrective intervention [111].

22.6.2.2 Etiology and Risk Factors

The etiology of UEAS is not completely known; however, according to the published data and expert opinions, *two factors may directly lead to this problem, namely ischemia of the implanted part of the ureter, and urinary leakage* at the anastomotic site with subsequent fibrosis around the ureter.

Several risk factors have been studied in few retrospective studies [10, 62, 100, 111, 112, 116, 117, 120, 121]. These risk factors include anti-reflux versus direct UEA, running versus interrupted sutures used for UEA, extensive dissection of the ureter, especially the left ureter, robot-assisted radical cystectomy (RARC) versus open radical cystectomy (ORC), intra-corporeal (ICUD) versus extra-corporeal urinay diversion (ECUD) performed with RARC, prolonged urinary leakage, and urinary tract infection.

22.6.2.3 Prevention

Although, the development of UEAS is inborn in the techniques of urinary diversion, yet prevention of this serious complication is definitely better than cure. The preventive strategies include preservation of the periureteral vascular network during ureteral dissection, dissection of a limited length of the ureter that is just sufficient to perform a tension-free anastomosis, and careful manipulation of the ureter with mostly athermal dissection and limited diathermy coagulation. In addition, wide ureteral spatulation, the use of soft silastic stents, water-proof, tension-free, mucosa-to-mucosa anastomosis, and the use of saline testing for a leaking anastomosis are among the recommendations [122]. Furthermore, with the advent of RARC, intraoperative indocyanine green (ICG) has been used to assess the vascularity of the ureter and to select the exact site of ureteral transection in an attempt to decrease the incidence of UEAS [123].

22.6.2.4 Presentation of UEAS

A big sector of the patients with UEAS is asymptomatic; therefore, a great sense of suspicion should be used to anticipate and diagnose this problem. Although, the diagnosis is usually made by imaging, patients with UEAS may present with loin pain, fever, and/or recurrent urinary tract infection. On imaging, hydronephrosis or back pressure changes are discovered. The kidney function, as assessed by serum creatinine or radioisotope renography, may be affected, especially if the resulting obstruction is bilateral.

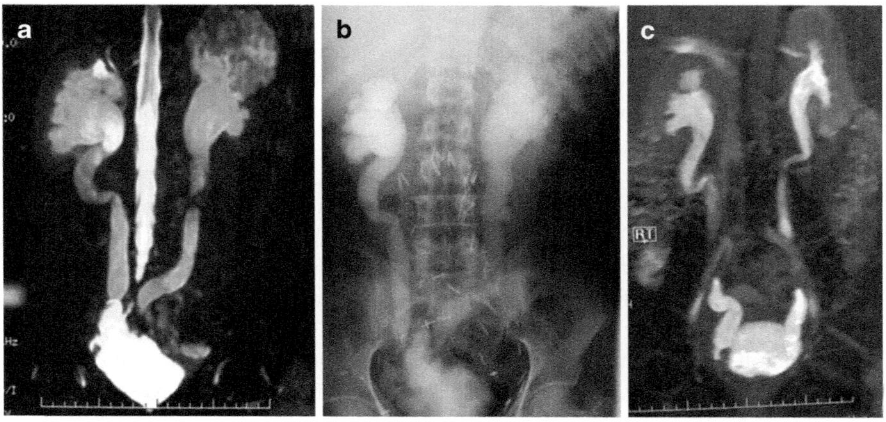

Fig. 22.18 (**a**) MRU one year after radical cystectomy and ileal "W" neobladder with serous-lined extramural tunnel, showing bilateral uretero-ileal anastomotic strictures. (**b**) IVU of the same patient showing the same finding. (**c**) Post-operative MRU, 6 months after open repair of bilateral UIAS, showing marked decompression of the pelvicaliceal system

22.6.2.5 Treatment

Open Revision

The treatment is always challenging. *So far, the gold standard is still the open revision* [10, 66, 100, 121, 124]. The open technique of revision of the UEA includes excision of the strictured part or ureteral transection proximal to it, and reimplantation of the ureter into the loop, pouch, or neobladder (Fig. 22.18). The open revision has been attended with the highest success rates on the long run, although it is challenging, and requires a very high surgical competence because of the extensive adhesions around the UEAS [10, 66, 100, 121, 124].

Minimally Invasive and Endourologic Approaches

Endourologic techniques have been used to treat UEAS, especially as a first-line treatment of strictures developing early after surgery, short strictures (1 cm or less), and when the patient is unfit for open revision [122, 125–127]. These procedures can be conducted in an antegrade fashion after PCN fixation, the usual scenario, or rarely in a retrograde fashion [125–127]. The endourologic intervention may be in the form of stent fixation, balloon dilation or endoureterotomy; the latter can be carried out with cold knife, electrocautery knife (hot knife), acuicise or laser [10, 100, 124, 125].

The success rate of endourologic techniques is not that high, and it ranges from 4% to 50% [125–128]. Nevertheless, the use of these minimally invasive procedures is attended with many advantages, including limited morbidity, faster technique, shorter hospital stay because of fast recovery, and cost-saving [128].

Morever, laparoscopic and robot-assisted approaches for repair of UEAS have recently been described in a highly selected cohort of patients [129, 130]. They were associated with high success rates, almost comparable to open surgery, with minimal morbidity and complications in early strictures and properly selected cases [129, 130].

22.6.3 Stone Disease

Stones may develop in the pouch or the upper tract after urinary diversion. The incidence of stone disease in the published studies ranges from *9% to 11% after Bricker conduit* [132, 133]. For Kock pouch urinary diversion, the incidence is relatively higher *(17–27%)*, because of the use of staples to stabilize the nipple valve [134, 135]. Apart from Kock pouch, the incidence of stone formation after *ONB and continent cutaneous* urinary diversion ranges from *2.9% to 13%* [66, 100, 135, 136].

All the treatment options for stone disease have been valid for the treatment of this disorder after various modes of urinary diversion [66, 100, 136–140]. These options include ureteroscopy, percutaneous nephrolithotomy, shock wave lithotripsy, open, and laparoscopic interventions; all of them have been used with good results (Fig. 22.19)

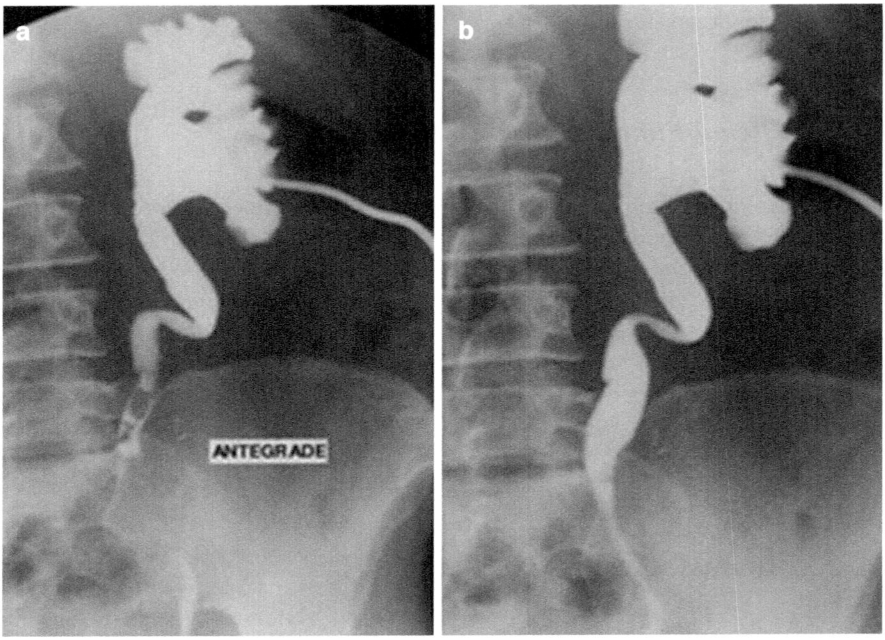

Fig. 22.19 Antegrade study in 1 woman with multiple ureteral stones, developing after radical cystectomy and Hautmann neobladder. (**a**) stones appeared as filling defects. (**b**) free passage of dye with absence of stones after removal by antegrade ureteroscopy. *Reproduced with permission from Ali-el-Dein et al.* [100]

[66, 100, 131, 136–140]. *The choice of either technique depends on patient criteria, the type of urinary diversion, location, and size of the stone, available facilities, and surgical skills* [131, 137, 141].

22.6.4 Urinary Tract Infection

Urinary tract infections are one of the most frequent and important complications after urinary diversion. These infections are commoner in the early versus late post-operative period, where their incidence ranges from 6% to more than 40%, in the early post-operative period [128].

The presentation of urinary tract infection may be vague and misleading, because this presentation may be in the form of abdominal discomfort, change in the smell of urine, and may be as severe as acute pyelonephritis and sepsis. Therefore, a high level of suspicion is needed to diagnose this post-diversion problem [128]. Appropriate and urgent anti-microbial treatment, based on culture and sensitivity testing, should be given to these patients [142–144]. The reported risk factors include diabetes, peri-operative blood transfusion, continent versus incontinent diversion, orthotopic versus heterotopic diversion, and urinary leakage [143, 144]. Multiple organisms are usually isolated, including gram-negative rods, fungi, and drug-resistant organisms [144].

22.6.5 Renal Function Deterioration

Newly developed chronic kidney disease, which may proceed to end-stage renal disease, has been reported after urinary diversion, with a rate of around 20% and a median onset of more than 2 years [110].

The main *risk factors include UEAS with subsequent hydronephrosis, chronic urinary tract infection, and possibly reflux of infected urine to the upper tract* [10, 100, 110, 128]. Therefore, meticulous surveillance of the upper tract and kidney function is mandatory after all forms of urinary diversion. However, this is a very important and serious problem, the details of which are not the subject matter of this chapter.

22.7 Minimally Invasive Technique

Because of the major advances in the field of minimally invasive techniques, laparoscopic and robot-assisted radical cystectomy (RARC) have been introduced in the last decade [101, 114–118, 145–150]. The first report of laparoscopic cystectomy came from the Cleveland Clinic in 2000, and was described by Gill et al. [145]; this is followed by the RAZOR trial, and other studies, which demonstrated some advantages of the RARC over open radical cystectomy (ORC) [146–150]. The reported advantages include less intra-operative blood loss and blood transfusion, and less post-operative complications, although the operative time was longer and the cost was higher [146–150]. Along with these advanges, in the recently published series, oncological outcome was comparable to ORC [149]. The diversion in RARC techniques may be performed intra-corporeally or extra-corporeally.

According to the available data, evidence is still insufficient to draw a solid conclusion on the improved peri-operative outcomes of the RARC, especially with the introduction of the enhanced recovery protocols. In addition, long-term functional outcome is still not well defined. Furthermore, the technique of RARC is technically challenging and needs high-volume surgeons, who are extremely competent in robotic surgery [151].

22.8 Future Perspectives "Tissue Engineering"

The potential to use autologus bladder grafts in augmentation cystoplasty was first introduced by Atala et al. in 2006 [152]. Thereafter, there have been multiple researches to investigate the possibility of tissue engineering to produce autologous bladder grafts to be used after radical cystectomy. The story starts with what is known as "bladder scaffold", which is seeded with the result of cell culture of both urothelial and smooth muscle cells, the expected product is bioartificial bladder tissue [153–156]. The preliminary data, on the first clinical application of autologous bioengineered urinary conduit in humans after radical cystectomy, has shown promising results [153]. However, the clinical data of this research is still to be announced.

22.9 Summary

The main indication of urinary diversion is radical cystectomy performed for bladder cancer. Many techniques of urinary diversion have been described, including continent, incontinent, orthotopic, and heterotopic diversions. Several of them have passed the test of time, and some of them had disappeared and became obsolete, such as continent rectal diversions.

Associated with these urinary diversions, there have been a lot of techniques to perform the uretero-enteric anastomosis (UEA), including direct and anti-reflux techniques. This step is very important and critical, because it may be followed by serious complications, such as uretero-enteric anastomotic stricture (UEAS) and subsequent upper tract deterioration. The current trend is to perform a direct uretero-enteric anastomosis in low-pressure reservoirs, because the direct anastomosis has lower rate of UEAS.

Instantaneous and proper treatment of the ureter-related complications following urinary diversion is of paramount importance to prevent renal function deterioration. Ureter-oenteric anastomotic stricture (UEAS) is the most important of these ureter-related complications of urinary diversion, because of its serious impact on the renal function. This problem is more frequent with anti-reflux than with direct UEA. A high level of suspicion and strict radiologic follow-up are mandated to make the early diagnosis of UEAS. The treatment of UEAS is essentially made by open revision, although minimally invasive techniques, such as endourologic, laparoscopic, or robot-assisted procedures have been used in highly selected cases with good results, especially in early and short strictures.

Tissue engineering and bioartificial bladder grafts are still under investigation in the field of urinary diversion.

Questions

1. **The basic mechanism associated with uretero-enteric anastomosis was first introduced by:**
   (a) Coffey
   (b) Bricker
   (c) Leadbetter
   (d) Hautmann
   (e) Lich-Gregoir
2. **What type of urinary diversion is almost obsolete nowadays?**
   (a) Sigmoid neobladder
   (b) Continent rectal diversion
   (c) Colon conduit
   (d) Ileo-cecal continent cutaneous urinary diversion
   (e) cutaneous ureterostomy
3. **The current trend is to use which of the following uretero-enteric anastomotic techniques in low-pressure urinary diversion reservoirs?**
   (a) Leadbetter and Clarke technique
   (b) Goodwin technique
   (c) Nipple valve technique
   (d) Le Duc technique
   (e) Direct anastomosis

4. **Which of the following statements best describes the conclusion of most studies comparing Bricker versus Wallace uretero-ileal anastomosis performed with ileal loop conduit?**
   (a) Bricker is inferior
   (b) Wallace is inferior
   (c) Both are comparable
   (d) Both are bad techniques
   (e) Bricker technique poses both upper tracts at danger.
5. **In Studer neobladder, the ureters are implanted:**
   (a) By Le Duc technique to the afferent tubular segment
   (b) By Le Duc technique to the pouch itself, not to the afferent segment.
   (c) By serous-lined extramural tunnel
   (d) By Nesbit technique to the afferent tubular segment
   (e) By Goodwin technique
6. **In Vesica Ileale Padovana (VIP) pouch:**
   (a) The isolated ileal segment is configured into a sideways "U".
   (b) The isolated ileal segment is configured into "W".
   (c) The isolated colonic segment is configured into a sideways "U".
   (d) The isolated colonic segment is configured into "W".
   (e) The isolated ileal segment is configured into a sideways "U" or "W".
7. **The gold standard treatment of uretero-enteric anastomotic stricture after urinary diversion is:**
   (a) Laser endoureterotomy
   (b) Balloon dilation and stenting
   (c) Acucise endoureterotomy
   (d) Open revision
   (e) Cold knife endoureterotomy
8. **The success rate of endourologic techniques used in treatment of uretero-enteric anastomotic stricture after urinary diversion ranges from:**
   (a) 10–90%
   (b) 15–72%
   (c) 40–80%
   (d) 50–70%
   (e) 4–50%

9. **One of the most important risk factors in deterioration of the renal function after urinary diversion is:**
   (a) Uretero-enteric anastomotic stricture with subsequent hydronephrosis
   (b) Urinary leakage
   (c) Hypertension
   (d) Stone disease
   (e) Urethral stricture

10. **The majority of uretero-enteric anastomotic strictures after urinary diversion are:**
   (a) Malignant
   (b) Both benign and malignant
   (c) Benign
   (d) Iatrogenic
   (e) Not determined

References

1. Pannek J, Senge T. History of urinary diversion. Urol Int. 1998;60:1–10.
2. Coffey RC. Physiologic implantation of the severed ureter or common bile-duct into the intestine. JAMA. 1911;LVI(6):397–403. https://doi.org/10.1001/jama.1911.02560060007002.
3. Goodwin WE, Harris AP, Kaufman JJ, Beal JM. Open, transcolonic ureterointestinal anastomosis; a new approach. Surg Gynecol Obstet. 1953;97(3):295–300.
4. Leadbetter WF, Clarke BG. Five years' experience with uretero-enterostomy by the combined technique. J Urol. 1955;73(1):67–82. https://doi.org/10.1016/s0022-5347(17)67368-3.
5. Bricker EM. Bladder substitution after pelvic evisceration. Surg Clin North Am. 1950;30(5):1511–21. https://doi.org/10.1016/s0039-6109(16)33147-4.
6. Warwick RT. Colonic urinary conduits. Proc R Soc Med. 1960;53(12):1032–4.
7. Bejany D, Suarez G, Penalver M, Politano V. Nontunneled ureterocolonic anastomosis: an alternate to the tunneled implantation. J Urol. 1989;142(4):961–3. https://doi.org/10.1016/s0022-5347(17)38953-x.
8. Helal M, Pow-Sang J, Sanford E, Figueroa E, Lockhart J. Direct (nontunneled) ureterocolonic reimplantation in association with continent reservoirs. J Urol. 1993;150(3):835–7. https://doi.org/10.1016/s0022-5347(17)35626-4.
9. Pantuck AJ, Han KR, Perrotti M, Weiss RE, Cummings KB. Ureteroenteric anastomosis in continent urinary diversion: long-term results and complications of direct versus nonrefluxing techniques. J Urol. 2000;163(2):450–5. https://doi.org/10.1016/s0022-5347(05)67898-6.
10. Shaaban AA, Abdel-Latif M, Mosbah A, Gad H, Eraky I, Ali-El-Dein B, Osman Y, El-Mekresh M, El-H I, El-Kappany H. A randomized study comparing an antireflux system with a direct ureteric anastomosis in patients with orthotopic ileal neobladders. BJU Int. 2006;97(5):1057–62. https://doi.org/10.1111/j.1464-410X.2006.06135.x.
11. Shigemura K, Yamanaka N, Imanishi O, Yamashita M. Wallace direct versus antireflux Le Duc ureteroileal anastomosis: comparative analysis in modified Studer orthotopic neobladder reconstruction. Int J Urol. 2012;19(1):49–53. https://doi.org/10.1111/j.1442-2042.2011.02870.x. Epub 2011 Oct 17.

12. Zhang Y, Ding H, Zhang Y, Tian J, Yang L, Dong Z, Wang J, Wang Y, Zhang Y, Wang Z. Is anti-reflux anastomosis an advantage in an orthotopic ileal neobladder? A systematic review and meta-analysis. Urol Int. 2022;107:1–14. https://doi.org/10.1159/000525017. Epub ahead of print.
13. Wallace DM. Ureteric diversion using a conduit: a simplified technique. Br J Urol. 1966;38(5):522–7. https://doi.org/10.1111/j.1464-410x.1966.tb09747.x.
14. Gigon C. Memoire sur l'ischurie ureterique et surl'ureterotomie ou taille de l'uretere. Union Med Paris. 1856;10:81.
15. Basic DT, Hadzi-Djokic J, Ignjatovic I. The history of urinary diversion. Acta Chir Iugosl. 2007;54(4):9–17. https://doi.org/10.2298/aci0704009b.
16. Burkhard FC, Wuethrich PY. Cutaneous ureterostomy: 'back to the future'. BJU Int. 2016;118(4):493–4. https://doi.org/10.1111/bju.13532.
17. Murphy LJT. Ureteric repair and replacement, urinary diversion, artificial bladders and allied subjects: cutaneous ureterostomy. In: Murphy LJT, editor. The history of urology. Charles C Thomas: Illinois; 1972. p. 301–3.
18. de Vries JK. Permanent diversion of urinary stream. J Urol. 1955;73(2):217–25. https://doi.org/10.1016/s0022-5347(17)67388-9.
19. Lusuardi L, Lodde M, Pycha A. Cutaneous ureterostomy. BJU Int. 2005;96(7):1149–59. https://doi.org/10.1111/j.1464-410X.2005.05837.x.
20. Feminella JG Jr, Lattimer JK. A retrospective analysis of 70 cases of cutaneous ureterostomy. J Urol. 1971;106:538–4.
21. Rodríguez AR, Lockhart A, King J, Wiegand L, Carrion R, Ordorica R, Lockhart J. Cutaneous ureterostomy technique for adults and effects of ureteral stenting: an alternative to the ileal conduit. J Urol. 2011;186(5):1939–43. https://doi.org/10.1016/j.juro.2011.07.032. Epub 2011 Sep 23.
22. Lee RK, Abol-Enein H, Artibani W, Bochner B, Dalbagni G, Daneshmand S, Fradet Y, Hautmann RE, Lee CT, Lerner SP, Pycha A, Sievert KD, Stenzl A, Thalmann G, Shariat SF. Urinary diversion after radical cystectomy for bladder cancer: options, patient selection, and outcomes. BJU Int. 2014;113(1):11–23. https://doi.org/10.1111/bju.12121.
23. Igel DA, Chestnut CJ, Lee EK. Urinary diversion and reconstruction following radical cystectomy for bladder cancer: a narrative review. AME Med J. 2021;6:4.
24. Leong CH. Use of the stomach for bladder replacement and urinary diversion. Ann R Coll Surg Engl. 1978;60(4):283–9.
25. Morrison CD, Kielb SJ. Use of bowel in reconstructive urology: what a colorectal surgeon should know. Clin Colon Rectal Surg. 2017;30(3):207–14. https://doi.org/10.1055/s-0037-1598162. Epub 2017 May 22.
26. Butcher HR Jr, Sugg WL, Mcafee CA, Bricker EM. Ileal conduit method of ureteral urinary diversion. Ann Surg. 1962;156(4):682–91. https://doi.org/10.1097/00000658-196210000-00015.
27. Riches EW, Jacobs A, Wallace DM, et al. Discussion on the treatment of carcinoma of the bladder. Proc R Soc Med. 1952;45:191–206.
28. Hendry WF. Morbidity and mortality of radical cystectomy (1971-78 and 1978-85). J R Soc Med. 1986;79(7):395–400. https://doi.org/10.1177/014107688607900706.
29. Wallace DM. Strategy of surgical management of bladder cancer. Proc R Soc Med. 1973;66(3):286–8.
30. Blandy JP, England HR, Evans SJ, Hope-Stone HF, Mair GM, Mantell BS, Oliver RT, Paris AM, Risdon RA. T3 bladder cancer--the case for salvage cystectomy. Br J Urol. 1980;52(6):506–10. https://doi.org/10.1111/j.1464-410x.1980.tb03101.x.
31. Wallace DM. Uretero-ileostomy. Br J Urol. 1970;42(5):529–34. https://doi.org/10.1111/j.1464-410x.1970.tb04498.x.
32. Kouba E, Sands M, Lentz A, Wallen E, Pruthi RS. A comparison of the Bricker versus Wallace ureteroileal anastomosis in patients undergoing urinary diversion for bladder cancer. J Urol. 2007;178(3 Pt 1):945–8. https://doi.org/10.1016/j.juro.2007.05.030. discussion 948-9. Epub 2007 Jul 16.

33. Evangelidis A, Lee EK, Karellas ME, Thrasher JB, Holzbeierlein JM. Evaluation of ureterointestinal anastomosis: Wallace vs Bricker. J Urol. 2006;175(5):1755–8. https://doi.org/10.1016/S0022-5347(05)01020-7. discussion 1758.
34. Davis NF, Burke JP, McDermott T, Flynn R, Manecksha RP, Thornhill JA. Bricker versus Wallace anastomosis: a meta-analysis of ureteroenteric stricture rates after ileal conduit urinary diversion. Can Urol Assoc J. 2015;9(5–6):E284–90. https://doi.org/10.5489/cuaj.2692.
35. Krafft U, Mahmoud O, Hess J, Radtke JP, Panic A, Püllen L, Darr C, Kesch C, Szarvas T, Rehme C, Hadaschik BA, Tschirdewahn S. Comparative analysis of Bricker versus Wallace ureteroenteric anastomosis and identification of predictors for postoperative ureteroenteric stricture. Langenbeck's Arch Surg. 2022;407(3):1233–40. https://doi.org/10.1007/s00423-021-02413-4. Epub 2021 Dec 23
36. Li Y, Zhuang Q, Hu Z, Wang Z, Zhu H, Ye Z. A modified ureteroileal anastomosis technique for Bricker urinary diversion. Urology. 2011;78(5):1191–5. https://doi.org/10.1016/j.urology.2011.07.001. Epub 2011 Sep 3.
37. Kavaric P, Eldin S, Nenad R, Dragan P, Vukovic M. Modified Wallace anastomotic technique reduces ureteroenteric stricture rates after ileal conduit urinary diversion. Int Braz J Urol. 2020;46(3):446–55. https://doi.org/10.1590/S1677-5538.IBJU.2019.0417.
38. Wang Q, Tang L, Bi L, Min J, Fang L, Sun W, Yu D. Ureteral distal ends combined and inserted into the ileum: a novel anastomotic technique for urinary diversion. BMC Urol. 2021;21(1):65. https://doi.org/10.1186/s12894-021-00835-2.
39. Croghan SM, Daniels AE, Kelly C, Fitzgibbon L, Shields WP, Cullen IM, Daly PJ. The pull-through anastomosis of ureter to enteric conduit (pautec): a novel technique for urinary diversion. Urology. 2021;157:263–8. https://doi.org/10.1016/j.urology.2021.07.003. Epub 2021 Jul 18.
40. Le Duc A, Camey M, Teillac P. An original antireflux ureteroileal implantation technique: long-term followup. J Urol. 1987;137(6):1156–8. https://doi.org/10.1016/s0022-5347(17)44433-8.
41. Bhojwani AG, Mellon JK. Contemporary cystectomy combined with ileal conduit or bladder substitution. Surg Oncol. 2002;11(1–2):65–75. https://doi.org/10.1016/s0960-7404(02)00011-7.
42. Schmidt JD, Hawtrey CE, Buchsbaum HJ. Transverse colon conduit: a preferred method of urinary diversion for radiation-treated pelvic malignancies. J Urol. 1975;113(3):308–13. https://doi.org/10.1016/s0022-5347(17)59469-0.
43. Altwein JE, Hohenfellner R. Use of the colon as a conduit for urinary diversion. Surg Gynecol Obstet. 1975;140(1):33–8.
44. Beckley S, Wajsman Z, Pontes JE, Murphy G. Transverse colon conduit: a method of urinary diversion after pelvic irradiation. J Urol. 1982;128(3):464–8. https://doi.org/10.1016/s0022-5347(17)52999-7.
45. Chang DT, Lawrentschuk N. Orthotopic neobladder reconstruction. Urol Ann. 2015;7(1):1–7. https://doi.org/10.4103/0974-7796.148553.
46. Qu LG, Lawrentschuk N. Orthotopic neobladder reconstruction: patient selection and perspectives. Res Rep Urol. 2019;11:333–41. https://doi.org/10.2147/RRU.S181473.
47. Kock NG. Intra-abdominal reservoir in patients with permanent ileostomy: preliminary observations on a procedure resulting in fecal continence in five ileostomy patients. Arch Surg. 1969;99:223–31.
48. Ghoneim MA, Kock NG, Lycke G, El-Din AB. An appliance-free, sphincter-controlled bladder substitute: the urethral Kock pouch. J Urol. 1987;138(5):1150–4. https://doi.org/10.1016/s0022-5347(17)43531-2.
49. Kock NG, Ghoneim MA, Lycke KG, Mahran MR. Replacement of the bladder by the urethral Kock pouch: functional results, urodynamics and radiological features. J Urol. 1989;141(5):1111–6. https://doi.org/10.1016/s0022-5347(17)41185-2.
50. Skinner DG, Boyd SD, Lieskovsky G. Clinical experience with the Kock continent ileal reservoir for urinary diversion. J Urol. 1984;132(6):1101–7. https://doi.org/10.1016/s0022-5347(17)50052-x.

51. Skinner DG, Boyd SD, Lieskovsky G, Bennett C, Hopwood B. Lower urinary tract reconstruction following cystectomy: experience and results in 126 patients using the Kock ileal reservoir with bilateral ureteroileal urethrostomy. J Urol. 1991;146(3):756–60. https://doi.org/10.1016/s0022-5347(17)37914-4.
52. Stein JP, Stenzl A, Esrig D, Freeman JA, Boyd SD, Lieskovsky G, Cote RJ, Bennett C, Colleselli K, Draxl H, et al. Lower urinary tract reconstruction following cystectomy in women using the Kock ileal reservoir with bilateral ureteroileal urethrostomy: initial clinical experience. J Urol. 1994;152(5 Pt 1):1404–8. https://doi.org/10.1016/s0022-5347(17)32431-x.
53. Ali-el-Dein B, El-Sobky E, Hohenfellner M, Ghoneim MA. Orthotopic bladder substitution in women: functional evaluation. J Urol. 1999;161(6):1875–80.
54. Lieskovsky G, Skinner DG, Boyd SD. Complications of the Kock pouch. Urol Clin North Am. 1988;15(2):195–205.
55. Studer UE, Ackermann D, Casanova GA, Zingg EJ. Three years' experience with an ileal low pressure bladder substitute. Br J Urol. 1989;63(1):43–52. https://doi.org/10.1111/j.1464-410x.1989.tb05122.x.
56. Studer UE, Varol C, Danuser H. Orthotopic ileal neobladder. BJU Int. 2004;93(1):183–93. https://doi.org/10.1111/j.1464-410x.2004.04641.x.
57. Rogers E, Scardino PT. A simple ileal substitute bladder after radical cystectomy: experience with a modification of the Studer pouch. J Urol. 1995;153(5):1432–8. https://doi.org/10.1016/s0022-5347(01)67422-6.
58. Skinner EC, Fairey AS, Groshen S, Daneshmand S, Cai J, Miranda G, Skinner DG. Randomized trial of Studer pouch versus T-pouch orthotopic ileal neobladder in patients with bladder cancer. J Urol. 2015;194(2):433–9. https://doi.org/10.1016/j.juro.2015.03.101. Epub 2015 Mar 28.
59. Bianchi G, Sighinolfi MC, Pirola GM, Micali S. Studer orthotopic neobladder: a modified surgical technique. Urology. 2016;88:222–5. https://doi.org/10.1016/j.urology.2015.11.020. Epub 2015 Nov 25.
60. Hautmann RE, Paiss T, de Petriconi R. The ileal neobladder in women: 9 years of experience with 18 patients. J Urol. 1996;155(1):76–81. https://doi.org/10.1016/s0022-5347(01)66546-7.
61. Hautmann RE. Ileal neobladder. BJU Int. 2010;105:1024–35. https://doi.org/10.1111/j.1464-410X.2010.09283.x.
62. Hautmann RE, de Petriconi RC, Volkmer BG. 25 years of experience with 1, 000 neobladders: long-term complications. J Urol. 2011;185:2207–12.
63. Lippert MC, Theodorescu D. The Hautmann neobladder with a chimney: a versatile modification. J Urol. 1997;158(4):1510–2.
64. Hollowell CM, Christiano AP, Steinberg GD. Technique of Hautmann ileal neobladder with chimney modification: interim results in 50 patients. J Urol. 2000;163(1):47–50. discussion 50-1.
65. Lee YS, Jung HB, Choi DK, Cho ST, Kim KK, Lee YG. Functional assessment of the Hautmann ileal neobladder with chimney modification using uroflowmetry and a questionnaire. Biomed Res Int. 2016;2016:8209589. https://doi.org/10.1155/2016/8209589. Epub 2016 Nov 29.
66. Abol-Enein H, Ghoneim MA. Functional results of orthotopic ileal neobladder with serous-lined extramural ureteral reimplantation: experience with 450 patients. J Urol. 2001;165(5):1427–32.
67. Hautmann RE, Egghart G, Frohneberg D, Miller K. The ileal neobladder. J Urol. 1988;139(1):39–42. https://doi.org/10.1016/s0022-5347(17)42283-x.
68. Shaaban AA, Gaballah MA, el-Diasty TA, Ghoneim MA. Urethral controlled bladder substitution: a comparison between the intussuscepted nipple valve and the technique of Le Duc as antireflux procedures. J Urol. 1992;148(4):1156–61. https://doi.org/10.1016/s0022-5347(17)36847-7.
69. Hautmann S, Chun KH, Currlin E, Braun P, Huland H, Juenemann KP. Refluxing chimney versus nonrefluxing LeDuc ureteroileal anastomosis for orthotopic ileal neobladder: a com-

parative analysis for patients with bladder cancer. J Urol. 2006;175(4):1389–93. https://doi.org/10.1016/S0022-5347(05)00709-3. discussion 1393-4.
70. Pagano F, Artibani W, Ligato P, Piazza R, Garbeglio A, Passerini G. Vescica Ileale Padovana: a technique for total bladder replacement. Eur Urol. 1990;17(2):149–54. https://doi.org/10.1159/000464024.
71. Thüroff JW, Alken P, Engelmann U, Riedmiller H, Jacobi GH, Hohenfellner R. The Mainz pouch (mixed augmentation ileum 'n zecum) for bladder augmentation and continent urinary diversion. Eur Urol. 1985;11(3):152–60. https://doi.org/10.1159/000472481.
72. Thüroff JW, Franzaring L, Gillitzer R, Wöhr M, Melchior S. Simplified orthotopic ileocaecal pouch (Mainz pouch) for bladder substitution. BJU Int. 2005;96(3):443–65. https://doi.org/10.1111/j.1464-410X.2005.05605.x.
73. Light JK, Engelmann UH. Le bag: total replacement of the bladder using an ileocolonic pouch. J Urol. 1986;136:27–31.
74. Reddy PK, Lange PH. Bladder replacement with sigmoid colon after radical cystoprostatectomy. Urology. 1987;29(4):368–71. https://doi.org/10.1016/0090-4295(87)90497-3.
75. Gilchrist RK, Merricks JW, Hamlin HH, Rieger IT. Construction of a substitute bladder and urethra. Surg Gynecol Obstet. 1950;90(6):752–60.
76. Skinner DG, Lieskovsky G, Boyd SD. Technique of creation of a continent internal ileal reservoir (Kock pouch) for urinary diversion. Urol Clin North Am. 1984;11(4):741–9.
77. Stein JP, Skinner DG. T-mechanism applied to urinary diversion: the orthotopic T-pouch ileal neobladder and cutaneous double-T-pouch ileal reservoir. Tech Urol. 2001;7(3):209–22.
78. Abol-Enein H, Salem M, Mesbah A, Abdel-Latif M, Kamal M, Shabaan A, Ghoneim M. Continent cutaneous ileal pouch using the serous lined extramural valves. The Mansoura experience in more than 100 patients. J Urol. 2004;172(2):588–91. https://doi.org/10.1097/01.ju.0000129437.33688.4d.
79. Thüroff JW, Alken P, Riedmiller H, Jacobi GH, Hohenfellner R. 100 cases of Mainz pouch: continuing experience and evolution. J Urol. 1988;140(2):283–8. https://doi.org/10.1016/s0022-5347(17)41584-9.
80. Rowland RG, Mitchell ME, Bihrle R, Kahnoski RJ, Piser JE. Indiana continent urinary reservoir. J Urol. 1987;137(6):1136–9. https://doi.org/10.1016/s0022-5347(17)44428-4.
81. Duckett JW, Snyder HM 3rd. Continent urinary diversion: variations on the Mitrofanoff principle. J Urol. 1986;136(1):58–62. https://doi.org/10.1016/s0022-5347(17)44725-2.
82. Lockhart JL. Remodeled right colon: an alternative urinary reservoir. J Urol. 1987;138(4):730–4. https://doi.org/10.1016/s0022-5347(17)43355-6.
83. Bejany DE, Politano VA. Stapled and nonstapled tapered distal ileum for construction of a continent colonic urinary reservoir. J Urol. 1988;140(3):491–4. https://doi.org/10.1016/s0022-5347(17)41699-5.
84. Smith T. An account of an unsuccessful attempt to treat extroversion of the bladder by a new operation. St Barth Hosp Rep. 1870;15:29.
85. Coffey RC. Transplantation of ureters into Large intestine by submucous implantation. JAMA. 1932;99:1320–3.
86. Jacobs JA, Young JD Jr. The Strickler technique of ureterosigmoidostomy. J Urol. 1980;124(4):451–4. https://doi.org/10.1016/s0022-5347(17)55492-0.
87. Ghoneim MA, Shehab-El-Din AB, Ashamallah AK, Gaballah MA. Evolution of the rectal bladder as a method for urinary diversion. J Urol. 1981;126(6):737–40. https://doi.org/10.1016/s0022-5347(17)54724-2.
88. Kock NG, Ghoneim MA, Lycke KG, Mahran MR. Urinary diversion to the augmented and valved rectum: preliminary results with a novel surgical procedure. J Urol. 1988;140(6):1375–9. https://doi.org/10.1016/s0022-5347(17)42049-0.
89. Fisch M, Wammack R, Hohenfellner R. The sigma rectum pouch (Mainz pouch II). World J Urol. 1996;14(2):68–72. https://doi.org/10.1007/BF00182560.
90. Leadbetter GW Jr, Zickerman P, Pierce E. Ureterosigmoidostomy and carcinoma of the colon. J Urol. 1979;121(6):732–5. https://doi.org/10.1016/s0022-5347(17)56973-6.

91. Ferris DO, Odel HM. Electrolyte pattern of the blood after bilateral ureterosigmoidostomy. J Am Med Assoc. 1950;142(9):634–41. https://doi.org/10.1001/jama.1950.02910270024006.
92. Rabinovitch HH. Ureterosigmoidostomy in children--revival or demise? J Urol. 1980;124(4):552. https://doi.org/10.1016/s0022-5347(17)55537-8.
93. Kristjánsson A, Mânsson W. Refluxing or nonrefluxing ureteric anastomosis. BJU Int. 1999;84(8):905–10. https://doi.org/10.1046/j.1464-410x.1999.00395.x.
94. Hohenfellner R, Black P, Leissner J, Allhoff EP. Refluxing ureterointestinal anastomosis for continent cutaneous urinary diversion. J Urol. 2002;168(3):1013–6. https://doi.org/10.1097/01.ju.0000025142.28876.be. discussion 1016-7.
95. Choi SY, Lim B, Chi BH, Kim JH, Lee W, You D, Kim CS. Hybrid ileal pouch with concomitant anti-refluxing and refluxing ureteroileal anastomosis. BMC Urol. 2021;21(1):92. https://doi.org/10.1186/s12894-021-00828-1.
96. Hassan AA, Elgamal SA, Sabaa MA, Salem KA, Elmateet MS. Evaluation of direct versus non-refluxing technique and functional results in orthotopic Y-ileal neobladder after 12 years of follow up. Int J Urol. 2007;14(4):300–4. https://doi.org/10.1111/j.1442-2042.2006.01716.x.
97. Song C, Kim SC, Park J, Moon DH, Ahn H. Renal function change after refluxing type orthotopic ileal substitution. J Urol. 2011;186(5):1948–52. https://doi.org/10.1016/j.juro.2011.07.012. Epub 2011 Sep 23.
98. Nichols WK, Krause AH, Donegan WL. Urinary fistulas after ureteral diversion. Am J Surg. 1972;124(3):311–6. https://doi.org/10.1016/0002-9610(72)90032-3.
99. Hensle TW, Bredin HC, Dretler SP. Diagnosis and treatment of a urinary leak after ureteroileal conduit for diversion. J Urol. 1976;116(1):29–31. https://doi.org/10.1016/s0022-5347(17)58660-7.
100. Ali-el-Dein B, Shaaban AA, Abu-Eideh RH, El-Azab M, Ashamallah A, Ghoneim MA. Surgical complications following radical cystectomy and orthotopic neobladders in women. J Urol. 2008;180(1):206–10. https://doi.org/10.1016/j.juro.2008.03.080. discussion 210. Epub 2008 May 21.
101. Nazmy M, Yuh B, Kawachi M, Lau CS, Linehan J, Ruel NH, Torrey RR, Yamzon J, Wilson TG, Chan KG. Early and late complications of robot-assisted radical cystectomy: a standardized analysis by urinary diversion type. J Urol. 2014;191(3):681–7. https://doi.org/10.1016/j.juro.2013.10.022. Epub 2013 Oct 4.
102. So A, Hickey L, Norman R. Late ureteral conduit urinary leak as a presentation of urothelial carcinoma of the ureter. Urology. 2002;59(6):946. https://doi.org/10.1016/s0090-4295(02)01554-6.
103. Yl Y, Ht L, Tan L, et al. Conservative treatment for urinary fistula following ileal conduit urinary diversion: a simple method. BMC Urol. 2019;19:131. https://doi.org/10.1186/s12894-019-0564-3.
104. Horenblas S, Kröger R, van Boven E, Meinhardt W, Newling DW. Use of balloon catheters for ureteral occlusion in urinary leakage. Eur Urol. 2000;38(5):613–7. https://doi.org/10.1159/000020340.
105. Forde JC, O'Connor KM, Fanning DM, Guiney MJ, Lynch TH. Management of a persistent ileo-ureteric anastomotic leak with bilateral ureteric occlusion using angioplasty balloon catheters. Can J Urol. 2010;17(5):5397–400.
106. Perimenis P, Burkhard FC, Kessler TM, Gramann T, Studer UE. Ileal orthotopic bladder substitute combined with an afferent tubular segment: long-term upper urinary tract changes and voiding pattern. Eur Urol. 2004;46(5):604–9. https://doi.org/10.1016/j.eururo.2004.07.009.
107. Studer UE, Burkhard FC, Schumacher M, Kessler TM, Thoeny H, Fleischmann A, Thalmann GN. Twenty years experience with an ileal orthotopic low pressure bladder substitute--lessons to be learned. J Urol. 2006;176(1):161–6. https://doi.org/10.1016/S0022-5347(06)00573-8.
108. Yang WJ, Cho KS, Rha KH, Lee HY, Chung BH, Hong SJ, Yang SC, Choi YD. Long-term effects of ileal conduit urinary diversion on upper urinary tract in bladder cancer. Urology. 2006;68(2):324–7. https://doi.org/10.1016/j.urology.2006.02.015.

109. Katkoori D, Samavedi S, Adiyat KT, Soloway MS, Manoharan M. Is the incidence of uretero-intestinal anastomotic stricture increased in patients undergoing radical cystectomy with previous pelvic radiation? BJU Int. 2010;105(6):795–8. https://doi.org/10.1111/j.1464-410X.2009.08835.x. Epub 2009 Sep 2.
110. Shimko MS, Tollefson MK, Umbreit EC, Farmer SA, Blute ML, Frank I. Long-term complications of conduit urinary diversion. J Urol. 2011;185(2):562–7. https://doi.org/10.1016/j.juro.2010.09.096. Epub 2010 Dec 18.
111. Anderson CB, Morgan TM, Kappa S, Moore D, Clark PE, Davis R, Penson DF, Barocas DA, Smith JA Jr, Cookson MS, Chang SS. Ureteroenteric anastomotic strictures after radical cystectomy-does operative approach matter? J Urol. 2013;189(2):541–7. https://doi.org/10.1016/j.juro.2012.09.034. Epub 2012 Dec 20.
112. Large MC, Cohn JA, Kiriluk KJ, Dangle P, Richards KA, Smith ND, Steinberg GD. The impact of running versus interrupted anastomosis on ureterointestinal stricture rate after radical cystectomy. J Urol. 2013;190(3):923–7. https://doi.org/10.1016/j.juro.2013.02.091. Epub 2013 Feb 27.
113. Shah SH, Movassaghi K, Skinner D, Dalag L, Miranda G, Cai J, Schuckman A, Daneshmand S, Djaladat H. Ureteroenteric strictures after open radical cystectomy and urinary diversion: the University of Southern California experience. Urology. 2015;86(1):87–91. https://doi.org/10.1016/j.urology.2015.03.014. Epub 2015 May 16.
114. Ahmed YE, Hussein AA, May PR, Ahmad B, Ali T, Durrani A, Khan S, Kumar P, Guru KA. Natural history, predictors and Management of Ureteroenteric Strictures after robot assisted radical cystectomy. J Urol. 2017;198(3):567–74. https://doi.org/10.1016/j.juro.2017.02.3339. Epub 2017 Mar 1.
115. Hosseini A, Dey L, Laurin O, Adding C, Hoijer J, Ebbing J, Collins JW. Ureteric stricture rates and management after robot-assisted radical cystectomy: a single-Centre observational study. Scand J Urol. 2018;52(4):244–8. https://doi.org/10.1080/21681805.2018.1465462. Epub 2018 Aug 14.
116. Ericson KJ, Thomas LJ, Zhang JH, Knorr JM, Khanna A, Crane A, Zampini AM, Murthy PB, Berglund RK, Pascal-Haber G, BHL L. Uretero-enteric anastomotic stricture following radical cystectomy: a comparison of open, robotic extracorporeal, and robotic intracorporeal approaches. Urology. 2020;144:130–5. https://doi.org/10.1016/j.urology.2020.06.047. Epub 2020 Jul 9.
117. Goh AC, Belarmino A, Patel NA, Sun T, Sedrakyan A, Bochner BH, Hu JC. A Population-based Study of Ureteroenteric Strictures After Open and Robot-assisted Radical Cystectomy. Urology. 2020;135:57–65. https://doi.org/10.1016/j.urology.2019.07.054. Epub 2019 Oct 13.
118. Faraj KS, Rose KM, Navaratnam AK, Abdul-Muhsin HM, Eversman S, Singh V, Tyson MD. Effect of intracorporeal urinary diversion on the incidence of benign ureteroenteric stricture after cystectomy. Int J Urol. 2021;28(5):593–7. https://doi.org/10.1111/iju.14521. Epub 2021 Feb 16.
119. Magnusson J, Hagberg O, Aljabery F, Hosseini A, Jahnson S, Jerlström T, Sherif A, Söderkvist K, Ströck V, Ullén A, Häggström C, Holmberg L, Kjölhede H. Cumulative incidence of ureteroenteric strictures after radical cystectomy in a population-based Swedish cohort. Scand J Urol. 2021;55(5):361–5. https://doi.org/10.1080/21681805.2021.1955967. Epub 2021 Jul 27.
120. Reesink DJ, Gerritsen SL, Kelder H, van Melick HHE, Stijns PEF. Evaluation of Ureteroenteric anastomotic strictures after the introduction of robot-assisted radical cystectomy with intracorporeal urinary diversion: results from a Large tertiary referral Center. J Urol. 2021;205(4):1119–25. https://doi.org/10.1097/JU.0000000000001518. Epub 2020 Nov 30.
121. Alonso Mediavilla E, Campos-Juanatey F, Azcárraga Aranegui G, Varea Malo R, Ballestero Diego R, Domínguez Esteban M, Ramos Barseló E, Zubillaga Guerrero S, Calleja Hermosa P, Gutiérrez Baños JL. Ureteroileal anastomosis stricture after urinary diversions performed by open, laparoscopic and robotic approaches. Incidence and management in a ter-

tiary care center. Actas Urol Esp (Engl Ed). 2022;46(1):49–56. https://doi.org/10.1016/j.acuroe.2021.06.010. English, Spanish. Epub 2021 Nov 25.
122. Lobo N, Dupré S, Sahai A, Thurairaja R, Khan MS. Getting out of a tight spot: an overview of ureteroenteric anastomotic strictures. Nat Rev Urol. 2016;13(8):447–55. https://doi.org/10.1038/nrurol.2016.104. Epub 2016 Jun 28.
123. Ahmadi N, Ashrafi AN, Hartman N, Shakir A, Cacciamani GE, Freitas D, Rajarubendra N, Fay C, Berger A, Desai MM, Gill IS, Aron M. Use of indocyanine green to minimise uretero-enteric strictures after robotic radical cystectomy. BJU Int. 2019;124(2):302–7. https://doi.org/10.1111/bju.14733. Epub 2019 Apr 11.
124. Ali-El-Dein B, Helmy T, Abdel-Latif M, et al. Treatment of ureteroileal anastomotic strictures after radical cystectomy and ileal W-neobladder. J Urol. 2006;175(Suppl):228. (abst V706). Annual AUA meeting, Atlanta, Georgia, May 20-25, 2006
125. Schöndorf D, Meierhans-Ruf S, Kiss B, Giannarini G, Thalmann GN, Studer UE, Roth B. Ureteroileal strictures after urinary diversion with an ileal segment-is there a place for endourological treatment at all? J Urol. 2013;190(2):585–90. https://doi.org/10.1016/j.juro.2013.02.039. Epub 2013 Feb 20.
126. Olson L, Satherley H, Cleaveland P, Zelhof B, Mokete M, Neilson D, Srirangam S. Retrograde Endourological Management of Upper Urinary Tract Abnormalities in Patients with Ileal Conduit Urinary Diversion: A Dual-Center Experience. J Endourol. 2017;31(9):841–6. https://doi.org/10.1089/end.2017.0271. Epub 2017 Jul 19.
127. Stuurman RE, Al-Qahtani SM, Cornu JN, Traxer O. Antegrade percutaneous flexible endoscopic approach for the management of urinary diversion-associated complications. J Endourol. 2013;27(11):1330–4. https://doi.org/10.1089/end.2012.0371. Epub 2013 Jun 12.
128. Tinoco CL, Lima E. Urinary diversions for radical cystectomy: a review of complications and their management. Mini-invasive Surg. 2021;5:28. https://doi.org/10.20517/2574-1225.2021.35.
129. Rosales A, Emiliani E, Salvador JT, Peña JA, Gaya JM, Palou J, Villavicencio H. Laparoscopic Management of Ureteroileal Anastomosis Strictures: initial experience. Eur Urol. 2016;70(3):493–8. https://doi.org/10.1016/j.eururo.2016.02.045. Epub 2016 Feb 28.
130. Scherzer ND, Greenberg JW, Shaw EJ, Silberstein JL, Thomas R, Krane LS. Robotic vs. open surgical management of ureteroenteric anastomotic strictures: technical modifications to enhance success. J Robot Surg. 2020;14(4):615–9. https://doi.org/10.1007/s11701-019-01027-9. Epub 2019 Oct 4.
131. Zhong W, Yang B, He F, Wang L, Swami S, Zeng G. Surgical management of urolithiasis in patients after urinary diversion. PLoS One. 2014;9(10):e111371. https://doi.org/10.1371/journal.pone.0111371.
132. Turk TM, Koleski FC, Albala DM. Incidence of urolithiasis in cystectomy patients after intestinal conduit or continent urinary diversion. World J Urol. 1999;17(5):305–7. https://doi.org/10.1007/s003450050151.
133. Terai A, Arai Y, Kawakita M, Okada Y, Yoshida O. Effect of urinary intestinal diversion on urinary risk factors for urolithiasis. J Urol. 1995;153(1):37–41. https://doi.org/10.1097/00005392-199501000-00016.
134. Ginsberg D, Huffman JL, Lieskovsky G, Boyd S, Skinner DG. Urinary tract stones: a complication of the Kock pouch continent urinary diversion. J Urol. 1991;145(5):956–9. https://doi.org/10.1016/s0022-5347(17)38499-9.
135. Terai A, Ueda T, Kakehi Y, Terachi T, Arai Y, Okada Y, Yoshida O. Urinary calculi as a late complication of the Indiana continent urinary diversion: comparison with the Kock pouch procedure. J Urol. 1996;155(1):66–8.
136. Arai Y, Kawakita M, Terachi T, Oishi K, Okada Y, Takeuchi H, Yoshida O. Long-term followup of the Kock and Indiana pouch procedures. J Urol. 1993;150(1):51–5. https://doi.org/10.1016/s0022-5347(17)35394-6.

137. Okhunov Z, Duty B, Smith AD, Okeke Z. Management of urolithiasis in patients after urinary diversions. BJU Int. 2011;108(3):330–6. https://doi.org/10.1111/j.1464-410X.2011.10194.x. Epub 2011 May 25.
138. Franzoni DF, Decter RM. Percutaneous vesicolithotomy: an alternative to open bladder surgery in patients with an impassable or surgically ablated urethra. J Urol. 1999;162(3 Pt 1):777–8. https://doi.org/10.1097/00005392-199909010-00042.
139. Delvecchio FC, Kuo RL, Iselin CE, Webster GD, Preminger GM. Combined antegrade and retrograde endoscopic approach for the management of urinary diversion-associated pathology. J Endourol. 2000;14(3):251–6. https://doi.org/10.1089/end.2000.14.251.
140. L'Esperance JO, Sung J, Marguet C, L'Esperance A, Albala DM. The surgical management of stones in patients with urinary diversions. Curr Opin Urol. 2004;14(2):129–34. https://doi.org/10.1097/00042307-200403000-00014.
141. Cohen TD, Streem SB. Minimally invasive endourologic management of calculi in continent urinary reservoirs. Urology. 1994;43(6):865–8. https://doi.org/10.1016/0090-4295(94)90154-6.
142. Clifford TG, Katebian B, Van Horn CM, Bazargani ST, Cai J, Miranda G, Daneshmand S, Djaladat H. Urinary tract infections following radical cystectomy and urinary diversion: a review of 1133 patients. World J Urol. 2018;36(5):775–81. https://doi.org/10.1007/s00345-018-2181-2. Epub 2018 Jan 25.
143. Ghoreifi A, Van Horn CM, Xu W, Cai J, Miranda G, Bhanvadia S, Schuckman AK, Daneshmand S, Djaladat H. Urinary tract infections following radical cystectomy with enhanced recovery protocol: a prospective study. Urol Oncol. 2020;38(3):75.e9–75.e14. https://doi.org/10.1016/j.urolonc.2019.12.021. Epub 2020 Jan 16.
144. Parker WP, Toussi A, Tollefson MK, Frank I, Thompson RH, Zaid HB, Thapa P, Boorjian SA. Risk factors and microbial distribution of urinary tract infections following radical cystectomy. Urology. 2016;94:96–101. https://doi.org/10.1016/j.urology.2016.03.049. Epub 2016 Apr 25.
145. Gill IS, Fergany A, Klein EA, Kaouk JH, Sung GT, Meraney AM, Savage SJ, Ulchaker JC, Novick AC. Laparoscopic radical cystoprostatectomy with ileal conduit performed completely intracorporeally: the initial 2 cases. Urology. 2000;56(1):26–9. https://doi.org/10.1016/s0090-4295(00)00598-7. discussion 29-30.
146. Shi H, Li J, Li K, Yang X, Zhu Z, Tian D. Minimally invasive versus open radical cystectomy for bladder cancer: a systematic review and meta-analysis. J Int Med Res. 2019;47(10):4604–18. https://doi.org/10.1177/0300060519864806.
147. Albisinni S, Veccia A, Aoun F, Diamand R, Esperto F, Porpiglia F, Roumeguère T, De Nunzio C. A systematic review and meta-analysis comparing the outcomes of open and robotic assisted radical cystectomy. Minerva Urol Nefrol. 2019;71(6):553–68. https://doi.org/10.23736/S0393-2249.19.03546-X. Epub 2019 Oct 10.
148. Parekh DJ, Reis IM, Castle EP, et al. Robot-assisted radical cystectomy versus open radical cystectomy in patients with bladder cancer (RAZOR): an open-label, randomised, phase 3, non-inferiority trial. Lancet. 2018;391(10139):2525–36. https://doi.org/10.1016/S0140-6736(18)30996-6.
149. Venkatramani V, Reis IM, Castle EP, et al. Predictors of recurrence, and progression-free and overall survival following open versus robotic radical cystectomy: analysis from the RAZOR trial with a 3-year Followup. J Urol. 2020;203(3):522–9. https://doi.org/10.1097/JU.0000000000000565. Epub 2019 Sep 24.
150. Lavallée E, Wiklund P. The Studer neobladder: an established and reproducible technique for intracorporeal urinary diversion. Eur Urol Open Sci. 2021;35:18–20. https://doi.org/10.1016/j.euros.2021.09.019.
151. Goh AC, Gill IS, Lee DJ, de Castro Abreu AL, Fairey AS, Leslie S, Berger AK, Daneshmand S, Sotelo R, Gill KS, Xie HW, Chu LY, Aron M, Desai MM. Robotic intracorporeal orthotopic ileal neobladder: replicating open surgical principles. Eur Urol. 2012;62(5):891–901. https://doi.org/10.1016/j.eururo.2012.07.052. Epub 2012 Aug 17.

152. Atala A, Bauer SB, Soker S, Yoo JJ, Retik AB. Tissue-engineered autologous bladders for patients needing cystoplasty. Lancet. 2006;367(9518):1241–6. https://doi.org/10.1016/S0140-6736(06)68438-9.
153. Sopko NA, Kates M, Bivalacqua TJ. Use of regenerative tissue for urinary diversion. Curr Opin Urol. 2015;25(6):578–85. https://doi.org/10.1097/MOU.0000000000000223.
154. Zhao Y, He Y, Guo JH, Wu JS, Zhou Z, Zhang M, Li W, Zhou J, Xiao DD, Wang Z, Sun K, Zhu YJ, Lu MJ. Time-dependent bladder tissue regeneration using bilayer bladder acellular matrix graft-silk fibroin scaffolds in a rat bladder augmentation model. Acta Biomater. 2015;23:91–102. https://doi.org/10.1016/j.actbio.2015.05.032. Epub 2015 Jun 3. Erratum in: Acta Biomater. 2016 Mar; 33: 324.
155. Shakhssalim N, Soleimani M, Dehghan MM, Rasouli J, Taghizadeh-Jahed M, Torbati PM, Naji M. Bladder smooth muscle cells on electrospun poly (ε-caprolactone)/poly (l-lactic acid) scaffold promote bladder regeneration in a canine model. Mater Sci Eng C Mater Biol Appl. 2017;75:877–84. https://doi.org/10.1016/j.msec.2017.02.064. Epub 2017 Feb 16.
156. Wang Y, Zhou S, Yang R, Zou Q, Zhang K, Tian Q, Zhao W, Zong L, Fu Q. Bioengineered bladder patches constructed from multilayered adipose-derived stem cell sheets for bladder regeneration. Acta Biomater. 2019;85:131–41. https://doi.org/10.1016/j.actbio.2018.12.016. Epub 2018 Dec 12.

Chapter 23
The Ureter and Renal Transplantation

John M. Barry and Bedeir Ali-El-Dein

Abstract In this chapter, the various methods of implantation of the ureter during renal transplantation are described. Included are discussions of the standard extravesical and transvesical ureteroneocystostomies, the indications for a ureteral stent, the management of the short ureter and the double ureter, and how to connect a transplant ureter to an intestinal conduit. The presentation, diagnosis and management of the most common ureteral complications after renal transplantation (urinary leakage, ureteral obstruction, vesicoureteral reflux, and calculi) are described along with the impact of these complications on graft function, graft survival, and patient survival.

Keywords Ureter · Ureteral · Ureteroneocystostomy · Pyeloureterostomy · Ureteroureterostomy · Stent · Transplant · Renal · Complications · Obstruction · Extravasation · Fluid collection · Lymphocele

Learning Objectives
The learning objectives for this chapter are

- To describe the methods of implantation of the transplant ureter, and
- To discuss the evaluation and treatment of early and late complications of the transplant ureter.

Test your learning and check your understanding of this book's contents: use the "Springer Nature Flashcards" app to access questions. To use the app, please follow the instructions in Chapter 1.

J. M. Barry (✉)
Departments of Urology and Surgery, Division of Abdominal Organ Transplantation, Oregon Health and Science University, Portland, OR, USA
e-mail: barryj@ohsu.edu

B. Ali-El-Dein
Urology Department, Urology and Nephrology Center, Faculty of Medicine, Mansoura University, Mansoura, Egypt

M. Abdel-Gawad et al. (eds.), *The Ureter*,
https://doi.org/10.1007/978-3-031-36212-5_23

23.1 Introduction

The factors that determine the type of urinary tract reconstruction during renal transplantation are the quality of the donor ureter, the condition of the recipient's bladder or bladder substitute, the condition of the recipient's ureter, and the familiarity of the surgeon with a technique.

Although many surgeons prefer the right iliac fossa for kidney transplantation, it's desirable to transplant the left kidney into the right iliac fossa and the right kidney into the left iliac fossa to place the renal pelvis and ureter of the kidney transplant as the most medial and superficial of the hilar structures. This simplifies urinary tract reconstruction if pyeloureterostomy, ureteroureterostomy or pyelovesicostomy are or become necessary. This principle is compromised in three instances: (1) the preferred iliac fossa is already occupied by another transplant, an ileostomy or a colostomy, (2) the recipient is obese (the skin-to-iliac vessel distance is less on the right than the left) or (3) the preferred iliac vessels are unsuitable for renal revascularization, for example, in a patient with iliac venous or arterial thrombosis, an iliac venous cannula or in a small child. [1].

Synthetic, absorbable sutures are preferred to non-absorbable sutures because of the risk of stone formation when non-absorbable suture material is exposed to urine. In vivo strength retention is better with absorbable synthetic materials than with natural fibers such as gut. Monofilament suture is preferred by many surgeons because it has less tissue drag than braided suture. Polydioxanone is commonly used; 4-0 or 5-0 for ureteric or renal pelvic anastomosis, and 3-0 for bladder closure.

23.2 Ureteroneocystostomy

Stented ureteroneocystostomy is the usual form of urinary tract reconstruction. It is several centimeters away from the vascular anastomoses, and the native ureter remains for the treatment of ureteric complications.

Although not practiced by all kidney transplant surgeons, it's reasonable to prevent transplant pyelonephritis from reflux of infected bladder urine by the formation of a one-way valve where the kidney transplant's ureter rests on bladder muscle in a 2- to 3-cm submucosal tunnel.

For either an extravesical or transvesical ureteroneocystostomy, the genitalia are prepared with an antiseptic solution, and a lubricated balloon retention catheter is passed into the urinary bladder or bladder substitute. The catheter is connected to a 3-way system which consists of a bag filled with an antibiotic solution on one line and a collection bag on the other. This allows the anesthetist to fill, irrigate, drain, and refill the bladder at the direction of the surgeon. The 3-way system is especially helpful when the bladder is difficult to identify because of pelvic scar tissue, recipient obesity or reduced capacity. After initially accommodating a small volume, a defunctionalized bladder, gravity-filled to its original small capacity, will often relax and accept more fluid 1 or 2 h into the transplant procedure.

23.2.1 Handling the Ureter before Ureteroneocystostomy

Delicate handling of the ureter, preservation of the periureteral vessels and avoidance of ureteric kinking are key elements. Ureteric length has to be as short as possible yet long enough to allow a tension-free ureteroneocystostomy. A short ureter sometimes necessitates a psoas hitch, bladder flap or transplant ureter to native ureteroureterostomy.

23.2.2 Techniques of Extravesical Ureteroneocystostomy

Extravesical techniques are based on the procedure described by Lich et al. [2]. This technique was adapted for renal transplantation in 1962 [3]. It is well illustrated in a publication by Konnak et al. [4] and has been modified by the addition of a stitch to anchor the toe of the spatulated ureter to the full thickness of the bladder to prevent proximal slippage of the ureter in the submucosal tunnel and loss of the antireflux mechanism (Fig. 23.1).

The bladder is prepared as described above, and its lateral surface is cleared of fat. To prevent post-transplant ureteric obstruction, the ureter is passed under the spermatic cord, and the round ligament in women is divided. A T-shaped or longitudinal oblique incision is made for approximately 3 cm until the bladder mucosa bulges into the incision. The bladder is drained partially, and the mucosa is dissected away from the muscularis to make a submucosal tunnel for the ureter. The bladder mucosa is grasped with forceps, the urinary bladder is partially drained, and a 5 mm incision is made in the medial portion of the exposed mucosa. The ureter is laid in the trough, spatulated and anastomosed to the bladder mucosa with running or interrupted fine absorbable sutures. If a double-pigtail stent is used, it is passed up the ureter and into the bladder before completing the second ureteric-to-bladder mucosa suture line. A suture is placed in the toe of the ureter, passed through the seromuscular layer of the bladder and tied about 5 mm distal to the cystotomy. The seromuscular layer is closed over the ureter with interrupted sutures so that the proximal one or two sutures can be removed if the ureteric lumen has been compromised by the closure.

The *one-stitch* [5] and *two-stitch* [6] extravesical ureteroneocystostomies are modifications of the Lich procedure in which one or two mattress sutures are placed full thickness through the spatulated ureter and the bladder without a deliberate mucosa-to-mucosa approximation. The disadvantage of these techniques has been reported to be significantly increased ureteric complications, most commonly, hematuria [7].

The parallel-incision extravesical ureteroneocystostomy is used by some [8]. The setup is the same as for a modified Lich procedure. Parallel incisions are made in the lateral bladder 2–3 cm apart until the bladder mucosa bulges into both incisions (Fig. 23.2). The bladder is drained partially, and a submucosal tunnel is created

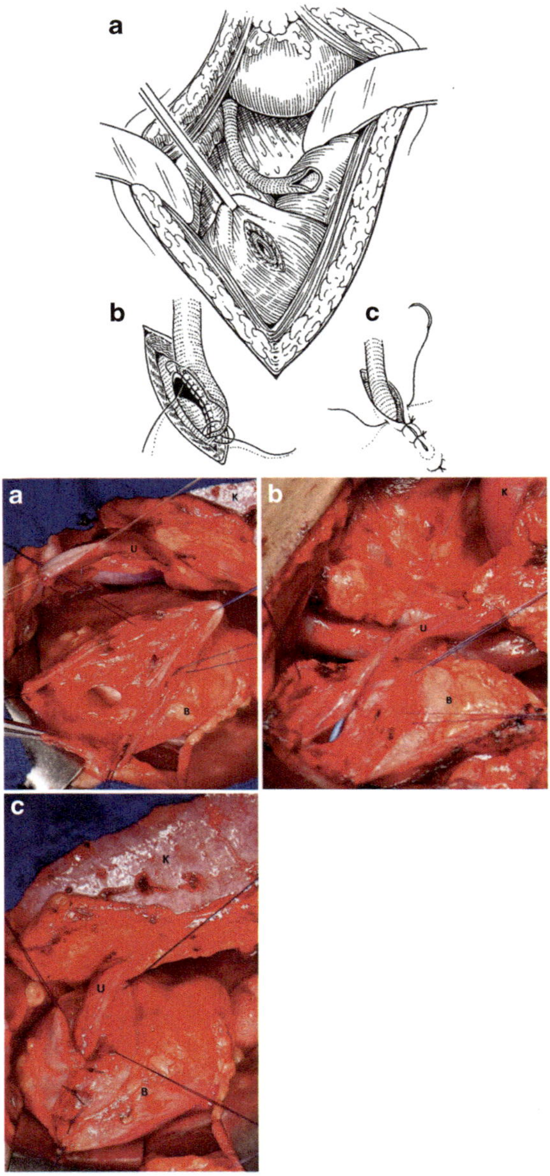

Fig. 23.1 Diagrammatic representation and intra-operative photos of extravesical ureteroneocystostomy. Top (**a**). The transplant ureter is prepared, spatulated for about 1.0 cm, the bladder mucosa is dissected off the detrusor and a button hole is made in the distal bladder mucosa. Top (**b**). A double-J ureteric stent is commonly placed before completion of the second suture line. Top (**c**). A toe stitch is added to anchor the ureter to the full thickness of the bladder of the submucosal tunnel (**a**–**c**) is reproduced with permission from Konnak et al. [4]. Bottom (**a**–**c**) are obtained from the courtesy of Dr. Bedeir Ali-El-Dein

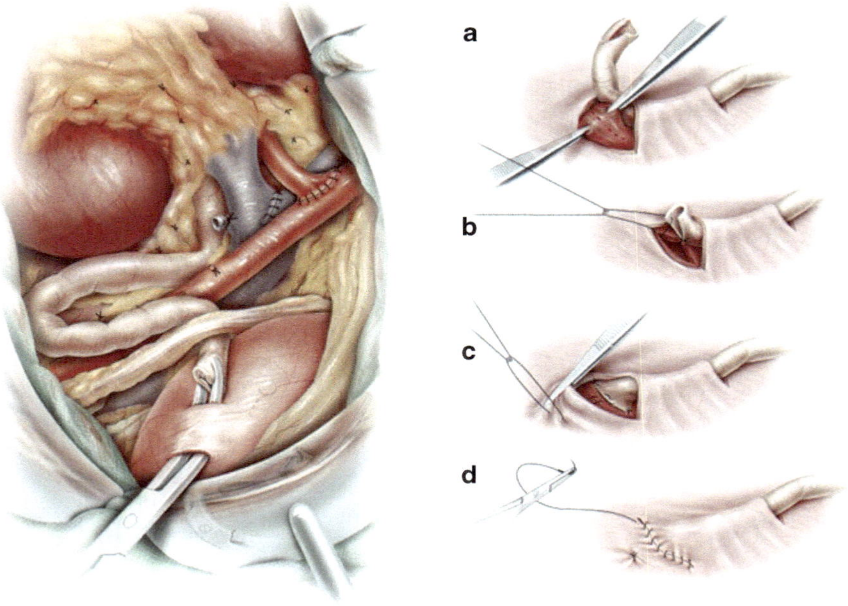

Fig. 23.2 Parallel incision extravesical ureteroneocystostomy. The sequence is (**a**–**d**). A double-J ureteric stent may be placed before completing the toe stitch. Reproduced with permission from Barry [8]

between the two incisions. The ureter is drawn through the tunnel, transected, spatulated and anastomosed to the bladder mucosa with interrupted, fine, absorbable sutures. A vertical or horizontal mattress suture is used to anchor the toe of the ureter to the urinary bladder. This suture is tied about 5 mm distal to the cystotomy. Finally, the distal cystotomy is closed with a running, fine absorbable suture. The parallel-incision extravesical ureteroneocystostomy has been slightly modified by Caparros and associates by application of the *one-stitch* principle with no suture approximation of the ureteric and bladder mucosal [9].

23.2.3 Technique of Transvesical Ureteroneocystostomy

The technique for transvesical ureteroneocystostomy is similar to that described by Merrill and colleagues in the first successful kidney transplant from a twin [10]; It is usually known as the Politano-Leadbetter technique [11, 12] (Fig. 23.3).

The dome of the bladder is cleared of fat, and stay sutures are placed on either side of a proposed vertical midline incision. The urinary bladder is drained, and an

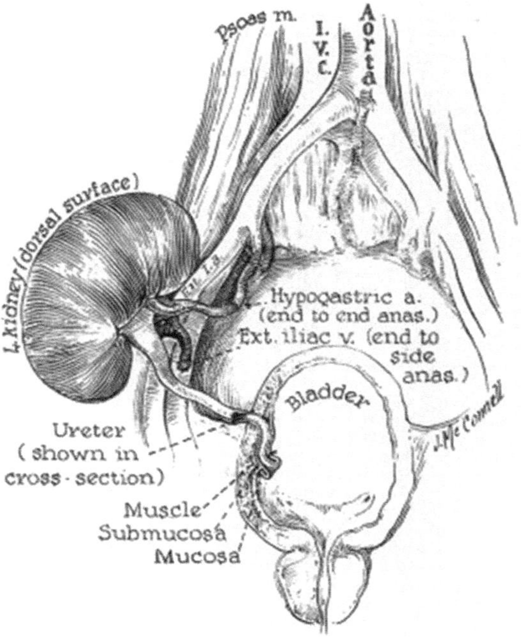

Fig. 23.3 Transvesical ureteroneocystostomy. Reproduced with permission from Starzl et al. [12]

incision is made through all layers of the anterior bladder wall. Retractors are placed in the dome and both sides of the bladder interior to expose the trigone. Cephalad to the native ureter, a transverse incision is made in the bladder mucosa. A submucosal tunnel is created with a right angle clamp or Thorek scissors for about 2 cm. The clamp is punched through the bladder, and the muscular opening is enlarged to accept the kidney transplant ureter. The ureter is drawn under the spermatic cord and into the bladder, where it is transected, spatulated, and sewn to the bladder mucosa with fine absorbable sutures. The inferior suture includes the bladder muscularis to anchor the ureter distally and prevent its movement in the submucosal tunnel. The retractors are removed, and the cystotomy is closed with a single layer of 3-0 absorbable suture. The bladder is refilled via the 3-way system to check for leaks. If present, they are closed with one or two interrupted sutures. Some surgeons use two bladder mucosal incisions about 2 cm apart and close the proximal bladder mucosa incision with fine absorbable suture.

23.2.3.1 Extravesical Versus Transvesical Ureteroneocystostomy

Compared with the extravesical procedures, the transvesical technique takes more time, a separate cystotomy is required, and more ureteral length is necessary. The extravesical modified Lich-Gregoire technique was reported by some authors to be associated with fewer overall complications than the transvesical Politano-Leadbetter technique; however, many investigators reported comparable rates of post-transplant ureteric complications for either technique [13–15].

23.2.4 Implantation of Double Ureters

Double ureters can be managed by leaving them in their common sheath to preserve blood supply, trimming them to appropriate length, spatulating them and either anastomosing the medial edges together with a running fine absorbable suture or by joining them, one on top of the other, with a single stitch from the toe of the upper one to the heel of the lower one [16]. The conjoined ureters can be treated as a single ureter by any of the previously described ureteroneocystostomy techniques. Some surgeons use a separate ureteroneocystostomy for each of the ureters.

These same techniques can be used for the *en bloc* transplantation of pediatric kidneys or the transplantation of two adult kidneys, stacked one on top of the other [17].

23.2.5 Technique of Pyeloureterostomy and Ureteroureterostomy

Pyeloureterostomy or ureteroureterostomy usually is done when (1) the transplant ureter's blood supply appears to be compromised, (2) the urinary bladder is difficult to identify because of pelvic scar, (3) the bladder does not distend enough for a ureteroneocystostomy, (4) the surgeon prefers one of them to ureteroneocystostomy, or (5) an orthotopic kidney transplant has been done. [18]. The techniques for pyeloureterostomy and ureteroureterostomy are similar. The posterior, or back wall anastomosis of the transplant renal pelvis or ureter to the end or side of the native ureter is completed first, a double-pigtail ureteric stent is placed, and the anterior suture line is completed (Fig. 23.4).

Ipsilateral native nephrectomy is not necessary with this technique. In the case of an iliac fossa kidney transplant, the proximal recipient ureter is managed by (1) leaving the native kidney in situ and using the side of the native ureter for the anastomosis, (2) removal of the ipsilateral native kidney and proximal ureter or (3) ligation of the proximal ureter and leaving the obstructed native kidney in situ. Although Schiff and Lytton [19] and Lord et al. [20] have described the safety of native ureteral ligation with kidney transplant urinary tract reconstruction, some surgeons prefer to leave the native ureter in continuity with its kidney and to anastomose the pelvis or ureter of the renal transplant to the side of the native ureter. This ensures a good blood supply to the native ureter and removes an obstructed kidney from the differential diagnosis of ipsilateral flank pain or postoperative fever.

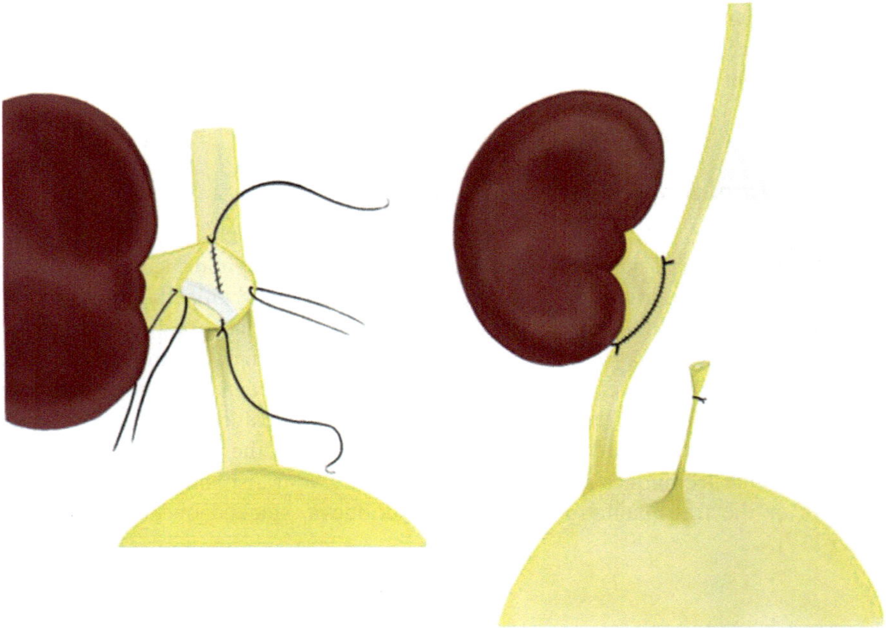

Fig. 23.4 Pyeloureterostomy. If the side of the recipient ureter is used, ureteral blood supply comes from above and below the anastomosis and ipsilateral native hydronephrosis is prevented. A double-J ureteric stent is placed before completion of the second suture line. Illustration by Poone Shoureshi, MD

23.2.6 Ureteroenterostomy

Ureteroenterostomy into an intestinal conduit or an intestinal pouch is accomplished by using one of the extravesical techniques (Fig. 23.5). Conduit or pouch identification is usually accomplished by slightly distending it with antibiotic irrigant, If it is difficult to identify the intestinal conduit or pouch because of surrounding intestines, a Foley catheter can be passed into it and the balloon inflated. If it still cannot be located, the conduit can be stained by adding methylene blue to the irrigant.

When the transplant ureter or the intestinal conduit is short, Urinary tract reconstruction can be performed by anastomosis of the transplant ureter to the side of the native ureter which is already connected to the conduit [15].

23.2.7 Ureteral Stents

Whether to use or not to use a ureteral stent is determined by transplant program policy or surgeon preference [21–24]. The rationale for routine ureteral stenting is that it can reduce the incidence of ureteral-related post-transplant complications,

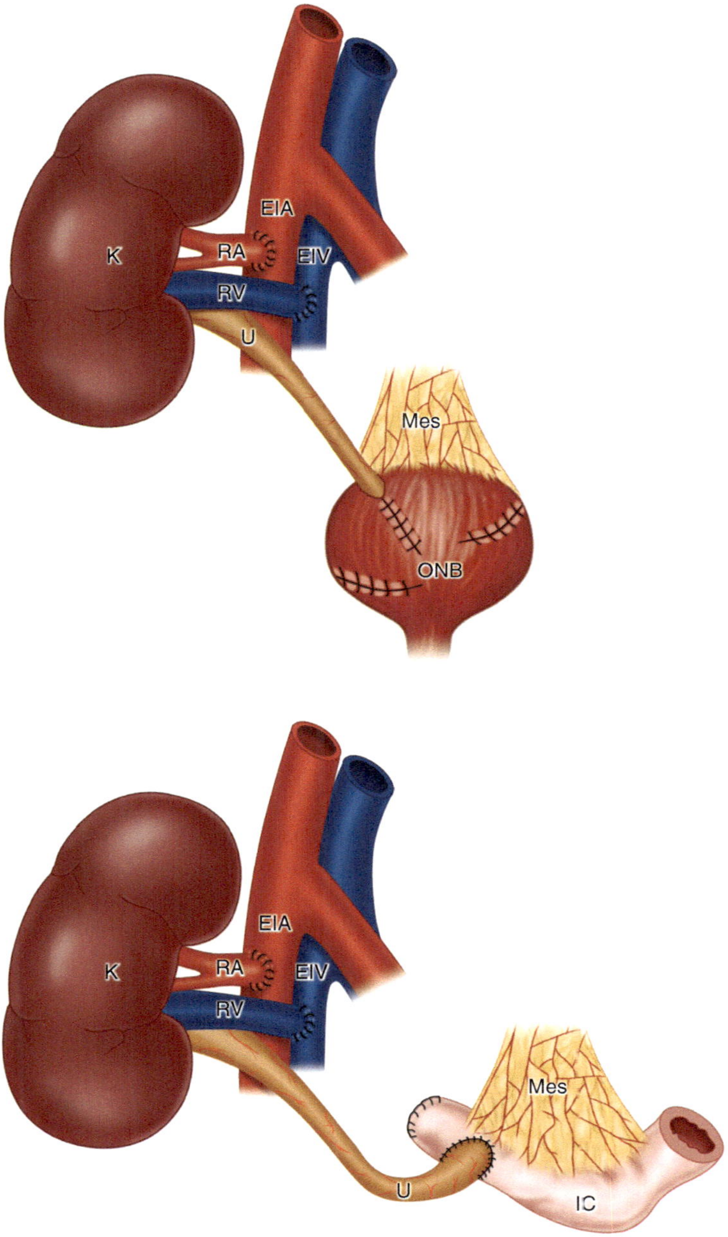

Fig. 23.5 (**a**) Ureteroenterostomy where the ureter (U) is anastomosed end-to-side to the ileal conduit (IC). (**b**) Renal transplantation with ureteroenterostomy (U) to orthotopic neobladder (ONB) by antireflux technique. K, kidney; RA, renal artery; RV, renal vein; EIA, external iliac artery; EIV, external iliac vein; Mes, mesentery

namely ureteral obstruction and urinary leakage [13, 22, 25]. However, the routine use of stents is criticized by some because of the higher incidence of some complications, such as urinary tract infection, stent migration, stent fragmentation, stones on forgotten stents, hematuria, bladder discomfort, and pain [21, 22, 26], and some transplant centers use ureteral stents selectively when the risk for development of ureteral complications is judged to be high [21, 27, 28]. Ureteral stenting in renal transplantation is recommended by the European Association of Urology Guidelines in order to prevent postoperative ureter-related complications [29].

23.2.8 Management of Catheter and Stent

The urinary bladder or bladder substitute's catheter usually is removed on the third to the seventh postoperative day after a urine specimen is tested at the bedside for nitrites and sent for bacterial culture. If the urine is shown to be infected, an antibiotic based on sensitivity results is prescribed for 10–14 days.

Stents are usually removed two to 6 weeks after transplantation, however, some authors recommend earlier stent removal to reduce the risk of stent-associated complications, especially urinary tract infections [26]. Some surgeons tie the stent to the indwelling Foley catheter, and it is removed when the catheter is pulled out.

23.3 Ureter-Related Complications after Renal Transplantation

Urologic complications after kidney transplantation have been well described. In the current era, it is unusual to lose a graft because of urological complications [14].

The commonest urologic complications after renal transplantation are those related to the transplant ureter, namely ureteral obstruction, urinary leakage, and vesicoureteral reflux [13, 14, 30–44]. The reported incidence of these complications ranges from 2.5% to more than 20% (Table 23.1).

23.3.1 Risk Factors ~~of~~ for Ureter-Related Complications

Risk factors associated with urological complications after renal transplantation are recipient age, multiple donor renal arteries, arterial reconstruction, some primary urinary reconstruction techniques such as the Taguchi reimplant or uretero-ureterostomy, delayed graft function, poor quality of the donor ureter, bladder abnormalities, repeat transplantation, recipient obesity, prolonged ischemia time, non-stented ureteral anastomosis, high glucocorticoid dose and recipient diabetes [14, 42–52]. Post-transplant ureteral complications are more common in pediatric

Table 23.1 The incidence and types of ureter-related complications after renal transplantation

Authors	Year	Incidence N0/ total (%)	Reported complications
Rigg et al. [30]	1994	189/1016 (14.1)	Ureteral obstruction, urine leak
Shoskes et al. [31]	1995	71/1000 (7.1)	Ureteral obstruction, urine leake, bladder outflow obstruction, reflux, ureteral stones
Salomon et al. [32]	1999	19/570 deceased donors (3.3)	Ureteral stenosis, urine leak, reflux
El-Mekresh et al. [14]	2001	100/1200 (8.3)	Ureteral obstruction, urine leake, clot anuria, obstructing lymphocele, ureteral stones
van Roijen et al. [33]	2001	42/695 (6.04)	The rate of revision of ureteroneocystostomy fo ureteral obstruction, urinary leak was 6.04%
Streeter et al. [34]	2002	141/1535 (9.2)	Ureteral stenosis, urine leak, stones, bladder outlet obstruction, hematuria causing obstruction
Kaskarelis et al. [35]	2008	21/250 (8.4)	Ureteral obstruction, urinary leaks
Pillot et al. [36]	2012	23/200 (11.5)	Ureteral obstruction, urinary leaks, reflux, stent complications, hematuria
Slagt et al. [37]	2014	118/566 (20.8) deceased donors	Mainly ureteral obstruction and urine leak
Duty and Barry [38]	2015	9% (review)	Ureteral obstruction, urinary leaks, vesicoureteral reflux
Krajewski et al. [39]	2016	58/460 (12.6)	Ureteral stenosis, lymphocele, ureteral stones, urethral stricture
Buggs et al. [40]	2019	36/1308 (2.75)	Report on urine leaks only
Carvalho et al. [41]	2019	184/3102 (5.93)	Ureteral obstruction, urinary fistula, infravesical obstruction, ureteral necrosis, reflux, stent obstruction

kidney transplant recipients than adults because of more frequent neurogenic or posterior urethral valve bladders in children [53]. If the kidney is transplanted in the lumbar region, a ureteroureterostomy or pyeloureterostomy may be necessary, and these techniques are associated with a higher incidence of urinary leakage [14]. A list of these risk factors is shown in Table 23.2.

23.3.2 Urinary Leakage

This is usually apparent within a month after transplantation and due to technical issues during donor nephrectomy, kidney graft preparation at the bench, or uretero-neocystostomy. [14, 39].

Table 23.2 Risk factors of ureter-related complications after renal transplantation

Risk factors	• old age • multiple arteries in the donor • arterial reconstruction • Taguchi or ureteroureteral anastomosis • early urinary tract infection • delayed graft function • poor quality of the harvested donor ureter • bladder abnormalities • repeat transplantations • obese recipients • prolonged ischemia time • non-stented anastomosis • high dose of steroids • diabetic recipients • Pediatric kidney transplantation

23.3.2.1 Presentation

In the early post-transplant period, urine leakage usually presents with as an excessive amount of fluid in the drain or as a wet wound dressing. After drain removal, it may present with pain or swelling in the transplant wound, oliguria, increasing serum creatinine, and/or fever. Leaking urine associated with urinary tract infection may result in a peri-graft abscess.

23.3.2.2 Management

Treatment will depend on the site, cause, amount, and the presence or absence of infection. Collections are initially diagnosed by ultrasound, and often further investigated with non-contrast computerized tomography (CT), magnetic resonance imaging (MRI) and/or radioisotope imaging.

Confirmation that the leaking fluid is urine is by detection of a high creatinine level on an aspirate or wet dressing. Additional diagnostic tests include culture of the fluid to select antibiotic treatment, a cystogram to detect a bladder or ureteroneocystostomy leak, and an antegrade nephro-ureterogram to detect a ureteral leak.

A retention catheter will decompress the bladder, and a percutaneous nephrostomy tube will decompress the kidney transplant (Fig. 23.6). If the urine leak doesn't significantly decrease within a week or two after decompression of the urinary tract, open repair is necessary.

If a transvesical ureteroneocystostomy had been done, and the leak is in the bladder incision, distension of the bladder via the 3-way system will identify the leak and confirm its repair after a stitch or two. If the leak is at the ureteroneocystostomy site and the ureter is viable, this can be repaired over a double-pigtail ureteral stent. If the primary ureteroneocystostomy is compromised, a new ureteroneocystostomy is performed.

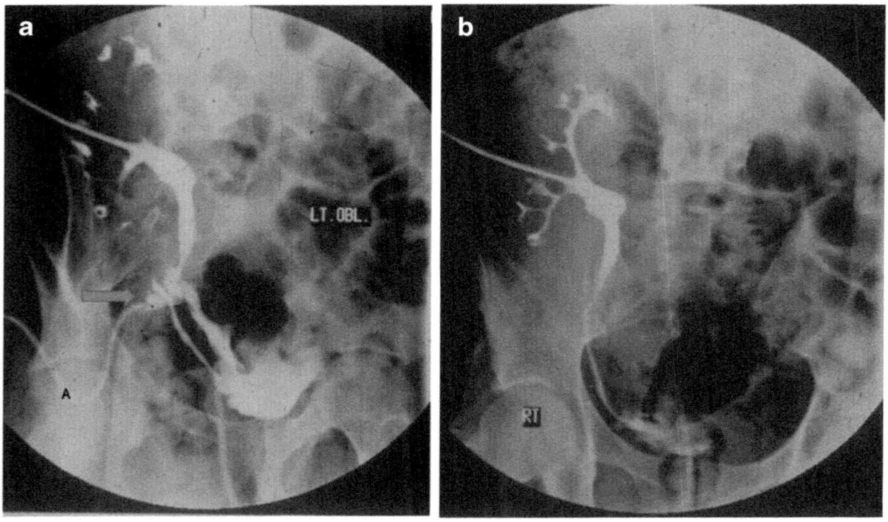

Fig. 23.6 (**a**) Urinary leakage of ureteral origin after renal transplantation, where PCN was placed and antegrade study showed leak. (**b**) Complete healing of the leakage after 10 days. Reproduced with permission from El-Mekresh et al. [14]

Ureteral necrosis is treated with fluid drainage, antibiotics, resection of the diseased ureter until a well-vascularized segment is reached, and surgical reconstruction. This is carried out by anastomosis of the debrided distal ureter or renal pelvis to the native ureter (ureteroureterostomy or pyelo-urerostomy) or to the bladder after creation of a bladder flap. A bladder flap can be created by transverse incision of the bladder, putting one's index finger in the dome to push a tongue of bladder up to the transplant's renal pelvis or proximal ureter and cutting down over the index finger. The transverse bladder incision is closed vertically after placement of a ureteral stent. An ileal ureter is a last resort in cases of total necrosis of the ureter when there is a large gap between the renal pelvis and the bladder and no suitable recipient ureter [14] (Fig. 23.7).

Figure 23.8 shows a management algorithm for urinary leakage after renal transplantation.

23.3.3 Ureteral Obstruction

23.3.3.1 Early Ureteral Obstruction

Transplant ureteral obstruction soon after the transplant procedure can be due to a technical issue, like a misplaced stitch during unstented ureteroneocystostomy, a perinephric hematoma or abscess, edema at the site of ureteroneocystostomy or ureteral torsion [54, 55]. The last usually becomes apparent right after ureteral stent removal.

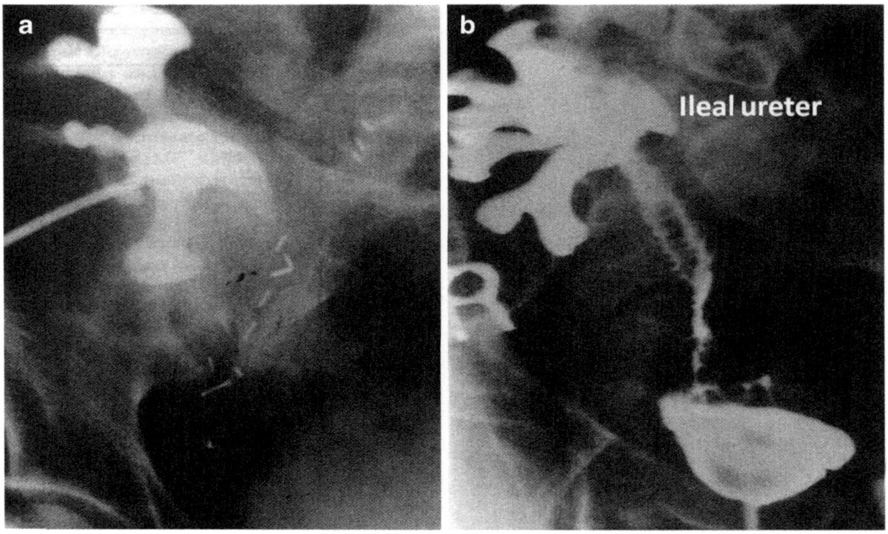

Fig. 23.7 (**a**) Percutaneous antegrade nephrostogram showing total necrosis of transplant ureter. (**b**) Antegrade nephrostogram demonstrates successful ileal ureter replacement of transplant ureter. Reproduced with permission from El-Mekresh et al. [14]

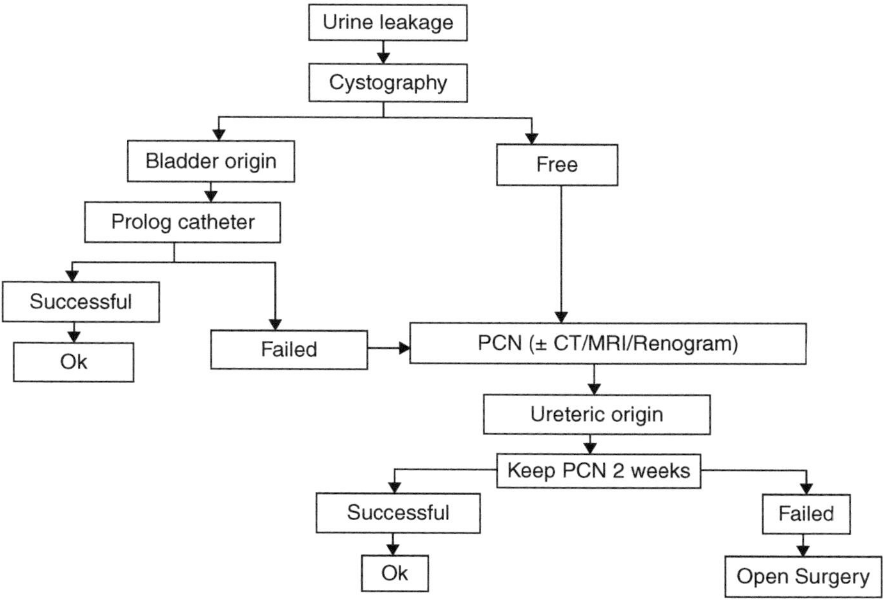

Fig. 23.8 Management algorithm for urinary leakage after renal transplantation

23.3.3.2 Late Ureteral Obstruction

Late ureteral obstruction may be due to a lymphocele, ureteral stone, sloughed papilla, ureteral ischemia or BK viral infection.

Infection with polyomavirus (BK) virus is important, but it rarely affects the ureter after renal transplantation [56–60]. BK virus can cause ureteral obstruction, fibrosis, or ulceration. It is usually asymptomatic and presents with progressive decline in urine output and deterioration of kidney graft function [59]. BK virus infection can be managed by reduction in maintenance immunosuppression and percutaneous nephrostomy or ureteral stent exchanges until the infection has resolved. Surgical treatment of subsequent stricture may be necessary.

23.3.3.3 Treatment of Ureteral Obstruction and Stricture

Treatment of ureteric obstruction/stricture should be started as soon as possible to avoid loss of graft function (Figs. 23.9 and 23.10). Although a transplant ureteral stricture due to chronic ischemia may respond to ureteral dilation and temporary stent placement with scheduled stent exchanges, open repair with anastomosis of the transplant ureter or renal pelvis to the native ureter or to a bladder flap is usually necessary.

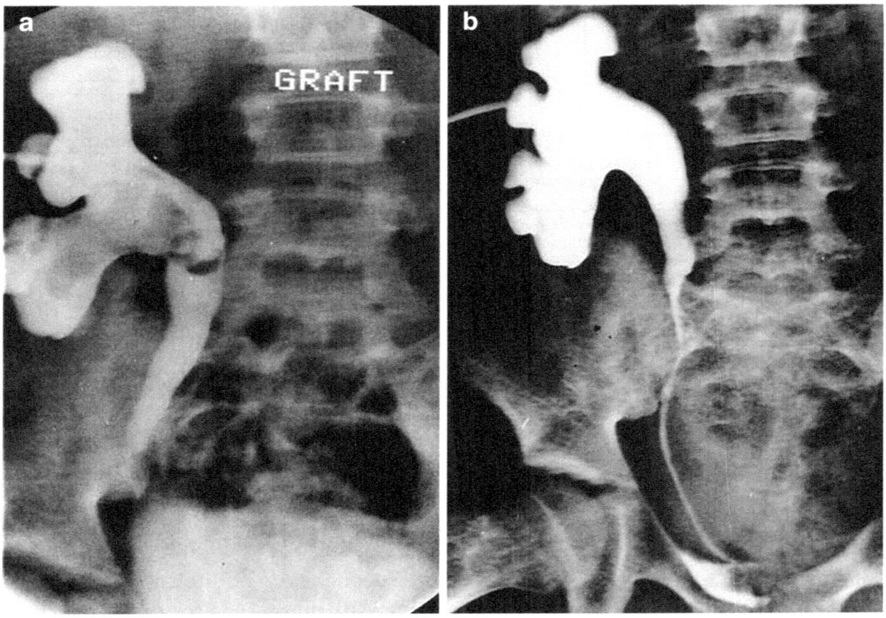

Fig. 23.9 (**a**) Antegrade nephrostogram demonstrates distal ureteral stricture after renal transplantation. (**b**) Antegrade nephrostogram after successful redo ureteroneocystostomy. Reproduced with permission from El-Mekresh et al. [14]

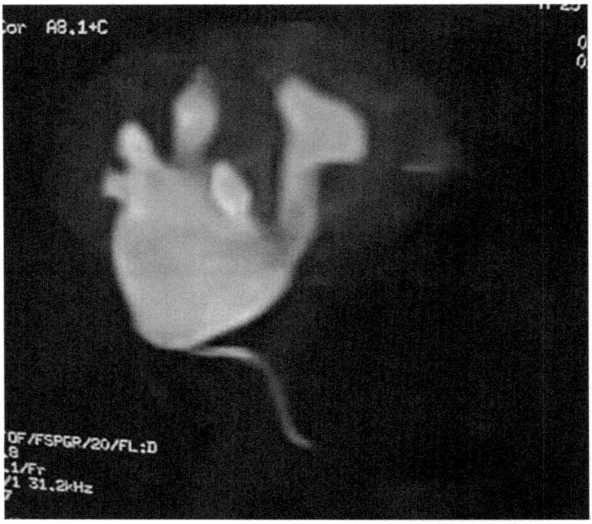

Fig. 23.10 Magnetic resonance urography (MRU) showing ureteropelvic junction obstruction (UPJO) after renal transplantation. Treatment was by pyeloureterostomy to the ipsilateral native ureter

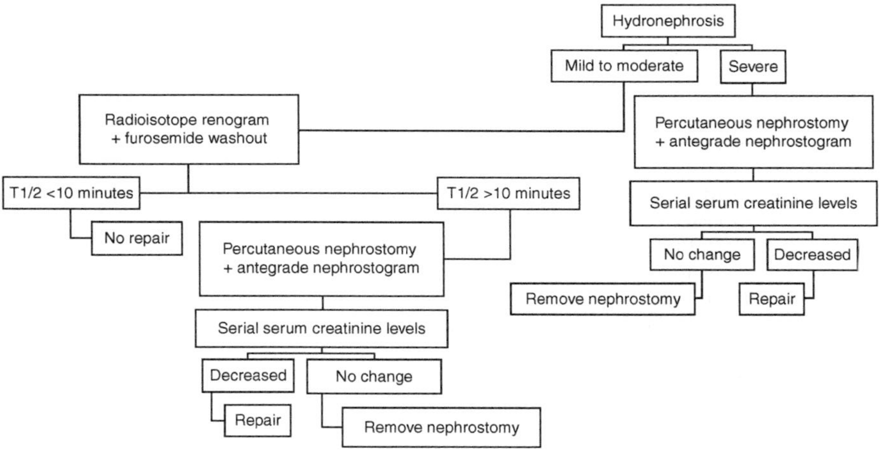

Fig. 23.11 Management algorithm for ureteral obstruction after renal transplantation. Pyelovesicostomy and ileal ureter are options for ureteropelvic junction (UPJ) obstruction when the native ureter is unavailable or unsatisfactory for UPJ repair

An algorithm for the management of ureteral obstruction is provided in Fig. 23.11. The treatment of ureteral strictures depends on the site and extent of the stricture. Figure 23.12 demonstrates different treatment options for renal transplant ureteral stricture.

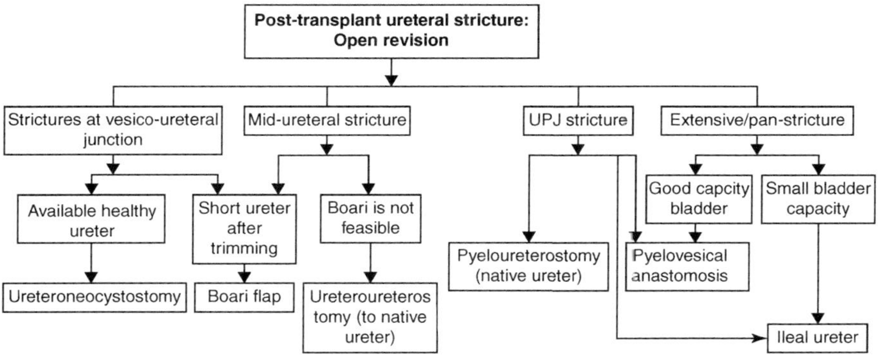

Fig. 23.12 Algorithm for surgical treatment of post-renal transplant ureteral strictures

23.3.4 Vesicoureteral Reflux

23.3.4.1 Incidence

The incidence of vesicoureteral reflux (VUR) after renal transplantation varies among transplant centers because most centers do not routinely do postoperative contrast cystography or voiding cystourethrography (VCUG). The prevalence of VUR has been reported to vary from 2% to more than 80% [39, 61–64].

23.3.4.2 Diagnosis

The clinical presentation of significant VUR is recurrent transplant pyelonephritis. Diagnosis is by VCUG, however, grade 4 or 5 reflux is usually present on a static cystogram. Voiding efficiency can be documented on a post-void film (Fig. 23.13). VUR as a risk factor for acute transplant pyelonephritis is controversial even though it is accepted as a risk factor for acute pyelonephritis in the general population, especially children [61]. There is no definite correlation between VUR and worsening of graft function or graft survival in most studies [61–65].

23.3.4.3 Treatment

Conservative therapy is with perineal hygiene in women or men with a perineal urethrostomy, single-dose daily or post-coital antibiotics, topical estrogen for post-menopausal women, reduction of voiding pressure with an oral alpha blocking agent in men or women, or 5-alpha reductase inhibitors to shrink the prostate. If present, urethral strictures and prostatic obstruction unresponsive to medical treatment can be managed with invasive procedures.

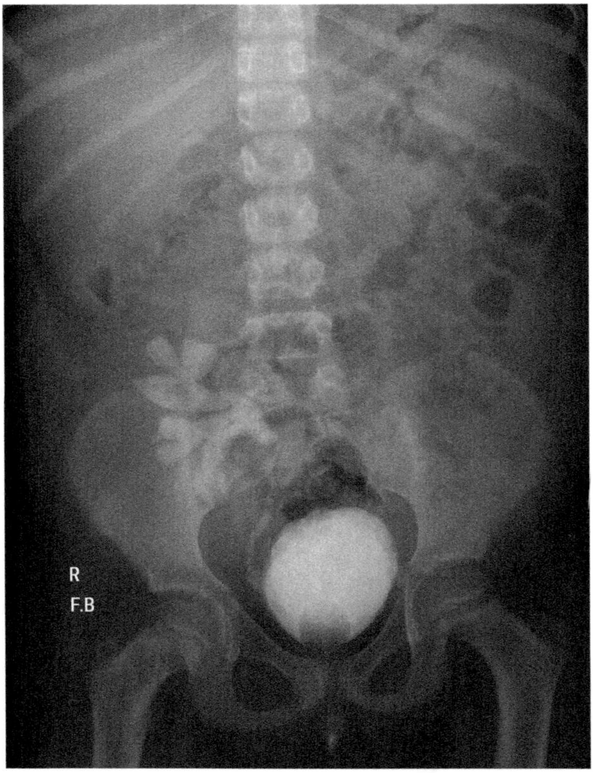

Fig. 23.13 Voiding cystourethrography (VCUG) showing vesicoureteral reflux to the graft

Endoscopic injection of a bulking material may be tried, however, it has limited success rates and may be followed by transient obstruction [62]. When more conservative measures fail or become unacceptable, especially with high grade reflux, the refluxing transplant ureteroneocystostomy can be repaired with an extravesical modification of the reimplant or anastomosis of the renal pelvis or proximal ureter of the kidney transplant to a non-refluxing native ureter.

23.3.5 *Obstructing Lymphocele*

23.3.5.1 Incidence and Causes

Post-transplantation fluid collections, including lymphoceles, around the kidney graft, have been reported to occur in more than 25% of renal transplant recipients [14, 66]. The majority of these collections are small and do not require treatment. The indications for treatment include symptomatic or obstructing lymphoceles and the incidence of these is less than 5% [14, 67–70].

The main cause of lymphoceles is considered to be due to incomplete ligation or fulguration of the lymphatics around the iliac arteries and veins or, in small children, the aorta and inferior vena cava. However, incomplete control of the lymphatic vessels of the donor kidney may also result in a recipient lymphocele. Meticulous dissection and ligation of lymphatics in both the recipient and donor is recommended to minimize the occurrence of lymphoceles.

Symptomatic lymphoceles have been associated with older recipient age, polycystic kidney disease, and the use of a drain [67, 69].

23.3.5.2 Diagnosis

Diagnosis is initially made by ultrasonography, with or without a non-contrast CT or MRI. Needle drainage of a lymphocele will result in confirmation of the diagnosis by the low concentration of creatinine in the fluid.

23.3.5.3 Treatment

Percutaneous aspiration a time or two may be all that is needed for treatment. If simple aspiration fails, the lymphocele can be treated with a sclerosing agent, such as povidone iodine or a tetracycline derivative [14, 67]. If the latter fails, the lymphocele can be unroofed into the peritoneal cavity by open or laparoscopic technique (Fig. 23.14).

23.3.6 Ureteral Stones

23.3.6.1 Incidence and Risk Factors

Stones after renal transplantation may be of donor or recipient origin. The de novo stones are rare and their incidence has been reported to be decreasing over the last decades [71, 72]. The causes include recurrent UTIs, persistent hyperparathyroidism, hypercalciuria, hyperuricemia, hypocitraturia, stagnant urine from obstructive uropathy, and uretero-enteric urinary tract reconstruction [71, 73].

23.3.6.2 Presentation and Diagnosis

Urolithiasis after renal transplantation, especially ureteral stones, constitute a serious problem because of the possibilities of obstruction, severe infection and deterioration of graft function. The presentation may be anuria, urinary tract infection, acute graft dysfunction and/or hematuria [14, 39, 70]. The typical colicky pain of ureteral stone is absent due to denervation of the graft and the ureter.

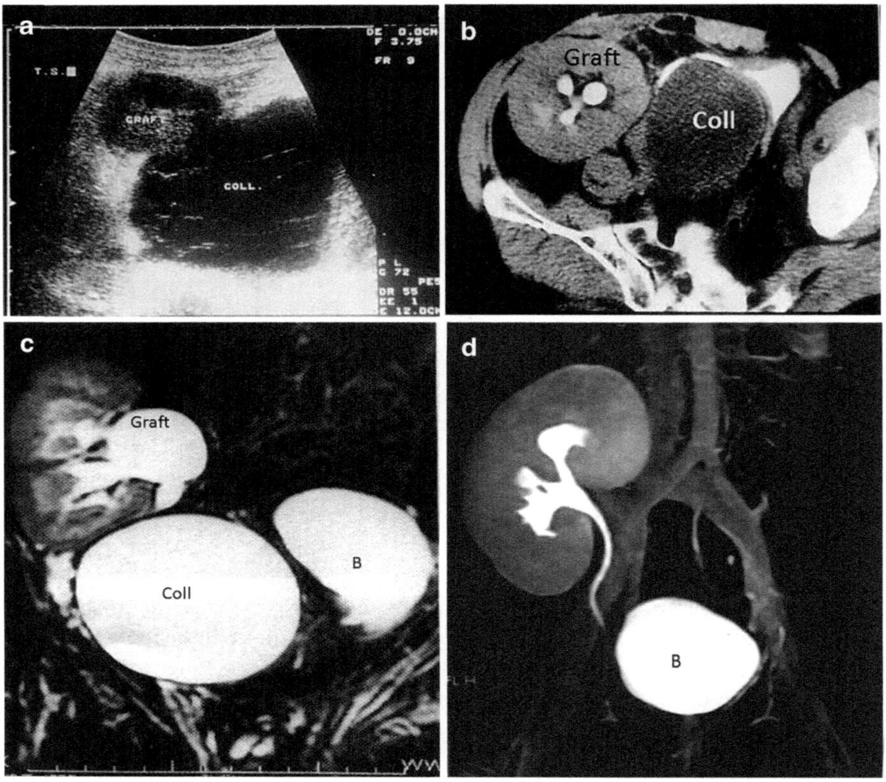

Fig. 23.14 (**a**) Ultrasound demonstration of an obstructing lymphocele (coll). (**b**) Nnoncontrast CT showing the same findings. (**c**) Noncontrast MRI showing the same findings with the bladder (B) displaced to the left. (**d**) MRU after lymphocele unroofed into peritoneal cavity; note decompressed kidney graft with no hydronephrosis. Reproduced with permission from El-Mekresh et al. [14]

23.3.6.3 Management

Ureteral stones can be managed by ureteroscopic extraction or lithotripsy; however, negotiating an intramural, redundant transplant ureter may be impossible, and a percutaneous nephroscopic approach with antegrade ureteroscopy is often necessary [14, 39] (Fig. 23.15).

23.3.6.4 Effect of Ureter-Related Complications on Graft and Patient Survival

When ureteral complications are diagnosed and managed in a timely manner, graft function and patient survival are reported to be preserved in most published series (Fig. 23.16).

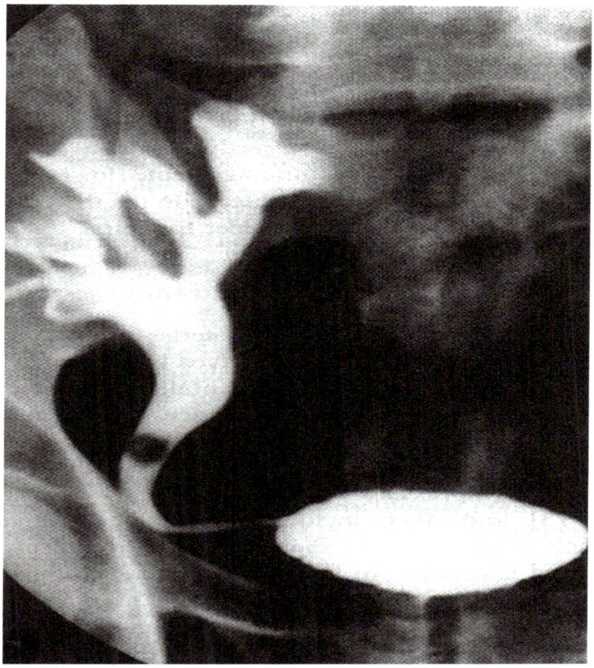

Fig. 23.15 Antegrade nephrostogram shows filling defect caused by ureteral stone Successful treatment was by antegrade ureteroscopy. Reproduced with permission from El-Mekresh et al. [14]

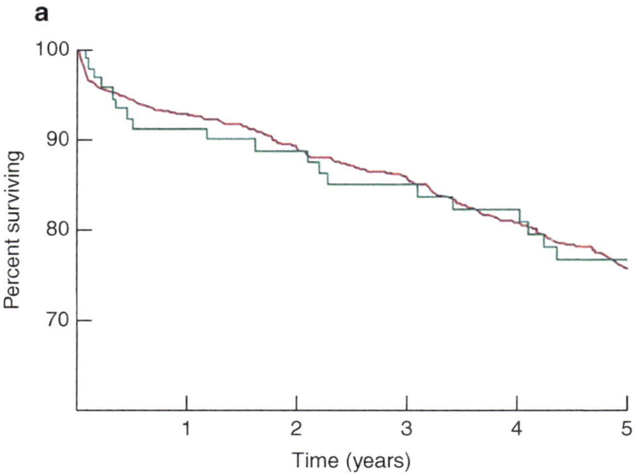

Fig. 23.16 (**a**) Patient survival and (**b**) Graft survival with (green) and without (red) urological complications; no significant difference was noted between the groups. Reproduced with permission from El-Mekresh et al. [14]

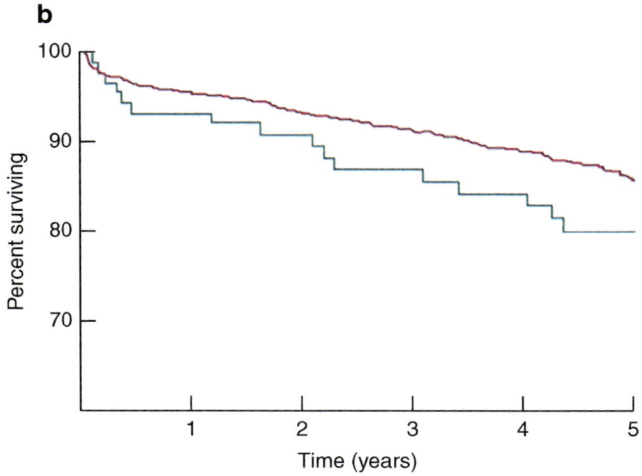

Fig. 23.16 (continued)

23.4 Summary

Kidney transplant urinary tract reconstruction is usually by stented extravesical ureteroneocystostomy, preferably with an antireflux procedure. When possible, the kidney transplant should be placed in the contralateral iliac fossa so the transplant's ureter and renal pelvis are easily available for secondary urinary tract reconstruction. Anastomosis of the renal transplant's pelvis or ureter to the native ureter is done when transplant ureteral blood supply is poor or when the bladder is unsuitable for ureteroneocystostomy. Double ureters can be joined together side-by-side or on top of one another and anastomosed to the bladder in the same submucosal tunnel or in separate submucosal tunnels. The current advances in renal transplant surgical techniques and immunosuppressive regimens together with strict surveillance have minimized the incidence of severe ureteral-related complications. Post-transplant ureteral complications present as ureteral obstruction, either intrinsic or extrinsic, and urinary leakage, most commonly from the distal ureter and the ureteroneocystostomy. Urinary tract obstruction and extravasation are diagnosed and initially treated with decompression of the urinary tract, drainage, laboratory examination of fluid collections, antegrade and retrograde imaging, selective antibiotic therapy, and subsequent definitive management. Endourological treatment has been successful in most cases of urinary leakage, but most of transplant ureteral strictures require open surgical repair. Kidney transplant function, graft and patient survival are usually maintained when ureteral complications are diagnosed and treated in a timely fashion.

Questions

Choose the best answer

1. Which of the following determines the type of urinary tract reconstruction during a kidney transplant?

   (a) Condition of the donor ureter
   (b) Condition of the recipient's bladder
   (c) Condition of the recipient's ureter
   (d) Surgeon's preference
   (e) All of the above

Answer: (e)

2. A left kidney transplant is preferentially placed in the right iliac fossa because

   (a) The skin to iliac vessel distance is less on the left
   (b) The skin to iliac vessel distance is less on the right
   (c) The ureter and renal pelvis of the kidney transplant are the most medial and superficial structures
   (d) A and C
   (e) B and C

Answer: (e)

The skin to iliac vessel distance is less on the right than on the left, and the kidney transplant's urinary tract is the most superficial and medial of the hilar structures.

3. Which of the following suture material is commonly used by surgeons for urinary tract reconstruction?

   (a) Polydioxanone
   (b) Polyglyconate
   (c) Polygalactine
   (d) Polyglycolic acid
   (e) Chromic catgut

Answer: (a)

Polydioxanone (PDS) is absorbable (removes the risk of stone formation when chronically exposed to urine), monofilament (less tissue drag than braided suture), synthetic (lasts longer than catgut), and is less stiff than other monofilament absorbable sutures (easier to tie).

4. Which one of the following statements about kidney transplantation is true?

   (a) Ureteral stents are rarely used
   (b) The commonest form of urinary tract reconstruction is ureteroneocystostomy
   (c) Transvesical ureteroneocystostomy is more common than extravesical ureteroneocystostomy
   (d) Thomas Starzl did first extravesical ureteroneocystostomy
   (e) Hematuria is not a problem with the one-stich ureteroneocystostomy

Answer: (b)

The commonest form of urinary tract reconstruction in kidney transplantation is ureteroneocystostomy, usually by a stented, extravesical procedure.

5. Urinary tract reconstruction for the first successful human-to-human kidney transplant was by

   (a) Ureteroureterostomy
   (b) Ureteropyelostomy
   (c) Transvesical ureteroneocystostomy
   (d) Extravesical ureteroneocystostomy
   (e) Ureterovesicostomy

Answer: (c)

Transvesical ureteroneocystostomy, commonly called a Politano- Leadbetter procedure.

6. Which of the following are done for ureteral necrosis?

   (a) Percutaneous nephrostomy
   (b) Operative site drainage
   (c) Antibiotics on the basis of culture and sensitivity
   (d) Surgical reconstruction
   (e) All of the above

Answer: (e)

7. A 10 cm diameter fluid collection between the bladder and a kidney transplant is aspirated. The creatinine level is 7 mmol/L. What is the most likely diagnosis?

   (a) Abscess
   (b) Urinoma
   (c) Lymphocele
   (d) Peritoneal cyst
   (e) Bladder diverticulum

Answer: (c)

Lymphocele. The creatinine level for a lymphocele is the same as that for serum. Normal serum creatinine values are between 2.5 mmol/L and 8.2 mmol/L.

8. Which of the following *is not* a treatment for a post-transplant lymphocele?

   (a) Ureteroureterostomy
   (b) Doxycycline sclerosis
   (c) Laparoscopic unroofing into the peritoneal cavity
   (d) Open surgical unroofing into the peritoneal cavity
   (e) A and B.

Answer: (a)

Ureteroureterostomy. This is only necessary if ureteral obstruction persists after lymphocele drainage.

9. Which of the following are possible treatment options for recurrent transplant pyelonephritis associated with vesicoureteral reflux?
   (a) Reduce bladder voiding pressure
   (b) Daily prophylactic low-dose antibiotic suppression
   (c) Repeat ureteroneocystostomy
   (d) Anastomosis of transplant ureter to non-refluxing native ureter
   (e) All of the above

Answer: (e)

10. Which of the following infections has been identified as a cause of ureteral obstruction in kidney transplant recipients?
    (a) BK virus
    (b) Cytomegalovirus
    (c) E. coli
    (d) Epstein-Barr virus
    (e) HPV

Answer: (a)

BK virus. It often responds to a reduction in immunosuppression and temporary decompression of the renal pelvis with percutaneous nephrostomy or an indwelling ureteral stent.

References

1. Watson CJE, Friend PJ, Marson LP. Surgical techniques of kidney transplantation. In: Knechtle SJ, Marson LP, Morris PJ, editors. Kidney transplantation - principles and practice. 8th ed. Elsevier; 2019. p. 157–72. ISBN 9780323531863,. https://doi.org/10.1016/B978-0-323-53186-3.00011-5.
2. Lich R Jr, Howerton LW, Davis LA. Childhood urosepsis. J Ky Med Assoc. 1961;59:1177–9.
3. Woodruff MFA, Robson JS, Nolan B, MacDonald MK. Renal transplantation in man: experience in 35 cases. Lancet. 1969;1:6.
4. Konnak JW, Herwig KR, Turcotte JG. External ureteroneocystostomy in renal transplantation. J Urol. 1972;108(3):380–1. https://doi.org/10.1016/s0022-5347(17)60747-x.
5. Shanfield I. New experimental methods for implantation of the ureter in bladder and conduit. Transplant Proc. 1972;4(4):637–8.
6. MacKinnon KJ, Oliver JA, Morehouse DD, Taguchi Y. Cadaver renal transplantation: emphasis on urological aspects. J Urol. 1968;99(5):486–90. https://doi.org/10.1016/s0022-5347(17)62737-x.
7. Veale JL, Yew J, Gjertson DW, Smith CV, Singer JS, Rosenthal JT, Gritsch HA. Long-term comparative outcomes between 2 common ureteroneocystostomy techniques for renal transplantation. J Urol. 2007;177(2):632–6. https://doi.org/10.1016/j.juro.2006.09.042.
8. Barry JM. Renal transplant-recipient surgery. BJU Int. 2007;99:701–17. https://doi.org/10.1111/j.1464-410X.2007.06785.x.
9. Caparrós J, Regalado RI, Sánchez-Martín F, Villavicencio H. A simplified technique for ureteroneocystostomy in renal transplantation. World J Urol. 1996;14(4):236–8. https://doi.org/10.1007/BF00182073.

10. Merrill JP, Murray JE, Harrison JH, Guild WR. Successful homotransplantation of the human kidney between identical twins. J Am Med Assoc. 1956;160(4):277–82. https://doi.org/10.1001/jama.1956.02960390027008.
11. Politano VA, Leadbetter WF. An operative technique for the correction of vesicoureteral reflux. J Urol. 1958;79(6):932–41. https://doi.org/10.1016/s0022-5347(17)66369-9.
12. Starzl TE, Marchioro TL, Brittain RS, et al. Problems in renal homotransplantations. JAMA. 1964;187:734–40. https://doi.org/10.1001/jama.1964.03060230062016.
13. Pleass HC, Clark KR, Rigg KM, Reddy KS, Forsythe JL, Proud G, Taylor RM. Urologic complications after renal transplantation: a prospective randomized trial comparing different techniques of ureteric anastomosis and the use of prophylactic ureteric stents. Transplant Proc. 1995;27(1):1091–2.
14. El-Mekresh M, Osman Y, Ali-El-Dein B, El-Diasty T, Ghoneim MA. Urological complications after living-donor renal transplantation. BJU Int. 2001;87:295–306.
15. Chaykovska L, Deger S, Wille A, Friedersdorff F, Kasper A, Dragun D, Liefeldt L, Miller K, Giessing M, Fuller TF. Kidney transplantation into urinary conduits with ureteroureterostomy between transplant and native ureter: single-center experience. Urology. 2009;73(2):380–5. https://doi.org/10.1016/j.urology.2008.07.069. Epub 2008 Nov 20.
16. Barry JM, Pearse HD, Lawson RK, Hodges CV. Ureteroneocystostomy in kidney transplants with ureteral duplication. Arch Surg. 1973;106:345–6.
17. Masson D, Hefty T. A technique for the transplantation of 2 adult cadaver kidney grafts into 1 recipient. J Urol. 1998;160(5):1779–80.
18. Gil-Vernet JM, Gil-Vernet A, Caralps A, Carretero P, Talbot-Wright R, Andreu J, Campos JA. Orthotopic renal transplant and results in 139 consecutive cases. J Urol. 1989;142(2):248–52. https://doi.org/10.1016/s0022-5347(17)38721-9.
19. Schiff M, Lytton B. Secondary ureteropyelostomy in renal transplant recipients. J Urol. 1981;126:723–6.
20. Lord RH, Pepera T, Williams G. Ureteroureterostomy and pyeloureterostomy without native nephrectomy in renal transplantation. Br J Urol. 1991;67(4):349–51. https://doi.org/10.1111/j.1464-410x.1991.tb15159.x.
21. Osman Y, Ali-El-Dein B, Shokeir A, Kamal M, El Din S. A.B.: routine insertion of ureteral stent in live-donor renal transplantation; is it worthwhile? Urology. 2005;65:867–71.
22. Harza M, Baston C, Preda A, et al. Impact of ureteral stenting on urological complications after kidney transplantation surgery: a single-Center experience. Transplant Proc. 2014;46:3459–62.
23. Liu S, Luo G, Sun B, et al. Early removal of double-J stents decreases urinary tract infections in living donor renal transplantation: a prospective, Randomized Clinical Trial. Transplant Proc. 2017;49:297–302.
24. Patel P, Rebollo-Mesa I, Ryan E, et al. Prophylactic ureteric stents in renal transplant recipients: a Multicenter randomized controlled trial of early versus late removal. Am J Transplant. 2017;17:2129–38.
25. Mangus RS, Haag BW. Stented versus nonstented extravesical ureteroneocystostomy in renal transplantation: a metaanalysis. Am J Transplant. 2004;4(11):1889–96.
26. Visser IJ, van der Staaij JPT, Muthusamy A, Willicombe M, Lafranca JA, Dor F. Timing of ureteric stent removal and occurrence of urological complications after kidney transplantation: a systematic review and meta-analysis. J Clin Med. 2019;8(5):689. https://doi.org/10.3390/jcm8050689.
27. Thompson ER, Hosgood SA, Nicholson ML, Wilson CH. Early versus late ureteric stent removal after kidney transplantation. Cochrane Database Syst Rev. 2018;1:Cd011455.
28. Sinangil A, Celik V, Barlas S, Akin EB, Ecder T. Should transplant ureter be stented routinely or not? Eur Rev Med Pharmacol Sci. 2014;18(23):3551–6.
29. Breda A, Olsburgh J, Budde K, Figueiredo A, LledóGarcía E, Regele H. EAU guidelines on renal transplantation. Edn. presented at the EAU Annual Congress Barcelona; 2019. https://uroweb.org/guideline/renal-transplantation/. Access June 2019.
30. Rigg KM, Proud G, Taylor RM. Urological complications following renal transplantation. A study of 1016 consecutive transplants from a single centre. Transpl Int. 1994;7(2):120–6.

31. Shoskes DA, Hanbury D, Cranston D, Morris PJ. Urological complications in 1,000 consecutive renal transplant recipients. J Urol. 1995;153(1):18–21. https://doi.org/10.1097/00005392-199501000-00008.
32. Salomon L, Saporta F, Amsellem D, Hozneck A, Colombel M, Patard JJ, Chopin D, Abbou CC. Results of pyeloureterostomy after ureterovesical anastomosis complications in renal transplantation. Urology. 1999;53(5):908–12. https://doi.org/10.1016/s0090-4295(98)00624-4.
33. van Roijen JH, Kirkels WJ, Zietse R, Roodnat JI, Weimar W, Ijzermans JN. Long-term graft survival after urological complications of 695 kidney transplantations. J Urol. 2001;165(6):1884–7. https://doi.org/10.1097/00005392-200106000-00010.
34. Streeter EH, Little DM, Cranston DW, Morris PJ. The urological complications of renal transplantation: a series of 1535 patients. BJU Int. 2002;90(7):627–34. https://doi.org/10.1046/j.1464-410x.2002.03004.x.
35. Kaskarelis I, Koukoulaki M, Georgantas T, Bairamidis E, Kokkinos C, Ieronymou M, Vougas V, Drakopoulos S. Ureteral complications in renal transplant recipients successfully treated with interventional radiology. Transplant Proc. 2008;40(9):3170–2. https://doi.org/10.1016/j.transproceed.2008.08.040.
36. Pillot P, Bardonnaud N, Lillaz J, Delorme G, Chabannes E, Bernardini S, Guichard G, Bittard H, Kleinclauss F. Risk factors for surgical complications after renal transplantation and impact on patient and graft survival. Transplant Proc. 2012;44(9):2803–8. https://doi.org/10.1016/j.transproceed.2012.09.030.
37. Slagt IK, Ijzermans JN, Visser LJ, Weimar W, Roodnat JI, Terkivatan T. Independent risk factors for urological complications after deceased donor kidney transplantation. PLoS One. 2014;9(3):e91211. Published 2014 Mar 7. https://doi.org/10.1371/journal.pone.0091211.
38. Duty BD, Barry JM. Diagnosis and management of ureteral complications following renal transplantation. Asian J Urol. 2015;2(4):202–7. https://doi.org/10.1016/j.ajur.2015.08.002.
39. Krajewski W, Dembowski J, Kołodziej A, Małkiewicz B, Tupikowski K, Matuszewski M, Chudoba P, Boratyńska M, Klinger M, Zdrojowy R. Urological complications after renal transplantation - a single centre experience. Cent European J Urol. 2016;69(3):306–11. https://doi.org/10.5173/ceju.2016.833. Epub 2016 Jul 11.
40. Buggs J, Gamarra V, Watson R, Sokolich J, Pearson H, Huang J, Rogers E, Kumar A, Bowers V. Repair of ureteral leaks post-kidney transplantation. Am Surg. 2019;85(8):e380–2.
41. Carvalho JA, Nunes P, Antunes H, Parada B, Tavares da Silva E, Rodrigues L, Roseiro A, Bastos C, Macário F, Figueiredo A. Surgical complications in kidney transplantation: an overview of a Portuguese reference Center. Transplant Proc. 2019;51(5):1590–6. https://doi.org/10.1016/j.transproceed.2019.05.001.
42. Alberts VP, Minnee RC, Bemelman FJ, van Donselaar-van der Pant KA, Laguna Pes P, Idu MM. Ureteral reconstruction after renal transplantation: clinical outcome and risk factors. Urol Int. 2012;88(3):333–7. https://doi.org/10.1159/000335329. Epub 2012 Jan 24.
43. Buttigieg J, Agius-Anastasi A, Sharma A, Halawa A. Early urological complications after kidney transplantation: an overview. World J Transplant. 2018;8(5):142–9. https://doi.org/10.5500/wjt.v8.i5.142.
44. Kumar A, Verma BS, Srivastava A, Bhandari M, Gupta A, Sharma R. Evaluation of the urological complications of living related renal transplantation at a single center during the last 10 years: impact of the double-J* stent. J Urol. 2000;164(3):657–60. https://doi.org/10.1097/00005392-200009010-00010.
45. Englesbe MJ, Dubay DA, Gillespie BW, Moyer AS, Pelletier SJ, Sung RS, Magee JC, Punch JD, Campbell DA Jr, Merion RM. Risk factors for urinary complications after renal transplantation. Am J Transplant. 2007;7(6):1536–41. https://doi.org/10.1111/j.1600-6143.2007.01790.x. Epub 2007 Apr 8.
46. Rahnemai-Azar AA, Gilchrist BF, Kayler LK. Independent risk factors for early urologic complications after kidney transplantation. Clin Transpl. 2015;29(5):403–8. https://doi.org/10.1111/ctr.12530. Epub 2015 Mar 6.
47. Shokeir AA, Osman Y, Ali-El-Dein B, El-Husseini A, El-Mekresh M, Shehab-El-Din AB. Surgical complications in live-donor pediatric and adolescent renal transplantation: study

of risk factors. Pediatr Transplant. 2005;9(1):33–8. https://doi.org/10.1111/j.1399-3046.2005.00244.x.
48. Angelico R, Pellicciaro M, Venza F, et al. Urological complications in kidney transplant recipients: analysis of the risk factors and impact on transplant outcomes in the era of "extended criteria donors". Transplantology. 2021;2:22–36. https://doi.org/10.3390/transplantology2010003.
49. Bessede T, Hammoudi Y, Bedretdinova D, Parier B, Francois H, Durrbach A, Benoit G. Preoperative Risk Factors Associated With Urinary Complications After Kidney Transplantation. Transplant Proc. 2017;49(9):2018–24. https://doi.org/10.1016/j.transproceed.2017.09.036.
50. Apel H, Rother U, Wach S, Schiffer M, Kunath F, Wullich B, Heller K. Transplant ureteral stenosis after renal transplantation: risk factor analysis. Urol Int. 2021;15:1–9. https://doi.org/10.1159/000519787. Epub ahead of print.
51. Ali-El-Dein B, Abol-Enein H, El-Husseini A, Osman Y, Shehab El-Din AB, Ghoneim MA. Renal transplantation in children with abnormal lower urinary tract. Transplant Proc. 2004;36:2968–73.
52. Kumar S, Ameli-Renani S, Hakim A, Jeon JH, Shrivastava S, Patel U. Ureteral obstruction following renal transplantation: causes, diagnosis and management. Br J Radiol. 2014;87(1044):20140169. https://doi.org/10.1259/bjr.20140169.
53. Zaontz MR, Hatch DA, Firlit CF. Urological complications in pediatric renal transplantation: management and prevention. J Urol. 1988;140:1123±8.
54. Krol R, Ziaja J, Chudek J, et al. Surgical treatment of urological complications after kidney transplantation. Transplant Proc. 2006;38:127–30.
55. Asadpour A, Molaei M, Yaghoobi S. Management of ureteral complications in renal transplantation: prevention and treatment. Saudi J Kidney Dis Transpl. 2011;22:72–4.
56. Coleman DV, Mackenzie EF, Gardner SD, et al. Human polyomavirus (BK) infection and ureteric stenosis in renal allograft recipients. J Clin Pathol. 1978;31:338–47.
57. Cavallo R, Costa C, Bergallo M, et al. A case of ureteral lesions in a renal transplant recipient with a co-infection of BK virus and JC virus. Nephrol Dial Transplant. 2007;22:1275.
58. Gaston KE, Gabriel DA, Lavelle JP. Rare cause of ureteral obstruction. Urology. 2005;66:1110.
59. Rajpoot DK, Gomez A, Tsang W, Shanberg A. Ureteric and urethral stenosis: a complication of BK virus infection in a pediatric renal transplant patient. Pediatr Transplant. 2007;11:433–5.
60. Krajewski W, Kamińska D, Poterek A, et al. Pathogenicity of BK virus on the urinary system. Cent European J Urol. 2020;73(1):94–103. https://doi.org/10.5173/ceju.2020.0034.
61. Ranchin B, Chapuis F, Dawhara M, et al. Vesicoureteral reflux after kidney transplantation in children. Nephrol Dial Transplant. 2000;15(11):1852–8. https://doi.org/10.1093/ndt/15.11.1852.
62. Wu HY, Concepcion W, Grimm PC. When does vesicoureteral reflux in pediatric kidney transplant patients need treatment? Pediatr Transplant. 2018;22(8):e13299. https://doi.org/10.1111/petr.13299. Epub 2018 Oct 15.
63. Sheth KR, White JT, Stanasel I, Janzen N, Mittal A, Koh CJ, Austin PF, Roth DR, Tu DD, Gonzales ET, Ryan S, Jorgez C, Seth A. Comparing treatment modalities for transplant kidney vesicoureteral reflux in the pediatric population. J Pediatr Urol. 2018;14(6):554.e1–6. https://doi.org/10.1016/j.jpurol.2018.07.006. Epub 2018 Jul 24.
64. Mastrosimone S, Pignata G, Maresca MC, Calconi G, Rabassini A, Butini R, Fandella A, Di Falco G, Chiara G, Caldato C, et al. Clinical significance of vesicoureteral reflux after kidney transplantation. Clin Nephrol. 1993;40(1):38–45.
65. Fontana I, Ginevri F, Arcuri V, Basile G, Nocera A, Beatini M, Bonato L, Barocci S, Bertocchi M, Manolitsi O, Valente R, Draghi P, Gusmano R, Valente U. Vesico-ureteral reflux in pediatric kidney transplants: clinical relevance to graft and patient outcome. Pediatr Transplant. 1999;3(3):206–9. https://doi.org/10.1034/j.1399-3046.1999.00017.x.
66. Khauli RB, Stoff JS, Lovewell T, Ghavamian R, Baker S. Post-transplant lymphoceles: a critical look into the risk factors, pathophysiology and management. J Urol. 1993;150(1):22–6. https://doi.org/10.1016/s0022-5347(17)35387-9.

67. Sevmis M, Aktas S, Alkara U, Kilercik H, Uyar M, Sevmis S Risk factors, diagnosis, and treatment of Lymphocele after renal transplantation: a retrospective study. Transplant Proc. 2021;53(3):1040–7. https://doi.org/10.1016/j.transproceed.2021.01.028. Epub 2021 Feb 8.
68. Fuller TF, Kang SM, Hirose R, Feng S, Stock PG, Freise CE. Management of lymphoceles after renal transplantation: laparoscopic versus open drainage. J Urol. 2003;169(6):2022–5. https://doi.org/10.1097/01.ju.0000063800.44792.61.
69. Joosten M, d'Ancona FC, van der Meijden WA, et al. Predictors of symptomatic lymphocele after kidney transplantation. Int Urol Nephrol. 2019;51:2161–7. https://doi.org/10.1007/s11255-019-02269-0.
70. Branchereau J, Karam G. Management of Urologic Complications of renal transplantation. Eur Urol Suppl. 2016;15(9):408–14.
71. Verrier C, Bessede T, Hajj P, Aoubid L, Eschwege P, Benoit G. Decrease in and management of urolithiasis after kidney transplantation. J Urol. 2012;187(5):1651–5. https://doi.org/10.1016/j.juro.2011.12.060. Epub 2012 Mar 14.
72. Harraz AM, Zahran MH, Kamal AI, El-Hefnawy AS, Osman Y, Soliman SA, Kamal MM, Ali-El-Dein B, Shokeir AA. Contemporary Management of Renal Transplant Recipients with De Novo Urolithiasis: a single institution experience and review of the literature. Exp Clin Transplant. 2017;15(3):277–81.
73. Lim JH, Cho JH, Lee JH, Park YJ, Jin S, Park GY, Kim JS, Kang YJ, Kwon O, Choi JY, Kim CD, Kim YL, Kim HK, Huh S, Park SH. Risk factors for recurrent urinary tract infection in kidney transplant recipients. Transplant Proc. 2013;45(4):1584–9. https://doi.org/10.1016/j.transproceed.2012.12.011.

Chapter 24
Ureteral Disorders During Pregnancy

Mahmoud Abdel-Gawad

Abstract Symptomatic maternal hydronephrosis is a common obstetric complaint during pregnancy and should be differentiated from non-symptomatic hydronephrosis. Renal colic due to obstructive ureteral stones during pregnancy is another medical problem that could be difficult in diagnosis and treatment. Many advanced diagnostic methods are available for the evaluation of renal colic and urolithiasis accurately and safely during pregnancy. The management of symptomatic hydronephrosis and urolithiasis is a challenge for obstetricians and urologists. A multidisciplinary medical team is often necessary for the evaluation and management of pregnant patients with acute urolithiasis and urinary tract obstruction. Conservative treatment usually is very successful in a higher proportion of cases, however, failed medical management requires an interventional procedure to relieve kidney obstruction, overcome the possibility of urosepsis and reduce obstetric complications. Many clinical algorithms have been proposed for the management of renal colic and urolithiasis during pregnancy. However, the clinician should intervene with minimally invasive surgical procedures at the proper time.

Keywords Ureter · Urolithiasis · Pregnancy · Renal colic · Magnetic resonance imaging

Abbreviations

CT	Computed tomography
DJ	Double J
MET	Medical expulsive therapy
MRI	Magnetic resonance imaging
MRU	Magnetic resonance urography

Test your learning and check your understanding of this book's contents: use the "Springer Nature Flashcards" app to access questions. To use the app, please follow the instructions in Chapter 1.

M. Abdel-Gawad (✉)
Toshka Urology and Endoscopy Center, Mansoura, Egypt

M. Abdel-Gawad et al. (eds.), *The Ureter*,
https://doi.org/10.1007/978-3-031-36212-5_24

PCNL	Percutaneous nephrolithotomy
RI	Resistive index
SWL	Shock wave lithotripsy
TVUS	Transvaginal ultrasound
URS	Ureteroscopy
US	Ultrasound
UTI	Urinary tract infection

Learning Objectives

- To explain the pathophysiological changes in the kidney and ureter during pregnancy.
- To discuss the possible theories of urinary stone formation during pregnancy.
- To understand the diagnosis and differential diagnosis of renal colic and symptomatic hydronephrosis.
- To detail the management of the pregnant woman with acute urolithiasis.

24.1 Introduction

The ureter is a thin, elastic tube that carries urine from the kidney down to the urinary bladder. It lies in the posterior abdominal wall behind the posterior peritoneum (retroperitoneum) and has many related organs and important structures. These unique features of the ureter make it susceptible to many pathological conditions, congenital disorders, trauma, and external compression. Obstructive ureteral pathology is usually reflected on kidney function with the associated signs and symptoms. Ureteral dilatation during pregnancy is usually considered a physiological event (gestational hydronephrosis), particularly in the primigravida unless it becomes symptomatic. The dilation of the ureter and renal calyces is due to many factors. Progesterone-induced smooth muscle relaxation, ureteral compression by the gravid uterus, and other hormonal and biochemical changes are involved. Ureteral dilatation is seen in approximately 80% of cases [1]. This dilatation is asymptomatic in many cases and accidentally discovered during the routine obstetric follow-up by ultrasound examination. However, in lots of cases, the dilatation becomes symptomatic and mimics renal colic. The rate of symptomatic maternal hydronephrosis is 0.2–3% [2]. The differential diagnosis of physiological dilatation from pathological obstruction is very important for the clinician. Symptomatic obstruction due to compression by the gravid uterus should also be differentiated from kidney and ureteral stones. Decompression of the obstructed urinary tract system is a multi-disciplinary approach that requires a prompt decision when conservative treatment fails. The best method for intervention depends on the symptoms, stage of pregnancy, and availability of medical, obstetric, and surgical care.

24.2 Morphological Changes in the Kidney and Ureter During Pregnancy

There are many anatomical, functional, and metabolic changes in the urinary system during pregnancy. The kidneys increase in size by 1–1.5 cm and volume increases by up to 30% during pregnancy. This is due to an increase in renal vascular and interstitial volume [3]. In pregnant women, physiological hydronephrosis (gestational hydronephrosis) occur in 90% on the right and 67% on the left side [4]. There are many definitions of hydronephrosis. Faundes et al. demonstrated the normal curve of dilatation of the urinary tract. The upper limit of calyceal dilatation is more than 15 mm in the mid-second trimester [5]. The right ureter is compressed by the uterus (dextrorotation) over the iliac vessels and the engorged ovarian plexus could also press on the ureter against the pelvic brim [6]. The left ureter is less liable to compression by the gravid uterus than the right side because of potential protection by the sigmoid colon. However, there is no association between the degree of maternal hydronephrosis and the severity of pain [7, 8]. The physiological dilatation of the ureter usually resolves within 4–6 weeks after delivery. Untreated symptomatic hydronephrosis can lead to pyelonephritis, urosepsis in the presence of urinary tract infection, and ultimately to many obstetric complications. Moreover, stone formation and acute urolithiasis during pregnancy is a medical dilemma. Therefore, prompt treatment of symptomatic hydronephrosis during pregnancy is very important to avoid maternal and fetal complications.

24.3 Urolithiasis During Pregnancy

Although an uncommon condition, urinary stone disease during pregnancy, represents a clinical challenge in diagnosis and management.

24.3.1 Epidemiology

Urolithiasis during pregnancy is one of the major urologic problems due to many considerations, most of the cases present in the second and third trimesters. Recurrence of renal calculi has been reported in 25% of pregnant patients [9]. Urolithiasis is more common in multiparous women than primipara [10]. There is a wide range in the incidence of renal colic due to many factors. Geographical differences, lack of communication, and unreported cases are the reasons for this variation. However, the overall incidence of urolithiasis during pregnancy ranges from 1: 88 to 1:14600. White women are more affected by urinary calculi than black. Calculi in black women are more likely to become infected than in white individuals [11]. This variation in race and stone composition may be due to dietary patterns, environmental factors, and socioeconomic status. Pregnant women with nephrolithiasis are more likely to be obese and have gestational diabetes than pregnant women without stones [12].

24.3.2 Pathophysiology and Etiology of Urolithiasis During Pregnancy

Many underlying factors contribute to stone formation during pregnancy. Several physiological, functional, and anatomical changes in the urinary system that occur all over the gestational period can promote urolithiasis. There are also biochemical alterations in the urine components and an increase in the lithogenic factors. The pH of urine is alkaline and favors the formation of stones [13]. Urinary excretion of sodium, calcium, and uric acid is subsequently increased [14]. Urinary tract dilatation, stasis, and decreased ureteral peristalsis due to the gravid uterus predispose also to urinary tract infection [10]. Moreover, the urinary stasis increases the contact time between lithogenic factors and promotes crystallization with subsequent stone formation. There is an imbalance between promoters and inhibitors of stone formation during pregnancy. There is also a decrease in the resistance of renal vessels and an increase in GFR by 40–65% [15]. This is due to an increase in the circulating volume and renal plasma flow by 80%. On the other hand, blood biochemical changes can help and promote stone formations during pregnancy. Hypercalcemia is one of the major etiological factors that lead to an increase in calcium excretion in urine (hypercalciuria). Therefore, it can lead to calcium oxalate stone formation [16]. However, the prevalence of stone formation during pregnancy does not differ from non-pregnant women [14]. Seventy-three percent of urinary stones during pregnancy are composed of calcium phosphate, and 26% of calcium oxalate [17]. The rate of calcium phosphate stones in pregnant women is high even when compared with non-pregnant women of similar age. Uric acid and oxalate excretion is increased due to increased GFR and fetal factors [16, 18]. Diabetes is considered an independent risk factor for the development of both primary and recurrent renal lithiasis [19]. Therefore, the combination of hypercalciuria, uricosuria, and oxaluria all contribute to renal stone formation. Additionally, calcium supplementation during pregnancy could augment calcium excretion.

24.3.3 Etiology and Types of Stones

The etiology of urolithiasis during pregnancy could be attributed to many underlying factors. Physiological changes and anatomical alterations during pregnancy lead to urinary stasis and an increase in lithogenic elements. There are also biochemical changes in the urine components, in addition to ureteral compression by the gravid uterus (discussed in the previous section). These factors contribute to stone formation. The urinary stones during pregnancy consist mainly of calcium phosphate (74%) and calcium oxalate (26%) [17]. This feature of urinary stones differs from other stones (calcium oxalate) in nonpregnant patients. The reason for the predominance of calcium phosphate has been discussed.

24.3.4 Presentation and Differential Diagnosis

Many conditions can mimic renal colic during pregnancy. The clinical presentation of ureteral stones during pregnancy can be misleading. History of stone disease (8%) helps in suspecting urolithiasis and should alert the clinician. However, 80% of women have no history of stone disease [20]. The symptoms include abdominal or flank pain in more than 85%. Acute flank pain and fever may indicate the possibility of acute pyelonephritis. Macroscopic hematuria in more than 15% and microscopic hematuria in 95% of pregnant women. However, microscopic hematuria is not specific to nephrolithiasis during pregnancy. Lower urinary tract symptoms can also occur in the form of frequency, dysuria, and pyuria. Other non-urinary symptoms such as pre-eclampsia and preterm labor could be the first presentation. Nausea and vomiting are common symptoms, but all are non-specific.

24.3.4.1 Differential Diagnosis of Non-obstetric Causes of the Acute Abdomen During Pregnancy

The diagnosis of the acute abdomen during pregnancy is difficult because there are many changes in the viscera due to the enlarged uterus. Appendicitis, cholecystitis, pyelonephritis, and diverticulitis can give symptoms similar to renal colic or abdominal pain. History of urolithiasis and clinical examination in addition to abdominal ultrasound can help in the correct diagnosis of renal colic. Urinalysis and CBC are particularly important, especially in febrile cases [21]. Third of urolithiasis cases during pregnancy could be misdiagnosed [22]. A high index of suspicion is essential, and all possible investigations should be carried out to make the correct diagnosis.

24.3.5 Locations of the Stones

During pregnancy, there is a physiological dilatation of the collecting systems, allowing migration of renal stones into the ureter, resulting in obstruction and/or pain. This could explain the reason for the observation that during pregnancy, stones are twice as likely to be found in the ureter than in the renal pelvis or calyces. This complicates the diagnosis of intramural obstruction during pregnancy. However, hydronephrosis due to pregnancy does not usually extend below the pelvic brim, and therefore dilatation below this level is more likely to be due to an intraluminal cause such as ureteral stones.

24.4 Metabolic Syndrome, Gestational Diabetes, and Infectious Stone

A higher incidence of urinary stones occurs in pregnant patients with obesity and hyperglycemia and metabolic syndrome [23]. Infectious stones are formed by urea-slitting bacteria [24]. Nowadays, it is uncommon during pregnancy. It could be formed in patients with previous congenital anomalies of the kidney and ureter. It consists of magnesium ammonium phosphate. The urine culture is necessary, and it usually reveals the type of organisms. Alkaline urine during pregnancy promotes uric acid stone formation.

24.5 Perinatal Complications of Acute Urolithiasis

There are many reported complications of acute urolithiasis during pregnancy. Preterm birth, low birth weight, and premature rupture of membranes have been reported in 7% of pregnant women [12]. However, in many countries, there are less reports of complications due to either lack of cooperation between obstetricians and urologists or incomplete registrations of such complications.

24.6 Laboratory Investigations

Initial laboratory tests should include CBC, urine analysis, electrolytes, and serum creatinine. Urine analysis is necessary to evaluate microscopic hematuria and pus cells. The presence of microscopic hematuria may indicate the presence of urinary stones. However, it is non-specific. Urine culture is mandatory in the presence of pyuria to select the proper and safe antibiotics. Up to 50% of pregnant women have appositive urine culture [25]. Alkaline pH may indicate the presence of infected stones. Conversely, acidic pH may indicate uric acid stones. Serum creatine and BUN should be evaluated to rule out renal insufficiency, particularly in patients with a solitary kidney or suspected chronic kidney diseases. Elevated serum uric acid may indicate hyperuricemia and hyperuricosuria. High calcium levels could provide a clue to the diagnosis in cases of primary or secondary hyperparathyroidism.

24.7 Radiological Evaluation of Renal Colic and Urolithiasis During Pregnancy

Renal colic is the most common non-obstetric cause of abdominal pain and subsequent hospitalization during pregnancy [24]. Physiological hydronephrosis can mimic obstructive uropathy. The diagnosis of ureterolithiasis during pregnancy is a challenging medical dilemma. It should be immediate, accurate and safe. There is an increased risk of obstetric complications such as premature rupture of membrane or preterm labor [12]. Furthermore, the use of ionizing radiation during pregnancy is a complicated and controversial issue. During early pregnancy, the fetal tissues are very sensitive to radiation effects specially during second and third trimesters. Conventional radiological techniques have been previously used (IVP and KUB). However, these techniques have some limitations and many adverse effects, such as the risk of hypersensitivity to contrast media, and fetal radiation exposure. The use of conventional CT imparts a higher risk due to higher doses of radiation [25]. CT is also associated with an increase of 2.4 times the risk of cancer in children and an increased incidence of fetal malformations. Recently, there are many regulations and recommendations for the use of low-dose CT in pregnancy [26].

24.7.1 *Ultrasound*

Ultrasound is usually the first method of diagnosis and evaluation of flank pain during pregnancy [27]. It is safe, widely available, and does not contain ionizing radiation. Ultrasound can show dilatation of the ureter without identifying the cause (Fig. 24.1). MRI is relatively the second safe line of diagnosis when ultrasound fails to define the cause of obstruction [28].

24.7.2 *Transabdominal Ultrasound*

Transabdominal ultrasound when compared to CT demonstrated sensitivity, specificity, and accuracy to be 40%, 84%, and 53%, respectively [29]. The differentiation between physiological dilatation of the ureter, due to compression of the gravid uterus and ureteral stones is challenging. Dilatation of the ureter below the iliac vessels indicates obstruction by a stone as compared to physiological hydronephrosis of pregnancy [30]. Identification of ureteral calculi is sometimes difficult by ultrasound especially if located in the middle of the pelvic ureter. However, the use of color Doppler ultrasound with twinkling can be extremely helpful in stone localization and identification [29, 31]. Other associated signs on ultrasound examination can indicate the presence of ureteric stone such as the abrupt cessation of the hydroureteronephrosis or presence of inflammatory signs, absent ureteral jet, and altered resistive index (RI). RI of 0.70 or greater is suggestive of ureteral obstruction. RI is not a

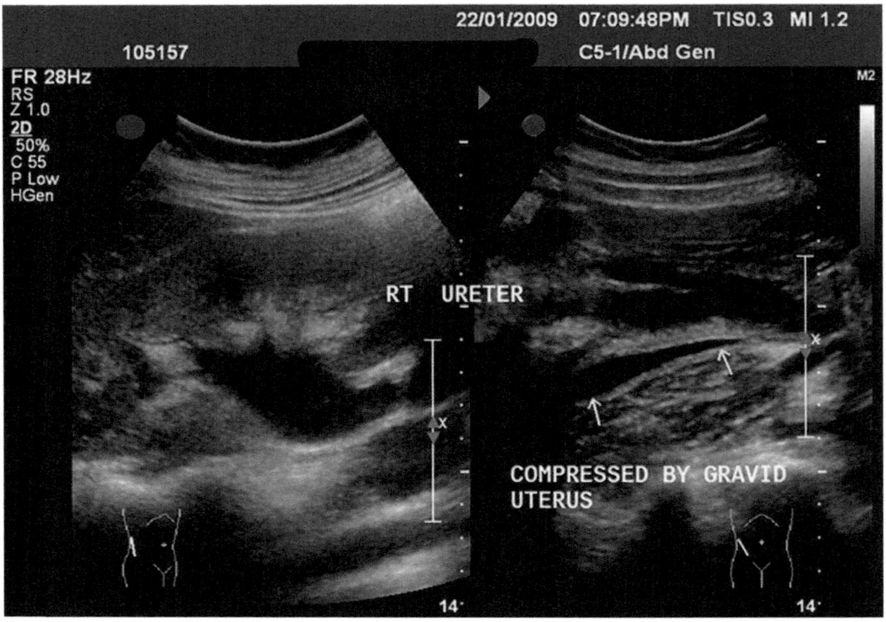

Fig. 24.1 Grey scale abdominal ultrasound shows dilated right ureter and associated hydronephrosis due to compression of the ureter by the gravid uterus

specific diagnostic test. The combination of the renal resistive index in addition to the absent ureteral jet increases the accuracy of ultrasound diagnosis of ureteral obstruction. However, these signs cannot identify the underlying reason for obstruction [32].

24.7.3 Transvaginal Ultrasound (TVUS)

Transvaginal ultrasound (TVUS) in pregnancy has shown superiority (94%) in the detection of lower ureteral stones compared to transabdominal (29%) [33]. Combined transabdominal and transvaginal ultrasound could be very helpful in the diagnosis of distal ureteral stones in pregnant women. It is well tolerated by pregnant patients and contraindicated in cases with ruptured membranes.

24.8 Nuclear Renal Scanning

The renal scan by using Tc 99 m DTPA (Technetium-99 Diethylene-Triamine-Pentaacetate) is an excellent study to determine kidney functions and obstruction. However, it does not allow anatomical visualization of the stones or the cause of obstruction.

24.9 Magnetic Resonance Image (MRI) and MR Urography (MRU)

MRI of the urinary system is safe and accurate in the diagnosis of many medical conditions associated with pregnancy (Fig. 24.2a–d). It is an excellent alternative to CT as it lacks ionizing radiation. However, MRI should be avoided in early pregnancy. Gadolinium agent can cross the placenta and cause teratogenesis (Category C) and should not be used during pregnancy. Furthermore, conventional MRI poorly visualizes calcium, and so does not visualize calcium stones. Alternatively, Magnetic resonance urography (MRU) is preferred as a second line of investigation of urolithiasis during pregnancy. MRU, Half-Fourier Acquisition Single Shot Turbo Spin Echo (HASTE), without contrast is safe during pregnancy. MRU using T2-weighted images can effectively differentiate physiological dilatation from ureteral stone [34]. Moreover, there are many signs indicating acute ureteral obstruction on MRI examination. Perinephric and periureteric fluid collection and perinephric stranding in addition to kidney edema. MRU can detect the ureteric stone as a filling defect (Fig. 24.3). Nevertheless, FSE (Fast Spin Echo] sequence has been reported to be of value in the identification of small stones [35]. However, there are many limitations of MRI. It is not available everywhere. The relatively high cost of the examination. MRI is not suitable for patients with metallic implants, in addition to the long duration of the scan. Some patients with claustrophobia cannot tolerate the procedure. Moreover, it cannot detect small stones. There are many signs in MRU suggesting the presence of stone and associated complications such as focal pyelonephritis, a rim of enhancement of renal capsule, and enlarged edematous kidney. MRI imaging at 1.5 Tesla is safe over the last two decades. However, the data on 3-T safety is not available.

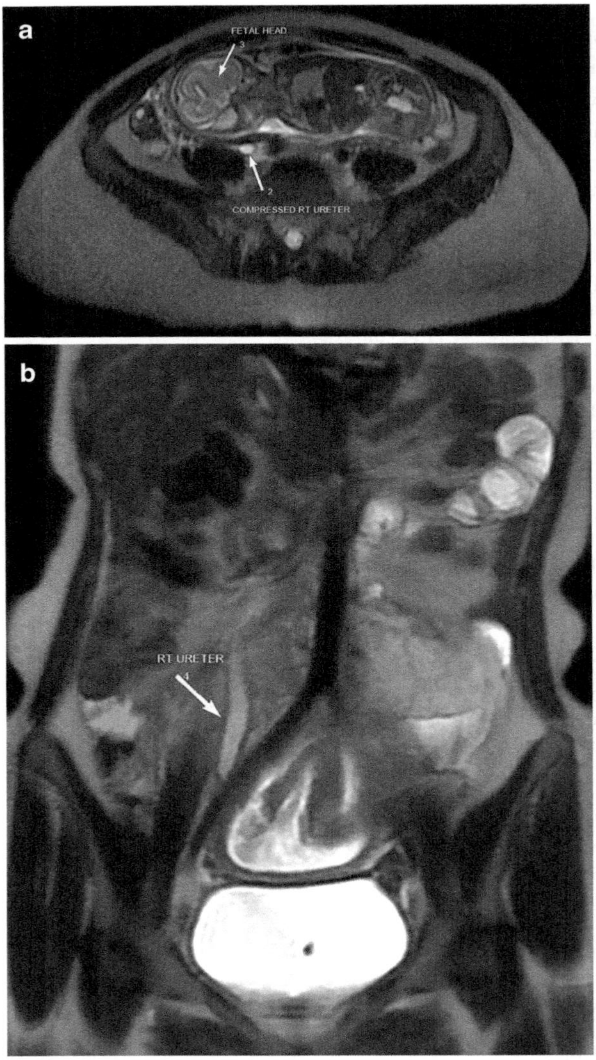

Fig. 24.2 (**a**) MRI Axial T2 showing gravid uterus compressing the right ureter against the right Psoas muscle. (**b**) MRI coronal T2 showing the dilated right lumbar ureter. (**c**) MRI with MIP (maximum intensity projection) showing the gravid uterus containing the fetal parts and the right hydroureteronephrosis down to level of uterus as well as the normal left kidney, left ureter and urinary bladder. (**d**) MRI, VR (Volume rendered) showing same findings in MIP image (image **c**) with more fetal anatomic details

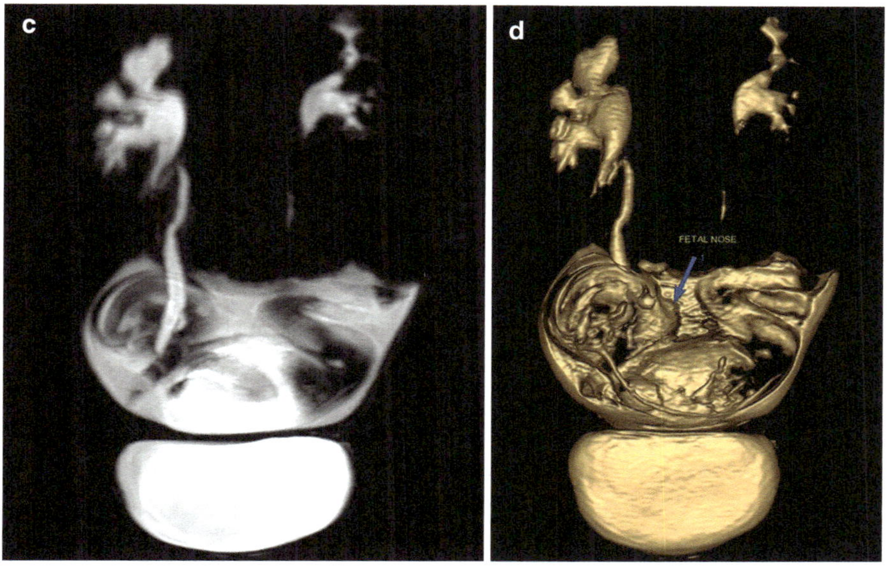

Fig. 24.2 (continued)

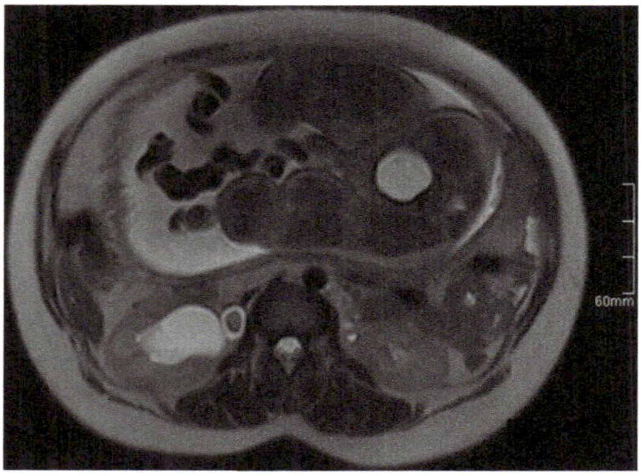

Fig. 24.3 A 33-year-old pregnant woman presented with acute right renal colic at 35 weeks of gestation. Axial T2 weighted MR image demonstrating stone (8 × 5 mm) at the level of right upper lumbar ureter with proximal hydronephrosis

24.10 Computed Tomography (CT)

Conventionally, KUB and IVP have been used in the past for the diagnosis of renal colic and ureteral obstruction. IVP has many disadvantages, including the risk of radiation exposure to the mother and fetus, allergy to contrast material, and inaccuracy of proper diagnosis of small stones. However, with modern radiological equipment and less radiation exposure such as low-dose CT and MRI techniques, the diagnosis of ureteral stones could be appropriate and safe. Conventional CT is contraindicated during pregnancy. The dose of radiation during CT examination ranges from 10 mGy to 50 mGy. This dose is hazardous and may result in fetal teratogenicity and childhood malignancy. However, when CT examination is necessary, the dose can be reduced by minimizing the duration of exposure time, changing the CT setting, and abdominal lead shielding. However, routine use of an abdominal lead shield is no longer advisable [36]. Low-dose CT is an alternative modality with high sensitivity (95%) and specificity (98%). Low-dose CT during pregnancy will lead to radiation exposure of 7.1 mGy [37]. The American Urological Association has recommended low-dose CT as a second line of imaging modality in pregnant women and should be reserved as the last line of investigation when there is no diagnostic alternative [38]. Studies of pregnant women evaluated with low-dose CT for urolithiasis have shown >95% specificity and positive predictive value [39].

24.10.1 Management of Symptomatic Hydronephrosis and Urolithiasis During Pregnancy

Symptomatic urolithiasis during pregnancy requires a collaborative management team that includes the urologist, obstetrician, anesthetist, and neonatologist. The initial management of urolithiasis should be conservative. Interestingly, most of the ureteral stones (64–84%) pass spontaneously with conservative treatment [40]. However, Burgess et al. 2011, reported that the percentage of spontaneous passage of stone during pregnancy is overestimated due to probable misdiagnosis [22]. Fifty percent of stones that do not pass during pregnancy will pass a few weeks postpartum [40]. Many algorithms have been proposed for the management of urolithiasis during pregnancy. Suggested management algorithm is given in Fig. 24.4. There are three options for the treatment of urolithiasis during pregnancy. Conservative treatment, medical expulsive therapy, and minimally invasive procedures. Conservative management remains the mainstay of the management of urolithiasis during pregnancy unless complications occur. However, the success rate of conservative treatment in pregnant women is often overestimated [41]. The AUA guidelines recommend the conservative treatment of ureteral stones in an uncomplicated pregnancy [42]. The urologist should decide when conservative treatment should be discontinued. There are many indications for the active intervention of ureteral stones during pregnancy. Bilateral ureteral obstruction or obstructed solitary kidney. Refractory pain to analgesia and vomiting by medications. Urinary sepsis, and deterioration of renal functions. Pre-eclampsia, pre-term labor, insufficient medical care, and poor medical accessibility. It should be noted that 20–30% of cases develop sepsis with conservative treatment, and 60–80% of patients will pass the stones [43]. The management of ureteral obstruction in pregnancy remains controversial. The options of the ureteral stent or percutaneous nephrostomy tube are intolerable to many patients and ureteroscopy is an alternative [44].

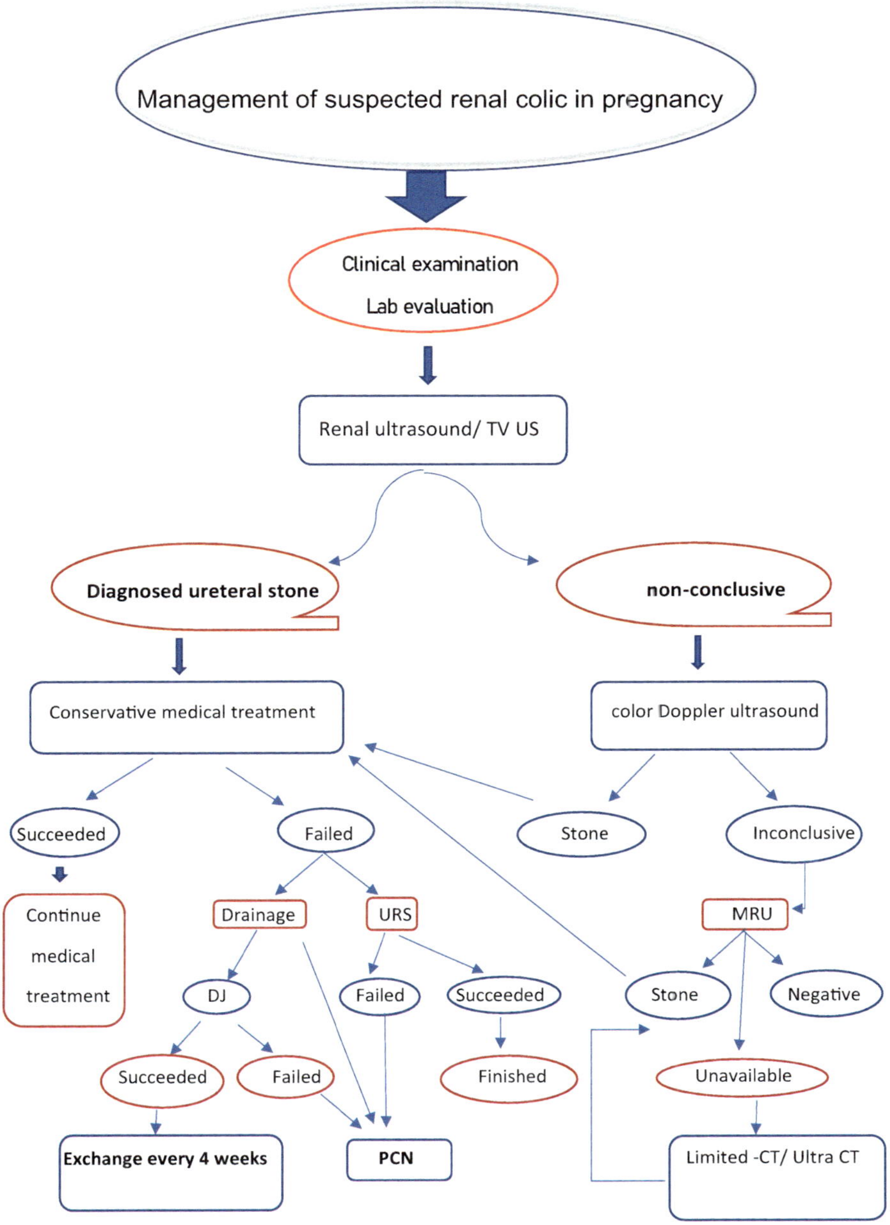

Fig. 24.4 Proposed Algorithm for management of pregnant patient with symptomatic hydronephrosis

24.11 Conservative Treatment

Conservative treatment remains the cornerstone in the management of renal colic and urolithiasis during pregnancy unless complicated. It is indicated to control pain, monitor vomiting, and correct dehydration, in addition, avoiding risks to mother and fetus [41]. Intravenous hydration therapy should be administered in cases of persistent vomiting, as repeated vomiting can lead to premature labor and disturbance in electrolytes and acid-base balance. Intravenous antibiotics are preferred when the infection is present to avoid septicemia. However, there are contraindications of many antibiotics during pregnancy. Sulfonamides, aminoglycoside, fluoroquinolones, tetracycline, and chloramphenicol are contraindicated. Pain control is particularly important and should be tailored. Pain medications should not affect the fetus or mother respiration. However, many narcotics and non-narcotics are safe and can be used during pregnancy to control pain. Oral acetaminophen alone or in combination with codeine could be given. Hydrocodone and Oxycodone are alternatives and available. NSAIDs should be avoided because of their complications. Paracetamol in therapeutic doses is safe and could be given intravenously as an antipyretic agent. Ibuprofen is contraindicated. If pain is intolerable despite oral medications, intravenous narcotics could be given. Meperidine and morphine sulfate could be given with close monitoring [45]. Hospital admission should be customized according to the pain severity, intractable vomiting, and close mother and fetal monitoring. Repeated administration of Morphine can induce dependence in the fetus and the risk-benefit relationship should be evaluated. Tramadol is contraindicated during all phases of pregnancy. Codeine is contraindicated in the third trimester. An epidural block is safe during pregnancy it could be used to control pain when needed [46]. Dietary modifications during pregnancy could reduce stone formation during pregnancy. Increase fluid intake and restriction of salt diets and excessive calcium in prenatal multivitamins. Pregnant women can also reduce their intake of oxalate-rich food and the nutritionist can help in the management of diet habits during pregnancy.

24.12 Medical Expulsive Therapy (MET)

Medical management by medications still has a role in the treatment of urinary stones during pregnancy. Many medications can be safely used to facilitate the passage of the ureteral stones. These drugs affect ureteral peristalsis and induce dilatation. Alpha-adrenergic blockers are safe during pregnancy. Tamsulosin has been used in many studies and is considered category B during pregnancy. Calcium channel blockers are also effective in the facilitation of stone passage. Nifedipine has been highly effective and safe in pregnancy. It also influences hypertension and reduces uterine contractions (tocolytic). MET is successful in 70–80% of patients [47]. Thiazide diuretics for calcium stones are contraindicated during pregnancy due to its side effects. Xanthine oxidase inhibitors for uric acid stones are also contraindicated during pregnancy. The size of the ureteral stone is one of the prognostic factors for successful conservative treatment. A ureteral stone larger than 8 mm is a risk factor for urological intervention [48].

24.13 Active Treatment (Minimally Invasive Procedures)

Many conditions necessitate active management of renal colic and urolithiasis during pregnancy. The indications for active interventions include failed conservative treatment, obstructed solitary kidney, urosepsis, bilateral obstructed kidneys, and impaired renal function. A nomogram for predicting surgical intervention is proposed by He et al. 2022. The nomogram is composed of four parameters. Fever: Body temperature over 37.5 °C, hydronephrosis (mm): was classified as none/mild and moderate/severe, Ureter stones: Ureteral stones size larger or smaller than 8 mm by ultrasound, Pain Duration (d): time from the beginning of pain to attendance at the emergency room. Each item has a range of points from 0 to 100. The predicted probability of surgical intervention ranges from 0.2 to 0.9 [49, 50].

24.13.1 Ureteroscopy During Pregnancy

Advances in ureteroscopy manufacture and improvements in endoscopic visualization made the procedure more comfortable than before. Ureteroscopy procedures should include a multidisciplinary team of different specialties for preoperative, intraoperative, and postoperative consultations and care. This team should involve obstetricians, urologists, anesthesiologists, and neonatologists. Approximately 20–30% of patients with ureteral stones during pregnancy require active treatment [50]. Ureteroscopy is relatively safe during pregnancy [51]. The overall obstetric complications rate of ureteroscopy is 4.3% [52]. The overall urological complication rate is 8.3% [53]. Ureteroscopy is usually performed under fluoroscopic guidance with radiation exposure. However, there are many ways to minimize the exposure of the mother and fetus to radiation. Some advocate low-dose fluoroscopy and lead shielding of the abdomen, positioning of the C-arm below the patient, and conning of the image to include only the renal area. Ureteroscopy could also be performed under ultrasound guidance [53]. The ACOG guidelines recommend URS be performed in the second trimester to reduce the risk of preterm uterine contractions, and the possibility of abortion [54]. The AUA guidelines recommend ureteroscopic stone treatment in those failing trial of conservative treatment options [44]. However, there are many contraindications of ureteroscopy. These include active infection and sepsis, associated abnormal anatomy, a large volume of stones, and a lack of adequate urological instruments [13]. In many studies, the stone-free rate after ureteroscopy is in the range of 63–93%. The complications of the ureteroscopy include UTIs, ureteral injury, and preterm labor [55, 56]. Insertion of a JJ stent after ureteroscopy is not preferable because it has many complications unless indicated in cases of residual stones or stricture ureter or anticipated obstruction due to other pathology. The procedure can be performed under both spinal and general anesthesia. Stone disintegration can be performed safely by using laser, pneumatic, and ultrasound disintegration. However, there are few reports on the side effects of ultrasound disintegration on fetal audition and induction of uterine contraction [57].

24.13.2 Temporizing Measures

In many conditions, drainage of the obstructed kidney is mandatory until the time of definitive management of the cause. One of the most reasonable indications is unsuccessful conservative treatment. There are many other indications for urinary decompression. The presence of active infection, sepsis, bilateral renal stones, solitary kidney, complex anatomy, transplanted kidney, and impending obstetric complications are reasons for immediate kidney drainage. Temporization is considered less invasive, potentially safe, and can be performed under local anesthesia with ultrasound guidance.

24.13.3 Insertion of the Double Pigtail (JJ) Ureteral Stent

Insertion of JJ stent is remarkably effective in the relief of symptomatic maternal hydronephrosis. Ureteral catheterization can be performed under local anesthesia and ultrasound guidance. Some authors advocate the use of limited fluoroscopy during the procedure. Intravenous sedation could also be used safely. However, general anesthesia should be avoided because of its risk to the mother and fetus [58]. There are many complications of DJ stents. Early complications include flank pain, bladder irritation, urinary tract infection, hematuria, and encrustation. It needs frequency changes every 4–6 weeks. Occasionally the stent can migrate to the bladder due to dilated ureter. Late complications include stent encrustation, stone formation, recurrent infection, fragmentation, and migration of the stent.

24.13.4 Percutaneous Nephrostomy (PCN)

Kidney drainage alone might be indicated when active surgical intervention is not available. Insertion of PCN tube during pregnancy is easy due to dilated system, it could be done under local anesthesia. Ultrasound-guided puncture could be easy and safe. In cases of urosepsis and pyonephrosis, PCN is a good option for adequate drainage with different sizes of tubes. The procedure also allows for urine collection and culture. There are many disadvantages of PCN tubes. Obstruction and encrustation are frequent problems of the PCN tube. Bacterial colonization, migration, and dislodgement can also occur. The PCN tube also affects the quality of life of the pregnant patient.

24.13.5 Percutaneous Nephrolithotomy (PCNL)

Percutaneous nephrolithotomy is not recommended during pregnancy. It is a lengthy procedure and requires fluoroscopy. The prone positioning makes the procedure high risk and discomfort to the patient. There are many reports on the success of PCNL during pregnancy. PCNL is suitable for staghorn stones or complex renal stones (>2 cm), and lower calyceal stones more than 1 cm or impacted stones in the upper ureter [59]. Modified PCNL has also been reported and supine PCNL and US-guided puncture have been described [60]. PCNL should be reserved, if possible, till after delivery.

24.14 Extracorporeal Shock Wave Lithotripsy (ESWL) and Pregnancy

ESWL is a non-invasive treatment method for urinary stones. However, it is contraindicated during pregnancy due to many considerations and fetal risks. Few animal studies have shown the effect of ESWL on the fetus. Low birth weight and bleeding in lungs, liver, and kidney tissues have been reported [61]. Nowadays, there is no justification for the use of ESWL during pregnancy.

24.15 Laparoscopy/Open Surgery During Pregnancy

Nowadays, open surgery is rare in cases of acute urolithiasis. However, it is indicated when the endoscopic treatment failed, or the endoscopic instruments are limited. Currently, there is no series on the use of laparoscopy for stone disease during pregnancy. However, laparoscopic cholecystectomy and appendicectomy have been successfully performed in the third trimester without increasing the risk of preterm labor or fetal demise [62, 63].

24.16 Surgical Risks and Complications During Pregnancy

Many risk factors are associated with increased morbidity during pregnancy. Thromboembolism is more common in pregnant than non-pregnant women. Decreased blood velocity and venous return due to the gravid uterus in addition to increased thrombotic blood factors during pregnancy can lead to venous thromboembolism and precipitate pulmonary embolism. There is also an increased risk of aspiration during induction of anesthesia due to pregnancy-related gastrointestinal dysfunction and low pH. Inhalation anesthesia can cross the placenta to the fetus. General anesthesia should be avoided in early pregnancy due to its complications [12]. Pre-term birth or low birth weight and premature rupture of the membrane, all can occur during the episodes of renal colic or due to manipulations of minimally invasive procedures.

24.17 Conclusion

The diagnosis of symptomatic hydronephrosis and acute urolithiasis during pregnancy is a complex medical condition. MRU examination and low-dose CT are safe during pregnancy. Management of acute urolithiasis during pregnancy is a multidisciplinary approach. There are no definite parameters (clinical and laboratory) that can be used to determine the optimal treatment option. However, the clinician should determine the best timing for a minimally invasive endoscopic procedure. All active management methods are accepted except PCNL and ESWL.

24.18 Future Perspective

Many important issues should be solved and need further study and investigation. What is the safest radiological examination during all phases of pregnancy? What is the appropriate and effective medical expulsive therapy during pregnancy? Proper and clear guidelines for medical and urological intervention based on controlled randomized trials.

Questions

1. The following medications are not contraindicated during pregnancy except:

   (a) Codeine
   (b) Nifedipine
   (c) Tamsulosin
   (d) Tramadol
   (e) Acetaminophen

Answer: (d)

2. The following are indications for the active invasive procedure during pregnancy except:
   (a) Obstructed solitary kidney
   (b) Urosepsis
   (c) Bilateral obstructed kidneys
   (d) Impaired renal function
   (e) Heavy pyuria

Answer: (e)

3. The following are not contraindicated radiological investigations during pregnancy except:
   (a) Transvaginal ultrasound
   (b) NCCT
   (c) MRU
   (d) Ultra-CT
   (e) KUB

Answer: (b)

4. The following procedure is could be done during pregnancy except:
   (a) PCN
   (b) URS
   (c) ESWL
   (d) PCNL
   (e) JJ stent

Answer: (c)

5. Which of the following statement is incorrect:
   (a) Gestational hydronephrosis is more common on the right side than on the left.
   (b) Hydronephrosis is a symptomatic in most pregnant patients
   (c) The left hydronephrosis usually indicates the presence of ureteral stone
   (d) Most symptomatic hydronephrosis can be managed conservatively
   (e) Most of the ureteral stones are in the upper ureter

Answer: (e)

References

1. Rasmussen PE, Nilsen FR. Hydronephrosis during pregnancy: a literature survey. Eur J Obstet Gynecol Reprod Biol. 1988;27(3):249–59.
2. Puskar D, Balagovic I, Filipovic A, et al. Symptomatic physiologic hydronephrosis in pregnancy: incidence, complications, and treatment. Eur Urol. 2001;39(3):260–3.

3. Baily RR, Rolleston GL. Kidney length and ureteric dilatation in the puerperium. J Obst Gynec Br Commonw. 1971;78(1):55–61.
4. Cherianchan D, Arianayagam M, Rashid P. Symptomatic urinary stone disease in pregnancy. Aust N Z J Obstet Gynaecol. 2008;48(1):34–9.
5. Faundes A, Bricola-Filho M, Pinto e Silva JL. Dilatation of the urinary tract during pregnancy: Proposal of a curve of maximal caliceal diameter by gestational age. Am J Obstet Gynecol. 1998;178(5):1082–6.
6. Grenier N, Pariente JL, Trillaud H, Soussotte C, Douws C. Dilatation of the collecting system during pregnancy: physiologic vs obstructive dilatation. Eur Radiol. 2000;10(2):271–9.
7. Farr A, Ott J, Kueronya V, et al. The association between maternal hydronephrosis and acute flank pain during pregnancy: a prospective pilot-study. J Matern Fetal Neonatal Med. 2017;30:2417–21.
8. Watson WJ, Brost BC. Maternal hydronephrosis in pregnancy: poor association of symptoms of flank pain. Am J Perinatol. 2006;23(8):463–6.
9. Charalambous S, Fotas A, Rizk DEE. Urolithiasis in pregnancy. Int Urogynecol J Pelvic Floor Dysfunct. 2009;20:1133–6.
10. Denstedt JD, Razvi H. Management of urinary calculi during pregnancy. J Urol. 1992;148(3 pt 4):1072–4.
11. Romero V, Akpinar H, Assimos DG. Kidney stones: a global picture of prevalence, incidence, and associated risk factors. Rev Urol. 2010;12(2-3):e86–96.
12. Lewis DF, Robichaux AG III, Jaekle RK, et al. Urolithiasis in pregnancy: diagnosis, management, and pregnancy outcome. J Reprod Med. 2003;48:28–32.
13. Semins MJ, Matlaga BR. Kidney stones during pregnancy. Nat Rev Urol. 2014;11:163–8.
14. Resim S, Ekerbicer HC, Kiran G, et al. Are changes in urinary parameters during pregnancy clinically significant? Urol Res. 2006;34:244–8.
15. Jeyabalan A, Lain KY. Anatomic and functional changes of the upper urinary tract during pregnancy. Urol Clin North Am. 2007;34(1):1–6.
16. Maikranz P, Holley JL, Parks JH, et al. Gestational hypercalciuria causes pathological urine calcium oxalate supersaturations. Kidney Int. 1989;36:108–13.
17. Ross AE, Handa S, Lingeman JE, et al. Kidney stones during pregnancy: an investigation into the stone composition. Urol Res. 2008;36:99–102.
18. Lindheimer MD, Katz AI. The renal response to pregnancy. In: Brenner BM, Rector RC, editors. The kidney. 2nd ed. Philadelphia: WB Saunders; 1981. p. 1762–819.
19. Knoll T. Epidemiology, pathogenesis, and pathophysiology of urolithiasis. Eur Urol Suppl. 2010;9:802–6.
20. Butler EL, Cox SM, Eberts EG, et al. Symptomatic nephrolithiasis complicating pregnancy. Obstet Gynecol. 2000;96:753–6.
21. Biyani CS, Joyce AD. Urolithiasis in pregnancy. I: pathophysiology, fetal considerations and diagnosis. BJU Int. 2002;89:811–8.
22. Burgess KL, Gettman MT, Rangel LJ, Krambeck AE. Diagnosis of urolithiasis and rate of spontaneous passage during pregnancy. J Urol. 2011;186(6):2280–4.
23. Wong P, Cook P, Roderick BK, Somani BK. Metabolic syndrome and kidney stone disease: a systemic review of literature. J Endourol. 2016;30(3):246–53.
24. Swanson SK, Heilman RL, Eversman WG. Urinary tract stones in pregnancy. Surg Clin North Am. 1995;75:123–42.
25. Srirangam SJ, Hickerton B, Van Cleynenbreugel B. Management of urinary calculi in pregnancy: a review. J Endourol. 2008;22(5):867–75.
26. Royal College Radiologists. 2009. http://www.rcr.ac.uk/system/files/publication/field_publication_files/HPA_preg_2nd.pdf
27. Masselli G, Weston M, Spencer J. The role of imaging in the diagnosis and management of renal stone disease in pregnancy. Clin Radiol. 2015;70(12):1462–71.
28. Meher S, Gibbons N, DasGupta R. Renal stones in pregnancy. Obstet Med. 2014;7:103–10.

29. Viprakasit DP, Sawyer MD, Harrell SD, Miller NL. Limitations of ultrasonography in the evaluation of urolithiasis: a correlation with computed tomography. J Endourol. 2012;26(3):209–13.
30. MacNeily AE, Goldenberg SL, Allen GJ, Ajzen SA, Cooperberg P. Sonographic visualization of the ureter in pregnancy. J Urol. 1991;146(2):298–301.
31. Abdel-Gawad M, Kadasne RD, Elsobky E, Ali-El-Dein B, Monga M. A prospective comparative study of color Doppler ultrasound with twinkling and noncontrast computerized tomography for the evaluation of acute renal colic. J Urol. 2016;196:757–62.
32. Shokeir AA, Mahran MR, Abdulmaaboud M. Renal colic in pregnant women: role of renal resistive index. Urology. 2000;55(3):344–7.
33. Bold MS, Boyum JH, Rose CH, et al. Detection of distal ureteral stones in pregnancy using transvaginal ultrasound. J Ultrasound. 2021;24:397–402.
34. Masselli G, Derme M, Bernieri MG, et al. Stone disease in pregnancy: imaging-guided therapy. Insights Imaging. 2014;5:691–6.
35. Masselli G, Derme M, Laghi F, et al. Imaging of stone diseases in pregnancy. Abdom Imaging. 2013;38:1409–14.
36. Marsh RM, Silosky M. Patient shielding in diagnostic imaging: discontinuing a legacy practice. Am J Roentgenol. 2019;212:755–7.
37. American College of Obstetricians and Gynecologists. Guidelines for diagnostic imaging during pregnancy and lactation. Committee opinions No. 723. Obstet Gynecol. 2017;130:e210–6.
38. Fulgham PF, Assimos DG, Pearle MS, Preminger GM. Clinical effectiveness protocols for imaging in the management of ureteral calculous disease: AUA technology assessment. J Urol. 2013;189:1203–13.
39. White WM, Johnson E, Zite NB, et al. Predictive value of current imaging modalities for the detection of urolithiasis during pregnancy: a multicenter, longitudinal study. J Urol. 2013;189:931–4.
40. Stothers L, Lee LM. Renal colic in pregnancy. J Urol. 1992;148(5):1383–7.
41. GL LI, Lim A, Hamoui N, et al. The use of medical expulsive therapy during pregnancy: a worldwide perspective among experts. J Endourol. 2016;30:354–8.
42. Assimos D, Krambeck A, Miller NL, et al. Surgical management of stones: American urological association/endourological society guidelines part II. J Urol. 2015;196:1161–9.
43. Martindale AD, Paisley AM. Surgical and urological problems in pregnancy. Curr Obstet Gynecol. 2004;14:350–5.
44. Turk C, Petrik A, Sarica K, et al. Eau guidelines on interventional treatment for urolithiasis. Eur Urol. 2016;69:475–82.
45. Irving SO, Burgess NA. Managing severe loin pain in pregnancy. BJOG. 2002;109:1025–9.
46. Peng X, Tu C, Wang K, Xiangbo W, Feng Y. Intracutaneous sterile water injection versus oral paracetamol for renal colic during pregnancy: a randomized controlled trial. Int Urol Nephrol. 2013;43:321–5.
47. Juan YS, Wu WJ, Chuang SM, et al. Management of symptomatic urolithiasis during pregnancy. Kaohsiung J Med Sci. 2007;23:241–6.
48. He M, Lin X, Lei M, Xu X, He Z. The identification of pregnant women with renal colic who may need surgical intervention. BMC Urol. 2022;22(1):30. https://doi.org/10.1186/s12894-022-00985-x.
49. Georgescu D, Multescu R, Geavlete B, et al. Ureteroscopy: first-line treatment alternative in ureteral calculi during pregnancy? Chirurgia (Bucur). 2014;109(2):229–32.
50. Scarpa RM, De Lisa A, Usai E. Diagnosis and treatment of ureteral calculi during pregnancy with rigid ureteroscopes. J Urol. 1996;155:875–7.
51. Johnson EB, Krambeck AE, White WM, et al. Obstetric complications of ureteroscopy during pregnancy. J Urol. 2012;188:151–4.
52. Semins MJ, Trock BT, Matlaga BR. The safety of ureteroscopy during pregnancy: a systematic review and meta-analysis. J Urol. 2009;181:139–43.
53. Deters LA, Belanger G, Shah O, et al. Ultrasound-guided ureteroscopy in pregnancy. Clin Nephrol. 2013;79:118–23.

54. Committee on Obstetric Practice and the American Society of anesthesiologists. Committee opinion No 696: nonobstetric surgery during pregnancy. Obstet Gynecol. 2017;129:777–8.
55. Ulvik NM, Bakke A, Høisaeter PA. Ureteroscopy in pregnancy. J Urol. 1995;154(5):1660–3.
56. Wang Z, Xu L, Su Z, Yao C, Chen Z. Invasive management of proximal ureteral calculi during pregnancy. Urology. 2014;83(4):745–9.
57. Song Y, Fei X, Song Y. Diagnosis and operative intervention for problematic ureteral calculi during pregnancy. Int J Gynaecol Obstet. 2013;121:115–8.
58. Jarrard DJ, Gerber GS, Lyon ES. Management of acute ureteral obstruction in pregnancy utilizing ultrasound-guided placement of ureteral stents. Urology. 1993;42:263–7.
59. Miller NL, Lingeman JE. Management of kidney stones. BMJ. 2007;334:468–72.
60. Fregonesi A, Dias FG, Saude RD, et al. Challenges on percutaneous nephrolithotomy in pregnancy: supine position approach through ultrasound guidance. Urol Ann. 2013;5:197–9.
61. Gümüs B, Lekili M, Kandiloglu AR, et al. Effects of extracorporeal shockwave lithotripsy at different stages of pregnancy in the rabbit. J Endourol. 1997;11(5):323–6.
62. Affleck DG, Handrahan DL, Egger MJ, et al. The laparoscopic management of appendicitis and cholelithiasis during pregnancy. Am J Surg. 1999;178:523–9.
63. Weiner E, Mizrachi Y, Keidar R, et al. Laparoscopic surgery performed in advanced pregnancy compared to early pregnancy. Arch Gynecol Obstet. 2015;292:1063–8.

Chapter 25
Radiological Signs and Syndromes of the Ureter

Doaa Sharaf and Haytham Shebel

Abstract Abnormalities of the ureter can give a clue to different pathologies that affect the urinary tract. Imaging plays a major role to characterize these abnormalities and identify the main pathology of the urinary tract. In this chapter, the commonest signs of ureteric abnormalities, the ways to their diagnosis by imaging, and the clinical significance of them are discussed.

Keywords Ureter · Comet tail sign · Goblet sign · Bergman sign · Bullet and bodkin sign: Curlicue ureter · Cobra head sign · Inverted J shaped ureter · Median waist deformity sign · Weigert-meyer law · Nutcracker syndrome

Learning Objectives

- After reading this chapter, the readers will be able to enlist the different radiological signs related to the ureter due to congenital, inflammatory, and neoplastic causes of the ureter, to describe imaging features of each sign and how to reach the diagnosis, to discuss causes, pathophysiology, and management of each disease, and to give an attention about the significance of each radiological sign.

25.1 Introduction

Precise diagnosis in radiology depends on signs we notice during practice. So, it is important to highlight these signs and deliver them to a urologist and uroradiologist. As we see what we know, this chapter is beneficial in describing and recognizing different radiological signs related to pathological diseases of the ureter. It contains nearly all the signs related to congenital, inflammatory, obstructive, neoplastic

Test your learning and check your understanding of this book's contents: use the "Springer Nature Flashcards" app to access questions. To use the app, please follow the instructions in Chapter 1.

D. Sharaf (✉) · H. Shebel
Radiology Department, Urology & Nephrology Center, Mansoura University, Mansoura, Egypt

M. Abdel-Gawad et al. (eds.), *The Ureter*,
https://doi.org/10.1007/978-3-031-36212-5_25

causes and signs related to tortuosity of the ureter. Each sign explains the diagnostic importance, causes, pathophysiology, clinical picture, and management of the corresponding disease.

25.2 Tissue Rim and Comet Tail Signs

Ureteral stone disease is a prevalent ailment that affects up to 10% of the population in developed countries [1]. The classical clinical symptoms of ureteric colic, such as loin pain that radiates to the groin, vomiting and microscopic hematuria, frequently overlaps with other clinical presentations such as pyelonephritis, appendicitis, gynecological problems or diverticulitis [2]. Radiological imaging is done, especially if the patient is admitted to the emergency room or if the clinical condition is unusual. Its role is to confirm the diagnosis, to determine the number, location, size and, if possible, the chemical composition of the calculus/calculi, to rule out complications, and to detect predisposing factors [1].

The 'gold standard' imaging for the identification of ureteric stones in the context of acute loin pain is computed tomography (CT). This technique is ideal for acute evaluations because it does not require any patient preparation and does not involve the use of oral or intravenous contrast injection [2]. When the stone is impacted within the ureter's lumen, it will be encircled by the edematous ureteral wall what is known as the soft tissue rim sign. (Figure 25.1a) It is typically defined as a 1–2 mm rim of soft tissue measuring 20–40 HU that surrounds the impacted stone in the ureter. It is considered as the direct sign [2].

The soft-tissue rim sign may be absent with stones larger than 4 mm due to the stone stretching the wall of the ureter, thus limiting the visibility of the edema or when a stone is impacted at the ureterovesical junction [3]. On the other hand ureteral stone should be differentiated from non-ureteral calcified structures such as arterial calcifications and phleboliths [1].

CT has 100% specificity and 65% sensitivity for differentiating phleboliths from a stone in the ureter with 100% positive predictive value of identifying a phleobolith [4].

The calcified phlebolith, which is the comet nucleus, and the surrounding, tapering, eccentric non-calcified segment of the vein, which is the comet tail, make up the comet tail sign [5] (Fig. 25.1b). The presence of indirect secondary signs of acute obstruction (perirenal stranding, renal enlargement, hydronephrosis) favors the diagnosis of ureteral stone. Indeed, 90% of stones with a diameter of 5 mm or less usually migrate spontaneously, aided by antispasmodic anti-inflammatory medication and also diuresis. In contrast, stones larger than 20 mm are resistant to ESWL [1].

Table 25.1 shows the differences between pelvic ureteral stone and phlebolith [1].

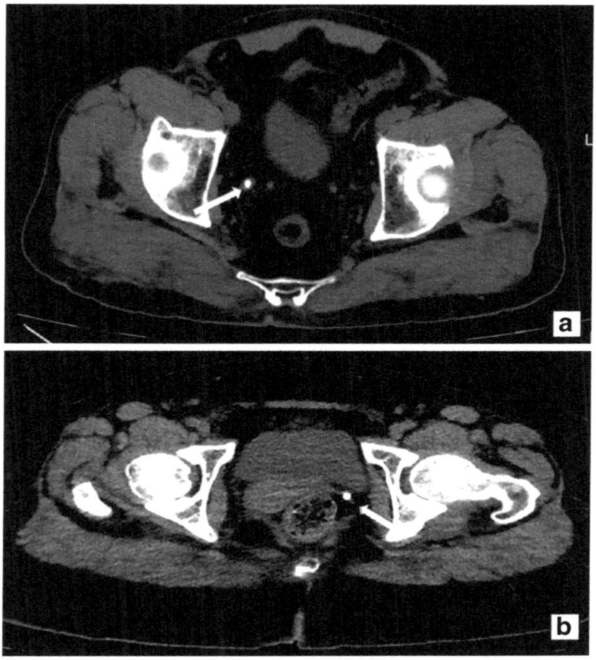

Fig 25.1 (**a**) Axial non contrast CT scan of the pelvis of 48-year-old man shows hyperdense stone right pelvic ureter associated with circumferential soft-tissue rim [arrow] indicating ureteral stone. (**b**) Another non contrast axial CT scan of 56-year-old male patient; shows hyperdense structure at the left pelvic region with posterior soft tissue attenuation [arrow] impressive of comet tail sign of a phlebolith

Table 25.1 The differences between pelvic ureteral stone and phlebolith on CT [1].

	Stone	Phlebolith
Mean attenuation	>300 Hu	<278 Hu
Central lucency	No	Yes (PPV 100%)
Bifid peak at profile analysis	No	Yes
Comet sign	No	Yes
Soft tissue rim sign	Yes (PPV 91%)	No
Shape	Geometric	Rounded

25.3 Bordeaux Glass Sign (Goblet Sign)

In the presence of a slow-growing intraluminal ureteral disease; the "goblet sign"describes the characteristic imaging aspect of a ureter as localized ureteric dilatation around and distal to the filling defect of a tumor [3]. As the mass slowly grows and expands the ureteral lumen, the resulting focally dilated ureter distal to the mass takes on a cup-shaped appearance when opacified with contrast material. The sides of the goblet correspond to the inflated ureteral wall, while the rim corresponds to the inferior contour of the mass (Fig. 25.2).

Presence of the goblet sign suggests a superficial i.e. less aggressive tumor [6].

The sign indicates that the filling defect was caused by a chronic process that allowed the ureter beneath the filling defect to accommodate to the lesion. The appearance is most likely the result of ureteral peristalsis-induced mechanical dilatation of the ureter below the filling defect [3]. Recently, the goblet sign can also be seen on several imaging modalities, including excretory urography, CT, and MR urography, however, it was described originally on retrograde ureteropyelography [6].

Ureteric transitional cell carcinoma [TCC] typically manifests as a single, polypoid-filled defect with ureteric dilatation proximal to the lesion. A diffuse ureteric wall infiltration from an intramural lesion may occasionally fix the ureter [7]. Retrograde pyelography is usually the best technique performed during cystoscopy as fluoroscopic monitoring allows this imaging modality to better visualize the pathology in the urinary tract. Repositioning of the patient can be done on the fluoroscopy head in order to obtain an optimal view of the problem as well as allow collection of a sample for cytologic examination [8].

The goblet sign was originally associated with ureteral transitional cell carcinoma, but it is now seen in a variety of diseases, including metastatic disease and endometriosis that has slowly spread into the ureteral lumen [6]. The ureter is unable to accommodate the obstructing process in the case of an acute obstruction, such as ureterolithiasis. Because no focal downstream ureteral dilatation occurs, a goblet sign is absent. In fact, reactive edema and ureteral spasm frequently narrow the distal ureter, resulting in an acute obstructive process. Because the proximal ureter can be dilated to varying degrees in both acute and chronic situations, depending on the extent of obstruction, it is not a reliable predictor of chronicity [9].

25.4 Bergman Sign [Coiled Catheter Sign]

The dilated ureteral segment below the filling defect provides a potential space that may allow coiling of a catheter within it, if retrograde catheterization is attempted. The appearance of the catheter in this setting has been referred to as the coiled catheter sign. At CT, the site of ureteral caliber transition should be closely inspected for the presence of an intraluminal soft tissue mass, as a reflection of the goblet appearance [3] (Fig. 25.2). Another frequent scenario, Bergman's sign could be identified with twisting *of the ureteral catheter in the dilate segement of the ureter due to presence of a tumor.*

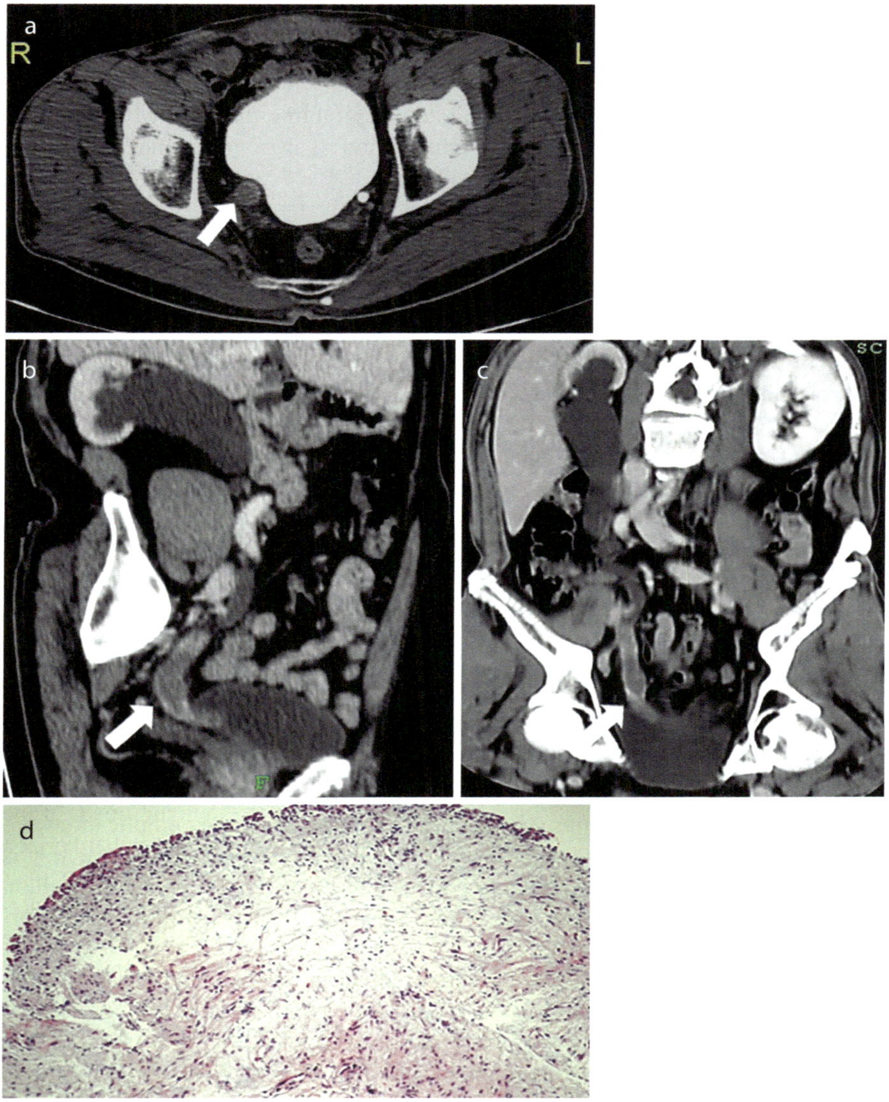

Fig. 25.2 (**a**) Contrast enhanced CT scan of the pelvis at the delayed phase of 57 years old male patient complaining of right loin pan and hematuria for 2 months, shows intraluminal right ureteric soft tissue mass [arrow]. (**b**) Sagittal & (**c**) Coronal reformatted contrast enhanced images at venous phase of the Ct study shows moderate right hydroureteronephrosis down to intraluminal soft tissue mass at the pelvic portion of the ureter giving the goblet appearance [arrows]. (**d**) Postoperative histopathology (Hx&E) X100 sections from the ureteric mass revealed papillary transitional neoplasm infiltrating the muscle layer. Diagnosis is GIII papillary TCC infiltrating the muscle layer of the right ureter

25.5 Curlicue *Ureter (Extraperitoneal Herniation of the Ureter)*

The "curlicue ureter," a ureteral configuration resembling the twist of a pig's tail. Ureteral inguinal herniation is a rare complication of inguinal hernias. It is more commonly caused by an indirect inguinal hernia (80% of cases) than a direct inguinal hernia (20%) [10].

In men in their fifth and sixth decades of life, ureteral inguinal hernias are more common. Furthermore, there are two types of ureteral herniation: para-peritoneal (80%) and extraperitoneal (20%) [11].

A peritoneal sac is thought to be involved in para-peritoneal hernias, in which the neighboring ureter is mechanically pulled through the defect. Extraperitoneal hernias, on the other hand, are characterized by high levels of retroperitoneal fat and are linked to nephroptosis [11]. It can be acquired or congenital in terms of aetiology. A retroperitoneal fat and ureter prolapse through the inguinal canal without a peritoneal sac is an acquired mechanism. However, a congenital cause is thought to be an embryologic abnormality in which the ureteral bud fails to detach from the Wolffian ducts, resulting in ureter development within the scrotum [12].

Patients with a history of renal transplantation are predisposed to this syndrome due to the position of the transplant ureter within the Retzius gap. Because the inferior portion of the Toldt fascia sits at the secondary root of the sigmoid mesocolon and tightens the retroperitoneum, the ureter is rarely herniated on the left; however, this anatomic reinforcement is missing on the right, which explains why the right side has a higher incidence of the finding [10, 13, 14].

Ureteral herniation is usually asymptomatic, and evidence of ureteral herniation is frequently discovered by chance. Strangulation is a rare occurrence. Obesity is still the single most dangerous risk factor [11]. Ureteral hernia complications are uncommon, and many cases go undiagnosed for years. If the ureteral obstruction is severe enough, it can lead to hydronephrosis and renal failure. A more common cause of complications is inadvertent ureter damage during inguinal hernia surgery [14].

Because diagnostic imaging is often not required prior to surgery for reducible inguinal hernias, many ureteral hernias go undetected until direct observation by the surgeon intraoperatively or when symptoms appear postoperatively [15, 16]. For imaging diagnosis, antegrade pyelography was traditionally used, but CT intravenous pyelography has recently been used. Retrograde pyelography can also be used to detect unilateral obstructive nephropathy. An anechoic structure that extends into the inguinal canal and scrotum and is devoid of vascular pulsatile flow will be revealed by colour Doppler sonography [14].

The use of retrograde ureteropyelography or a CT urogram to delineate the course of the ureter, can reveal the classic "curlicue" or "loop the loop" ureter (Fig. 25.3). The ureter should be simply reduced unless absolutely necessary; unnecessary manipulation can jeopardize ureteral blood supply and necessitate additional interventions. If the ureter is damaged or otherwise compromised, a

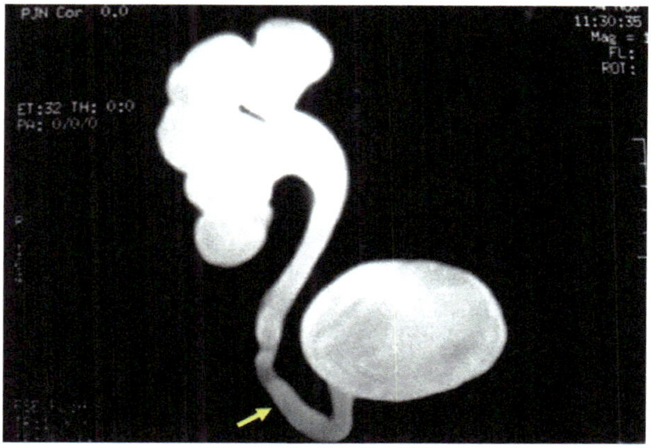

Fig. 25.3 Magnetic resonance urography showing moderate hydroureteronephrosis of the graft with downward displacement of a loop of the lower third ureter [yellow arrow] in the region of a sliding inguinal hernia after renal transplantation. "Reproduced with permission from: Osman et al. [13]

ureteroneocystotomy can be performed [11]. An open surgical technique was used to repair a ureteral inguinal hernia; some authors have claimed that a laparoscopic repair is implausible [17].

25.6 Nutcracker Syndrome

The physical compression of the left renal vein [LRV] can occur between the superior mesenteric artery [SMA] and the aorta ("anterior nutcracker") or between the aorta and an underlying vertebral body ("posterior nutcracker") if the LRV has a retroaortic or circumaortic course [18]. A short aorto-mesenteric distance [AMD] caused by steep angulation of the SMA relative to the aorta can predispose to nutcracker syndrome [19, 20].

The majority of affected patients are young or middle-aged, and more common in females. Any disease that results in rapid weight loss and loss of retroperitoneal fat is considered predisposing factor for nutcracker syndrome [18]. Patients with nutcracker syndrome had a significantly lower AMD of 3 mm and an aortomesentric angle AMA of less than 16° as reported before [21].

Symptoms are caused by increased pressure in the LRV as a result of a restriction in its venous outflow into the inferior vena cava (IVC). This results in the formation of intrarenal and extrarenal hypertensive valveless venous collateral veins, as well as gonadal vein reflux, which is most commonly seen on the left side. The symptoms range from mild to severe, and physical activity may aggravate them. Some of the symptoms include mild microhematuria to severe gross hematuria (which can cause anaemia), mild to severe orthostatic proteinuria, and left flank pain caused by the passage of ureteral blood clots [18, 22].

Multidetector CT or MR imaging in the venous phase after iodinated contrast material injection allows for simultaneous depiction of mesoaortic anatomy as well as focal midline LRV compression and its hemodynamic consequences (prestenotic dilatation; hilar, periureteric, and pelvic varices; dilated gonadal veins). The AMA and AMD are best seen on sagittal MPR images, while varices and dilated gonadal veins are best seen on coronal MPR images (Fig. 25.4). In the age of multidetector CT, IVU is no longer used to rule out suspected nutcracker syndrome. Excretory or retrograde urography can reveal indentations and scalloping of the renal pelvis or ureter caused by increased retroperitoneal varices [18].

A gradient of more than 3 mm Hg has been reported to be hemodynamically important in patients with LRV compression, though a wide range of gradient values has been described. For example, nutcracker syndrome is still a clinical diagnosis that should be made only when specific symptoms are present. Observations of LRV compression on multidetector CT or MR imaging in the absence of varices or symptoms show the nutcracker phenomenon, not nutcracker syndrome [19, 23].

Intervention is recommended for patients who are severely symptomatic. The main goal is to reduce LRV outflow obstruction and hypertension. Numerous surgical approaches have been used, including LRV transposition to the inferior IVC,

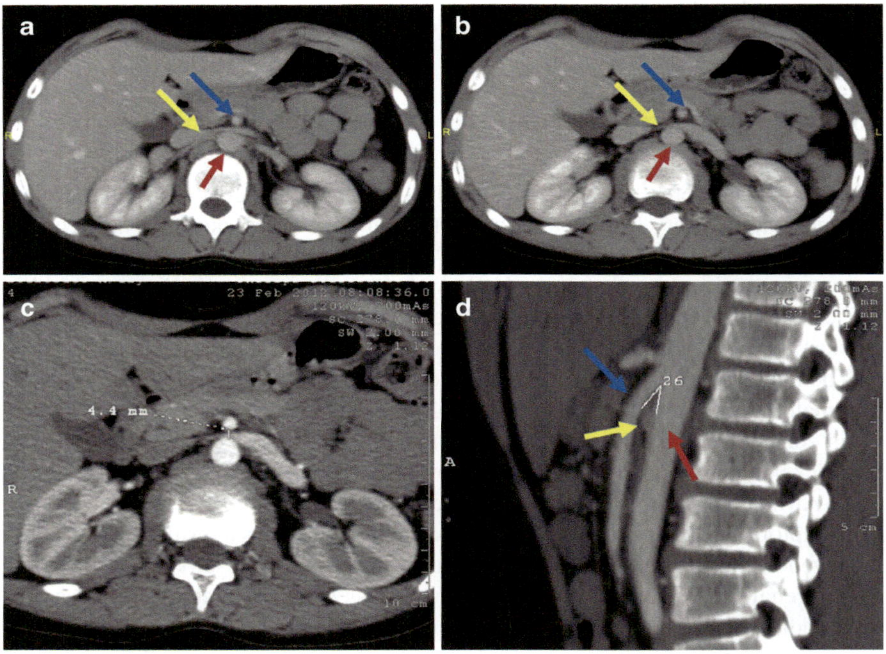

Fig. 25.4 Nutcracker syndrome in a 23-year-old woman with progressive left flank pain, as well as microscopic hematuria. (**a, b**) Axial post contrast enhanced CT of the abdomen at the venous phase shows compression of the LRV [yellow arrow] between the SMA [blue arrow] and the aorta [red arrow] with significant post stenotic dilatation. (**c**) Axial post contrast enhanced CT of the abdomen at the arterial phase shows the distance in between the aorta and superior mesenteric artery = 4 mm. (**d**) Midline sagittal reformatted post contrast enhanced image at the arterial phase shows steep angulation of the SMA with compression of the LRV in the narrowed aortomesenteric angle = 26. LRV [yellow arrow], SMA [blue arrow], aorta [red arrow]

external venous stent placement, LRV bypass surgery, renal autotransplantation to the iliac fossa, and left nephrectomy [19, 23, 24, 25].

25.7 Bullet and Bodkin Sign

The "bullet on bodkin" sign describes the imaging appearance of a sudden transition of ureteral caliber due to extrinsic encasement. A bodkin is a type of mediaeval arrowhead that tapers to a sharp point. The sign denotes ureteral dilation proximal to an abrupt site of ureteral narrowing at the level of the pathologic process. As a result, the radiographic appearance resembles a bullet with its "business end" balanced on the bodkin's tip [26].

The ureter may be encased, resulting in an abrupt change in ureteral caliber (Fig. 25.5). The dilated ureter (the bullet) may appear to be perched precariously on the nondilated, encased ureter (the bodkin, defined as a sharp, slender instrument). Metastatic disease, extension from an adjacent tumour, lymphoma, and, in rare cases, benign inflammatory conditions such as retroperitoneal fibrosis can all cause the bullet and bodkin appearance [3].

This appearance can be caused by both benign and malignant conditions, such as the extension of an adjacent primary tumour into the ureter, metastatic ureter involvement, and encasement by lymphoma or retroperitoneal fibrosis. Each of these disease processes can cause the ureter to narrow to varying degrees. The appearance of a bullet on bodkin in the ureter is important to recognise because it reliably indicates external ureteral encasement, as opposed to narrowing caused by a process intrinsic to the ureter, such as an infiltrating transitional cell carcinoma or stricture caused by infection, trauma, or irradiation [26, 27, 28].

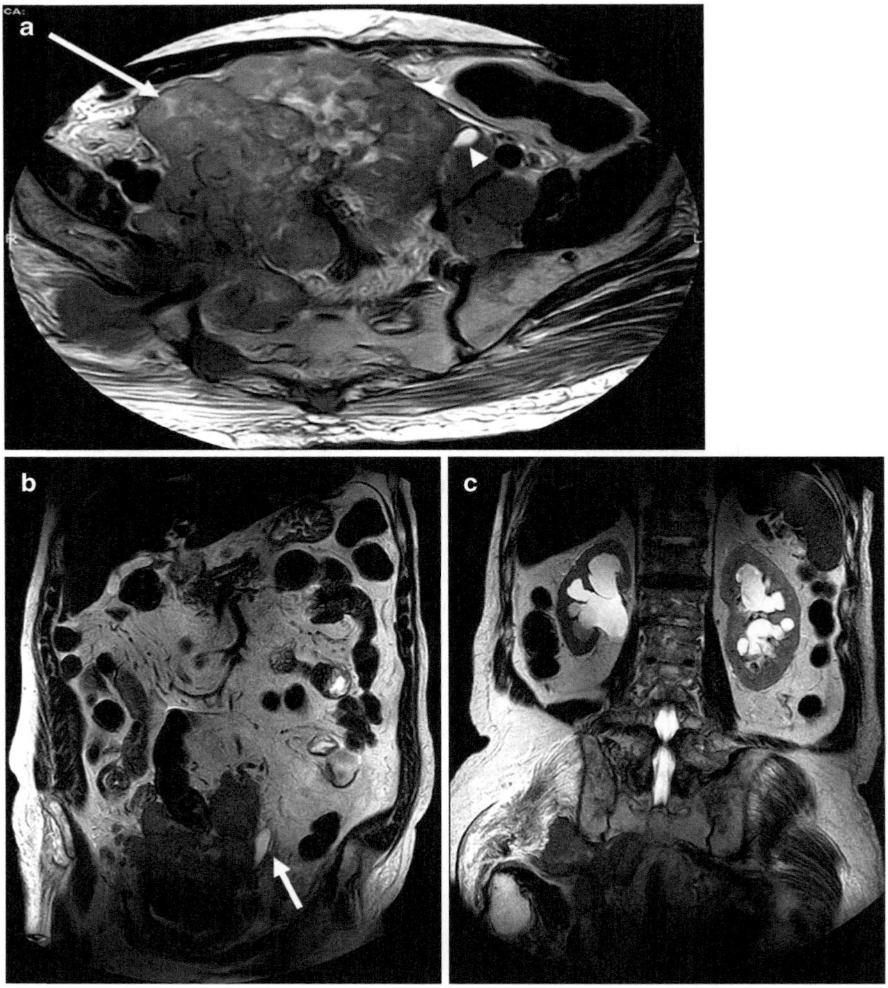

Fig. 25.5 (**a**) Axial T2wi MRI of male patient aged 73 Years old complaining of obstructive LUTS for 2 years shows large well defined lobulated and amalgamated pelvic soft tissue mass [arrow] compressing the left pelvic ureter [arrow head]. (**b**) Coronal T2wi of the abdomen & pelvis shows the abrupt transition of ureteral calibre due to extrinsic encasement and tapers to a sharp point [arrow] giving the appearance of budkin sign. (**c**) Coronal T2WI of the abdomen shows bilateral renal hydronephrosis

25.8 Cobra Head Sign

A ureterocele is a cystic dilatation of the intravesical segment of the distal ureter [1].

The cobra head sign, also known as the spring onion appearance, refers to dilatation of the distal ureter surrounded by a thin lucent line seen in patients with

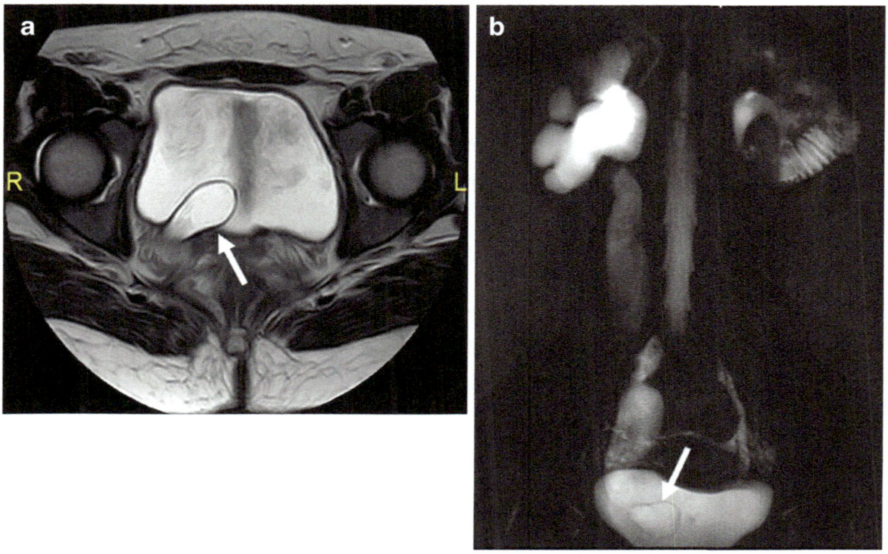

Fig. 25.6 (**a**) Axial high resolution T2WI of the pelvis shows well defined cystic structure inside the urinary bladder surrounded by hypointense halo giving the appearance of copra head sign [arrow] suggesting the presence of ureterocele. (**b**) Coronal single shot MRI of the abdomen and pelvis shows moderate right hydroureteronephrosis down to the ureterocele (Orthotopic ureterocele) [arrow]

adult-type (orthotopic) ureteroceles (Fig. 25.6) [3]. Females have roughly twice the incidence of males. In children, ureterocele can be associated with reflux or an obstructed kidney in a duplicated system [1].

The most common symptoms in adults are pain and, in males, symptoms related to sexual activity (pain during ejaculation, epididymitis). Females are more likely to experience recurring UTI. Incontinence is unusual in males and is uncommon in adult females. The goals of imaging are to demonstrate the significance of upper moiety parenchyma obstruction and/or destruction, the site of ectopic ureter implantation, and, if present, the type of ectopic ureter (intravesical or extravesical) [1].

The upper segment frequently functions poorly, indicating parenchymal destruction and/or dysplastic changes. It appears as a multilocular pseudocystic mass on ultrasonography with dropping Lili sign of the lower moiety. A thorough pelvic examination, possibly via the transrectal or transvaginal route, can reveal the dilated ureter and its ectopic orifice [1]. A CT scan can also show if the upper pole is hypoplastic or hydronephrotic. The dilated ureter can also be followed to the pelvis, but determining the exact position of the ectopic orifice and the presence or absence of ureterocele may be difficult. Multiplanar reconstruction may reveal more about the distal ureter. With fast, heavily T2-weighted or contrast-enhanced sequences, MR urography allows for accurate imaging and multiplanar visualization of the urinary tract from the upper pole to the pelvis (Fig. 25.7). As a result, it may be extremely useful after ultrasonography [29].

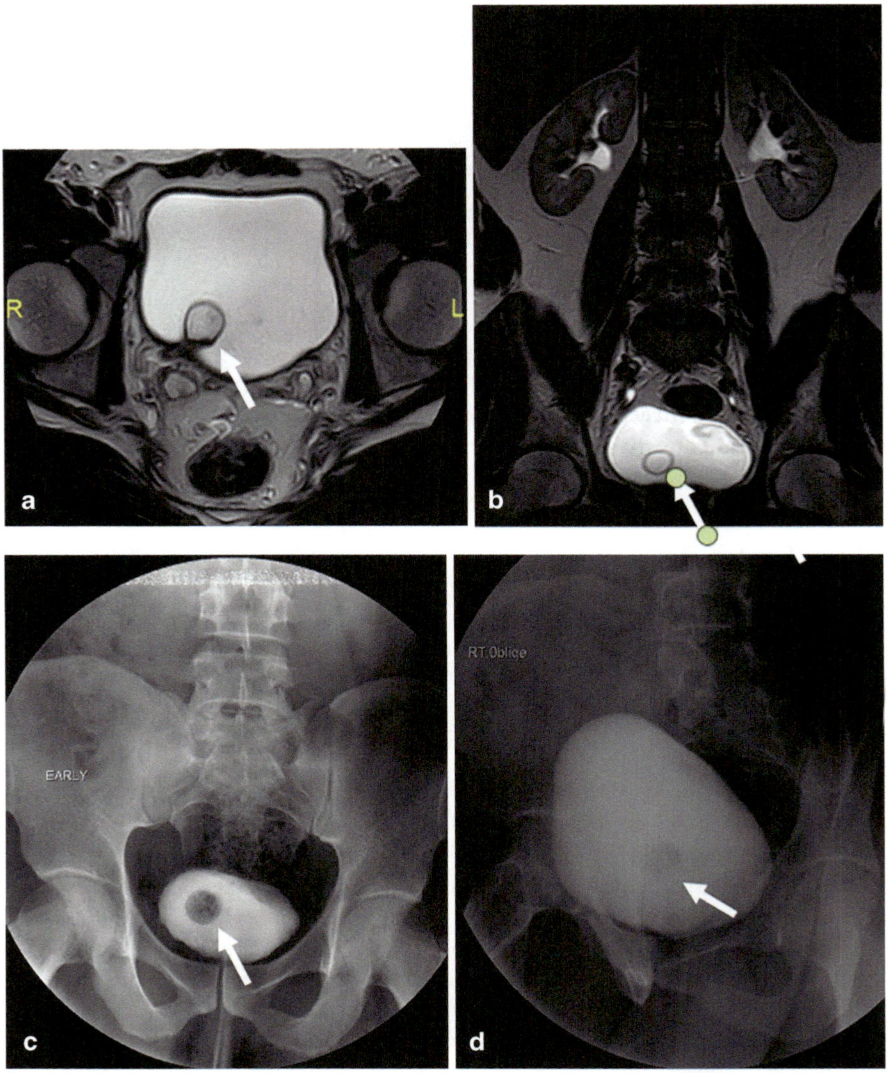

Fig. 25.7 (**a**) Axial High resolution T2WI MRI pelvis shows well defined cystic structure inside the urinary bladder to the right side surrounded by Hypointense halo [arrow] giving the appearance of cobra head sign suggesting the presence of ureterocele. (**b**) Coronal T2WI MRI of the abdomen and pelvis shows mild distended PCSs of both kidneys with evidence of the urinary bladder ureterocele. [arrow]. (**c**) Ascending cystography of the same patient (Early film) shows ureterocele as a rounded smooth filling defect inside the urinary bladder [arrow]. (**d**) Right oblique view of ascending cystography shows the location of ureterocele on the right side [arrow]

A VCUG is always required to rule out a VUR. Treatment is determined by the functional status of the affected kidney: upper moiety and ureter removal, ureteroneocystostomy, or transurethral ureterocele incision [1]. The distal ureter dilates when the flow at the ureteral opening in the bladder is restricted. The combined thickness of the ureteral wall and prolapsed bladder mucosa is represented by the lucent hood, which is delineated by contrast material within the bladder lumen. This lucent line should be thin and well defined. If the cobra's hood thickens, becomes uneven, or loses definition, the presence of a pseudoureterocele should be suspected. A pseudoureterocele can be caused by oedema caused by stone impaction or recent stone passage, or, more importantly, by tumour enlargement of the ureteral orifice. If the appearance is not classic, a cystoscopic examination should be performed [3].

25.9 Weigert-Meyer Law

Complete duplication occurs when two independent ureteral buds emerge from the mesonephric duct. The ureter that drains the upper pole of the kidney has an ectopic distal insertion caudal and medial to the ureter that drains the lower pole. The latter inserts into the bladder either normally in the trigone or more cranially and laterally, making it vulnerable to VUR. The Weigert-Meyer law expresses the two ureters' relationships [1].

The most common congenital abnormality of the upper urinary tract is collecting system duplication, which has an incidence of 0.8–2%. Unilateral duplication is more common than bilateral duplication [30]. Some people may complain of urinary tract infections, haematuria, and, in rare cases, continuous incontinence due to ureteral insertion distal to the urethral sphincter complex [31].

The diagnosis of a duplicated renal collecting system in adulthood is uncommon because the majority of these anomalies are discovered in childhood. When there is complete polar ureteral duplication, both the upper and lower moiety ureters drain into the bladder separately, each with its own orifice. According to the Weigert-Meyer law, the anatomy of the duplex collecting system is as follows: The upper moiety ureter has an ectopic insertion (inferomedially) that is prone to obstruction, which is frequently caused by a ureterocele. The lower moiety ureter has an orthotopic insertion but is susceptible to vesicoureteral reflux (Fig. 25.8) [32, 33]. This is frequently associated with vesicoureteral reflux due to a lack of sufficient submucosal tunnel, which causes pyelonephritis, scarring, and a "drooping lily" appearance on IVPs [34, 35].

Partial duplication is typically diagnosed on examination under anesthesia, while complete duplication is often symptomatic (antenatal diagnosis, urinary tract infection, incontinence) and much more common in females [1]. MRU also provides diagnostic information, which is particularly useful in complex duplex systems. The use of ultrasound to evaluate ectopic ureteral implantation may be difficult. MRU can detect ectopic extravesical implantation even when the upper pole parenchyma is minimal or not functioning properly. MRU can show dysplastic or hypoplastic

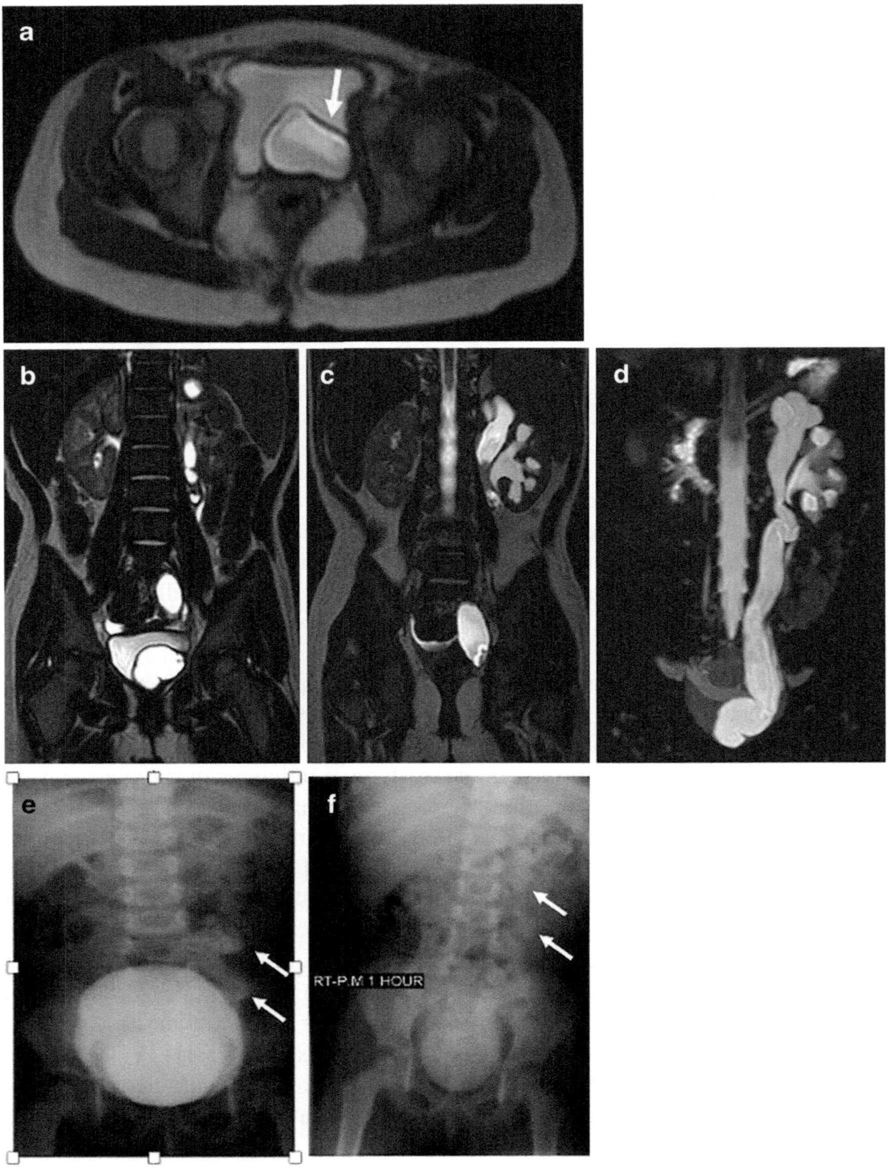

Fig. 25.8 (**a**) Axial high resolution T2WI MRI of the pelvis shows large well defined ureterocele inside the urinary bladder to the left side filled with the high SI as the bladder [arrow]. (**b, c**) Coronal MRU shows duplicated left kidney with dysplastic hydronephrotic upper moiety [due to obstruction] and hydronephrotic of the lower moiety [due to reflux]. (**d**) Coronal single shot MRU shows marked hydronephrotic upper moiety of left renal duplex down to ureterocele. (**e**) Ascending cystogram shows two lumens with different densities of the bladder and ureterocele with grade V VUR at the ureter of lower moiety of left renal duplex. (**f**) Post micturition film about (1 h) shows persistence of the contrast at both ureterocele as well as lower moiety of left renal duplex [arrows]

poles with no or little function due to the natural contrast produced by urine on precontrast T2-weighted images, which is a significant advantage [36]. Surgical correction is sometimes indicated in patients in order to preserve renal function and prevent complications, like infection [37].

25.10 Inverted J Shaped Ureter

Hochstetter identified retrocaval ureter (also known as circumcaval ureter) as a rare congenital defect in 1893. Males have a 2.8-fold higher prevalence than females [38].

Despite the fact that the condition is congenital, patients rarely exhibit symptoms until their third or fourth decade of life. Flank pain, recurring urinary tract infections, calculi above the obstruction, and microscopic or extensive haematuria are all common symptoms [39].

The retrocaval ureter [RCU] develops in response to the maldevelopment of the infrarenal vena cava. RCU is caused by abnormal persistence of the right cardinal vein [40].

Retrocaval ureters are classified into two types based on their radiographic appearance and the location of ureteral narrowing. In Type I, the ureter usually crosses behind the IVC at the level of the third or fourth lumbar vertebra, and IVU examination reveals a *typical* 'fish-hook' shaped ureter deformity (Fig. 25.9). Type II is less common, and the ureter's retrocaval segment crosses higher at the level of the renal pelvis. CT scans and magnetic resonance imaging are both effective methods of confirming the diagnosis, and surgical intervention is frequently required [41].

Ultrasonography, antegrade and retrograde pyelography with inferior venocavography, and intravenous urogram (IVU) were frequently used to diagnose circumcaval ureter. Because they are the least invasive and have the inherent ability to depict the lesion in three dimensions, CT scans and magnetic resonance imaging (MRI) are currently thought to be the most effective means of verifying the diagnosis [40]. Treatment of the retrocaval ureter includes open or laparoscopic surgery. Surgical correction is not required in individuals with no subjective symptoms or hydronephrosis, and therapeutic abstinence is justified [41].

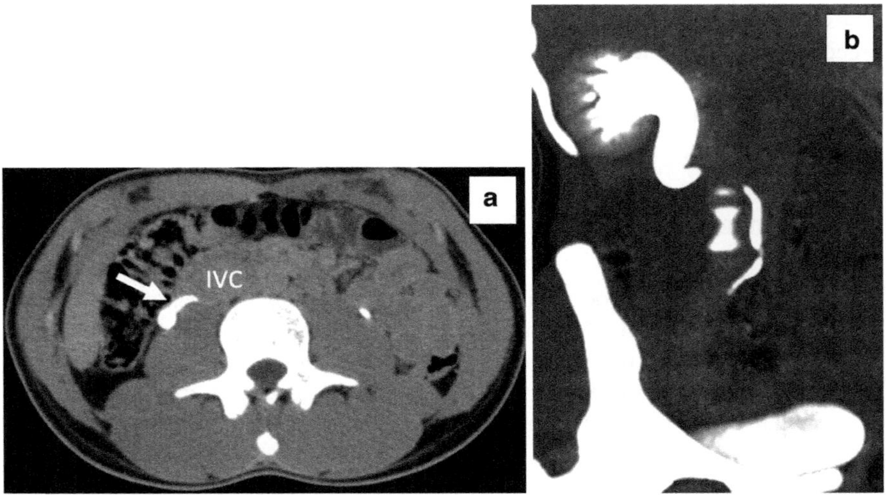

Fig. 25.9 (**a**) Axial post contrast CT scan of the abdomen at the delayed phase shows the course of right ureter [arrow] behind the IVC. (**b**) CTU of the abdomen and pelvis shows right moderate hydroureteronephrosis with kinked ureter passing midline behind the IVC giving J shaped ureter of the retrocaval course

25.11 Median Waist Deformity Sign

The fibrotic plaque associated with retroperitoneal fibrosis (RPF) is usually centered at the lumbosacral junction, often encircling the abdominal aorta, inferior vena cava, and iliac vessels [42]. The fibrotic process can also affect the ureters, causing them to be drawn medially and altering the normal ureteral course. When both ureters are involved, the more medial position of the opacified mid to lower ureters seen on excretory urography (EXU), CT or MR urography is said to ascribe the "figure" of *a narrow-waisted maiden* [43].

Aside from medial deviation, the fibrotic plaque may cause tapered narrowing of one or both ureter lumens in the lower lumbar or upper sacral region (Fig. 25.10). The ureteral narrowing is associated with varying degrees of unilateral or bilateral hydroureteronephrosis, which is frequently accompanied by delayed excretion of contrast material [3].

The vast majority of RPF cases are idiopathic, and the condition is sometimes referred to as Ormond's disease. Certain drugs, malignancy, infection, vascular and autoimmune disease have all been linked to the development of RPF. If diagnosed and treated promptly, the condition has a good prognosis. RPF has traditionally been treated surgically, but after initial relief of urinary tract obstruction, medical strategies involving steroids, Tamoxifen, and immunosuppression have shown promising results [43].

Retroperitoneal fibrosis (RPF) is a rare but serious condition characterized by chronic nonspecific inflammation of the retroperitoneum that can entrap and

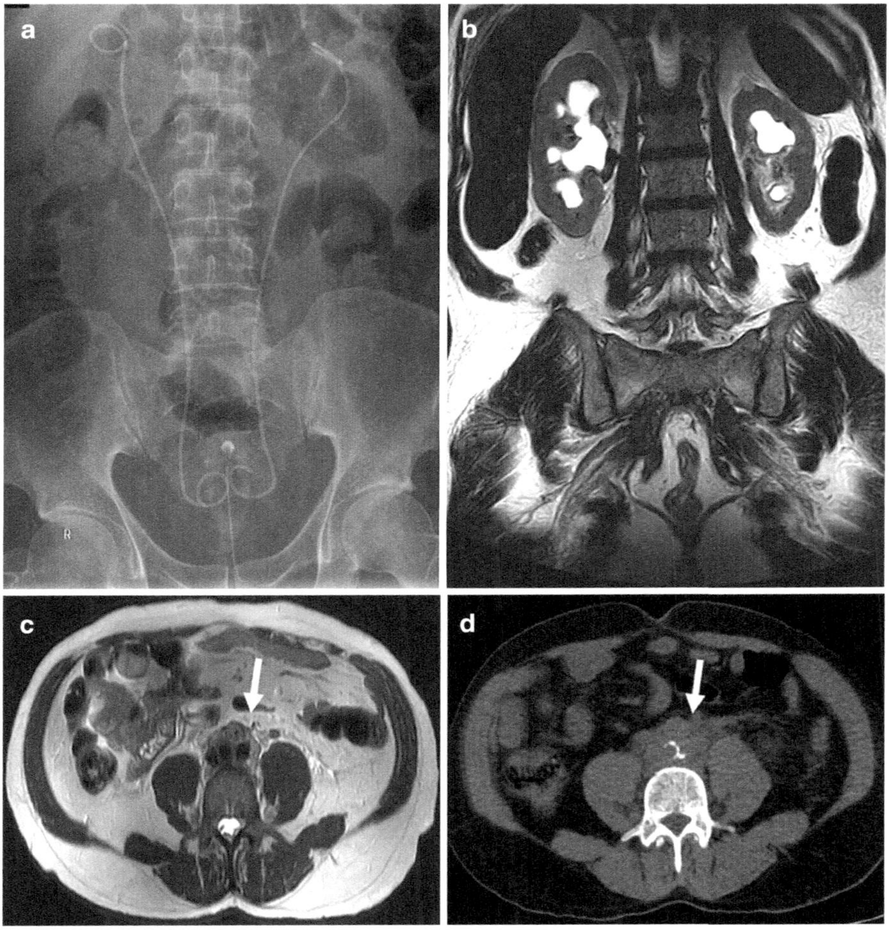

Fig. 25.10 (**a**) plain X ray of the abdomen and pelvis (KUB) shows evidence of bilateral renal double J stents with medicalization of their course opposite L4&5 levels. (**b**) Coronal T2WI shows bilateral renal hydronephrotic changes. (**c**) Axial T2WI of the abdomen shows evidence of intermediate soft tissue intensity encircling the both common iliac vessels as well as both ureters. (**d**) Axial non contrast CT scan of the abdomen shows, soft tissue density [arrow] at the encircling the level of common iliac vessels and ureters. Biopsy was taken proved retroperitoneal fibrosis

obstruct retroperitoneal structures, most notably the ureters. More than two-thirds of all cases of RPF are idiopathic, with the remainder being secondary to various causes such as tumors, infections, radiotherapy, and drugs. Tobacco use is a risk factor for RPF. RPF symptoms include flank pain, unexplained systemic symptoms (fatigue, weight loss), and less frequently, lower extremity swelling, oliguria or anuria, and testicular pain. Inflammatory markers in the blood, such as erythrocyte sedimentation rate (ESR) and C-reactive protein, are usually elevated [44].

In the last few years, an association with IgG4 related disease has been shown and serum IgG4 levels are often elevated [45]. Because of the vague symptoms, diagnosis is often delayed. Diagnosis of RPF relies primarily on imaging studies. Histopathology is useful to rule out malignancy. Historically, treatment has focused on relieving the ureteral obstruction with cystoscopy assisted placement of ureteral stents followed by more definitive resolution of ureteric obstruction with open or laparoscopic ureterolysis. However, recently, medical measures—steroids and immunosuppressive agents are preferred. Currently, treatment in the acute phase rests on steroids with a tapering schedule, variably combined with immunosuppressive agents in the later period. Surgical measures are reserved for patient's refractory to medical management or those with advanced fibrosis requiring relief of ureteral obstruction.

Diagnosis and management of RPF represent a challenge for clinicians. Because of the non-specific nature of the symptoms and the lack of sensitive and specific laboratory tests, RPF is frequently detected only after severe renal failure has been established. Furthermore, if promptly diagnosed and treated, most benign forms of RPF have a good prognosis, whereas malignant RPF carries a very poor prognosis, with a mean survival of less than 6 months [46].

Questions

1. Which is the most diagnostic CT feature of a phlebolith?
   (a) Mean attenuation above 1000 Hu.
   (b) Display soft tissue rim sign.
   (c) Elliptical in shape.
   (d) Have central lusceny (Central Umbilication).

Answer: (d)

2. Which of the following is associated with the goblet sign?
   (a) Metastasis of the ureter.
   (b) Transitional cell carcinoma of the ureter.
   (c) Endometriosis of the ureter.
   (d) All of the above.

Answer: (d)

3. Select the most appropriate statement describing the Nut-cracker phenomenon.
   (a) Asymptomatic dilatation of the left renal vein due to compression between the aorta and superior mesenteric artery.
   (b) More common I children.
   (c) Dilatation of left renal vein in patients with hematuria, proteinuria and hypertension.
   (d) Needs interventional management by repositioning of the left renal vein most inferior to the IVC.

Answer: (a)

4. Select the most appropriate statement describing Bullet and bodkin sign.
   (a) Occurs with malignant conditions as primary ureteric tumor, metastatic ureteric involvement, and infiltration by TCC.
   (b) Not occur with benign conditions.
   (c) Change in the ureter caliber due to extrinsic encasement.
   (d) More common in children.

Answer: (c)

5. Regarding Copra head sign, which statement is correct?
   (a) Means dilatation of the pelvic ureter.
   (b) Better seen on excretory phase of IVU.
   (c) More common in males
   (d) There is no radiological difference between ureterocele and pseudo ureterocele.

Answer: (b)

References

1. Joffre F, Otal PH, Soulie M, editors. Radiological imaging of the ureter. Berlin: Springer; 2003. p. 63–100.
2. Wah TM. Unenhanced CT in the evaluation of renal/ureteric colic. Imaging Med. 2013;5(4):371–82.
3. Dyer RB, Chen MY, Zagoria RJ. Classic signs in uroradiology. Radiographics. 2004;24(Suppl 1):S247–80. https://doi.org/10.1148/rg.24si045509. PMID: 15486245.
4. Boridy IC, Nikolaidis P, Kawashima A, Goldman SM, Sandler CM. Ureterolithiasis: value of the tail sign in differentiating phleboliths from ureteral calculi at nonenhanced helical CT. Radiology. 1999;211(3):619–21. https://doi.org/10.1148/radiology.211.3.r99ma44619. PMID: 10352582.
5. Guest AR, Cohan RH, Korobkin M, Platt JF, Bundschu CC, Francis IR, Gebramarium A, Murray UM. Assessment of the clinical utility of the rim and comet-tail signs in differentiating ureteral stones from phleboliths. AJR Am J Roentgenol. 2001;177(6):1285–91. https://doi.org/10.2214/ajr.177.6.1771285. PMID: 11717067.
6. Morgan WJ, Dyer RB. The goblet sign. Abdom Imaging. 2015;40(4):931–3. https://doi.org/10.1007/s00261-014-0273-z. PMID: 25331566.
7. Browne RF, Meehan CP, Colville J, Power R, Torreggiani WC. Transitional cell carcinoma of the upper urinary tract: spectrum of imaging findings. Radiographics. 2005;25(6):1609–27. https://doi.org/10.1148/rg.256045517. PMID: 16284138.
8. Inman BA, Blute ML, Hartman RP. Urothelial cell carcinoma of the upper urinary tract: introduction. Imag Oncol Urol. ch 11. 2009:121–44.
9. Daniels RE 3rd. The goblet sign. Radiology. 1999;210(3):737–8. https://doi.org/10.1148/radiology.210.3.r99mr04737. PMID: 10207475.
10. Yahya Z, Al-Habbal Y, Hassen S. Ureteral inguinal hernia: an uncommon trap for general surgeons. BMJ Case Rep. 2017;2017:bcr2017219288. https://doi.org/10.1136/bcr-2017-219288. PMID: 28275027; PMCID: PMC5353493.
11. Pucheril D, Chun B, Dalela D, Abdollah F, Laker SA, Rogers CG. Robot-assisted laparoscopic repair of extraperitoneal ureteral inguinal hernia with mesh placement. J Endourol Case

Rep. 2017;3(1):97–100. https://doi.org/10.1089/cren.2017.0046. PMID: 28894843; PMCID: PMC5587904.
12. Giuly J, François GF, Giuly D, Leroux C, Nguyen-Cat RR. Intrascrotal hernia of the ureter and fatty hernia. Hernia. 2003;7(1):47–9. https://doi.org/10.1007/s10029-002-0091-z. Epub 2002 Nov 1. PMID: 12612799.
13. Osman Y, Ali-El-Dein B, El-Leithy R, Shokeir A. Sliding hernia containing the ureter--a rare cause of graft hydroureteronephrosis: a case report. Transplant Proc. 2004;36(5):1402–4. https://doi.org/10.1016/j.transproceed.2004.05.008. PMID: 15251343.
14. Epps JC, Close TP. Extraperitoneal herniation of the ureter. Appl Radiol. 2019;48(2):44–5.
15. Falidas E, Gourgiotis S, Veloudis G, Exarchou E, Vlachos K, Villias C. Asymptomatic extraperitoneal inguinoscrotal hernia involving ureter: a case presentation and review of the literature. J Nat Sci Biol Med. 2015;6(Suppl 1):S153–5. https://doi.org/10.4103/0976-9668.166126. PMID: 26604607; PMCID: PMC4630751.
16. Berger D. Evidence-based hernia treatment in adults. Dtsch Arztebl Int. 2016;113(9):150–7. https://doi.org/10.3238/arztebl.2016.0150. quiz 158. PMID: 26987468; PMCID: PMC4802357.
17. Ghielmini E, Julita L, Cerantola Y, Matter M, Zingg T. Inguinal bladder hernia with acute ureteral obstruction 14 years after kidney transplantation: a case report. Transplant Proc. 2017;49(7):1593–5. https://doi.org/10.1016/j.transproceed.2017.04.003. PMID: 28838448.
18. Lamba R, Tanner DT, Sekhon S, McGahan JP, Corwin MT, Lall CG. Multidetector CT of vascular compression syndromes in the abdomen and pelvis. Radiographics. 2014;34(1):93–115. https://doi.org/10.1148/rg.341125010. Erratum in: Radiographics. 2015 May-Jun; 35(3): 973. PMID: 24428284.
19. Menard MT. Nutcracker syndrome: when should it be treated and how? Perspect Vasc Surg Endovasc Ther. 2009;21(2):117–24. https://doi.org/10.1177/1531003509338402. Epub 2009 Aug 23. PMID: 19703821.
20. Kurklinsky AK, Rooke TW. Nutcracker phenomenon and nutcracker syndrome. Mayo Clin Proc. 2010;85(6):552–9. https://doi.org/10.4065/mcp.2009.0586. PMID: 20511485; PMCID: PMC2878259.
21. Fu WJ, Hong BF, Xiao YY, Yang Y, Cai W, Gao JP, Guo G, Wang XX. Diagnosis of the nutcracker phenomenon by multislice helical computed tomography angiography. Chin Med J. 2004;117(12):1873–5. PMID: 15603725.
22. Scultetus AH, Villavicencio JL, Gillespie DL. The nutcracker syndrome: its role in the pelvic venous disorders. J Vasc Surg. 2001;34(5):812–9. https://doi.org/10.1067/mva.2001.118802. PMID: 11700480.
23. Reed NR, Kalra M, Bower TC, Vrtiska TJ, Ricotta JJ 2nd, Gloviczki P. Left renal vein transposition for nutcracker syndrome. J Vasc Surg. 2009;49(2):386–93. https://doi.org/10.1016/j.jvs.2008.09.051. discussion 393–4. PMID: 19216958.
24. Rudloff U, Holmes RJ, Prem JT, Faust GR, Moldwin R, Siegel D. Mesoaortic compression of the left renal vein (nutcracker syndrome): case reports and review of the literature. Ann Vasc Surg. 2006;20(1):120–9. https://doi.org/10.1007/s10016-005-5016-8. PMID: 16374539.
25. Ali-El-Dein B, Osman Y, Shehab El-Din AB, El-Diasty T, Mansour O, Ghoneim MA. Anterior and posterior nutcracker syndrome: a report on 11 cases. Transplant Proc. 2003;35(2):851–3. https://doi.org/10.1016/s0041-1345(02)04026-5. PMID: 126441630.
26. Hanley-Knutson K, Dyer RB. The bullet on bodkin sign. Abdom Radiol (NY). 2016;41(2):338–9. https://doi.org/10.1007/s00261-015-0566-x. PMID: 26867918.
27. El-Ghar MA, Farg H, Sharaf DE, El-Diasty T. CT and MRI in urinary tract infections: a spectrum of different imaging findings. Medicina (Kaunas). 2021;57(1):32. https://doi.org/10.3390/medicina57010032. PMID: 33401464; PMCID: PMC7824127.
28. Shebel HM, Al-Natour MS, Elsamaloty H. Cross-sectional imaging of the kidney. In: Elsayes KM, editor. Cross-sectional imaging of the abdomen and pelvis. New York: Springer; 2015. https://doi.org/10.1007/978-1-4939-1884-3_25.

29. Engin G, Esen T, Rozanes I. MR urography findings of a duplicated ectopic ureter in an adult man. Eur Radiol. 2000;10(8):1253–6. https://doi.org/10.1007/s003300000319. PMID: 10939484.
30. Lenton J, Wah T. Pelvo-ureteric junction obstruction in the lower pole moiety of a duplex kidney with an associated intraparenchymal abscess: a case report. J Med Case Rep. 2008;2:241. https://doi.org/10.1186/1752-1947-2-241. PMID: 18652665; PMCID: PMC2494999.
31. Mishra K, Elliott CS. A violation of the Weigert-Meyer law – an ectopic ureter arising from the lower renal pole. J Clin Urol. 2017;10(3):202–4.
32. Başdaş C, Çelebi S, Özaydın S, Karaaslan B, Alim ER, Güvenç Ü, Sander S. Unusual presentation of duplex kidneys: ureteropelvic junction obstruction. Ther Adv Urol. 2016;2016:7960794. https://doi.org/10.1155/2016/7960794. Epub 2016 Oct 18. PMID: 27829833; PMCID: PMC5088327.
33. Scantling D, Ross C, Altman H. A 52-year-old male with bilaterally duplicated collecting systems with obstructing ureteral stones: a case report. Curr Urol. 2013;7(2):104–6. https://doi.org/10.1159/000356257. Epub 2013 Oct 30. PMID: 24917767; PMCID: PMC4017758.
34. Esfahani SA, Close C, Yousefzadeh DK. Side-to-side and interpolar renal duplications: the nonpolar variety. Int Urol Nephrol. 2013;45(2):333–8. https://doi.org/10.1007/s11255-013-0383-5. Epub 2013 Feb 5. PMID: 23381502.
35. Zamani R, Martinez R, Reddy MP. Duplicated collecting system: not following Weigert-Meyer rule as a result of renal stone obstructing the lower ureteropelvic junction. Clin Nucl Med. 2004;29(6):386–7. https://doi.org/10.1097/01.rlu.0000127098.63372.30. PMID: 15166891.
36. Adeb M, Darge K, Dillman JR, Carr M, Epelman M. Magnetic resonance urography in evaluation of duplicated renal collecting systems. Magn Reson Imaging Clin N Am. 2013;21(4):717–30. https://doi.org/10.1016/j.mric.2013.04.002. Epub 2013 Aug 9. PMID: 24183522.
37. Rathbun JAR, Buatsi EM. Weigert-Meyer Law violation with lower pole obstruction and ectopia. Surg Case Rep. 2020;3(2):3–4.
38. Hsu HL, Huang KH, Liu KL. Retrocaval ureter. QJM. 2011;104(1):65–6. https://doi.org/10.1093/qjmed/hcq010. Epub 2010 Feb 15. PMID: 20156989.
39. Kanojia RP, Bawa M, Handu AT, Naredi BK, Menon P, Rao KL. Retrocaval ureter with stone in the retrocaval segment of the ureter. Pediatr Surg Int. 2010;26(8):863–5. https://doi.org/10.1007/s00383-010-2607-4. Epub 2010 Apr 30. PMID: 20431890.
40. Al-Hajjaj M, Aljool AA. Retrocaval ureter with ureteral calculus: case report. Urol Case Rep. 2020;33:101288. https://doi.org/10.1016/j.eucr.2020.101288. PMID: 32518758; PMCID: PMC7270211.
41. Acharya SK, Jindal B, Yadav DK, Singha S, Bagga D. Retrocaval ureter: a rare cause of hydronephrosis in children. J Pediatr Surg. 2009;44(4):846–8. https://doi.org/10.1016/j.jpedsurg.2008.11.053. PMID: 19361652.
42. Caiafa RO, Vinuesa AS, Izquierdo RS, Brufau BP, Ayuso Colella JR, Molina CN. Retroperitoneal fibrosis: role of imaging in diagnosis and follow-up. Radiographics. 2013;33(2):535–52. https://doi.org/10.1148/rg.332125085. Erratum in: Radiographics. 2014 Jan-Feb; 34(1): 15a. PMID: 23479712.
43. Ponnatapura J, Dyer RB. The "maiden waist" sign of the ureters. Abdom Radiol (NY). 2019;44(5):1940–1. https://doi.org/10.1007/s00261-018-01890-4. PMID: 30603883.
44. Jadhav KK, Kumar V, Punatar CB, Joshi VS, Sagade SN. Retroperitoneal fibrosis-clinical presentation and outcome analysis from urological perspective. Investig Clin Urol. 2017;58(5):371–7. https://doi.org/10.4111/icu.2017.58.5.371. Epub 2017 Aug 4. PMID: 28868510; PMCID: PMC5577335.
45. Khosroshahi A, Stone JH. A clinical overview of IgG4-related systemic disease. Curr Opin Rheumatol. 2011;23(1):57–66. https://doi.org/10.1097/BOR.0b013e3283418057. PMID: 21124086.
46. Scheel PJ Jr, Feeley N. Retroperitoneal fibrosis. Rheum Dis Clin N Am. 2013;39(2):365–81. https://doi.org/10.1016/j.rdc.2013.02.004. Epub 2013 Mar 9. PMID: 23597969.

Chapter 26
Ureteral Fistulae

Yasser Osman and Mohamed Elawdy

Abstract The three main types of ureteral fistulae are ureterogenital, ureteroenteric, and ureteroarterial. A ureterogenital fistula is a communication between the lower ureter and the genital tract. It is usually due to iatrogenic ureteral injury during hysterectomy. If discovered early, simple insertion of a ureteral stent may suffice. If that fails, a percutaneous nephrostomy to divert the urine may give the fistula a chance to close. If those conservative measures fail, ureteroneocystostomy is usually curative. Ureterocolonic fistula is usually communication between the left ureter and the sigmoid colon due to a diverticular abscess. A contrast enema is usually diagnostic, and management usually requires surgery. Ureteroarterial fistula is a communication between a ureter and one of the iliac arteries. A previous vascular procedure is the major risk factor. The diagnosis is made by arteriography and retrograde pyelography. Most patients are treated with endovascular embolization or an endovascular stent. Ureteropancreatic, ureteroduodenal, ureteroperitoneal and, ureterolymphatic fistulae are extremely rare.

Keywords Ureteral fistulae · Ureterovaginal · Ureterouterine · Ureteroarterial fistula · Ureterocolic fistula · Iatrogenic ureteral injuries

Abbreviations

CS	Cesarean section
CT	Computed tomography

Test your learning and check your understanding of this book's contents: use the "Springer Nature Flashcards" app to access questions. To use the app, please follow the instructions in Chapter 1.

Y. Osman
Mansoura Urology and Nephrology Center, Mansoura University, Mansoura, Egypt

M. Elawdy (✉)
Consultant Urologist, Ministry of Health, Muscat, Oman

M. Abdel-Gawad et al. (eds.), *The Ureter*,
https://doi.org/10.1007/978-3-031-36212-5_26

CTU	Computed tomography urography
DJ	Double J
ERCP	Endoscopic retrograde cholangiopancreatography
IUIs	Iatrogenic ureteral injuries
MRU	Magnetic resonance urography
UAF	Ureteroarterial fistula
UCF	Ureterocolic fistula
UF	Ureteral fistula
UUF	Ureterouterine fistula
UVF	Ureterovaginal fistula

Learning Objectives
After reading this chapter, the readers are expected to know:

- The major types of ureteral fistulae
- The pathophysiology and risk factors for the development of each type of fistula
- The clinical presentations, the diagnostic studies of choice, and management of each type of fistula

26.1 Introduction

Ureteral fistula is generally a rarely reported urologic disorder with no definite guidelines in its management in view of limited data in the literature which is mostly derived from short case reports or series. This topic has rarely been addressed in urology books and in most cases, it is difficult to find a thorough review. For that reason, we aimed in this concise chapter to introduce a comprehensive review as a source in discussing topics on ureteral fistulae. Details on the surgical procedures of the ureter, such as ureteroneocystostomy, are out of the scope of this chapter and can be found in other resources.

26.2 Ureteral Fistulae

A fistula is a pathological communication between two epithelized surfaces. The ureter is lined by transitional cell epithelium, and a fistula can form between the ureter and the skin or internal organs with an epithelial lining. Formation of a ureteral fistula requires exposure of the ureteral lumen with subsequent urinary extravasation which is mainly a sequence of ureteral injuries that can be traumatic (blunt, penetrating or iatrogenic), or as a consequence of the invasion of the ureteral wall by neoplastic conditions.

When the ureter is involved in traumatic injury alone with subsequent urinary extravasation, and if left untreated, urine can find its way through the wound to the skin forming a ureterocutaneous fistula. The fistula may also develop internally between the ureter and another epithelized structure. The internal structure can be a hollow organ with epithelial linings, such as the uterus, intestine or colon, or a tubal epithelized structure, such as a vessel and the Fallopian tube. The internal fistula could form when both the ureter and internal structure are injured at the same time with exposure of both epithelial surfaces.

The ureter is a delicate structure with special anatomical considerations; having a small caliber and being situated deeply in the retroperitoneal space gives it relative protection from being involved in external traumatic injuries. On the other hand, the lower ureter has an immediate relationship to important abdominal and pelvic structures, such as the female genital organs, colonic mesentery, and iliac vessels. That makes the lower ureter more prone to iatrogenic injuries. So, iatrogenic ureteral injuries (IUIs) are the most common causes of ureteral fistulae. Obstetrics, gynecology, colorectal, and vascular surgeries are the most common surgeries associated with IUIs [1]. Knowing the anatomical course of the ureter and its relationship to the pelvic organs and vessels is of paramount importance, so blind mass clamping at the anatomical sites of the ureter may result in IUIs with deleterious effects.

The ureter takes its blood supply from different abdominal and pelvic arteries. The ureter also has an extensive anastomotic network of arterial supplies and venous drainage that runs within its adventitia. So, excess ureterolysis with adventitial stripping results in segmental ureteral ischemia and necrosis that could end with a fistula if passed unnoticed and left untreated.

In a case series of ureteral injuries, including 33 patients, all had urinary incontinence at presentation while only 7 (21%) presented with flank pain due to an affected ipsilateral renal unit. The vast majority (28/33, 84%) of ureteric injuries from surgical misadventures contributed from the obstetric 17 (60%) and gynecological procedures 11 (40%) [2].

The incidence of iatrogenic ureteral injuries (IUIs) that have resulted from endourological procedures was initially high, but has subsequently decreased [3]. With the development of small caliber ureteroscopes, improved optics and experience with the advent of flexible ureteroscopy (URS) and durable access sheaths, ureteral injury is now a rare event, and most injuries are not severe, detected early, and stented [4]. However, the incidence of IUIs in other surgical specialties has been rising. This is due to the increase in the rate of cesarean section, the wide use of laparoscopy, minimally-invasive procedures, and robotic surgeries in gynecological, colorectal surgeries, and endovascular cover stent graft.

In all forms of acute iatrogenic ureteral injury, such as ligation, thermal coagulation, and partial or complete transection, the onset of the ureteral fistula is acute. So, all precautions should be taken to avoid IUIs; prevention is better than a cure. On the other hand, the onset of ureteral fistula could be insidious and takes a longer time to develop which is the case in those injuries that induce erosion of the ureteral wall inducing gradual ischemia, such as ureteroarterial fistula which results from arterial synthetic graft or as a consequence of radiotherapy.

The symptoms of UF vary based on its onset, location, and the involved structures. Ureteral fistula that accompanies IUIs could present early in the postoperative period with symptoms of urinary extravasation, fever, unexplained abdominal pain, abdominal distention, delayed healing of the wound, urinary leakage, intra-abdominal urinoma, and elevated serum creatinine. If these symptoms are mild and pass unnoticed, the fistula may form within a few days to weeks. The symptoms of UF are either due to the passage of urine to another epithelized structure, inducing urinary leakage, or the passage of the contents of the epithelized structure to the urine. That depends on the nature of the contents and relative intraluminal pressure inside the ureter and the other structure.

Because urinary production is a continuous process, continuous urinary leakage in the presence of voided urine is the hallmark of ureterocutaneous fistulae and ureterogenital fistulae. On the other hand, when there is a fistula between the ureter and an artery, the blood passes to the ureter owing to the high pressure and continuous blood flow. Similarly, the gas pressure inside the intestine and colon makes the ureteroenteric fistulae associated with the passage of air with intestinal or fecal contents with urine. In some instances, and if the ureteral fistulae are associated with ureteral stenosis, it could develop progressive hydronephrosis which ends in renal loss if undetected and untreated early. Flank pain from kidney obstruction could be the first manifestation of ureteral fistulae.

The diagnosis of the ureteral fistula is quite straightforward. It accounts principally on the clinical picture and presentation. The presence of one of the previous symptoms with a recent surgical history of pelvic surgery involving colorectal, female genital or vascular surgeries, is highly suspicious for a ureteral fistula. Continuous urinary leakage may induce soreness, infection, and excoriation to the skin or external genitalia. Despite this negative impact, urinary leakage is in fact protective of the kidney. This may explain why most patients maintain ipsilateral renal function despite having a fistula for a long duration. Urine may show abnormal findings, such as haematuria, air, intestinal or fecal matter based on the type of fistula.

Even with an obvious clinical picture of a fistula, imaging studies are ordered to determine the exact location, extent, and any associated other fistulae—all guiding the decision of proper surgical approach and plan. Intravenous urography (IVU) was the traditional method of imaging modality that has been nearly replaced with CT urography. If the diagnosis is unconfirmed with CT urography, retrograde urography can be performed, and it is a prerequisite step if endoscopic management, such as stenting, is planned. Additional imaging modalities can be ordered based on the type of the fistula; angiography for ureteroarterial fistula and barium studies with a barium enema or barium small bowel follow-through for ureteroenteric fistulae.

The treatment of ureteral fistulae depends on many factors: patient, kidney, and the condition of the both ureter and the other structure. Patient factors include age, associated comorbidities, previous radiotherapy, and the presence of active malignancy. Performing reconstructive surgery on the ureter requires good renal function;

otherwise, regular exchange of ureteral stent or nephrectomy is indicated. The location of the fistula and its extent, the condition of the other structures (intestine, colon, etc.), all these parameters determine which modality is appropriate in treating the fistula.

There are different ways to minimize ureteral fistula formation: good knowledge of the ureteral anatomy, preserving its blood supply by keeping ureteral adventitia and avoiding excessive ureterolysis, and the electrocauterization should be away from the ureteral wall. Surgeons should be fully aware of the anatomical course of the ureter and the common sites of ureteral injuries, especially when it is crossed by the uterine artery. For any suspected ureteral injury intraoperatively, early identification and management based on the nature of the injury are mandatory. Minimally invasive laparoscopic or robotic procedures depend usually on visual cues with a lack of tactile indicators of the ureter and its identification. Subsequently, these procedures are expected to be associated with a higher incidence of ureteral injury [5, 6]. Different prophylactic measures were reported in the literature, and intra-ureter indocyanine green with subsequent visualization of near-infrared fluorescence was attempted and had a promising outcome [7].

Prophylactic ureteral catheters, which are used to help identification of the ureters intraoperatively, were also found to have questionable value in the prevention of intraoperative ureteral injury. In a review of 3071 major gynecologic surgeries by Kuno et al., in which 15% of patients underwent bilateral prophylactic ureteral catheterization, they concluded that prophylactic ureteral catheterization did not eliminate the risk of ureteral injuries that can be avoided only by meticulous surgical techniques.

On the other hand, in a systematic review, it has been concluded that prophylactic ureteral catheter placement has the advantage of reducing ureteral injury, shortening the operative time, and reducing the amount of bleeding. It might be a good option for laparoscopic gynecological surgery with pelvic adhesion [8].

It is certainly a debate; Schimpf et al. recommended ureteral catheterization as a cost-saving procedure when the rate of ureteral injury during benign abdominal hysterectomy or radical hysterectomy is greater than 3.2% [9].

The timing of the reconstructive surgery to correct a urinary fistula is variable. However, there is an agreement to wait for a minimum of 3 months or longer. All ureteral fistulae can be managed electively except for ureteroarterial fistula which can present with massive hematuria and should be treated urgently. The delay in repair is aimed to perform the surgery after subsiding the inflammation, tissue edema, and stabilization of the fistulous tract. Before any fistula repair, the associated infection should be treated, and the source of infection should be eradicated. Also, nutritional deficiency should be corrected if present. Despite different modalities and approaches, the general principles of surgical correction of the fistula should be followed intraoperatively: identification, excision of the whole fistulous tract, and excision of devitalized tissues. Moreover, it is necessary to have adequate separation of the involved structures, water-tight anastomosis, multiple-layer closure of both sides, putting well-vascularized interpositional tissue flaps if available, and non-overlapping of the suture lines. After surgery, urine should be diverted away from the anastomotic site for a few weeks.

In this chapter, the most frequent types of ureteral fistulae will be discussed:

26.3 Ureterogenital Fistulas

A fistula can occur between the ureter and one of the female genital tract organs; vagina, uterus, and fallopian tube. Ureterovaginal fistula (UVF) is unusual, uretero-uterine fistula (UUF) is rare, and ureterofallopian fistula is extremely rare. Almost all ureterogenital fistulas are linked to an iatrogenic lesion which usually follows gynecologic and obstetric surgeries [10, 11].

26.3.1 Ureterovaginal Fistula (UVF)

It is quite uncommon in comparison to vesicovaginal or vesicouterine fistulas, but it is the most common ureterogenital fistula. Hysterectomy is the most common surgical procedure that could induce UVF, and with the recent use of minimally invasive techniques, robotic/laparoscopic assisted hysterectomy is the most frequent one, followed by open and vaginal hysterectomy (Fig. 26.1).

The risk factors of iatrogenic ureteral injuries (IUIs) in these cases are pelvic inflammatory diseases, endometriosis, and previous radiotherapy. These conditions are associated with friable tissues, and dense adhesions that make ureteral identification difficult with possible injury. Neglected vaginal pessaries or foreign bodies were reported as risk factors for UVF in a few cases. In a series that included 17 cases of UVF, 60% of them were discovered after hysterectomies, and the rest were after CS [12].

Paradoxical urinary incontinence which is incontinence of urine in the presence of normal voiding is a common presentation of ureterogenital fistulas, and it could be severe enough that requires the usage of pads. Chronic fistula may induce recurrent vaginal infection and soreness of the vulval skin. Rarely, ureterogenital fistula could be silent, possibly leading to progressive loss of the ipsilateral renal unit.

26.3.2 Ureterouterine Fistula (UUF)

It is most commonly following CS; especially emergent CS. Emergent CS is a major risk factor for IUIs with subsequent vesicouterine fistula and UUF [12]. This can be explained by the added stress to save the fetus, the non-availability of expert surgeons, the presence of massive intraoperative bleeding from placental anomalies or impending rupture of the uterus. All the above-mentioned causes could be

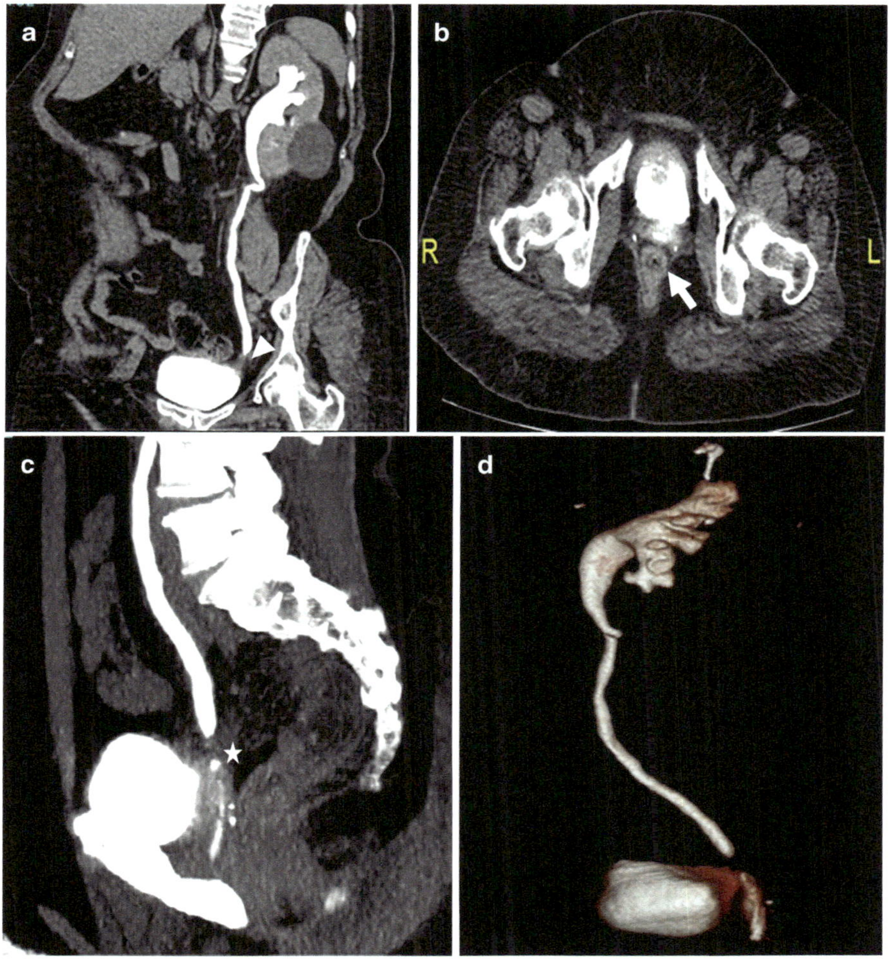

Fig. 26.1 (**a**) CTU shows mild left hydroureteronephrosis down to abrupt cut off at the pelvic ureter (Arrow head). (**b**) Axial contrast enhanced CT image of the pelvis at the excretory phase shows opacification of the vagina posterior to the bladder (Arrow). (**c**) Sagittal contrast enhanced CT image of the pelvis at the excretory phase shows connection between the left ureter and vagina (Asterisk) posterior to the bladder. (**d**) Volume rendering reconstructing CTU image at the sagittal plane shows evidence of left ureterovaginal fistula

associated with massive clamping that may accidentally involve the ureter. The rate of ureteral injury in the UK in 1997 was reported to be 0.27 cases/1000 CS [13, 14].

In the presence of inadvertent ureteral injury that has passed unnoticed, urine extravasation occurs and urine can find its way to the uterine suture line-inducing a fistula. This kind of fistula that accompanies iatrogenic ureteral injury usually

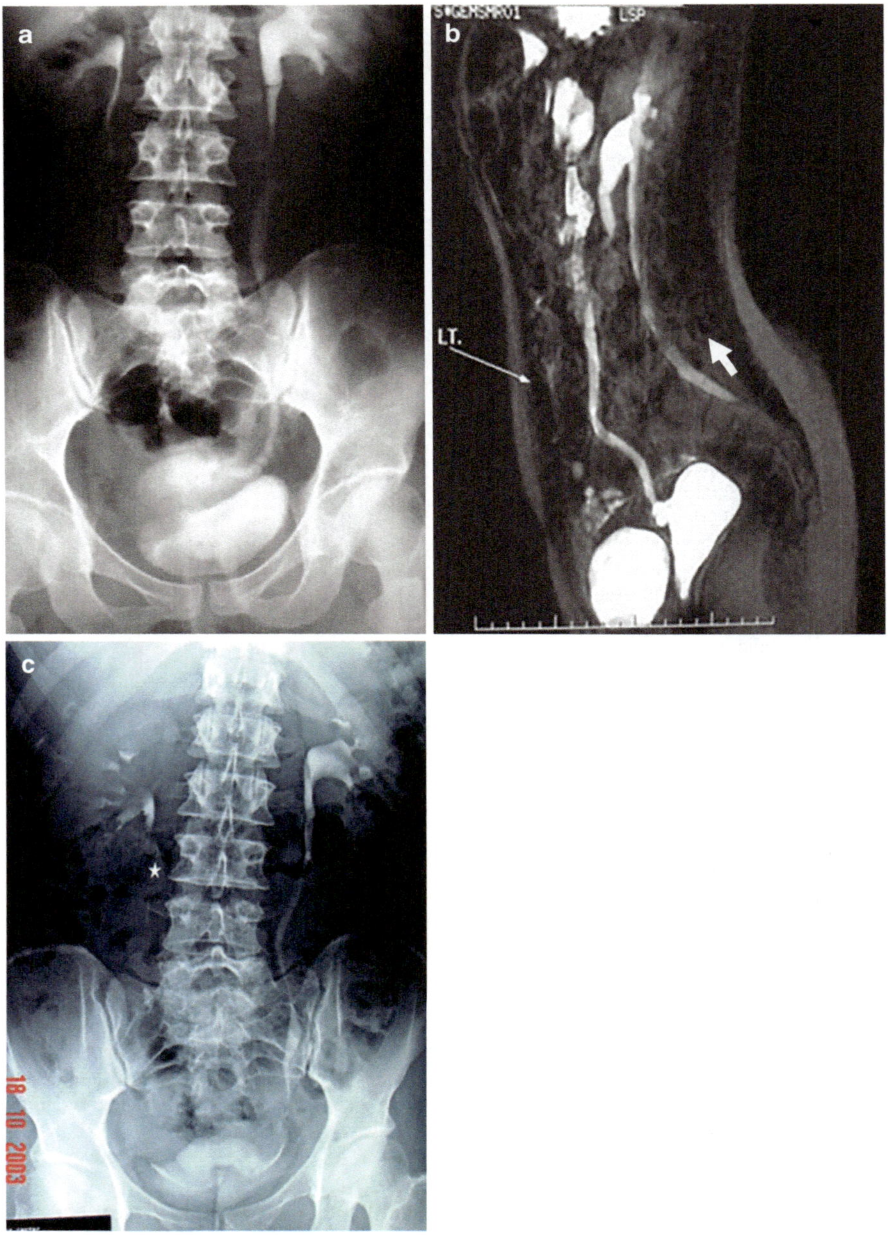

Fig. 26.2 Left ureterovaginal fistula post hysterectomy as shown by IVU (**a**) and by MRU (**b**). IVU 6 months later (**c**) shows normal upper tract after ureterovesical reimplantation. Reproduced with permission from El-Tabey et al. Urological trauma after gynecological and obstetric surgeries. Scan J Urol Nephrol. 2006;40(3):225–231

manifests early, within days to a few weeks postoperatively. The symptoms of UUF are quite similar to UVF (Fig. 26.2).

26.3.3 Ureterofallopian Fistula

It is extremely rare, and very few cases have been reported in the literature after endometriosis surgery, fallopian tube embolization for birth control or other surgeries [15, 16].

Patients with ureterogenital fistulae have varying degrees of urinary leakage which makes UUF or UVF fistulae not only a pathological problem but also a cause of psychological stress in those patients. Continuous urinary leakage induces excoriation to the vaginal and vulval skin. In view of limited medical centers and expertise that provide complex reconstructive surgeries, most of these patients are kept for months on waiting lists, which adds to the burden of fistulae diseases. So, in the event of injury, several authors have demonstrated that early detection and treatment are associated with less morbidities, and better short-term and long-term outcomes.

If the fistula is discovered early in the vicinity of IUIs, many series in the literature advise early intervention with trial retrograde stenting and, if it fails, performing urinary diversion via percutaneous nephrostomy and antegrade DJ stent "if possible". Cystoscopy is recommended to exclude accompanying vesicovaginal fistula. Large intraabdominal or pelvic urinoma requires drainage with a tube drain that can be inserted with ultrasound guidance. Early management and urinary diversion minimize urinary leakage, could save the ipsilateral kidney in presence of a distal ureteral stricture, and could heal a small fistula and minimize the number of patients requiring surgical intervention. After a period of at least 3 months, a formal retrograde or antegrade ureterography can be repeated, and the extension of the ureteral injury and the fistula to be evaluated again. Endoureterotomy can be done at this time for a ureteral stricture "if amenable". If a ureteral fistula is discovered late and well-established, if it is not amenable to stenting or if it persists after urinary diversion, or after an unsuccessful endourologic procedure, surgery is the optimal management. In certain instances, like patients who are very risky for anesthesia, patients with short survival, and when the function of the affected kidney is poor, urinary diversion could be the option. In such cases, urinary diversion will only improve the quality of life rather than a definitive cure.

Surgery is the ultimate option for UVF and can be performed through open surgery, laparoscopically, or robotically. Through the transperitoneal approach, the ureter has to be carefully dissected because it is usually surrounded by dense fibrosis. The majority of the ureterogenital fistulae involve the distal part of the ureter, and performing direct ureter-to-ureter anastomosis (ureteroureterostomy) at this location could yield unsuccessful results. For that reason, most of the published series recommend ureteroneocystostomy as the standard treatment. The ureter has to be cut above the level of injury or stenosis, and the presence of a healthy distal ureter is mandatory for a successful outcome. Ureterovesical reimplantation can be done with a psoas hitch, and for a longer ureteral gaping, the Boari flap is the method of choice [16, 17].

In a case series that consisted of 17 UVF patients, retrograde insertion of DJ stent was successful in only 2, and the remaining patients had a percutaneous nephrostomy tube inserted. Antegrade insertion of DJ stent was successful in two of them. The remaining 13 patients required ureterovesical reimplantation (11 with direct ureteroneocystostomy and 2 required Boari flap). Of all patients, two had ureteral strictures, one after antegrade double-J stenting and the other after open repair. The recommendation is routine periodic follow-up with imaging studies after the removal of a ureteral stent [18].

26.4 Ureteroenteric Fistulae

A fistula could develop between a part of the urinary system and the digestive system. The majority of the urinary-enteric fistulae were reported between the colon and urinary bladder. Approximately 2% of the patients with diverticulitis will eventually develop vesicoenteric fistula secondary to the disease, and those patients account for approximately 70% of all diagnosed colovesical fistulae [19].

The incidence of ureteroenteric fistulae is very rare. The stomach has no direct relationship with the ureters, and the entire small intestine, except the intraperitoneal part of the duodenum,. The majority of the duodenum is a retroperitoneal structure and lies posteriorly to the hilum and the right of the kidney and to the right upper part of the ureter. The left ureter lies posteriorly to the mesosigmoid. The incidence of ureteroenteric fistulae is extremely rare and the literature accounts only on case reports. Ureterocolic fistula (UCF) is the most common form of ureteroenteric fistulae and it forms between the ureter mainly the left side and the sigmoid colon.

Ureterocolic fistula (UCF) fistula is quite different from ureterogenital fistulae in many aspects. Inflammatory conditions, especially diverticulitis, contribute more to the risk for fistula formation, as well as neoplastic, traumatic, and idiopathic causes. The symptoms are also quite different. The higher pressure inside the colon relative to the intra-ureteral pressure makes the passage of air and gases to the ureter more frequent than the passage of urine from the ureter to the colon. So, patients with ureterocolic fistula may present with pneumaturia and fecaluria. If urine passes to the colon, it could induce watery stool [20, 21].

The presentation of UCF could be vague, with non-specific abdominal pain, and recurrent urinary tract infection. The symptoms are usually insidious rather than acute. Barium enema diagnoses the fistula with a reliability of 75% in comparison to IVU (33%) and retrograde pyelography (25%). Air pyelography and/or opacification of the ureter with barium enema is highly diagnostic of UCF.

In a review of 18 cases of urinary-enteric fistulae, 3 were ureterocolic and 1 was ureteroileal, 15/18 (83%) were corrected surgically. So, surgery seems to be the primary option in treating UCF [19].

Ureteroduodenal fistula is an extremely rare condition with few case reports in the literature. Risk factors may include chronic peptic ulcer and chronic obstruction or infection of the upper urinary tract. The fistula may develop between the renal pelvis/upper ureter and the third part of the duodenum [22, 23].

26.5 Ureteroarterial Fistula

Ureteroarterial fistula (UAF) is an abnormal communication between a major artery and the ureter. The common arteries affected are the external iliac arteries and the most commonly affected site of the ureter is the mid to distal portion. In the majority of patients, the anatomic localization of the fistula has been at the arterial crossing in the pelvic brim; that is between the ureter and common iliac artery.

UAF is relatively uncommon, and most of the available data in the literature is either case reports or case series with a limited number of cases. The types of UAF can be classified into primary and secondary. Primary UAF is less often than secondary UAF and is associated with an aortoiliac aneurysm in the vast majority of cases [24]. The secondary UAF is more common and constitutes for nearly 85% of the UAF. Causes that may induce secondary UAF are numerous; however, previous pelvic surgeries with radiotherapy constitute more than 60%, and the median time between the surgery and hematuria is 2 years (2 m–30y). Previous vascular reconstructive surgeries are the second common cause of secondary UAF (20%), which are associated with more delay in presentation as compared to patients with pelvic surgeries, a median of 10 y (3 m–25 y).

The advances in cancer management, radiotherapy, and vascular reconstructive surgeries have increased the use of ureteral stents and could explain the increased incidence and reporting of UAF cases. The exact pathophysiology of UAF is unknown. The formation of dense inflammatory adhesion between the ureter and the artery and necrosis, either ischemic or pressure necrosis could explain the development of UAF [25]. Ureteral strictures may manifest as hydroureteronephrosis, and recurrent urinary tract infections that may be complicated by pyelonephritis. Ureteral strictures in those patients are usually managed with ureteral stents because of their special situations (elderly, previous cancer surgeries, and under chemoradiotherapy). The presence of stents, especially if left for a longer time, may facilitate the establishment of the fistula [26].

The diagnosis of UAF requires a high degree of suspicion, and history is the clue to the diagnosis. Hematuria can be intermittent, continuous or brisk hematuria [24]. Severe hematuria at the time of ureteral stent exchange or removal is a common presentation. Sometimes, it is life-threatening and requires urgent intervention [27]. Hematuria with a history of previous pelvic surgeries, radiotherapy for pelvic cancer, vascular reconstructive surgeries or prolonged ureteral stents, raises the risk of UAF occurrence. Because the fistula could be intermittent and could be occluded with a clot, sometimes the fistula is not obvious on CT. CT angiogram could be quite normal or could show non-specific findings as arterial pseudoaneurysm, a stricture at the site of the crossing of ureter over the common iliac. If CT angiogram is not conclusive, catheter angiography is highly diagnostic for UAF. Ureteropyelography can be performed either retrograde or antegrade and could be of a high diagnostic value. The presence of stricture with proximal hydroureteronephrosis, holding of the dye at the anatomical site of the crossing of the ureter to the common iliac artery with failure to pass a guidewire, raise the suspicion of the UAF. Escape of the contrast from the ureter to the artery is diagnostic for UAF.

The management of UAF depends on both the patient's and fistula's factors and the management includes the arterial and ureteral parts, so it is a multidisciplinary approach that includes different teams; vascular surgery, interventional radiology and urology. There has been a paradigm shift in the management of UAF from open to minimally-invasive surgeries (MIS) due to multiple reasons [25]. Patients who present with UAF are usually elderly, of poor physical performance, with previous radical surgeries for cancers, and with a history or currently receiving radiochemotherapy, all encourage the intent of MIS. Immediate exploration for life-threatening hematuria due to UAF is associated with a mortality of 64%. However, elective management with a proper diagnosis of the fistula and its location lowers the mortality to 8%. That is due to the advantages of MIS.

The management of the arterial component is vital in the management of UAF. An open approach includes a variety of techniques, such as arteriography, partial closure, grafting, and bypass surgeries. Nowadays, with the advent of interventional radiology, more than 85% of the UAF are treated with endovascular embolization or an endovascular-covered stent graft. The ureteral component also depends on the severity of the lesion and the condition of the kidney. In a patient with an expected long survival, if the stricture of the ureter is limited, and the function of the kidney is accepted, ureteroureterostomy can be performed, if possible. Otherwise, ureteroneocystostomy with the preservation of the kidney or nephroureterectomy can be performed in poorly-functioning kidney. However, in patients with poor performance and short survival, minimal procedures are advised, such as nephrostomy with proximal urine diversion or ureterostomy with cutaneous stoma. Ureteral ligation can be performed in a poorly-functioning kidney.

26.6 Ureteropancreatic Fistula

Ureteropancreatic fistula is extremely rare with few case reports in the literature. A fistula can form between the main pancreatic duct and other secondary epithelial strictures, such as the ureter. Persistent leakage of pancreatic secretion from the distal tubal pancreatic duct to the urinary tract ultimately results in chronic inflammation, erosion and fistula formation between the pancreatic duct and the ureter (usually the left ureter).

Urologic manifestations due to pancreatic fistula may be due to the escape of pancreatic secretions to the ureter that results in alkaline urine, cystitis, urethritis, frequent UTI, and haematuria.

Different modalities can be used for the diagnosis of uretero-pancreatic fistula, such as endoscopic retrograde cholangiopancreatography (ERCP), resonance cholangiopancreatography (MRCP), contrast-enhanced CT, and retrograde pyelography. ERCP has been found to be 100% sensitive and specific in the diagnosis of pancreatic duct rupture and is considered superior to CT.

Up to 70–90% of external pancreatic fistulas may heal with conservative measures; broad-spectrum antibiotics, enteral nutrition, fluid, and correction of electrolytes imbalance [28]. If conservative measures fail, or the fistula becomes complicated, endoscopic surgeries are warranted. ERCP can be considered as the first-line therapy in the management of pancreatic fistulae [29]. Three cases of ureteropancreatic fistulae were reported in the literature and blunt, penetrating traumatic injuries and chronic pancreatitis were the predisposing factors for formation of the fistulae. Two of them were closed successfully with conservative management and one required insertion of a proximal nephrostomy tube [30, 31].

26.7 Ureteroperitoneal Fistula

Ureteroperitoneal fistula is a very rare with few cases reported in the literature. It could result from injury to the ureter during laparoscopic or open surgeries. The previous cases were decades ago, and the most recent case was reported after laparoscopic tubal sterilization with the ureter most likely injured during electrocauterization. The problem passed unnoticed, and the patient was treated for pelvic inflammatory disease until the patient returned 1 month later with free fluid in the pelvic peritoneum and mild hydroureteronephrosis. The case was diagnosed with retrograde pyelography when contrast passed to the Douglas pouch. Laparotomy revealed a hole at the posterior parietal peritoneum, and the pathology was corrected by ureteroureterostomy. Follow-up IVU after 2 months revealed a normal ureter [32].

Questions

1. *What is the main risk factor for ureteroarterial fistula?*
   (a) Caesarean section
   (b) Endovascular intervention
   (c) Diverticulitis
   (d) Laparoscopic hysterectomy
   (e) Ureteroscopy

Answer: (b)

2. *Which is the main risk factor(s) for ureterovaginal fistula?*

   (a) Caesarean section
   (b) Endovascular intervention
   (c) Diverticulitis
   (d) Laparoscopic hysterectomy
   (e) A and D

Answer: (e)

3. *What is the main symptom of ureterovaginal fistula?*

   (a) Hematuria
   (b) Urinary leakage
   (c) Vague abdominal pain and recurrent UTI
   (d) Fecaluria
   (e) Heavy menstrual period

Answer: (b)

4. *What is the diagnostic study of choice for ureteroarterial fistula?* The following are the choices:

   (a) Arteriography
   (b) Barium enema
   (c) Barium small-bowel follow through
   (d) Plain CT
   (e) Cystoscopy

Answer: (a)

5. *Which of the following surgeries is associated with the highest incidence of iatrogenic ureteral injuries?*

   (a) Obstetrics and gynecology surgeries
   (b) Plastic surgeries
   (c) Vascular surgeries
   (d) General surgeries
   (e) Open urologic surgeries

Answer: (a)

6. *On the third day after laparoscopic hysterectomy*, a patient developed abdominal pain, mild abdominal distention, and a slightly elevated serum creatinine (1.8 mg/dL).

   Ultrasonography revealed a 7 × 8 cm pelvic fluid collection and a CT with intravenous contrast showed mild left hydroureteronephrosis and a urine leak from the distal left ureter into the pelvic fluid collection. The findings were highly suggestive of an iatrogenic left ureteral injury, and trial insertion of a left DJ stent was tried but failed, what is the appropriate next step in the management?

   (a) No management is required at this time
   (b) Ureteroneocystostomy

(c) Insertion of percutaneous nephrostomy tube
(d) Left nephrectomy
(e) Ureterostomy

Answer: (c)

References

1. Elawdy MM, Osman Y, Awad B, El-Mekresh M, El-Halwagy S. Iatrogenic ureteral injuries: a case series analysis with an emphasis on the predictors of late ureteral strictures and unfavorable outcome in different surgical specialties. Int Urogynecol J. 2021;32(11):3031–6.
2. Wanjala A, Mwangi H, Mabeya H. Pattern of ureteric pathology presenting to a fistula Centre in Western Kenya. Ther Adv Urol. 2018;2018:5056049.
3. Brandes S, Coburn M, Armenakas N, McAninch J. Diagnosis and management of ureteric injury: an evidence-based analysis. BJU Int. 2004;94(3):277–89.
4. Stern JM, Yiee J, Park S. Safety and efficacy of ureteral access sheaths. J Endourol. 2007;21(2):119–23.
5. Palaniappa NC, Telem DA, Ranasinghe NE, Divino CM. Incidence of iatrogenic ureteral injury after laparoscopic colectomy. Arch Surg. (Chicago, Ill: 1960). 2012;147(3):267–71.
6. Parpala-Spårman T, Paananen I, Santala M, Ohtonen P, Hellström P. Increasing numbers of ureteric injuries after the introduction of laparoscopic surgery. Scand J Urol Nephrol. 2008;42(5):422–7.
7. Lee Z, Kaplan J, Giusto L, Eun D. Prevention of iatrogenic ureteral injuries during robotic gynecologic surgery: a review. Am J Obstet Gynecol. 2016;214(5):566–71.
8. Feng D, Tang Y, Yang Y, Wei X, Han P, Wei W. Does prophylactic ureteral catheter placement offer any advantage for laparoscopic gynecological surgery? A urologist' perspective from a systematic review and meta-analysis. Transl Androl Urol. 2020;9(5):2262–9.
9. Schimpf MO, Gottenger EE, Wagner JR. Universal ureteral stent placement at hysterectomy to identify ureteral injury: a decision analysis. BJOG. 2008;115(9):1151–8.
10. Akman RY, Sargin S, Ozdemir G, Yazicioğlu A, Cetin S. Vesicovaginal and ureterovaginal fistulas: a review of 39 cases. Int Urol Nephrol. 1999;31(3):321–6.
11. Li X, Wang P, Liu Y, Liu C. Minimally invasive surgical treatment on delayed uretero-vaginal fistula. BMC Urol. 2018;18(1):96.
12. Murtaza B, Mahmood A, Niaz WA, Akmal M, Ahmad H, Saeed S. Ureterovaginal fistula--etiological factors and outcome. J Pak Med Assoc. 2012;62(10):999–1003.
13. el-Mahgoub S, el-Zeniny A. Ureterouterine fistula after cesarean section. Diagnostic procedures. Am J Obstet Gynecol. 1971;110(6):881–2.
14. Rajasekar D, Hall M. Urinary tract injuries during obstetric intervention. Br J Obstet Gynaecol. 1997;104(6):731–4.
15. Crochet P, Savoie PH, Agostini A, Zaritsky E, Lechevallier E, Coulange C. Uretero-fallopian fistula after gynecological surgery for endometriosis: a case report. J Minim Invasive Gynecol. 2008;15(1):108–9.
16. Zhang Y, Ma T, Shao G, Xiao Z. Uretero-fallopian fistula after hysteroscopy fallopian tube embolization: a case report. BMC Urol. 2018;18(1):70.
17. Dmitry F, Ambereen S. Ureterovaginal fistula linked to a retained pessary. Int Urogynecol J. 2014;25(9):1283–5.
18. Elabd S, Ghoniem G, Elsharaby M, Emran M, Elgamasy A, Felfela T, et al. Use of endoscopy in the management of postoperative ureterovaginal fistula. Int Urogynecol J Pelvic Floor Dysfunct. 1997;8(4):185–90.
19. Najjar SF, Jamal MK, Savas JF, Miller TA. The spectrum of colovesical fistula and diagnostic paradigm. Am J Surg. 2004;188(5):617–21.

20. Almerie MQ, Culverwell A, Gill J, Harrison JD. Spontaneous right-sided ureterocolic fistula: a rare complication of colonic diverticular disease. BMJ Case Rep. 2015;2015:bcr2015211282.
21. Bensouda A, El Hader K, Sbihi L, Benkabbou A, Karmouni T, Tazi K, et al. Entero-urinary fistula. Tunis Med. 2010;88(11):814–9.
22. Patel B, Yande S, Kumar S, Talaulikar A. Ureteroduodenal fistula. J Surg Case Rep. 2015;2015(7):rjv065.
23. Wu ST, Lee SS, Ma CP, Chang SY, Yu DS. Ureteroduodenal fistula: a rare complication of duodenal ulcer. J Urol. 2000;163(2):546.
24. Bergqvist D, Pärsson H, Sherif A. Arterio-ureteral fistula--a systematic review. Eur J Vasc Endovasc Surg. 2001;22(3):191–6.
25. Madoff DC, Gupta S, Toombs BD, Skolkin MD, Charnsangavej C, Morello FA Jr, et al. Arterioureteral fistulas: a clinical, diagnostic, and therapeutic dilemma. AJR Am J Roentgenol. 2004;182(5):1241–50.
26. Batter SJ, McGovern FJ, Cambria RP. Ureteroarterial fistula: case report and review of the literature. Urology. 1996;48(3):481–9.
27. Andreasen JJ, Fahrenkrug L, Madsen PV. Massive hematuria due to iliac artery-ureteral fistula. Case report. Eur J Surg. 1991;157(3):223–4.
28. Ĉeĉka F, Jon B. Pancreatic fistula. Curr Treat Options Gastroenterol. 2002;5(5):1–24. https://doi.org/10.1007/S11938-002-0023-0.
29. Alexakis N, Sutton R, Neoptolemos JP. Surgical treatment of pancreatic fistula. Dig Surg. 2004;21(4):262–74. https://doi.org/10.1159/000080199.
30. Wolf JH, et al. Pancreaticoureteral fistula following penetrating abdominal trauma. JOP. 2007;8(5):613–6.
31. Toporoff B, et al. Percutaneous antegrade ureteral stenting as an adjunct for treatment of complicated ureteral injuries. J Trauma. 1992;32(4):534–8. https://doi.org/10.1097/00005373-199204000-00019.
32. Machuca J, de La Martinez Ossa R, Camara M. Ureteroperitoneal fistula secondary to tubal sterilization by laparoscopy. Br J Urol. 1996;78(6):953–4. https://doi.org/10.1046/j.1464-410x.1996.131531.x.

Chapter 27
Miscellaneous Ureteral Diseases

Mahmoud Abdel-Gawad and Ahmed M. Eliwa

Abstract There are many rare radiological ureteral abnormalities and uncommon pathological conditions. The urologist and radiologist should be aware of such findings during clinical and radiological investigations.

Keywords Ureter · Ureteritis · Intussusception · Hernia · Diverticulosis

Abbreviations

CC	Cystitis cystica
CT	Computed tomography
IVU	Intravenous urography
MRI	Magnetic resonance image
UC	Ureteritis cystica
UI	Ureteral intussusception

Learning Objectives

- The objectives of this chapter are familiarize the reader the uncommon disorders of the ureter, and to describe the causes, symptoms, signs, diagnosis and treatment of these conditions.

Test your learning and check your understanding of this book's contents use the "Springer Nature Flashcards" app to access questions. To use the app, please follow the instructions in Chapter 1.

M. Abdel-Gawad (✉)
Toshka Urology and Endoscopy Center, Mansoura, Egypt

A. M. Eliwa
Urology and Andrology, Urology Department, Zagazig University, Zagazig, Egypt

M. Abdel-Gawad et al. (eds.), *The Ureter*,
https://doi.org/10.1007/978-3-031-36212-5_27

27.1 Ureteritis

27.1.1 *Definition*

Acute inflammatory processes can involve the ureteral mucosa due to many causes. It could be specific inflammation such as chronic inflammatory disease (discussed in Chap. 11), or acute nonspecific inflammation. The latter is called "*primary Ureteritis*" and is associated with infection of the urinary tract including ipsilateral pyelonephritis and cystitis.

27.1.2 *Etiology*

Impacted ureteral stone, ureteral obstruction, and vesicoureteral reflux could result in an acute inflammatory process especially if the bacterial infection is present. E. coli is the most offending cause of acute bacterial inflammation. The latter may be due to ascending infection from the urinary tract or direct spread of infection from adjacent organs like appendicitis, diverticulitis, and inflammatory bowel disease. Hematogenous spread is also possible. Chronic ureteritis can be caused by a ureteral stent.

27.1.3 *Symptoms and Signs*

Acute flank pain associated with dysuria and with macroscopic hematuria is a common presentation. Fever and suprapubic pain are also associated symptoms. Microscopic hematuria and pyuria are frequent findings. Sloughing of the ureteral mucosa could be seen during microscopic examination.

27.1.4 *Diagnosis*

Radiological signs of acute ureteritis are nonspecific but can give clues to diagnosis in combination with clinical presentation and laboratory investigations. Abdominal ultrasound could detect thickening of the bladder mucosa and ureteral wall edema (Fig. 27.1). CT examination will show ureteral wall edema, thickened wall, and occasional segmental wall edema with periureteral stranding of the surrounding fat. Ureteral edema is usually unilateral, and it could be bilateral. Ureteritis should be differentiated from other lesions of the ureter, especially ureteral malignancy. Longstanding ureteritis will eventually lead to a ureteral stricture (stenosing ureteritis).

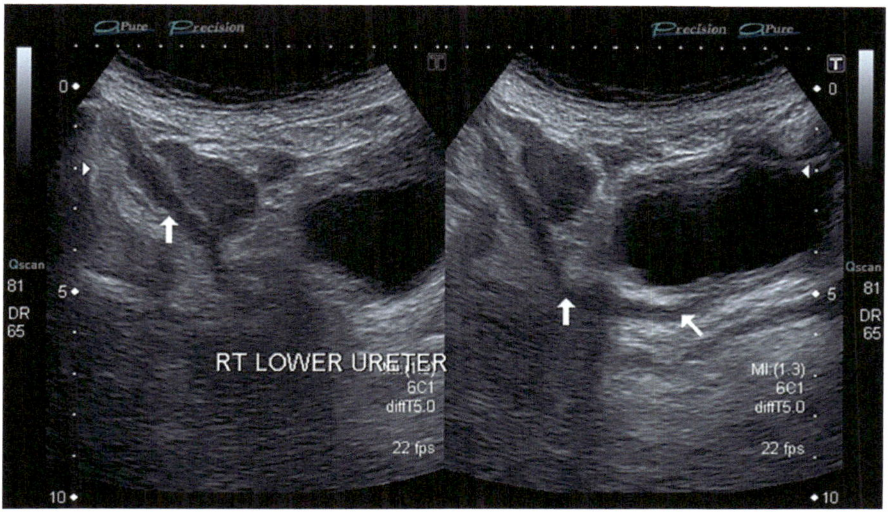

Fig. 27.1 Greyscale ultrasound shows thickened ureteral wall and edematous tissue of the lower third of the ureter associated with acute cystitis

Treatment: Medical treatment of associated urinary tract infections is mandatory in addition to anti-inflammatory medications. If there is associated obstruction by stone, kidney drainage or insertion of DJ stent is a temporary procedure till resolution of the obstruction by the appropriate surgical procedure.

27.2 Ureteritis Cystica (UC)

27.2.1 Definition

This is a benign cystic lesion of the ureteral wall. It is submucosal cysts of small size. It could be unilateral or bilateral in 50%. It is common in females over 50 years of age.

27.2.2 Etiology

The ureteritis cystica is usually secondary to chronic inflammatory conditions and chronic irritation of the ureteral mucosa, especially by ureteral stones. Infection with many organisms has been confirmed. These organisms are E. coli (common), M. tuberculosis, Enterococcus, Proteus spp., and schistosomiasis. [1].

27.2.3 Symptoms and Signs

Ureteritis cystica is not a pre-malignant lesion and is usually a symptomatic. However, few cases of ureteral obstruction have been reported due to large ureteral cysts. It could be associated with pyelitis cystica or cystitis cystica. It appears as multiple filling defects during examination by IVP and contrast CT (Fig. 27.2). It also can be seen during antegrade or retrograde pyelography. Under light microscopy, it appears as white cystic areas with glandular metaplasia associated with chronic inflammatory cells and intact umbrella cells (Fig. 27.3). It should be differentiated from other conditions like transitional cell carcinoma, ureteral stones, air bubbles, vascular impressions, and blood clots. There is no specific treatment for UC [2].

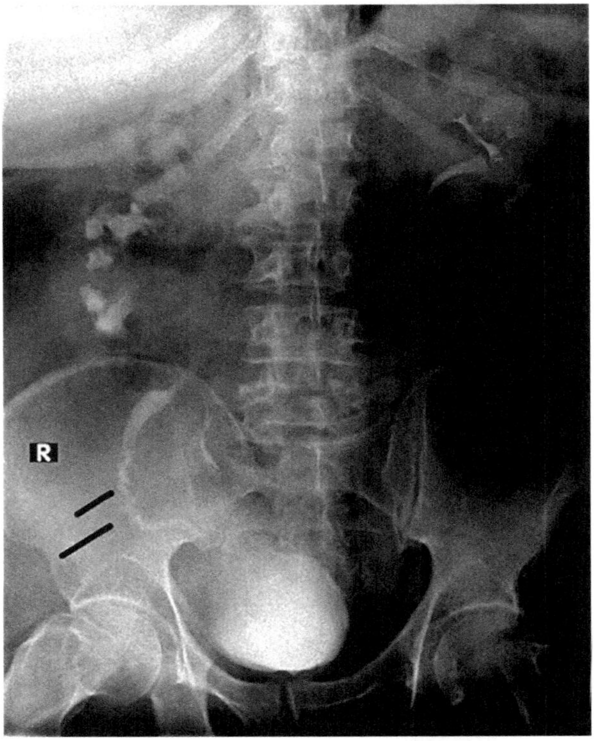

Fig. 27.2 IVU in a bilharzial patient shows multiple submucosal fillings at the right iliac ureter (ureteritis cystica)

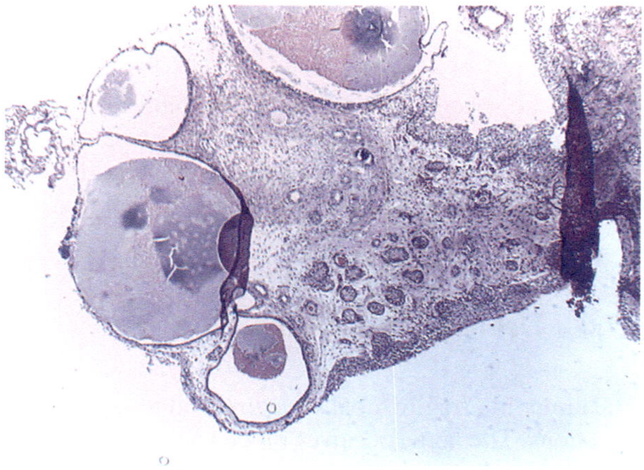

Fig. 27.3 Histopathological examination of ureteritis cystica by light microscope. Cystically dilated lumens or cystic cavities filled with eosinophilic fluid (ureteritis cystica), HX&Ex100

27.3 Ureteral Amyloidosis

27.3.1 Definition

Amyloidosis is an extracellular deposition of protein aggregates (Amyloid). Primary deposition of the amyloid substance in the ureter is rare. Amyloidosis could be also localized in the kidney or bladder. Few cases of ureteral amyloidosis have been reported. Secondary ureteral amyloidosis occurs due to systemic chronic inflammatory conditions, rheumatoid arthritis, immune disorders, and tuberculosis. Localized ureteral amyloidosis could be found in 10–20% of cases.

27.3.2 Symptoms and Signs

The common symptoms are flank pain and painless hematuria. It is more common in females than males. The left ureter is more affected than the right, and the lower ureter is more than the upper one.

27.3.3 Radiological Diagnosis

Unfortunately, there is no specific radiological sign for amyloidosis. Localized amyloidosis has been described by using MRI T2 weighted imaging. It appears as a hypointense lesion without an obvious mass effect. This characteristic can differentiate amyloidosis from carcinoma. However, amyloidosis macroscopically can mimic urothelial carcinoma. Ureteroscopy, ureteral biopsy, staining with Congo red, and examination under light microscopy will show apple-green birefringent under polarized light. Intraoperative frozen section can also be helpful in the diagnosis of amyloidosis.

27.3.4 Treatment

There is no specific treatment for amyloidosis. Localized amyloidosis of the ureter has a good prognosis. Conservative treatment follow-up by serial imaging is the classic treatment option. Medical treatment in the form of oral colchicine and topical Dimethyl Sulphoxide (DMS) has been reported. [see also Chap. 11].

27.4 Ureteral Ischemia

The ureter is a fragile tubal structure, and its blood supply is liable to injury in many situations. The ureter receives blood supply from many sources. The most common site of ureteral ischemia is the lower end of the ureter which usually results in ureteral stenosis.

27.4.1 Etiology

The conditions that can lead to ureteral ischemia include traction on the ureter during surgical dissection, stripping of the ureter from its adventitia and/ or the use of cauterization close to the ureteral wall. Severe ureteral edema can jeopardize the blood supply of the ureter. Nevertheless, chronic ureteral obstruction can also affect the blood supply of the ureter and result in chronic ischemia and ends up with ureteral stenosis. Ureteral access sheath has been reported as a cause of injury of the lower ureter and can lead to ischemia and stricture. Ureteral ischemia may also be venous ischemia. Shaul and coworkers have described clinically and experimentally ureteral necrosis after renal transplantation due to venous congestion and subsequent venous ischemia [3]. One of the earlier reports regarding ureteral complications after renal transplantation was by Salvatierra et al. they emphasized the importance of the vascular dissection during donor nephrectomy, and they stated that "interruption of venous blood supply can be as lethal as interruption of arterial blood supply " [4].

27.5 Ureteral Hernia and Ureteral Herniation

The herniated ureter is a potential source of serious renal and ureteral complications, especially in renal allograft recipients. Ureteral herniation is an uncommon urological problem.

Types: Ureteral hernia includes the following locations:

- Ureteral inguinal hernia
- Ureteral femoral hernia

- Ureteral herniation through the lumbar triangle
- Ureteral obturator hernia
- Ureteral sciatic hernia
- Ureteral diaphragmatic hernia
- Internal hernia of the ureter

More than 150 cases have been reported. In many instances, the condition is discovered accidentally during radiological investigations or intraoperative repair of the hernia. Ureteral herniation can be associated with unexplained hydronephrosis or renal failure if it is bilateral. Recurrent urinary tract infection can be a symptom of ureteral herniation. Clinically, a large-size inguinal hernia should alert the surgeon for possible ureteral during preoperative assessment. CT urography and retrograde pyelography can easily diagnose ureteral herniation. The condition has also been reported in many cases after kidney transplantation [5, 6].

Ureteral inguinal hernias are mostly indirect inguinal hernias (80%) and can be classified into two anatomical types, paraperitoneal and retroperitoneal types (Fig. 27.4). A paraperitoneal type is diagnosed when the ureter slides alongside the peritoneal sac and forms part of the hernia wall [80% of cases]. On the other hand, an extraperitoneal type occurs in 20% of cases, where the ureter and extraperitoneal

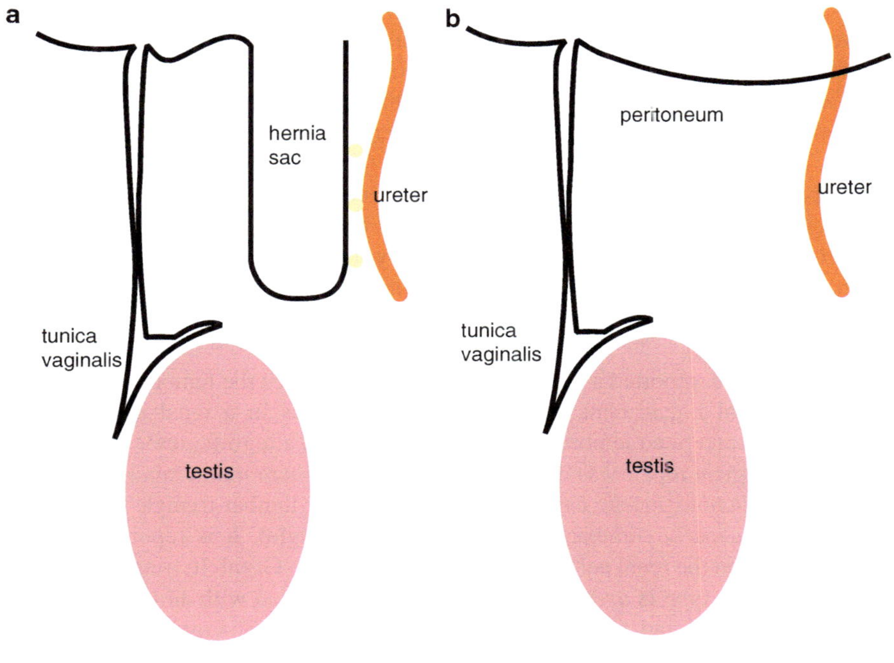

Fig. 27.4 Paraperitoneal (**a**) involves adhesion of the ureter to the peritoneal hernial sac, approaching the inguinal canal and scrotum. (**b**) The extraperitoneal inguinal ureteral hernias, the ureter approaches the inguinal canal without a peritoneal sac

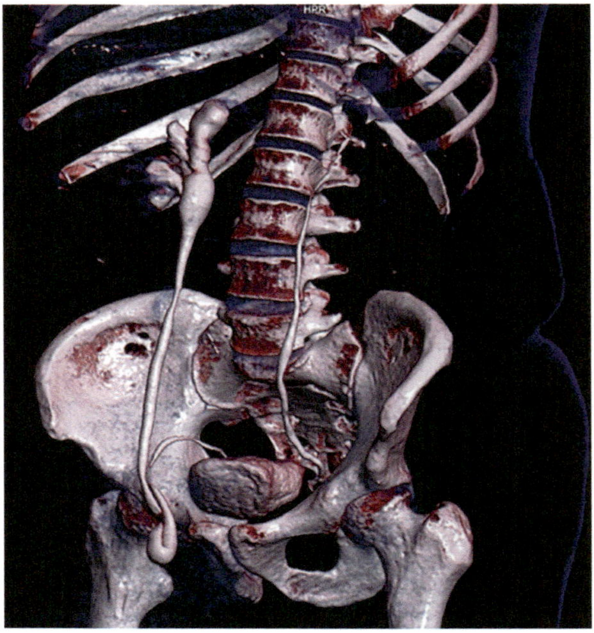

Fig. 27.5 3-D reconstruction of enhanced CT of both kidneys and ureter shows herniated right ureter in the inguinal region (Loop-shaped "Curlicue sign" ureter with mild hydroureteronephrosis

fat reach the inguinal canal with no peritoneal sac present. There is a radiological sign "Curlicue" which is characteristic of ureteral herniation [7, 8] (Fig. 27.5).

Ureterosciatic hernia [Lindbom hernia]: This hernia is classified as suprapiriformis or infrapiriformis hernia of the pelvic ureter, in which the ureter slides into the pelvic fossa, fovea, or greater or lesser sciatic foramina. This type of hernia may cause pain, obstructive uropathy, urosepsis, or renal failure [9–11].

Ureteral obturator hernia is a rare condition. The clinical manifestations include abdominal pain, hydroureteronephrosis, urinary tract infection, kidney stones, and even uremia. Diagnosis is difficult to reach based on physical examination alone. Intravenous contrast studies may aid in diagnosis and surgical correction can avoid complications [12].

Esposito et al. reported a case of ureteral hernia through the femoral ring associated with renal impairment and hydroureteronephrosis in a renal allograft. CT showed an incarcerated femoral hernia with a distended allograft ureter in the femoral canal. Surgical repair was done for the incarcerated femoral hernia [13].

Acquired lumbar hernia can arise from the inferior lumbar triangle (Petit triangle) and the superior lumbar triangle (Grynfeltt triangle). It is reported that the upper ureter and the renal pelvis can herniate through the Grynfeltt triangle [14, 15].

Another rare type is *ureteral thoracic hernia* associated with an idiopathic diaphragmatic hernia and incarcerated proximal ureter. Open surgical repair of the diaphragmatic hernia, reduction, resection, and anastomosis of the redundant proximal incarcerated ureter are carried out [16].

An internal hernia of the ureter was described by Page in 1955. During the exploration of the hydroureter, the ureter disappeared into a pocket between the iliac vessels and the psoas muscle at the brim of the pelvis [17].

27.6 Ureteral Intussusception (UI)

Ureteral intussusception is a rare urological condition but can happen after either rigid or flexible ureteroscopy. There are many reported cases in the literature. The symptoms are flank pain and hematuria. There are many causes of ureteral intussusception, the most common is ureteral tumors, ureteral polyp, or iatrogenic.

Ureteral intussusception during ureteroscopy is rare. It can occur in antegrade or retrograde directions (Fig. 27.6). Antegrade ureteral intussusception can occur during basketing ureteral stones. It has also been reported with polypoid ureteral masses transitional cell carcinoma or fibroepithelial polyps. In rare situations, ureteral intussusception is caused by a ureteral stone or antegrade endopyelotomy [18–20]. Retrograde intussusception was reported with retrograde pyelography [21]. Also, retrograde ureteral intussusception was reported after ureteroscopy [22]. The mechanism of intussusception is the telescoping of the ureteral proximal part into the distal part.

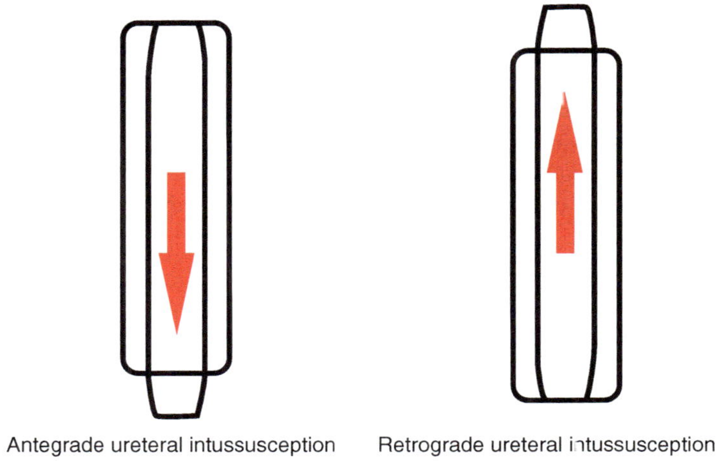

Fig. 27.6 Diagrammatic representation of the antegrade and retrograde ureteral intussusception

27.6.1 Diagnosis

The condition can be diagnosed during intraoperative retrograde pyelography or intravenous pyelography (IVP). CT with contrast is very helpful in diagnosis. Coronal CT with contrast can reveal the intussusception [23]. MRI can be alternatively used if the patient is hypersensitive to the contrast material. In a CT scan, it appears as a V-shaped sign or called "Stalk of-corn-sign or target sign. The intussusception appears like a filling defect or tongue-like shape. Diagnosis and management of ureteral intussusception should be immediate without delay. Surgery is the best option for repair. Few cases have been corrected (reversed) by using hydrostatic pressure [24].

27.7 Spontaneous Rupture of the Ureter

Spontaneous rupture of the ureter is a very rare condition (Fig. 27.7). It was described as a consequence of trauma, urinary calculi, obstruction, malignancy, idiopathic retroperitoneal fibrosis, or previous urinary tract surgery [25, 26]. Other rare causes of this condition include idiopathic retroperitoneal fibrosis [27], posterior urethral valves or bladder outlet obstruction [28], Klinefelter syndrome [29], during kidney biopsy [30], as a complication of extracorporeal shock wave lithotripsy [31], and increased urine flow from a fluid bolus [23].

Clinically it can present with acute abdomen mimicking other causes of acute abdominal pain. To be described as a 'spontaneous' rupture Schwartz et al. described the following conditions: (1) no external trauma; (2) no endoscopic ureteral manipulation; (3) no external compression; (4) absent destructive kidney disease; and (5) no history of any previous surgery [32, 33].

Treatment options include ureteric stenting, percutaneous nephrostomy, or surgical repair. The choice of treatment should be individualized.

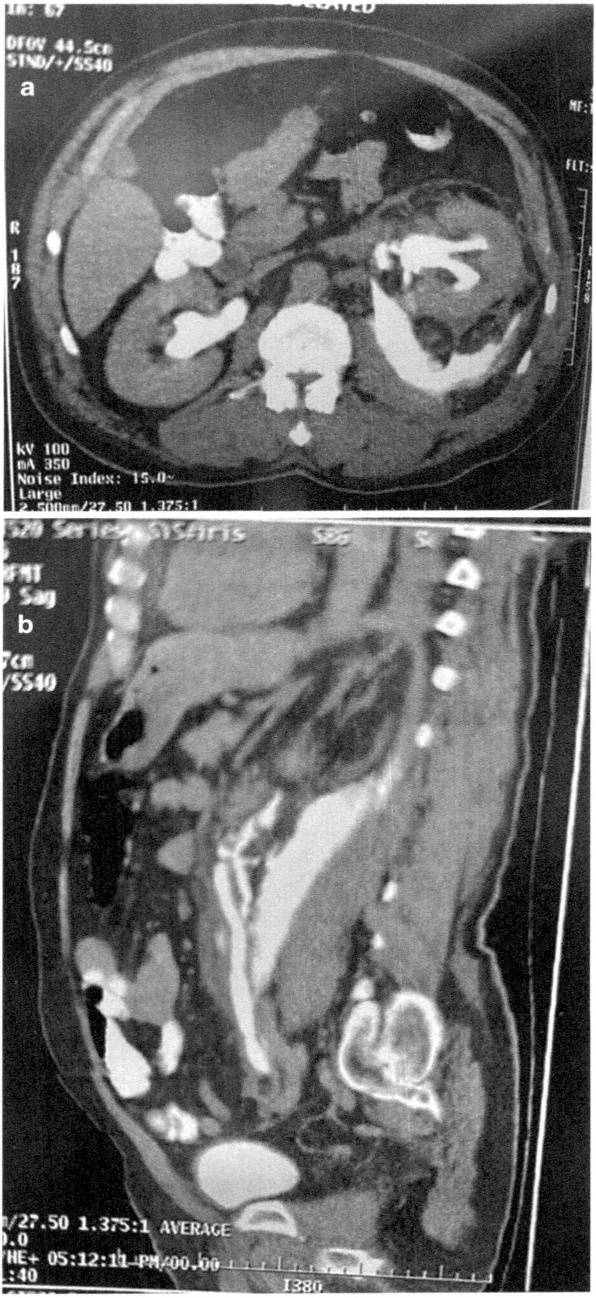

Fig. 27.7 (**a**) and (**b**) Enhanced CT of both kidneys and ureters (axial and coronal sections) shows fluid collection around the ureter and pelvicalyceal system due to spontaneous rupture of the ureter

27.8 Ureteral Diverticulum and Pseudodiverticulosis

It is an uncommon ureteral disorder. The condition was first described by Holly and Sumcad in 1957 [34]. It occurs due to herniation of the ureteral epithelium through the muscularis layer. It appears as small and multiple small pouches. It can be congenital, acquired, or abortive ureteral duplication [35].

Congenital diverticulum is the true diverticulum containing all the layers of the ureter while acquired condition does not contain the muscle layer and is called false diverticulum. The predisposing conditions are chronic urinary tract infection, chronic obstruction of the ureter, and urothelial tumors. Abortive diverticulum is the most common type and it's caused by abnormal ureteral budding. It can be diagnosed by conventional IVP or during enhanced multidetector CT. Retrograde and antegrade pyelography can also show irregular pouches along the wall of the ureter [36].

27.9 Spontaneous Subepithelial Hemorrhage

Spontaneous subepithelial ureteral hemorrhage is a rare cause of abdominal pain and hematuria [37–39]. It is usually accompanied by bleeding diathesis due to anticoagulant drugs or hemophilia [40]. "Antopol-Goldman lesion" is a mass-like hematoma of the renal pelvis or ureter [39]. Non-contrast abdominal computed tomography is important in making the diagnosis as it shows spontaneously hyperattenuating thickening of the renal pelvis and/or ureteral wall. In contrast-enhanced abdominal CT, it can be mistakenly seen as an enhanced lesion [similar to urothelial neoplasms] making non-contrast CT of great importance in diagnosis to avoid unnecessary nephrectomy [41, 42].

27.10 Ureteral Foreign Bodies

Foreign bodies are a challenging condition facing the physician in diagnosis and treatment. They usually calcify and are mistakenly diagnosed as stones. Foreign bodies of the upper urinary tract can have the following routes:

- External trauma including bullets or shrapnel of explosives or penetrating sharp objects.
- Eroded foreign bodies from surgical procedure [clips, threads…]
- Migration from the gastro-intestinal canal, from which foreign bodies can penetrate

In Table 27.1 the different types of ureteral foreign bodies, different presentations, and treatment options are shown [43–52].

Table 27.1 The types of ureteral foreign bodies, different presentations, and treatment options are shown

Author	FB	Location	Cause	Presentation	Treatment
Wang et al. [44]	Migrating IUD	Ureter	IUD migration	Hydronephrosis	Minimally invasive surgeries
Kurz et al. [45]	Metal surgical clip and suture material eroding ureter	Upper ureter	Open pyeloplasty	Flank pain Hematuria	Retrieved with a basket
Finley et al., [46]	Lapra-Ty suture clips	Upper ureter	Laparoscopic pyeloplasty	Extravasation, bacteriuria, and funguria pseudodiverticulum	Nephoscopy Then ureterocalicostomy
Brusky [47]	Migrated Lapra-Ty	Lower ureter	Laparoscopic pyeloplasty	Flank Pain, fever	Ureteroscopy
Dursun et [48]	Non-absorbable sutures	Lower ureter	Misplaced sutures in the ureter during laparotomy caused by stab wound injury	Lumber pain, dysuria, and hematuria	Retrograde semirigid ureterorenoscopy
Silva et al. [49]	Embolization coils	Mid ureter	Percutaneous nephrolithotomy followed by angioembolization	Fever and right flank pain.	RIRS
Chen et al. [50]	N-butyl Cyanoacrylate glue	Upper ureter	Transarterial embolization of a renal pseudoaneurysm secondary to percutaneous nephrostomy	Persistent hydronephrosis Urinary tract infections and hematuria	URS PCN Open ureterotomy Spontaneous passage
Gondos B [43]	Fishbone	Ureter	Swallowed and perforated opening of the ureteral	Pain, fever, and chills	Nephrectomy
Miguel et al. [51]	Swallowed wooden toothpick	Ureterovesical junction	Migrated from the digestive tract the left ureter	Frequency, dysuria, and urgency repeated Urinary tract infections	Endoscopic treatment
Aso et al. [52]	Acupuncture needle	Upper ureter	Penetrating by a part of an acupuncture needle	Macro hematuria and Back pain.	Spontaneously passed

27.11 Vascular Impression of the Ureter and Ovarian Vein Syndrome

Abnormal vessels can cross over the ureter. These vessels can occasionally cause vascular impressions that can appear during radiological investigations as filling defects. When the ovarian vein is engorged or extremely dilated, it can lead to obstruction of the ureter and symptomatic hydronephrosis.

27.12 Emphysematous Ureteritis

Diabetic Mellitus is one of the reasons for infection with gas-forming organisms. Immunocompromised patients are also susceptible to such conditions. Isolated emphysematous ureteritis is rare. The condition is associated usually with emphysematous pyelonephritis and cystitis. Elderly females are more affected than males. KUB can show the delineation of the ureteral wall by gases. In many cases, the intestinal gases can mask the emphysematous wall of the ureter. Renal ultrasound can reveal hydroureteronephrosis and evidence of obstruction by a stone. CT without contrast is diagnostic and can reveal the gases within the lumen of the ureter and gas within the urinary bladder as well as the pelvicalyceal system.

Questions

1. In ureteritis cystica, which of the following statements is incorrect?
   - (a) Is a premalignant lesion.
   - (b) Is a benign ureteral lesion.
   - (c) Is due to chronic infection.
   - (d) Commonly seen in bilharzial patients.
   - (e) Usually, a symptomatic.

Answer: (a)

2. In ureteral amyloidosis, which statement is incorrect?
   - (a) Can cause painful hematuria.
   - (b) Is a premalignant ureteral condition.
   - (c) MRI imaging is the best diagnostic modality.
   - (d) The best treatment option is resection re-anastomosis.
   - (e) Colchicine and DMS can be used as medical treatment.

Answer: (a)

3. In ureteral ischemia, which statement (s) is correct?
   (a) Can be inflicted by using a ureteral access sheath.
   (b) Is due to interruption of venous blood supply.
   (c) Is due to interruption of arterial blood supply.
   (d) Is a complication after renal transplantation.
   (e) All of the above.

Answer: (e)

4. In ureteral intussusception, which statement is incorrect?
   (a) Can occur after ureteroscopy.
   (b) Can be due to ureteral tumor.
   (c) Can occur in an antegrade fashion.
   (d) Can occur in a retrograde fashion.
   (e) NCCT is the best diagnostic radiologic modality.

Answer: (e)

5. In ureteral herniation, which statement is incorrect?
   (a) Common with direct inguinal hernia.
   (b) Usually runs in paraperitoneal space.
   (c) Commonly runs in the retroperitoneal space.
   (d) Is common after renal transplantation.
   (e) "Curlicue" radiological sign is characteristic of ureteral hernia.

Answer: (c)

References

1. Hugosson C. Striation of the renal pelvis and ureter in bilharziasis. Clin Radiol. 1987;38(4):407–9.
2. Petersen UE, Kvist E, Friis M, Krogh J. Ureteritis Cystica Scan J Urol Nephrol. 1991;25:1–4.
3. Shaul DB, Xie HW, Shimada H, Hardy BE, Anderson KD. Venous ischemia as a cause of ureteral necrosis in transplanted ureters. J Pediatr Surg. 1999;34(11):1725–7.
4. Salvatierra O Jr, Kountz SL, Belzer FO. Prevention of ureteral fistula after renal transplantation. J Urol. 1974;112(4):445–8.
5. Lu A, Burstein J. Paraperitoneal inguinal hernia of ureter. J Radiolo Case Rep. 2012;6:22–6.
6. Odisho AY, Freise CE, Tomlanovich SJ, et al. Inguinal herniation of a transplant ureter. Kidney Int. 2010;78:115.
7. Giuly J, François GF, Giuly D, et al. Intrascrotal hernia of the ureter and fatty hernia. Hernia. 2003;7:47–9.
8. Yahya Z, Al-habbal Y, Hassen S. Ureteral inguinal hernia: an uncommon trap for general surgeons. BMJ Case Reports. 2017;2017:bcr2017219288.
9. Whyburn JJ, Alizadeh A. Acute renal failure caused by bilateral ureteral herniation through the sciatic foramen. Urology. 2013;81(6):e38–9.

10. Sechrist E, Elmaoued A, Ong CJ, et al. Ureterosciatic hernia with concomitant Amyand hernia: case report and review of the literature. Radiol Case Rep. 2021;16(10):3134–8.
11. Gandhi J, Lee MY, Joshi G, et al. Ureterosciatic hernia: an up-to-date overview of evaluation and management. Transl Res Anat. 2018;11:5–9.
12. Hong Y, Zhang S, Kong X, et al. Case report of ureter obturator hernia and literature review analysis. BMC Urol. 2021;21(1):86.
13. Esposito M, Ratnasekera A, Sebastian E, et al. Femoral herniation of transplanted ureter after deceased-donor kidney transplantation. Int J Surg Case Rep. 2015;10:115–7.
14. Cabello R, Cancho MJ, Monzó JI, et al. Herniation of renal pelvis and ureteropelvic junction resulting from superior lumbar triangle hernia. Scand J Urol Nephrol. 2008;42(1):81–2.
15. Mehrabi S, Yavari Barhaghtalab MJ, Babapour M. Renal pelvis and ureteropelvic junction incarceration in a Grynfeltt-Lesshaft hernia: a case report and review of the literature. BMC Urol. 2020;20(1):74.
16. Lin FC, Lin JS, Kim S, Walker JR. A rare diaphragmatic ureteral herniation case report: endoscopic and open reconstructive management. BMC Urol. 2017;17(1):26.
17. Page BH. Obstruction of ureter in internal hernia. Br J Urol. 1955;27(3):254–5.
18. Compton JS, Drummond M. Intussusception of the ureter by a polypoid transitional cell carcinoma. Br J Urol. 1986;58:725.
19. Sewell J, Blecher G, Tsai K, et al. Calculus-related ureteral intussusception: a case report and literature review. Int J Surg Case Rep. 2015;12:63–6.
20. Chiong E, Consigliere D. Antegrade ureteral intussusception: a rare complication of percutaneous endopyelotomy. Urology. 2004;64(6):1231.e12–4.
21. Park J, Siegel C, Moll M, Konnak J. Retrograde ureteral intussusception. J Urol. 1994;151:997.
22. Bernhard RH, Reddy PK. Retrograde ureteral intussusception: a rare complication. J Endourol. 1996;10:349–51.
23. Chao CH, Fong TC, Tiffany C. Ureteral intussusception: a case report and literature review. J Comput Assist Tomogr. 2012;36(2):261–4.
24. Liu DM, Torreggiani WC, Rowley VA. Hydrostatic reduction of iatrogenic intussusception of the ureter secondary to percutaneous nephrostomy catheter exchange. J Vasc Interv Radiol. 2000;11(8):1076–8.
25. Ay D, Yencilek E, Celikmen MF, Akkas M, et al. Spontaneous rupture of ureter: an unusual cause of acute abdominal pain. Am J Emerg Med. 2012;30(390):e1–2.
26. Liu S, Lin J, Huang C, Tsai I. Spontaneous rupture of the ureter mimicking acute appendicitis: two case reports. JACME. 2011;1:61–3.
27. Caruso Lombardi A, Rinaldi MF, Bartalena T. Urinary ascites due to retroperitoneal fibrosis: a case report. Acta Radiol. 2007;48:119–21.
28. Akpinar H, Kural AR, Tüfek I, et al. Spontaneous ureteral rupture: is immediate surgical intervention always necessary? Presentation of four cases and review of the literature. J Endourol. 2002;16:179–83.
29. Reva S, Tolkach Y. Spontaneous pelvic rupture as a result of renal colic in a patient with Klinefelter syndrome. Case Rep Urol. 2013;2013:374973.
30. Chen SC, Liu WC, Wang CS, et al. Iatrogenic rupture of the ureter during kidney biopsy. Kaohsiung J Med Sci. 2010;26:502–5.
31. Trottmann M, Tritschler S, Graser A, et al. Injuries of the renal pelvis and ureter. Diagnosis and management. Urologe A. 2007;46:927–s34. German.
32. Huang E, Sayegh R, Craigo S, et al. Rupture of the renal pelvis associated with intravenous fluid bolus. J Matern Fetal Neonatal Med. 2002;11:345–6.
33. Schwartx A, Caine M, Hermann G, et al. Spontaneous renal extravasation during intravenous urography. Am J Roentgenol Radium Ther Nuclear Med. 1966;98:27–40.
34. Holly LE 2nd, Sumcad B. Diverticular ureteral changes; a report of four cases. Am J Roentgenol Radium Therapy, Nucl Med. 1957;78(6):1053–60.
35. McLoughlin LC, Davis NF, Dowling C, et al. Ureteral diverticulum: a review of the current literature. Can J Urol. 2013;20:6893–6.

36. Mehra K, Sreerag KS, Manikandan R, et al. Rare entity of proximal ureteral diverticulum managed by robotic resection and Ureteroureteral anastomosis. J Endourol Case Rep. 2020;6(1):39–41.
37. Gayer G, Desser TS, Hertz M, et al. Spontaneous suburothelial hemorrhage in coagulopathic patients: CT diagnosis. AJR Am J Roentgenol. 2011;197(5):W887–90.
38. Eccher A, Brunelli M, Gobbo S, et al. Subepithelial pelvic hematoma (Antopol-Goldman lesion) simulating renal neoplasm: report of a case and review of the literature. Int J Surg Pathol. 2009;17(3):264–7. Review.
39. Antopol W, Goldman L. Subepithelial hemorrhage of renal pelvis simulating neoplasm. Urol Cutan Rev. 1948;52(4):189–95.
40. Sahin TK, Aladag E, Setterzade E, et al. Spontaneous subepithelial hemorrhage of renal pelvis and ureter (Antopol-Goldman lesion) in hemophilia a patient with inhibitor: case report and review of the literature. Medicine (Baltimore). 2020;99(26):e20851.
41. Kossol JM, Patel SK. Suburothelial hemorrhage: the value of preinfusion computed tomography. J Comput Assist Tomogr. 1986;10(1):157–8.
42. Fonseca EKUN, Torres RVA, Scoppetta LRPD, et al. Spontaneous subepithelial hemorrhage: the Antopol-Goldman lesion. Einstein (Sao Paulo). 2021;19:eAI5829.
43. Gondos B. Foreign body in the left kidney and ureter. J Urol. 1955;73(1):35–8. https://doi.org/10.1016/s0022-5347(17)67363-4.
44. Wang L, Li Y, Zhao XP, et al. Hydronephrosis caused by intrauterine contraceptive device migration: three case reports with literature review. Clin Exp Obstet Gynecol. 2017;44:301–4.
45. Kurz DA, Mucksavage P. The endoscopic removal of eroded foreign bodies in the ureter. J Endourol Case Rep. 2016;2(1):30–2.
46. Finley DS, Perer E, Eichel L, Clayman RV. Ureteral pseudodiverticulum associated with absorbable suture clips after laparoscopic pyeloplasty: case report. J Endourol. 2005;19:726–9.
47. Brusky JP, Tran VQ. Resorbable clip migration resulting in ureteral obstruction and sepsis after laparoscopic pyeloplasty. J Endourol. 2010;24(10):1563–4.
48. Dursun M, Danis E, Otunctemur A, et al. Foreign body stone of the ureter originated from the suture thread: a case report. Prague Med Rep. 2014;115(3–4):141–4.
49. Lopez Silva M, Sanguinetti H, Battiston S, et al. Simultaneous ureteral and renal foreign bodies. J Endourol Case Rep. 2019;5(1):1–3.
50. Chen WJ, Wang SC, Chen SL, et al. Foreign body in the ureter: a particle of glue after transarterial embolization of a renal pseudoaneurysm during percutaneous nephrostomy. J Chin Med Assoc. 2012;75(4):183–6.
51. Di Migueli R, De La Roca R, Korkes F. Mysterious ureteral migration of a wooden toothpick from the digestive tract: case report and diagnostic considerations. Einstein (Sao Paulo). 2022;20:eRC5743.
52. Aso Y, Murahashi I, Yokoyama M. Foreign body stone of the ureter as a complication of acupuncture. Eur Urol. 1979;5(1):57–9.

Index

M. Abdel-Gawad et al. (eds.), *The Ureter*,
https://doi.org/10.1007/978-3-031-36212-5

V

W

GPSR Compliance

The European Union's (EU) General Product Safety Regulation (GPSR) is a set of rules that requires consumer products to be safe and our obligations to ensure this.

If you have any concerns about our products, you can contact us on ProductSafety@springernature.com

In case Publisher is established outside the EU, the EU authorized representative is:

Springer Nature Customer Service Center GmbH
Europaplatz 3
69115 Heidelberg, Germany

Batch number: 10726032

Printed by Printforce, the Netherlands